Physiotherapy and the Growing Child

Physiotherapy and the Growing Child

Edited by

YVONNE R BURNS MPhty PhD
Associate Professor, Head of Department of Physiotherapy,
University of Queensland, Australia

JULIE MACDONALD BPhty MA
Associate Lecturer, Department of Physiotherapy,
University of Queensland, Australia

Foreword by
MICHAEL O'CALLAGHAN
Director of Neurology and Child Development,
Mater Children's Hospital, Brisbane, Australia

WB Saunders Company Ltd
London • Philadelphia • Toronto • Sydney • Tokyo

WB Saunders Company Ltd 24–28 Oval Road
London NW1 7DX, UK

The Curtis Center
Independence Square West
Philadelphia, PA 19106–3399, USA

Harcourt Brace & Company
55 Horner Avenue
Toronto, Ontario M8Z 4X6, Canada

Harcourt Brace & Company, Australia
30–52 Smidmore Street
Marrickville, NSW 2204, Australia

Harcourt Brace & Company, Japan
Ichibancho Central Building, 22–1 Ichibancho
Chiyoda-ku, Tokyo 102, Japan

A catalogue record for this book is available from the British Library

ISBN 0–7020–1942–9

Design by Landmark Design Associates

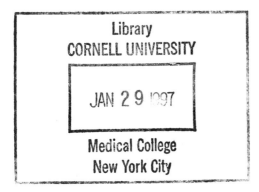
Typeset by J&L Composition Ltd, Filey, North Yorkshire

Printed and bound in Great Britain by The Bath Press, Avon

Contents

SECTION G   PHYSIOTHERAPY PRACTICE IN NEUROLOGICAL, NEUROMUSCULAR AND DEVELOPMENTAL CONDITIONS FROM INFANCY TO ADOLESCENCE

Prologue: Yvonne Burns

SECTION H   DEALING WITH LIVING

Prologue: Yvonne Burns

Contributors

Yvonne R Burns MPhty, PhD
Associate Professor, Head of Department of Physiotherapy, University of Queensland, Brisbane, Queensland, Australia

Geertruida Bekker Dip Phty
c/o LYNX/DR-Santiago, PO Box 5600, Ft Lauderdale, Florida, USA

Brenda Button Dip Phty, MAPA
Senior Cardiorespiratory Physiotherapist, Royal Children's Hospital, Melbourne, Victoria, Australia

Joan Cole DipPT, BPT, MSc, MEd, PhD
Acting Deputy Vice-Chancellor, Division of Health Services and Head, Department of Physiotherapy, Curtin University of Technology, Perth, Western Australia, Australia

Amanda Croker BPhty
Senior Policy Officer, Physiotherapy Services, Department of Education, Queensland, Australia

Prue Galley BPhty, B Ed, M Ed St, MAPA
Lecturer, Department of Physiotherapy, University of Queensland, Brisbane, Queensland, Australia

John Gilmour BPhty
Senior Physiotherapist, Mater Children's Hospital, Brisbane, Queensland, Australia

Melissa Hewitt BPhty
Private Practitioner, Graduate of University of Queensland, Brisbane, Queensland, Australia

Catherine Higgins BPhty
Education Adviser for Therapy Services, Department of Education, Queensland, Australia

Megan Kentish BPhty
Coordinating Physiotherapist, Spinal Disabilities Clinic, Royal Children's Hospital, Brisbane, Queensland, Australia

Julie MacDonald BPhty, MA
Associate Lecturer, Department of Physiotherapy, University of Queensland, Brisbane, Queensland, Australia

Margaret Masel B Soc Wk, BA
Social Work Department, Mater Mothers' Hospital, Brisbane, Queensland, Australia

Heather Mohay BSc (Hons), Dip App Psych (Clinical), PhD
Associate Professor, Director, Centre for Applied Studies in Early Childhood, Queensland University of Technology, Brisbane, Queensland, Australia

Kym Morris BPhty, MPhty, MAPA
Senior Physiotherapist, Mater Mothers' Hospital, Brisbane, Queensland, Australia

Jennifer Paratz MPhty, FACP, Grad Cert Ed, PhD
Lecturer, Cardiothoracic Physiotherapy, University of Queensland, St Lucia, Queensland, Australia

Susan Sawyer MBBS, FRACP
Respiratory Paediatrician and Adolescent Specialist, Royal Children's Hospital, Melbourne, Victoria, Australia

Karin Shepherd MBBS, MRCP (UK), FAFRM
Consultant Paediatrician and Director of Paediatric Spinal Unit at Royal Children's Hospital, Brisbane, Queensland, Australia

Susan Sienko Thomas, BSc Kinesiology, MA Health Services Administration
Clinical Research Coordinator, Shriners Hospital for Crippled Children, Portland, Oregon, USA

David Ian Tudehope MBBS, MRACP, FRACP
Director of Neonatology at Mater Mothers' Hospital, Brisbane, and Associate Professor in Neonatal Paediatrics, Department of Child Health, University of Queensland, Brisbane, Queensland, Australia

Pauline Watter BPhty, MPhty, MAPA
Lecturer, Department of Physiotherapy, University of Queensland, St Lucia, Australia

Ann Wright BPhty (Hons), MAPA
Education Adviser: Physiotherapy, Therapy Services, Low Incidence Support Centre, Department of Education, Annerley, Queensland, Australia

Foreword

MICHAEL O'CALLAGHAN

A physiotherapist has the potential to make a unique and invaluable contribution to children with neurological impairment or chronic physical disorder and to their families. As a therapist involved in an ongoing relationship with the child and family, it is important not only to apply the theoretical knowledge and practical skills of physical therapy, but also to do this in an individualized way that respects and empowers the child and family, and facilitates their overall development and growth as people. By focusing initially on the child and family, followed by issues of assessment and then individual fields of paediatrics, this book will assist physiotherapists with the knowledge and skills to achieve these goals.

Through the work of many authors with excellent and integrated contributions, the overall philosophy and approach of this book reflects the beliefs of Dr Yvonne Burns. In addition to her extensive academic and research contributions, Dr Burns has been intimately involved in the clinical practice of physiotherapy with children who have neurological impairments, deviations in development or chronic physical illness. Her theoretical knowledge, clinical practice and her teaching, coupled with a deep respect for children, have led to a keen ability to devise and implement individualized management programmes that meet the needs of the child and family.

This book will be helpful not only to physiotherapists working with children and adolescents but also to other members of multidisciplinary teams working alongside the physiotherapist. An understanding of the approach and philosophy of another discipline facilitates multiprofessional team function.

In writing this text Dr Burns and her associated authors have made an important contribution to children and their families.

Dedication

We dedicate this book to the hundred and thousands of infants, children, young people, parents, students and colleagues who have taught us so much.

Acknowledgements

A book such as this cannot happen without the willingness of others to share the vision and work involved in writing. Experienced physiotherapy practitioners find it much easier to express their expertise in practise rather than in writing. Although currently, throughout the world there is a wealth of medical information and research being published, work relevant to physiotherapy particularly in paediatrics is often sparse and difficult to locate. Our sincere thanks to all contributors for the way in which they undertook the task and to their many colleagues who offered much needed advice, ideas and practical assistance.

Preface

The aim of this book is to provide student and graduate physiotherapists as well as those involved in teaching physiotherapy, with an up-to-date resource which addresses the unique and special characteristics of working as a health professional with children and their families.

No infant, child or adolescent presents with a typical condition, but each brings their own individual personality, experience and combination of other factors. Furthermore, in many situations the diagnosis or cause of the developmental or movement disorder is not known for some time. It is the individual person who presents for physiotherapy not the condition. It is important therefore that the physiotherapist in paediatrics has a clear understanding of the basic principles of growth and development in all areas and systems relevant to disorders of posture, movement and respiratory dysfunction as well as a knowledge of approach, assessment, problem-solving and management.

Case studies have been used to illustrate specific points or developmental aspects of long-term conditions. Although fictitious, these case studies have been drawn from a combination of clinical experiences. Some stories demonstrate the changing nature of the problems and challenges and offer possible management and/or treatment strategies, others pose the problem and guide the reader to consider their own options while still others highlight a particular caution that needs to be considered. It is hoped that the reader's interest will be captured to encourage thoughtful learning and understanding.

Typical of the world today, the range and type of work requiring the skills of the physiotherapist is constantly changing. In some areas, war or poverty are rife, in other areas conditions such as human immunodeficiency virus (HIV), leprosy or blindness are major causes of disability or shortened life span, while in others, there is an increase in physical abuse of children or the possible re-emergence of conditions such as tuberculosis, whooping cough and poliomyelitis due to reduced public acceptance of the importance of immunization against infectious diseases. This text introduces the reader to a wide range of situations and conditions from the very preterm infant in a highly specialized tertiary intensive care unit to the child in a country with minimal or no resources for either physiotherapists or basic equipment.

The book is divided into eight sections containing one or more chapters. In each section or chapter the special characteristic strengths or needs of the infant and children through to adolescence are addressed. The scene is set in the opening section (A) through the stories of four young people, their families and physiotherapists. Aspects of growth and development particularly pertinent to the understanding of physiotherapy assessment, diagnosis and management as well as a brief overview of developmental anomalies of infancy are considered in the second section (B). The next two sections (C and D) address the principles of assessment, outcome evaluation and clinical practice including the context in which these are undertaken.

Physiotherapy in the management of cardiorespiratory, musculoskeletal, developmental and neurological problems are covered in Sections E, F and G respectively. The final section (G) entitled 'Dealing with Living' looks at a range of issues such as children with a severe or multiple disability, children with a short life expectancy, the abused child and living with disability in countries with minimal resources.

Yvonne R. Burns
Julie MacDonald

Section A:

Setting the Scene

PROLOGUE: HEATHER MOHAY

Prologue

HEATHER MOHAY

Movement disorders, congested chests, fractured limbs and so on do not occur in the abstract. They occur in people who live in families, which belong to networks of extended family and friends, and operate within a community and social setting which has particular beliefs, conventions, laws and policies. The later chapters of this book will describe the physiotherapy management of many paediatric conditions. This section of the book explores the psychosocial milieu in which paediatric physiotherapists work and attempts to alert practitioners to factors, other than the principles of physiotherapy treatment, which need to be considered when implementing treatment programmes.

Providing physiotherapy services for children with a variety of paediatric conditions is complex and multifaceted. Paediatric physiotherapists must not only have expert professional knowledge and skills within their discipline, they must also have an understanding of child development, an awareness of family dynamics and an ability to communicate effectively with children, parents and professional colleagues.

These requirements place heavy demands on practitioners, especially the young and inexperienced.

All children have the right to receive the best possible treatment for their condition; however, what constitutes the best treatment will be influenced by a multitude of factors many of which will not be directly related to the child's physical condition. These will include, factors within the child, such as attention span or intellectual abilities; factors within the family such as needs of siblings or financial resources; and factors within the environment such as availability of space, equipment and services. The therapist must be sensitive to the personality and psychological needs of the child and aware of the impact which the child's disability, injury or illness may have on members of the immediate family, the extended family and the support network of neighbours and friends. They must also be aware of the ways in which the introduction of therapists can distort previously established social networks.

Compliance with intervention programmes is dependent upon the programme being 'user friendly'.

3

Therapy programmes must therefore not only meet the child's physical needs but also be compatible with the circumstances in which he or she lives.

Physiotherapists rarely work in isolation. Therefore, in addition to considering the needs of the child and the family they should also take into consideration the way in which the therapy team operates. Each member of the team must be able to identify their role within the team, be aware of the roles of other team members and be conscious of each person's relationship with the patient and his or her family.

In addition to all the above, therapists need to pay some attention to their own well-being. Working with children who have disabilities or chronic illness can be extremely exacting and at times daunting. Therapists therefore need to protect themselves from excessive stress.

The factors within the child, the family and the environment which impact upon the design and implementation of intervention programmes, and upon the ability of families to comply with treatment will be explored in the following pages. This will be achieved by considering, from a number of different perspectives, the cases of four children who present for physiotherapy.

1

Focus on the Child, Family and Therapist

HEATHER MOHAY

Focus on the Child
•
Focus on the Family
•
Focus on the Therapist
•
Focus on the Intervention Programme

Focus on the Child

There are a multitude of reasons why a child may require physiotherapy. Problems may be short-term, transient difficulties which will get better (for example, movement problems resulting from fractures), or long-term, permanent problems which cannot be cured (for example, cerebral palsy). Problems may be severe or mild, they may improve over time or deteriorate or may even be life threatening (for example, cystic fibrosis or Duchenne muscular dystrophy). They may be congenital or acquired, due to genetic factors or environmental factors. They may result from a disability, a chronic or acute illness or an injury. The type of problem, cause, and age of onset, are all factors which will influence how the child and family respond to the condition and its treatment.

Every child, irrespective of colour, creed or social class, has the right to the best treatment available. Each child is unique both in terms of personal characteristics and home environment, and what constitutes 'best treatment' for one child may be inappropriate for another. This discussion will focus on factors within the child and individual differences between children which influence the structure of intervention programmes.

Although the degree and type of problem are likely to be the primary factors affecting the therapy programme which will be implemented, other factors such as the child's sex, age and developmental stage, personality, attention span, abilities, likes and dislikes, needs for independence, self-esteem, self-efficacy and acceptance by the peer group all need to be considered if an effective and acceptable intervention programme is to be put in place. In designing an intervention programme the physiotherapist must therefore not only assess disabilities and limitations but must also consider abilities and interests, developmental needs and a myriad other factors from within the child which will influence his or her response to the condition and to the therapy programme (Becker 1979, Eiser 1993, Garrison and McQuiston 1989, Pless and Nolan 1991).

The following four children will be used to illustrate the impact of individual differences on the design of therapy programmes. The case histories are fictitious, but are typical of the children who could be on the case load of a physiotherapist working in a hospital or in the community.

Kim

Kim was born 12 weeks preterm. He was a sick baby who required care in the neonatal intensive care unit for 3 months before he was allowed to go home. He is now a slightly built, black haired, 2-year-old who has spastic quadriplegia, with his lower limbs more affected than his arms and hands. He can sit in a high chair with some support and can take some weight on his legs, but is not yet walking. He makes sounds, but does not produce any clear speech, although his mother feels that he understands what she says to him. It is difficult to assess his intellectual abilities because of his lack of speech and his impaired fine and gross motor coordination which interfere with his performance on test items. Furthermore, as the language of the home is Vietnamese he may not understand instructions which are given in English. He is rather a shy little boy who tends to cling to his mother at first, but, as he gets used to people he relaxes and becomes quite sociable. He has an endearing smile.

Kim is beginning to get frustrated about not being able to communicate his needs and not being able to reach things or manipulate them in the way he wants to. This can result in severe temper tantrums during which he gets distressed and is difficult to settle. Loud noises also upset him. Kim responds well to visual forms of praise and encouragement such as smiling, clapping and hugging.

COMMENTARY

Kim's disability is clearly stressful for him as it is preventing him from doing things that he wants to do and from gaining the autonomy and independence which children normally strive to achieve at his age. It is interfering with his acquisition of self-help skills such as feeding, toileting and dressing, and his lack of mobility is restricting his choice of activities and hence the range of cognitive stimulation which is available to him. His delayed language development may reflect a global developmental delay, or an aspect of his cerebral palsy (i.e. poor control of the oral musculature), or the effects of his bilingual home environment, or any combination of these factors. Whatever the cause, his inability to express his needs is also causing him to be frustrated and is interfering with his social interactions.

Sarah

Having repeated a year in preschool Sarah, aged 8, is now in grade 2 at a small, local, church school. She is tall for her age and somewhat overweight, but she has a pretty face and beautiful curly strawberry-blonde hair. Her intellectual abilities are slightly below average and she is struggling with her school work. She also has low muscle tone and poor postural control, which make it difficult for her to sit still for any length of time and adversely affects her written work. During therapy sessions Sarah is always cooperative. She likes to get ticks, positive comments and stars or stickers on her work. Star charts are also a successful form of reward as she enjoys seeing the visual record of her progress and the sense of accomplishment when she obtains the prize at the end.

Sarah tries hard to please, and always does her best, but she rarely smiles and presents as an anxious, depressed girl. Sarah is acutely aware of the difficulties she is having with her school work and very self-conscious about her height and weight. At school she is a bit of a loner with only one special friend, a girl who also has some motor problems and with whom she went to preschool. She does not like having time off school to attend therapy sessions as she feels this draws atten-

tion to her problems. Sarah is not involved in any out of school activities and spends a lot of time watching television. She is responsible for feeding and grooming her pet dog, Shandy, and enjoys playing with him and taking him for a walk.

COMMENTARY

Although both Kim and Sarah have motor coordination problems the intervention programmes they require will be quite different as their pattern of abilities and disabilities is different and they are at vastly different development stages. Activities suitable for a 2-year-old are clearly not appropriate for an 8-year-old. Like Kim, Sarah's problems are causing her considerable stress, but whilst Kim externalizes his frustration in the form of temper tantrums Sarah internalizes her feelings and manifests them as anxiety, depression and low self-esteem.

At Sarah's stage of development the acquisition of positive self-esteem is crucial as this will have long-term effects on her self-confidence and hence on her willingness to attempt new tasks and engage in social activities.

John

John is 12-years-old. Four months ago he was cycling along the pavement near his home when he diverged on to the road and into the path of a car. He was not wearing a helmet and sustained head injuries, a broken collarbone, severe bruising and lacerations to his face and upper body. Following the accident he was admitted to the intensive care ward of a major metropolitan hospital where he regained consciousness after 2 days. Subsequently he received a range of therapy programmes from the multidisciplinary rehabilitation team and made significant progress. He is now felt to be ready to be discharged from hospital although there are a number of residual problems. He still has limited mobility and needs to use a wheelchair to cover any distance, his intellectual abilities appear to have deteriorated, his attention span is very short and he is often verbally aggressive, abusive and uncooperative. It is anticipated that his recovery will continue but he will require ongoing therapy as an outpatient.

It is difficult to predict what John's ultimate functioning level will be. Before his accident he was in grade 7 at the local state school where his school achievements were described as average. He was a good athlete and an especially keen football player and avid fan of the local football team. His doctor has told him that because of his head injury, even when he does become mobile he will not be allowed to play football again for some time. This has caused him considerable distress and interfered with his motivation to regain his motor skills.

COMMENTARY

John's situation is different to that of the previous two children. His motor impairment has been acquired as the result of a traumatic event. Unlike the other children who are attempting to gain skills which they had not previously acquired, he has lost, and must now attempt to regain, functions which he previously had. He is likely to feel frustrated, confused and angry at his inability to do things which he could previously do with ease; annoyed and embarrassed by his increased dependency on others (at a stage in his development when he would normally be seeking increased independence); upset and angry about his inability to participate in many peer group activities and worried about seeming inferior to his peers (at a stage in his development when it is important not to be different from the peer group). In summary, he is likely to be in an emotional turmoil; angry and frustrated about his current limitations and anxious and uncertain about the future. His brash and uncooperative behaviour may be his defence against these unpleasant and undesirable feelings. It may, however, also be a manifestation of personality changes resulting from his head injury.

He may not be enthusiastic about participating in the

therapy programme, especially with a female therapist, because it highlights his inadequacies in motor control and because boys at this age typically do not think it is 'cool' to have females showing them how to do things. Like Sarah, John needs to be integrated into peer group activities and may benefit from some group therapy sessions. John has to learn to cope with his limitations and to establish positive self-esteem and a positive self-image despite the loss of some skills and the restrictions on his activities.

Jane

At nearly 15 years of age Jane is a late-developing adolescent. She is extremely thin and has a pale complexion. Her fine brown hair is tied up in a pony tail. She has cystic fibrosis and has just been admitted to hospital for the third time this year. Her chest is severely congested and she is losing a lot of weight. The doctors suspect that she is not complying with treatment well and they fear she may not survive for much longer if this continues. Over the years Jane has been aware of the deaths of several of the children in the Cystic Fibrosis Society. She has recently become embarrassed about the increased clubbing of her hands and feet as she feels that it is unattractive.

Jane is in grade 10 at a private coeducational school. She has always worked hard and her school achievements have been in the average range. Her school achievements, however, have deteriorated dramatically in the past few months. Jane enjoys reading and swimming and has been an active member of the local youth club. Recently she seems to have lost interest in everything.

COMMENTARY

Adolescence is a vulnerable stage of development when people are acutely aware of their weaknesses and of any differences between themselves and their peers. Jane is self-conscious about the changes in shape of her hands and feet although other people might scarcely notice them. Teenagers need to feel attractive, competent and accepted by others. Jane may not wish to acknowledge the seriousness of her medical condition or the need for special diets, medication, exercise and chest percussion because these set her apart from her peers. On the other hand she is likely to be intensely aware of the deaths of other adolescents with cystic fibrosis. Thus, at a time when her friends are planning their future in terms of careers and boyfriends, she must question what the future holds for her. At present she appears to be quite depressed and disinterested in life. This will need to be carefully addressed as part of her overall therapy programme.

Jane's medical condition is stressful for her because it makes her different to her peers and causes anxiety about the future. Her treatment may also be stressful because it again highlights the differences between herself and her peers and consumes a significant proportion of each day, which she might prefer to devote to other activities such as listening to music, watching television or talking to her friends on the telephone. It will not be possible to impose a treatment regimen on Jane because she is at a stage in her development when she must decide whether she will comply. At 15, Jane is seeking independence but her illness and the therapy required may make her dependent upon others. As she is just beginning to develop physically she may be self-conscious about her body and may be embarrassed about other people (even immediate family) carrying out chest physiotherapy.

If there is a real fear that Jane may not live for long it is important to acknowledge this but not to abandon her or give up on intervention programmes. She will need a great deal of psychological and emotional support and counselling but she will also need to be as physically comfortable as possible, and as intellectually stimulated and socially involved as possible right to the end of her life. All the research suggests that patients, even young ones, prefer to know the prognosis for their condition rather than being shielded with lies and denials. They can then make appropriate plans and face their death with dignity.

Summary

These four vignettes have been used to give an impression of the range of different problems which face paediatric physiotherapists. They also highlight the need to recognize and respect the individuality of each child. It is important for therapists to recognize that disabilities and chronic illness can create considerable stress for the children. The source and form of the stress will vary from child to child, but tends to increase as they get older, reaching a peak in adolescence. The impairment itself may be a source of stress because it prevents the child from doing things and thus causes frustration. The response of the parents to the child's condition may be a further source of stress as the child has to cope with parental guilt, uncertainty and anxiety and their resultant overprotection, lowered expectations or rejection (Weiss 1994).

The reactions of other people to the condition and restrictions on opportunities to socialize with peers may lead to distortions in social relationships that are likely to cause additional stress. Therapy itself may be a significant source of stress and frustration to the child. It may be painful or boring or prevent the child from participating in more interesting activities. Furthermore, it may draw attention to the child's problems and force them to miss school thus singling them out from their classmates and adversely affecting their school achievements. Many disabled children have low school achievements which may be directly due to the disability or more indirectly related to frequent absence from school or lowered expectations of teachers and parents. Whatever the cause there is ample evidence to show that failure at school is a source of anxiety and is related to low self-esteem and reduced long-term job prospects.

In planning a therapy programme, consideration must be given to all of these factors within the child and to the transactions which occur between the child and his or her physical and psychosocial environment. We will now move on to examine some of the environmental factors which have a significant effect upon the management of a child's medical condition as well as his or her development, attitudes and beliefs, psychological adjustment and well-being.

Focus on the Family

Children do not live in isolation. They live within a family which is supported by (and in turn supports) a network of extended family and friends and operates within a community with a set of cultural beliefs, laws, policies and institutions.

These relationships can be schematized, in a rudimentary way, by placing the child at the hub of a series of concentric circles (see Figure 1). The first circle represents the immediate family, the next represents people who have considerable influence upon, and operate in mutual support relationships with the family (for example, grandparents, relatives, neighbours and friends). The third and outermost circle represents general community services and formalized relationships such as those with teachers, doctors, priests and therapists. Access to these community resources usually has to be initiated by the parents and most families have little contact with them. The structure of a family's social network is not static but changes over time as needs and interests change and people come into or leave the network. This figure is, of course, simplistic as all members of a particular circle will not have the same degree of closeness with the child and family. This will be influenced by factors such as geographical proximity, interests, personalities and needs. The figure serves, however, to illustrate the

Figure 1   A schematic representation of the social network surrounding the family of a non-disabled child.

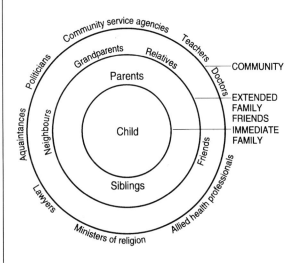

different types of relationships within a normal social support network and demonstrates graphically the degree of affinity which families have with different formal and informal networks within society (Schilling et al. 1984).

When there is a disabled or sick child in the family the nature of the network changes significantly (see Figure 2). The presence of the disabled child impacts on all members of the family leading to changes in roles and relationships (Calderon and Greenberg 1993). Typically the mother adopts a leading role in the care of the disabled child and takes responsibility for carrying out the therapy programme, taking the child to appointments and negotiating with various community agencies. Hence she becomes the family's expert on the child's condition and care, and all other members of the family receive information second hand from her (Eiser 1990, Traustadottir 1991). Fathers assume even less responsibility for the care of disabled children than for non-disabled children (McConachie 1986, Bristol et al. 1988, Hornby 1992) and able-bodied siblings may feel rejected, neglected and left out as their parents are forced to spend a disproportionate amount of time with their disabled brother or sister (Brett 1988, Knafl and Deatrick 1990, Eiser 1993). Relationships between the family and their relatives and friends also become distorted. A number of studies have found that mothers of disabled or chronically sick children become reliant upon their own mothers for support and advice and may feel

that their mothers-in-law hold them responsible for the children's problems (Gallagher et al. 1983, Brown and Hepple 1989, Seligman 1991). Frequently, the demands of caring for the disabled child are so great that parents become isolated from their former friends and extended family (Quine and Pahl 1985) and experience feelings of loneliness and abandonment.

Of particular interest to the readers of this book are the changes which occur in the outer circle which is made up of certain institutions within the community and members of those institutions, such as doctors, teachers and therapists. Under normal circumstances these community resources have little impact upon family functioning. However, when there is a disabled child in the family services are often thrust upon them with little consideration of their needs, readiness or capacity to cope with them. Ironically, at the same time, these families are frequently unable to access all the community resources that they require, and to which they are entitled (Schilling et al. 1984, Baxter 1989, Meltzer et al. 1989, Beresford 1994).

Thus, when a family has a disabled or chronically ill child their contact with health and other services in the community is greatly increased. Consequently these service providers can come to have a substantial influence on family functioning and child-rearing practices. In some cases professional relationships replace or merge with the network of extended family and friends. The relationship with a professional is, however, very different to that with a friend. With a professional the relationship is one way, i.e. the professional gives advice and support to the family, but does not request advice or support in return. In a friendship the relationship is more symmetrical with both partners seeking or giving advice, support and comfort at different times. The loss of these reciprocal relationships and their replacement with more formalized relationships can leave parents with feelings of inferiority and powerlessness (Burden and Thomas 1986b). Therapists need to be acutely aware of their impact on the family and sensitive to the fact that parents have the right to make decisions about the care and upbringing of their child, even if these are contrary to the therapist's recommendations.

Figure 2   A schematic representation of the social network surrounding the family of a disabled or chronically sick child.

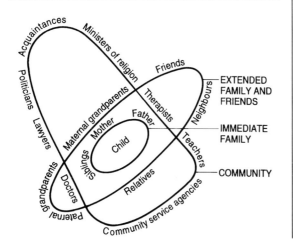

Parents enter their child's therapy situation having already well-established personalities, interests, knowledge, beliefs and expectations. They vary widely along these dimensions depending upon their previous experience and upbringing. They also differ in terms of age, education, occupation, financial resources, stability of the marriage, availability of a support network and so on. They live in a variety of different family structures including extended families, single-parent families, step families, families with other natural children and families with adopted or fostered children, and differ in terms of their housing, the amount of space available and the ease with which they can access community resources. All of these factors, and many more, influence how parents cope with the disabled or sick child and how they respond to intervention programmes (Frey et al. 1989, Kampfe 1989, Wallander et al. 1990, Eiser 1990, 1993).

Just as there is no single best way to bring up a child there is no one way in which all parents will respond to their child's disablement. In the past, parental responses were often conceptualized in terms of a grief model which suggested that parents needed to grieve for the loss of their expected normal child. The processes involved in this were seen to be akin to those of bereavement, i.e. shock, denial, bargaining, anger, sorrow and finally adjustment. However, in the case of a disabled child it was believed that parental sadness was ongoing and recurrent. Olshansky (1962) described this as 'chronic sorrow'. Whilst the grief model served an important role in alerting professionals to the emotional needs of parents, it is now generally regarded as somewhat simplistic and linear.

More recent evidence has suggested that parents respond in a variety of different ways to the diagnosis and care of their disabled child. Although many experience emotional turmoil at the diagnosis of their child's disability, some are extremely resilient and adapt in positive ways to meet the special needs of their child (Burden and Thomas 1986a, 1986b, Trute and Hauch 1988). Thus, there has been a move away from pathologizing the families of handicapped children and seeing them as 'handicapped families' (McMichael 1971) and a trend towards a more positive approach of seeking to understand the coping strategies used by these families. More modern theories have therefore focused on the factors which enable families to adjust successfully to caring for a disabled or chronically sick child.

The process model of stress and coping, proposed by Lazarus and Folkman (1984) and the transactional model suggested by Wallander et al. (1990) are both concerned with the interaction of a wide array of factors which affect the degree to which families are able to cope with the stress of caring for a child with special needs. These factors include the nature and severity of the disability, parental personalities and previous experience with the condition, demands on parents from other sources, financial resources, accessibility of a support network and stability of the marriage. Contrary to popular belief, parents of disabled children are no more likely to separate or divorce than parents of non-disabled children (Freeman et al. 1975, Baldwin 1985, Cooke et al. 1986, Beresford 1994).

Parents are primary caretakers of their child and therapists must remain non-judgemental and respectful of parental choices and child-rearing practices as long as they are not harmful to the child. Therapists must also remember that although they are the expert in their professional area, parents know more about their child than anyone else and they are the experts in terms of the child's behaviour and his or her likes and dislikes. Because of their expert knowledge and experience therapists can easily (and unintentionally) make parents feel inadequate (Burden and Thomas 1986b). For example, a physiotherapist should know good strategies for relieving discomfort and settling a child when he or she is distressed, this can however make a mother feel incompetent when she has been trying to calm her child for some time. It is therefore important to share knowledge with the family rather than show them what they were doing wrong.

We will now explore some family factors which may affect the design and implementation of physiotherapy programmes, by considering the family circumstances of the four children described previously.

Kim's family

Kim's parents, Mr and Mrs T are a young Vietnamese couple who were married in a refugee camp in Thailand and migrated to Australia 3 years ago. Kim is their first child and Mrs T is expecting another baby. They have no relatives in Australia but live in a part of town where there are many Vietnamese families. They are devout Catholics and active members of the local church, which has a large Vietnamese congregation. They are currently running a 'corner store' and live in the small flat above the shop. There is a small backyard with a clothes hoist but very little space where Kim could play. Whenever it is necessary for Kim to leave the flat he has to be carried down a steep flight of stairs. As he is getting bigger and heavier this is becoming increasingly difficult for Mrs T to manage, especially at this late stage in her pregnancy. Kim's lack of mobility is therefore becoming a major problem which could force the family to seek alternative (less convenient and more expensive) housing. The shop is open for long hours every day, including weekends.

Mrs T does not speak good English and communication with her is often difficult. Mr T, who has a better command of English, is rarely able to attend therapy sessions because of his long working hours. The Ts do not own a car and public transport to the hospital is both costly and inconvenient. Mrs T sometimes uses public transport but often relies upon friends to drive her to appointments. Despite these problems Mrs T rarely misses Kim's therapy sessions. Two weeks ago Mrs T showed Kim's physiotherapist a magazine article describing a child with cerebral palsy who had been helped by an alternative intervention programme. She stated that her friend gave the article to her and suggested that she should take Kim to a similar programme operating in a nearby suburb. The congregation at the church have agreed to raise the funds to pay for Kim's therapy in this programme.

Mr and Mrs T have had no previous experience with child rearing and are unsure about what to expect children to do at different ages. They have no direct support from their own parents and family members. Indeed, although they have tried to explain about Kim's problems, the families at home in Vietnam do not seem to understand and often ask if Kim is 'better' now, or offer advice which is contrary to that being given by the therapists. As Mrs T does not speak fluent English she finds going to the hospital quite threatening and often feels confused and anxious. Because of their circumstances the Ts are vulnerable and dependent upon the Vietnamese community. They are working hard to make a success of life in their new country. They feel that it is important for their business to succeed so that they are financially secure. The attention which Kim requires limits the assistance Mrs T is able to give to her husband in their joint business venture. She feels guilty about this but at the same time is worried about Kim. There is therefore considerable conflict in terms of how she divides her time between Kim and the business. She is also anxious about her current pregnancy and concerned that nothing should go wrong. She doesn't know how she will manage all the conflicting demands on her time when the new baby arrives.

COMMENTARY

This vignette shows you some of the problems that the T family face as they attempt to deal with the challenge of caring for their physically disabled child. Other families live in different circumstances and face quite different problems. To be successful, therapy programmes must be designed around the needs and resources of the family as well as the specific treatment requirements of the child. In the case of the T family, cultural and language factors will need to be considered as well as transportation problems, space and time limitations and financial constraints. One of the potential strengths of this family is the support that they have from their local ethnic community

We will now look at Sarah's family and consider their circumstances and factors which may influence the design and implementation of a therapy programme to help her.

Sarah's family

Sarah's parents both have university degrees and have senior professional appointments. They both work long hours and are committed to their careers. Sarah has a younger brother, Adam, who recently started school and is rapidly catching up with her in terms of academic skills. This is threatening to Sarah's self-esteem. The family live in a large comfortable house with a big garden in an outer suburb. Because of Mr and Mrs G's long working hours the children go to their grandparents' home after school and are collected by their parents on the way home. Mrs G is conscious of Sarah's problems and anxious to help her. However, because of her commitments at work it is often difficult for her to attend therapy sessions and when she gets home at night she is tired and there is little time to work with Sarah. Mr G has less insight into Sarah's difficulties and tends to get impatient with her. He feels that she is lazy and that if she tried harder she would be more successful.

COMMENTARY

The Gs have difficulty attending therapy sessions and, in addition, Sarah does not like being taken out of school. Moreover, Mr G has little understanding of Sarah's difficulties and may see therapy as unnecessary. The family's attitude towards the physiotherapy programme is therefore likely to be ambivalent. Sarah's problems could be considered as subtle and minimal. In some circumstances they might almost go unnoticed. However, in this high-achieving family

their adverse impact on Sarah's school achievements is likely to be conspicuous and may have a profound effect on her self-esteem and her psychological well-being. On these grounds continued intervention is warranted.

There are no significant financial constraints that might interfere with Sarah's attendance at therapy or with the purchase of equipment that might help her. There are, however, major time pressures affecting the family's motivation and capacity to follow through with interventions.

John's family

John is the youngest of five children who live with their mother on the outskirts of a small country town about 360 km from the major metropolitan hospital where he was cared for following his accident, and 50 km from a small country hospital in a neighbouring town. The family moved to this town about 4 years ago and live in a rented high-set house with a flight of stairs at both the front and the back. John shares a bedroom with his two brothers. They have no relatives and few close friends in the town. Ms K (John's mother) drives an old and unreliable car.

John's parents separated 5 years ago and he has had little contact with his father since then. His father did, however, visit him in hospital and it was clear that he blamed John's mother for the fact that John was not wearing a helmet at the time of his accident. John's elder brother has finished school and is currently unemployed. His other three siblings attend the local state high school (the school which John had anticipated attending next year). John's mother had little education. She supplements her single parent allowance by working, on a casual basis, at a nearby farm and doing some cleaning for local families.

Ms K describes her fears at the time of the accident and her relief when John regained consciousness and was obviously going to survive. She feels guilty about the fact that he was not wearing a helmet at the time of the accident, but also feels helpless in controlling the behaviour of her headstrong teenage children. She wants to be with John in hospital but is also conscious of the fact that she is needed at home to care for the other children. As a result she has been travelling back and forth from home to the hospital on a regular basis. This has placed a substantial financial burden on her, adding to the stress associated with John's accident and her worries about the welfare of the rest of the family. She is emotionally and physically drained and is anxious to have John home as soon as possible, as she feels this will ease some of the pressure on her. Her major concern at present is John's changed, and often very difficult behaviour and the effect that this will have on his siblings. She is also worried about how she will get him in and out of the house and about the changes which may need to be made to accommodate a wheelchair. She is contemplating moving house but doubts if she will be able to find anything suitable at a rent that she can afford. She does not want to leave the area because of the children's schooling and their friendships. John's condition is expected to continue to improve, hence he is unlikely to require a wheelchair indefinitely and it can be anticipated that he will eventually manage the stairs unaided. The problem is the uncertainty about the rate at which his progress will occur and about any residual long-term problems.

COMMENTARY

Both John's behaviour and his limited mobility are likely to present problems when he returns home. The house will require some reorganization to meet his needs and his siblings will have to adjust to his changed behaviour and physical abilities (Martin 1988, Waalander and Kreutzer 1988). The location of the family home is likely to be the major factor influencing John's ongoing therapy programme. Access to therapy services in rural areas is problematic and Mrs K has transport problems and limited financial resources. As John is the youngest child in the family it may be possible to mobilize his older siblings to assist with his therapy programme.

Jane's family

Jane is the only child of Mr and Mrs D. When they discovered she had cystic fibrosis they decided that they would not have any further children and would do everything in their power to enable Jane to have as happy and as normal a life as possible. Mr D has a fairly senior clerical position in a large electrical company. He has been offered promotions on several occasions but these have always involved moving to country towns where he felt that optimal treatment for Jane's condition would not be available. As a result he has rejected these offers and has not made the career progressions which might have been expected. Prior to Jane's birth Mrs D earned a good salary as a cook in a local restaurant. She planned to return to this job but as the hours were long and somewhat unpredictable she decided to remain at home in order to be available to care for Jane when needed. Mrs D generates a small income by working from home to provide catering for occasional functions. Mrs D also helps out at the tuck shop at Jane's school and is heavily involved in the Women's Guild at the local church. The D's income is modest but by carefully budgeting they manage quite well. They live in a small comfortably furnished suburban home which is on the bus route to the hospital where Jane receives her treatment. Like so many parents of disabled children Mr and Mrs D bear not only the obvious additional costs associated with their child's special needs, such as medication, but also a huge hidden financial burden created by restrictions on career and work opportunities and limitations on where they can live (Baldwin 1985, Smith and Robus 1989, Parker 1990).

Mrs D has read everything she can find on cystic fibrosis and is quite an authority on the subject and a great support for other parents in the Cystic Fibrosis Association. She ensures that Jane always attends appointments at the clinic, she carefully supervises Jane's medication and diet and carries out the daily physiotherapy programme. In addition, she encourages Jane to take adequate exercise by going for a brisk walk with her every morning and by involvement on the school swimming club (for which Mr D is the treasurer).

COMMENTARY

Adolescence is not only a difficult time for children it is also a difficult time for parents and especially for parents of children who have disabilities or chronic illness. After all the years of caring for and protecting their child they must gradually relinquish control and allow the child to take responsibility for themselves. This is a major step for parents. They are fearful about how well the child can manage alone and without their supervision. Often they are left with a feeling of rejection and of not being wanted or needed any more. This can leave a void in their lives which may be difficult to fill. In addition, there is often a renewed sadness about the child's condition as they watch their friends' children leave home, get married and produce children. These are poignant reminders of the difficulties facing their child and of the fact that they are unlikely to experience the joy of becoming grandparents.

The D's life has revolved around Jane and it is easy to see the emptiness that could be created if she no longer needed their care and attention and even more so if she was to die. It is possible that they have been overly involved in Jane's condition and in her activities, to a point where she has felt stifled and deprived of independence. The current poor control of her condition may be her way of rebelling against this overprotection and lack of freedom. It is, however, a dangerous strategy and one which will almost certainly result in even further deterioration of her health if she persists with it.

A great deal of tact is going to be needed in managing this case. From a medical point of view Jane's parents' management of her condition has been exemplary and it is understandable if they feel somewhat cheated and angry about the sudden deterioration in her health. On the other hand, from a psychological point of view their involvement may have been overbearing and has not adjusted to meet Jane's growing need for independence and control over her own well-being. The Ds may need to be encouraged to step back a little and encourage Jane to take more responsibility for her health, whilst at the same time giving her the support and encouragement to continue with activities that she enjoys. Jane may also be depressed at present and this may need to be treated. If, despite all efforts, Jane is likely to die in the near future, Mr and Mrs D will need to be prepared for this and given adequate support by members of the cystic fibrosis team.

Summary

These brief descriptions of the family circumstances of the four paediatric patients described in the first part of the chapter provide some insights into the complex factors which influence parental responses to their child's disability and their capacity to carry out intervention programmes. With the best will in the world, and with considerable insight into the benefits which the therapy may hold for the child, parents may have major problems in following through with an intervention programme. It is important for therapists to be aware of family circumstances and parental beliefs and expectations and to adjust their programmes to cater for these, rather than perceive the parents as inadequate or disinterested when they fail to comply with treatment.

Focus on the Therapist

Physiotherapists come to their job with years of professional training and expert knowledge about the treatment of a wide range of physical conditions. They are not, however, automatons. Even assuming they all have the same level of professional expertise in all aspects of paediatric physiotherapy (which is unlikely) they come in a range of different shapes and sizes with different interests, personalities, beliefs, values, prejudices, expectations and so on which are borne of their life experiences. These individual differences impinge upon the ways in which they relate to professional colleagues and clients, and influence the decisions which they make about treatment.

Look around at your colleagues and classmates and notice how different they are. Ask yourself honestly whether you like all of them and whether you would be equally comfortable with any of them as your therapist? This is an important lesson to learn. There may be nothing wrong with a therapist's skills but they may not be the right person to deal with a particular patient. A second important lesson to learn is that no one is equally skilled in all areas of their discipline. It is critically important to recognize the limits of your expertise and to know when to ask for help or to refer a patient to a colleague. A willingness to make referrals for these reasons is not an indication of professional inadequacy but a sign of maturity and professional responsibility.

Therapists not only have a professional life, but they also have a personal life, which is likely to vary as much as their personal characteristics. They have membership of at least one family, participate in community activities and have a range of friendships, all of which bestow upon them a variety of responsibilities. Thus, in addition to their workload they have to carry with them the stress associated with the minor hassles and major crises of everyday life. The degree of personal stress will vary from person to person and will be influenced by factors such as personal and family health, financial security and marital stability amongst others. These external stresses may influence a therapist's ability to cope professionally. It is therefore important to monitor stress levels and to develop mechanisms to separate personal worries from professional responsibilities.

Physiotherapists (and other health professionals) are in a privileged role in relation to the client and their family. The patient's problem may be acute and the therapist's contact may be short lived. Such contact, however, frequently occurs at a time of maximum stress for the child and parents, for example, during a period of illness or following surgery or an accident, when anxiety and concern for the child's well-being is likely to be running high. In this situation therapists frequently find themselves being forced into a support role in addition to providing a physiotherapy programme.

When the child has a long-term disability or chronic illness the therapist's role with the family is ongoing over many years so that close bonds are formed and therapists sometimes become family friends and confidants. If care is not taken this can interfere with the professional relationship which must exist and may affect the therapist's ability to make unbiased judgements about treatment programmes and progress. Therapists are frequently privy to parental concerns and family problems and need to consider whether it is appropriate for them to adopt a counselling role or whether a colleague with greater skills and training in this area should be involved. Under all circumstances therapists must respect the confidentiality of both parents and children.

Physiotherapists come into the profession for a variety of reasons. For example, they may have selected physiotherapy as a second choice if they failed to get into medical school, or they may have chosen it because of its intrinsic interest and intellectual challenges, or because they felt a desire to help people, or because it would provide a financially secure career which could easily be combined with family responsibilities, or because of pressure from family members or the observation of physiotherapists working with a disabled relative. Physiotherapists need to examine their motivation carefully in order to minimize the effects this may have on the ways in which they respond to clients and the management decisions they make.

Whatever the initial motivation, no one would remain a physiotherapist for very long if the work was not intrinsically interesting, intellectually challenging, rewarding and, for the most part, enjoyable. However, it would be foolish to deny the job-related stresses. This is a topic that is rarely discussed during training and is generally ignored in textbooks, although it clearly has an impact on the day-to-day work of the practitioner. The case load and pressure of work can be high and managing the demands of both work and home can be problematic. Working with children with disabilities or chronic illness can be frustrating as progress is often extremely slow and the condition can never be cured. Furthermore, parents may have unrealistic expectations about what the interventions will achieve and thus vent their discontent upon the therapists when the expected 'cure' does not occur. This can arouse reciprocal feeling of anger towards the parents or can cause the therapist to feel insecure and to question his or her skills. Sometimes, despite the best efforts of doctors and therapists, patients die. Often therapists have spent many hours working with these patients and have formed attachments to them. Their loss can create feelings of failure and leave a gap in the therapist's life. It is important for therapists to recognize that they too have a need to grieve at these times and that this shared grief can be a great support to the family.

Sometimes children can be severely disfigured due to congenital malformations or trauma. The general public frequently experience feelings of fear and a sense of repulsion when they encounter these children. Health professionals are no different (Newson and Hipgrave 1982). In order to work effectively with these children it is important to look beyond physical appearances and to seek their special qualities. Asking parents about the particular endearing behaviours of the child or their special skills can often quickly provide insights into the positive side of the child's personality. Irrespective of the condition, children must be seen as children who require assistance and not as conditions to be treated.

At times therapy may be painful for the child and they may cry and want to terminate the session. When intervention causes the child to become distressed parental anxiety also increases and they too may become apprehensive about therapy sessions and show some avoidant behaviour or disapproval of the therapist. Inflicting pain on another person is equally stressful for the therapist even if they firmly believe that in the long run it is for the child's benefit. Explaining to the child and parent exactly what is about to happen and why it is necessary and, where possible, allowing the child to assist, will usually lead to fewer complaints and greater compliance from the child (Bush et al. 1986, Mohay in press).

Physiotherapists frequently find themselves working in interdisciplinary teams. Whilst the team structure can be a source of great strength, it can also be a source of great conflict. It is extremely important for members of the team to negotiate carefully, and review regularly, their roles in relation to each patient as these will vary from patient to patient and may change over time, depending on the personal rapport which each therapist has with the child and family. It is critically important for parents and patients to see the team as united and working together for the child's good. If disharmony is perceived, further disruption can be caused by parents (or patients) playing off one member of the team against another. Furthermore, if the team and the therapy plan are not well coordinated this can be a major cause of stress to the parents, as they may be presented with conflicting, and even incompatible, advice making it impossible for them to implement a cohesive therapy programme. Team meetings are therefore crucial to good management as they enable a regular review of progress, assessment and revision of the existing intervention programme and careful planning of future interventions. They should also provide opportunities for team members to discuss problems and gain support from each other.

As many physiotherapy assessments are based upon clinical judgement, it is essential for physiotherapists to maintain regular contact with non-disabled children to prevent distortion of the standard against which their judgements are made. In addition, they should allow themselves time to attend workshops and seminars to update their skills so that they can feel confident about their ability to provide the best possible service to their clients.

The four children and their families described earlier in the chapter will be used to illustrate some of the dilemmas which may face their physiotherapists.

Kim's physiotherapist

Kim was referred to the physiotherapy department by his paediatrician when he was 6-months-old and cerebral palsy was first suspected. Mary has been Kim's physiotherapist since then. She is 25 years old and single. She grew up on a property in the outback and during her high school years attended a boarding school in a country town. After obtaining her qualifications in physiotherapy she returned to work as a physiotherapist in the town's small general hospital. Nearly 2 years ago she decided to take an appointment in a large metropolitan hospital in order to specialize in paediatric physiotherapy. Kim's family were the first Vietnamese people she had ever met. She knew nothing about their culture or their language. Her father was very conservative and did not fully approve of Asian immigration. Mary found the communication problems difficult to deal with and, when she made a home visit, was taken aback by the cramped conditions in which the family lived. Initially she felt uncomfortable with the family but over the months she became very fond of Kim and established good rapport with Mrs T. Kim was making good progress and she felt confident that he would start to walk within the next few months.

Mary was shocked when Mrs T informed her that they would be attending the alternative therapy programme. She felt hurt and rejected and believed that the family's decision was a reflection of their dissatisfaction with her and with the therapy programme she had developed. She also felt angry that after all her hard work the other programme, which she regarded as totally inappropriate, would probably get the credit for Kim starting to walk.

COMMENTARY

Mary needs to talk about her feeling with her colleagues and come to a more realistic appraisal of the reasons for the T's decisions. This is important both in terms of restoring her self-confidence and enabling her to assure the parents of her continuing support and her willingness to provide therapy for Kim in the future if they should decide to discontinue the alternative programme.

Sarah's physiotherapist

Amanda works in a private physiotherapy practice in a suburb adjacent to the one in which Sarah lives. She took over as Sarah's physiotherapist when Louise left the practice 6 months ago to have a baby. Amanda is married and has three school-age children all of whom are high achievers and are involved in numerous out-of-school activities. Her husband works long hours and often has to be away from home on business. As a result she has a hectic schedule involving work, children's activities and household duties. She finds it difficult to schedule Sarah's sessions late in the afternoon and gets annoyed by Mrs G's continual requests for late appointments, frequent lack of punctuality and regular cancellation at short notice. She reflects upon her own busy life style and finds it difficult to relate to Mrs G's problems. She also feels frustrated with the lack of follow-through with the programme at home and questions whether it is legitimate to pursue a therapy programme for a child who has only subtle problems. She is, however, aware of the damage that can be done to Sarah's self-esteem if she continues to fail both at school and in the eyes of her father.

COMMENTARY

As a physiotherapist in private practice Amanda may have few opportunities to discuss her concerns with colleagues at work. Ideally she needs to have a supervisor with whom she can meet regularly to discuss her case load and air her concerns. Failing this it is important for her to maintain contact with her colleagues through meetings of the professional association and attendance at conferences, workshops and seminars.

John's physiotherapist

John's physiotherapist is Fiona. She is 29 years old and recently married. She was educated at a coeducational state high school in a lower middle class area of the city. She has four brothers and grew up in a family in which sport played an important role and where there was always a lot of rough-and-tumble play. She is currently studying part-time for a postgraduate degree. Two weeks ago her father had a heart attack and was admitted to a hospital close to the one in which she works. Her mother is staying with her so that she will be closer to the hospital. Although her father is now out of danger Fiona attempts to visit him every day. During this difficult time her colleagues have been very supportive and have taken over part of her case load so that she can have some time off.

John's difficult behaviour and verbal abuse have not particularly worried her although she has been aware of the effect they have had on many of the other staff. She has been able to gain his confidence and cooperation more than anyone else in the rehabilitation team and his progress has been excellent. She has also established a good relationship with John's mother and is conscious of the hardships imposed on her, and other members of the family, by her frequent trips between home and the hospital, and of her desire to be with John and give him her support. Fiona is aware that John tends to rely on her (although he would not openly admit this) and that she is one of the few members of staff whom he completely trusts. In view of this she feels that it would be detrimental to his progress if she was to ask one of her colleagues to take over his treatment. As a result she has elected to maintain him on her case load, although at times it has been difficult to fit in his sessions with all the other demands on her in the past 2 weeks.

COMMENTARY

Fiona works in a multidisciplinary rehabilitation team which has regular weekly meetings to discuss the programmes for the children they are working with. Initially Fiona took a leading role in the team as John required intensive physiotherapy to regain his motor skills and also because she could cope with his behaviour better than most other people. Like many head injury patients he made quite rapid progress in this area after regaining consciousness. This progress can be expected to continue although at a slower rate and the more subtle intellectual, emotional and language deficits are emerging as his primary problems. The roles of the team members will therefore require some careful revision. Detailed planning and liaison with local therapists will also be required to maintain his rehabilitation programme when he returns home. Fiona feels that John might respond better to a male therapist and that his older brother could possibly be persuaded to assist with the therapy programme. She, and other members of the team, will have to prepare John for his return home and for the change of therapists.

Jane's physiotherapist

Monica, Jane's physiotherapist, is in her late thirties. She is married and has two teenage children. She has a twin brother who has cerebral palsy and she remembers how much she resented the time her mother spent with him when they were children and how guilty she was made to feel whenever she complained about this. Monica has worked in the cystic fibrosis clinic for over 15 years and has known Jane since she was a baby. She knows the family very well and often sees them at social functions, as her daughter attends the same school as Jane.

Monica is distressed by the deterioration in Jane's condition. She has seen the same thing happen to other children but had not anticipated it with Jane as her cystic fibrosis had always been so well managed.

COMMENTARY

Monica needs to consider how her personal experiences and close, long-term involvement with the family will influence her management decisions. For example, suggesting to the family that they give Jane more autonomy in the management of her health may be difficult for her as she may see this as a criticism of the parents (who are by now her friends) or it may arouse feelings of guilt related to how she felt about her own mother during her childhood. Monica is able to talk over her feelings with the hospital counsellor, which helps her to view Jane's situation more objectively.

These thumbnail sketches aim to raise awareness of the conflicts which may arise for therapists as the result of their previous experience or current circumstances and the ways in which these may impinge upon treatment decisions.

The final part of this chapter will attempt to pull together all the psychosocial factors influencing the structure of intervention programmes which have been discussed. It aims to develop an overall strategy for planning paediatric interventions which is equally applicable to all forms of therapy. Specific interventions will not be discussed as these will be dealt with in the later chapters of the book by people who have much greater expertise in their management.

Focus on the Intervention Programme

When a child is referred for a physiotherapy programme a diagnosis has frequently already been made, or at the very least the referral letter should contain a description of the difficulties which the child is experiencing. The physiotherapist can therefore begin to plan the intervention programme.

The planning process should include the following steps:

1. **Review existing knowledge** about the condition and the form of intervention required. Check in the library and/or with the referring agency if further information is needed.

2. **Assess the child as a whole.** This includes taking into consideration the child's age, sex, developmental stage and developmental needs, personality, interests, likes and dislikes, intellectual abilities and any other relevant factors as well as his or her physical abilities and disabilities.

3. **Appraise the structure and functioning of the family,** including amongst others, the child's ordinal position in the family, the family's home environment, financial circumstances, job demands, attitudes, beliefs, expectations, support network, coping strategies, existing knowledge about and experience with the particular condition and capacity and motivation to participate in an intervention programme.

4. **Identify other intervention programmes which the child is involved in,** including those implemented by other members of the interdisciplinary team, of which the physiotherapist may be a member, and those conducted by community agencies such as remedial education programmes, and parenting programmes.

5. **Evaluate the position of the physiotherapy programme within the total intervention programme** and, with the permission of the parents, liaise with other professionals providing services for the child.

6. **Re-evaluate knowledge about management of the child's condition and develop an individualized intervention programme** catering for both the physical and psychosocial needs of the child and family. The programme must develop the child's abilities whilst at the same time strengthening areas of weakness. It must emphasize the development of functional skills by linking the development of motor skills to other areas of development such as the acquisition of self-help skills or involvement in peer group activities.

Except for the relatively short periods of time when children are hospitalized the majority of physiotherapy programmes will be carried out by untrained parents in the home environment. It is therefore essential for programmes to be easily learnt and implemented by lay people, and designed to be carried out in a normal home environment, and within the constraints of normal family life. Furthermore, programmes should be both motivating and enjoyable if parents and children are to persist with them.

Factors influencing the design and implementation of physiotherapy programmes for the four children described in this chapter will be used to illustrate the points listed above.

Kim's Physiotherapy Programme

When assessing Kim's development his physiotherapist must make allowance for the fact that he was born 12 weeks preterm. This number of weeks must therefore be deducted from his chronological age to gain an accurate impression of his rate of development. Furthermore, the principles guiding the management of cerebral palsy and the type of intervention programmes suitable for young children with this condition need to be reviewed (see Chapter 21).

Kim will need a physiotherapy programme to increase his mobility and improve the quality of his movements. It is vitally important, however, that this programme is functional and allows Kim to develop the skills which will enable him to make progress not only in his motor development but also in his cognitive, social and language development. He is at a developmental stage where he needs to gain some control over his environment, to be able to do some things for himself and to make some choices about the activities he will engage in. His physiotherapy programme might therefore include a feeding or dressing programme which would increase his sense of independence in these areas. It might also include some games which involve social interaction (for example, ball games, or peekaboo), some activities which provide cognitive stimulation (for example, form boards or simple puzzles), and some activities to encourage language development, such as action songs.

Kim is a quiet child who needs time to adjust to new environments, so it will be necessary to schedule a 'warm up' period into the therapy session. Given this, and the transport problems and time constraints experienced by Mrs T, it might be appropriate to schedule less regular but somewhat longer therapy sessions. He is only 2 years old so his attention span will be short and activities will need to be changed frequently. Consideration of his daily routine will also be necessary in order to schedule a time for his appointments when he will be alert and able to get the greatest benefit from the therapy sessions. As noisy toys are known to upset him their use should be kept to a minimum. They will cause disruption to the sessions and may lead Kim to associate unpleasant experiences with therapy sessions, thus reducing his level of cooperation. Choosing quiet colourful toys which he enjoys playing with and introducing new toys as he masters each skill, is likely to be more successful. As Kim's knowledge of English is limited, praise and rewards for achievements should be given not only in words but also in a visual form (for example, smiling, clapping, patting him, or giving him a little hug).

Similarly, as Mrs T and Kim do not have English as a first language they will need to be shown how to do things rather than being given verbal instructions: Mrs T should be encouraged to participate in activities to demonstrate that she has understood what is required. Arrangements should also be made for an interpreter to attend the sessions to ensure that Mrs T understands what she is told. It is unwise (and unprofessional) to rely on a friend or family member to act as an interpreter. This may lead to breaches of confidentiality or may limit what the patient, or parent, is willing to divulge. In addition, an unqualified interpreter may not be familiar with the technical language used and this may lead to a lot of misunderstanding and misinformation.

A home visit to ascertain what space and facilities are available for carrying out a therapy programme is often valuable as it is pointless to design a programme which cannot be implemented because of the family's living arrangements. The flat where the T family lives is quite small and there is not much room for special equipment or for boisterous activities. The flat is above the shop and the only access is via a steep flight of stairs. Mrs T is finding it difficult to carry Kim up and down the stairs in her advanced stage of pregnancy. In view of this Kim may need to be taught some strategies for managing the stairs at an earlier stage than would normally be considered in a developmental programme.

Mrs T feels under considerable pressure to assist her husband in the shop and cannot therefore devote a lot of time to working with Kim. A home therapy programme consisting of a number of short activities which can easily be slotted into the daily routine would therefore be ideal.

When Kim's family heard about the alternative therapy programme it sounded like a miracle. Their Vietnamese friends also thought it sounded wonderful. The Centre is close to their home so there would be fewer transport problems and the programme sounded quite simple and routine so that lots of friends could help Mrs T which would allow her to spend more time working in the shop. In addition, having read the magazine article, the members of the local church were so convinced about the programme that they were willing to pay for Kim's therapy. The offer seemed too good for the Ts to refuse.

Although most trained professionals would not see the alternative therapy programme as valid or acceptable. It is important to understand that the lay public have no way of judging the validity of these programmes or of evaluating their claims of success. Parents merely perceive the promise and the hope that the programmes hold out for them and they, and not the therapists, must make the decisions about what is best for their child. Parents are the ones who will continue to live with the child, and it is they who will bear the guilt if they feel that they have not tried everything possible to help their child.

Kim's physiotherapist feels, understandably, hurt, rejected and let down when Kim's parents decide to enrol him in an alternative therapy programme. She will gain little by trying to persuade the family against this decision and may run the risk of losing their respect and confidence if she tries to dissuade them. She should, however, be willing to give them her professional opinion about the programme. It would be inadvisable to continue with the conventional programme alongside the alternative therapy programme. The two programmes would be too time-consuming and would frequently be incompatible,

causing confusion, conflict and divided loyalties for the parents. Kim's therapist needs to explain this to Mr and Mrs T and to assure them of her continued interest in Kim. In order to maintain contact she may offer to reassess Kim in 6 months time and she must affirm her willingness to work with Kim again if they decide that the alternative therapy programme is unsuitable. Essentially the therapist must not make the parents feel guilty about trying a different form of therapy and must make it possible for the family to return to the conventional therapy programme without embarrassment or loss of face.

Sarah's Physiotherapy Programme

Sarah's motor problems are subtle but they are adversely affecting her school achievements, and this in turn is lowering her self-esteem and having a detrimental effect on her relationship with both her peers and her father. Sarah's physiotherapist will need to consider what is known about the management of minor coordination dysfunction (MCD) and the relationship between this condition and school achievement (see Chapter 22). Sarah will need an intervention programme which aims not only to improve her motor coordination and postural control but also to increase her self-esteem and self-confidence.

Sarah's motor problems are most apparent at school therefore the intervention programme needs to target skills that will allow her to function more effectively in this environment. However, as Sarah's self-esteem is low, she is somewhat depressed and rarely experiences success at school, the therapy programme should also incorporate activities which Sarah particularly enjoys and which she can successfully complete. Sarah thrives on praise and this needs to be given for improved performance as well as successful completion of tasks. Verbal praise will help, but concrete indicators of her achievements such as ticks, stars, stamps and certificates are likely to be more rewarding.

Sarah is conscientious and motivated to succeed. She has reached an age where she could take some responsibility for carrying out her intervention programme at home. This could increase her self-confidence and give her a feeling of self-efficacy and control over what happens to her. A star chart could be used to monitor this programme with a small prize or certificate if she carries out the activity at least four times a week.

She has few hobbies but does enjoy looking after her dog. It might therefore be possible to incorporate some activities in which she could play with the dog and at the same time improve her motor skills.

Sarah's low self-esteem and feelings of failure are also causing her to withdraw from her peer group. She needs to gain self-confidence and have some positive experiences with other children. In a private practice, group therapy sessions are unlikely to be feasible but it might be possible to include her in a vacation programme at a local community health centre or the children's hospital.

Taking Sarah out of school for therapy sessions is inadvisable as this draws attention to her problems and also causes her to miss lessons which she can ill afford to do as she is struggling academically. In addition, Sarah's mother's busy work schedule makes it difficult for her to keep daytime appointments. As Sarah's attention span is good and she is cooperative, one fairly long session with follow-up telephone calls to check on the home programme may be preferable to two, or more, short therapy sessions. It may also be possible to involve Sarah's grandparents in her therapy programme if her parents are agreeable. In addition, the physiotherapist should, with parental permission, liaise with Sarah's teacher to give her a greater understanding of Sarah's difficulties and some strategies for classroom management.

It is very important that Sarah's physiotherapist does not allow her irritation with Sarah's mother to jeopardize her relationship with Sarah, as this would add to Sarah's feelings of worthlessness. Sarah needs to perceive her physiotherapist as her friend and advocate.

John's Physiotherapy Programme

Following his accident, John's physiotherapy programme focused on helping him to regain the motor skills which he had lost. It aimed not only to increase his mobility but also to give him skills that enabled him to be as independent as possible. This included such things as getting in and out of bed, toileting and other self-help skills as well as skills which enabled him to entertain himself, for example the fine motor skills required to play computer games.

Because of John's difficult behaviour it was not easy to establish rapport or to gain his cooperation with therapy. Knowledge of his interests was valuable in this regard and the incorporation of discussions about the previous weekend's football games and the use of a videotapes of football games as a reward for cooperation were quite effective.

Like many children suffering brain injury, John made rapid progress in the first few months after his accident and regained some basic skills. These skills will now require refinement and the focus of therapy will have to shift to the mastery of the fine motor, cognitive, language and behavioural skills required for re-integration into school. This is likely to be a long-term programme which can be more appropriately conducted on an outpatient basis. In any case his mother is anxious for him to return home because of the problems that his hospitalization is creating for the family.

Because of the family's circumstances John will not be able to return regularly to the metropolitan hospital, where he has been cared for during the acute recovery stage, for continuing therapy. It is therefore necessary for the hospital rehabilitation team to plan not only for his discharge from hospital but also for the hand over of the rehabilitation programme to community-based therapists.

It is unlikely that there will be a rehabilitation team, as such, in John's local area so there will probably need to be liaison with a number of different agencies for the provision of ongoing care. John's physiotherapist believes that, in view of his behaviour, he may relate better to a male therapist. This person may also be able to involve John's older brother in the therapy programme. She knows of a young man, who went through university with her, who is currently working in John's home area. He has not had a lot of experience in paediatrics but she feels that he would be able to work with John if she provided him with some guidance and support. John will not be able to return to school for some time but provisions need to be made for him to continue with his schooling and have social contact with his peers. A social worker may need to be involved to help the family make whatever arrangements are necessary to meet John's needs, and a psychologist may be required to provide counselling and a behaviour modification programme to manage John's unacceptable behaviour. These services will all need to be coordinated. Before John leaves the hospital an appointment should be made for him to attend for review and reassessment in approximately 3 months so that there is no sense of abandonment and any problems with the continuity of the programme can be resolved.

Jane's Physiotherapy Programme

Jane has been attending the cystic fibrosis clinic and having twice-daily chest physiotherapy at home since she was a baby. She has had a number of admissions to hospital over the years but never as many as in the past year. In general, her condition has been extremely well controlled and she has remained healthy. She knows the staff in the clinic well and is on first-name terms with many of them. She is particularly fond of Monica, the physiotherapist whom she has known all her life.

Jane has been over-protected by her parents who have organized her life for her. She has had to make few decisions but she has had little freedom.

The content of the physiotherapy programme will have changed little over the years; however, at this stage it may be valuable to encourage Jane to take more responsibility for her health by giving her the knowledge and skills to take control of her physiotherapy programme. This will give her some degree of independence.

Jane appears to be depressed and it will also be important to rekindle some of her previous interests and develop new interests. For example, an interest in cooking could help her to plan her diet in more varied ways and an interest in grooming, make-up or dressmaking might help to increase her self-confidence and self-esteem.

It will also be important to assist Jane in negotiating increased independence from her parents, and perhaps to assist her parents in finding new avenues for their energies so that they do not resent losing control of Jane's therapy. Furthermore, the possibility of Jane's death needs to be addressed and Jane, her parents and the members of the therapy team need to be given the support and counselling necessary to confront this issue.

Summary

These examples have been used to illustrate the fact that physiotherapy programmes involve much more than simply the mechanical treatment of physical abnormalities. To be effective they must address the well-being of the child as a whole and must be compatible with the needs and resources of the family. The physiotherapy programme is frequently only one component of a much broader rehabilitation programme and therefore must not only fulfil the needs of the child and family, but also be carefully crafted to fit in with the other aspects of the programme. To be an expert therapist it is not sufficient to be a good technician, it is also necessary to be sensitive to the needs and circumstances of the families whom you serve and the colleagues with whom you work.

REFERENCES

Baldwin, SM (1985) *The Cost of Caring*, 210 pp. London: Routledge and Kegan Paul.

Baxter, C (1989) Parental access to assistance from services: social status and age related differences. *Australian and New Zealand Journal of Developmental Disabilities* 15(1): 15–25.

Becker, MH (1979) Understanding patient compliance: the contributions of attitudes and other psychological factors. In: Cohen S (ed.), *New Directions in Patient Compliance*, pp 1–31. Lexington, MA: Lexington Books.

Beresford, BA (1994) Resources and strategies: how parents cope with the care of a disabled child. *Journal of Child Psychology and Psychiatry* 33(1): 171–209.

Brett, KM (1988) Sibling responses to chronic childhood disorders: research perspectives and practice implications. *Issues in Comprehensive Pediatric Nursing* 11: 43–57.

Bristol, MM, Gallagher, JJ, Schopler, E (1988) Mothers and fathers of young developmentally disabled and nondisabled boys: adaptation and spousal support. *Developmental Psychology* 24(3): 441–451.

Brown, A, Hepple, S (1989) *How Parents Cope*. Hertford: Barnardo's.

Burden, R, Thomas, D (1986a) Working with parents of exceptional children: the need for more careful thought and more positive action. *Disability, Handicap and Society* 1: 165–171.

Burden, R, Thomas, D (1986b) A further perspective on parental reaction to handicap. *Exceptional Child* 33(2): 140–145.

Bush, JP, Melamed, BG, Sheras PL *et al.* (1986) Mother–child patterns of coping with anticipatory medical stress. *Health Psychology* 5: 137–157.

Calderon, R, Greenberg, MT (1993) Considerations in the adaption of families with school age deaf children. In: Marschark, M, Clark, D (eds) *Psychological Perspectives on Deafness*, pp 27–47. Hillsdale, NJ: Lawrence Erlbaum.

Cooke, K, Bradshaw, J, Lawton, D *et al.* (1986) Child disablement, family dissolution and reconstitution. *Developmental Medicine and Child Neurology* **28**: 610–616.

Eiser, C (1990) *Chronic Childhood Disease: An Introduction to Psychological Theory and Research*, 174 pp. Cambridge: Cambridge University Press.

Eiser, C (1993) *Growing up with a Chronic Disease. The Impact on Children and their Families*, 255 pp. London: Jessica Kingsley.

Freeman, RD, Malkin, SF, Hastings, JO (1975) Psychosocial problems of deaf children and their families. *American Annals of the Deaf* **120**: 391–405.

Frey, K, Greenberg, M, Fewell, R (1989) Stress and coping amongst parents of handicapped children: a multidimensional approach. *American Journal of Mental Retardation* **94**: 240–249.

Gallagher, JJ, Beckman, P, Cross, AH (1983) Families of handicapped children: sources of stress and its amelioration. *Exceptional Children* **50**: 3–14.

Garrison, WT, McQuiston, S (1989) *Chronic Illness During Childhood and Adolescence. Psychological Aspects*, 160 pp. Newbury Park: Sage.

Hornby, G (1992) A review of fathers' accounts of their experiences of parenting children with disabilities. *Disability, Handicap and Society* **7(4)**: 363–374.

Kampfe, C (1989) Parental reaction to a child's hearing impairment. *American Annals of the Deaf* **134**: 255–259.

Knafl, KA, Deatrick, JA (1990) Family management style: concept analysis and development. *Journal of Pediatric Nursing* **5(1)**: 4–14.

Lazarus, RS, Folkman, S (1984) Coping and adaption. In: Gentry, WD (ed.) *Handbook of Behavioural Medicine*, pp 282–325. New York: Guilford Press.

Martin, DA (1988) Children and adolescents with traumatic brain injury: impact on the family. *Journal of Learning Disabilities* **21**: 464–470.

McConachie, H (1986) *Parents and Young Mentally Handicapped Children: A Review of Research Issues*. London: Croom Helm.

McMichael, JK (1971) *Handicap: A Study of Physically Handicapped Children and their Families*, 208 pp. London: Staples Press.

Meltzer, H, Smyth, M, Robus, N (1989) *OPCS Surveys of Disability in Great Britain, Report 6, Disabled Children, Services Transport and Education*. London: HMSO.

Mohay, H (in press) Interviewing children. In: Sanders, M, Mitchell, C, Byrne, G (eds), *Medical Consultation Skills: A Practical Handbook*. Sydney: Addison Wesley.

Newson, E, Hipgrave, T (1982) *Getting Through to Your Handicapped Child*, 134 pp. Cambridge: Cambridge University Press.

Olshansky, J (1962) Chronic sorrow: a response to having a mentally deficient child. *Social Casework* **43**: 190–193.

Parker, G (1990) *With Due Care and Attention*, 2nd edn. London: Family Policy Studies Centre.

Pless, B, Nolan, T (1991) Revision, replication and neglect in research on maladjustment in chronic illness. *Journal of Child Psychology and Psychiatry* 32: 347–365.

Quine, L, Pahl, J (1985) Tracing the causes of stress in families with severely mentally handicapped children. *British Journal of Social Work* **15**: 501–517.

Schilling, RF, Gilchrist, LD, Schinke, SP (1984) Coping and social support in families of developmentally disabled children. *Family Relations* **33**: 47–54.

Seligman, M (1991) Grandparents of disabled grandchildren: hopes fears and adaptations. *Families in Society: Journal of Contemporary Human Services* **72(3)**: 147–152.

Smith, M, Robus, N (1989) *The Financial Circumstances of Families with Disabled Children Living in London*. London: HMSO.

Traustadottir, R (1991) Mothers who care. Gender, disability and family life. *Journal of Family Issues* **12(2)**: 211–228.

Trute, B, Hauch, C (1988) Building on family strengths: a study of families with positive adjustment to the birth of a developmentally disabled child. *Journal of Marital and Family Therapy* **14(2)**: 185–193.

Waalander, PK, Kreutzer, JS (1988) Family response to childhood traumatic brain injury. *Journal of Head Trauma Rehabilitation* **3**: 51–63.

Wallander, JL, Pitt, LC, Mellins, CA (1990) Child functional independence and maternal psychosocial stress as risk factors threatening adaptation in mothers of physically or sensorally handicapped children. *Journal of Consulting and Clinical Psychology* **58(6)**: 818–824.

Weiss, M (1994) *Conditional Love. Parents' Attitudes Towards Handicapped Children*, 296 pp. Westport, Conn: Bergin and Garvey.

SELECTED READING

Baldwin, SM (1985) *The Cost of Caring*, 210 pp. London: Routledge and Kegan Paul.

Beresford, BA (1994) Resources and strategies: how parents cope with the care of a disabled child. *Journal of Child Psychology and Psychiatry* **33(1)**: 171–209.

Eiser, C (1993) *Growing Up with a Chronic Disease. The Impact on Children and their Families*, 255 pp. London: Jessica Kingsley.

Garrison, WT, McQuiston, S (1989) *Chronic Illness During Childhood and Adolescence. Psychological Aspects*, 160 pp. Newbury Park: Sage.

Section B:

The Growing and Developing Child

PROLOGUE: YVONNE BURNS

Prologue

YVONNE BURNS

Growth and maturation begin in utero and continue throughout childhood into adolescence. While in utero there is an orderly development of the various structures and systems basic to survival and function. As physiotherapists it is important to recognize that the continuum of growth and development throughout childhood is influenced by external input and experience gained from the environment through which one moves. Sensation and movement are closely intertwined at both the automatic and volitional levels as one learns to move and moves to learn.

The first three chapters of Section B follow the development of movement in three stages: from birth through the first 2 years; in early childhood from 2 to 6 years; and through the school-aged period of around 6 years to puberty. Rather than considering development as purely age related, the authors address the importance of recognizing individual differences and alternative perspectives on development. In addition, the importance of an efficient postural background for effective volitional motor control; the significance of the development, integration and interpretation of input from the various senses in coordination and the performance of motor skills; and the role of motivation and experience are discussed.

Knowledge and understanding of motor development in the first few years after birth is not enough: important changes continue to occur throughout childhood and puberty. These chapters attempt to provide a baseline for the paediatric physiotherapist responsible for the assessment and treatment of children at any age with a wide, and often complex, variety of conditions.

Chapter 5 addresses the sequential development, interdependence and maturation in utero, of neuromuscular and skeletal systems relevant to the development of movement. Chapter 6 follows logically in that it considers the factors that adversely affect brain growth or cause other abnormalities of growth and development during pre-, peri- and early postnatal periods.

2

Development of Movement – Birth to 2 Years

YVONNE BURNS

Development
•
Theoretical Basis of Movement
•
Motor Control
•
Development of Movement: Basis for Effective Performance

The first 2 years after birth represents a time of dramatic change in the growth and development of a child. Although during the first few weeks after birth the infant can respond to touch, taste, sound, movement and visual images, especially the human face, they are totally dependent on a carer for nourishment, protection, support against gravity and movement through the environment. By 2 years most children have a basic appreciation of the environment in which they live, motor independence in locomotion, functional ability in feeding and assisting with dressing/undressing and some verbal communication. They can hold and manipulate objects and are aware of basic differences in size, feel and use but their movement and coordination lacks precision and dexterity. In comparison to a child of 6 years, the movement of the 2 year old could be considered clumsy. The process of change which occurs throughout childhood and adolescence is called development.

Development

Development is a complex interactive process of change involving all aspects of growth and maturation of body systems. The pattern of development of each child is unique as inherent characteristics are influenced by the constant chain of transactions between the child and the environment (Ausubel and Sullivan 1970, Sameroff 1980). During the first few years developmental progress tends to follow a broad but orderly sequence which allows a certain amount of age-related predictability about the expected abilities and performance of a child. Although there is considerable individual variability within and between children at various ages, there are particular characteristics that allow some broad judgements about level and quality of performance to be made. It is on the basis of these more expected and repeatable characteristics that the development of a particular infant or child can be compared with that of age-related peers or against selected criteria. Assessment of infants and children is addressed in Chapter 7.

In order to assess infants or children at any age it is imperative to have a clear understanding and knowledge of development. It is important to be able to recognize the individual characteristics of performance as well as the expected age-related abilities and responses to specific inputs. The borderline between variations of the normal motor development and 'real' deviations, which are often subtle or minor in presentation, is difficult to derive unless the assessor has a detailed knowledge of normal development (Flehmig 1992). When examining the posture and movement of an infant or child it is essential that the way in which the child performs a task or responds to a situation is considered in some detail, not just the achievement of a goal or milestone. When dealing with such a complex interactive process as development, defects in any part of the system are likely to influence performance in a number of ways. Furthermore, each child has their own personality, ability to react to stimuli from the environment, respond to possibilities provided through sensory receptive systems and a freedom of choice. The observer therefore requires an extensive background knowledge of all aspects of development in the areas of cognition — reasoning and learning; hearing, speech and language; vision and eye—hand coordination; motor performance; and social and emotional development.

Table 1 provides a broad framework of aspects of development over the first 5 years; there are a number of texts available which provide details of age-appropriate expectations and these will complement this text.

Individual Differences in Development

Some differences in development relate to inherited characteristics, others to neural and physiological maturation, while differences in performance can be due to the level and efficiency in sensorimotor feedback systems (Williams *et al.* 1983). According to Ayres (1972), Martenuik (1979) and Smyth and Wing (1984), successful movement relies on effective and efficient feedback. In a 5-year longitudinal study Burns *et al.* (1984) found that children at any age exhibit expressions of development that are charac-

teristic of their particular age, but vary individually according to various inherited attributes, the influence of previous experiences or events, the present situation, the special demands of assessment test items, and the continual transactions which occur between the child and people and objects within the immediate environment. Structural and growth factors, particularly age-related proportional changes, also influence development of posture and movement (Sinclair 1989). For example, the centre of gravity in the young child is much higher than in the older child and adult. Some social and cultural customs, such as infant positioning, may result in minor postural differences, but have little effect on the overall development of movement. It is important to consider also the motivation that lies behind the action since motor performance is often determined not so much by ability as by the motivation to achieve.

Infants born prematurely several weeks before term will often present with minor variations in later development. The age of infants born 6 or more weeks before term should be corrected for the number of weeks early for at least the first 2 years and possibly longer, depending on the nature and precision of the test. When the age of the infant born preterm is adjusted for the number of weeks born before term their motor development generally follows the expected sequence of age-related abilities (Burns *et al.* 1984, Mandich *et al.* 1994). Some qualitative differences in performance, however, have been noted and the incidence of both minor and major problems of movement is higher than average in a population of children very preterm and/or who have required prolonged neonatal intensive care (Drillien *et al.* 1980, MacDonald *et al.* 1991). Even problems that appear to be minor in terms of disability, but interfere with the quality of performance, can adversely affect performance at school. Signs of neurological, motor and/or behavioural difficulties need to be recognized and acted upon as early as possible (Drillien *et al.* 1988).

The development of infants who have experienced numerous problems during the neonatal period may appear to be delayed, particularly in the first 6 months after term. Often this is a reflection of their health status and is transitory. By 8 months post-term the

Table 1

Development from 1 Month to 6 Years: An Overview Indicating Progress in Aspects of Functioning

Age	Postural/motor	Social/emotional/behavioural	Hearing/vocalization/speech/language	Visual/eye—hand manipulative	Performance
1/12	Overall flexor posture of limbs Reflex response to specific sensory stimuli	Consolability [when picked up] Alertness — to sound and visual input response to mother Self quieting 6/52 — smiles and cuddliness	Startled by sound vocalization 6/52 — listens to sound	Follows a ball visually: horizontally [4/52], vertically [6/52], circle [8/52] Grasp reflex Tactile grasp [12/52]	Hand to mouth Active movement of legs Some movement of arms
4/12	Held in sit — head up and balanced Prone — rests on elbows and hands; may roll from back to side In prone — head above midline Supported prone — head in line with body	Plays with mother Anticipates being picked up Aware of new situations	Vocalizes two different sounds Turns towards sound source	Ulnar—palmar grasp Watches object pulled by string Visually explores room Eyes follow all movement Eyes converge and fix on specific object	Holds toy Plays with own fingers Attempts to reach for toy held at appropriate distance
8/12	Landau, present Placing/supporting Takes weight All righting reaction Protects forward and to side parachute Sits alone, rolls, creeps, may crawl	Knows strangers from friends, but wary. Stretches to be lifted Reacts to own image in mirror Cries if toy removed	Listens to speech Babbles MM da da, four different sounds Drinks from cup Cup held by 'M'	Grasps dangling object Transfers/takes hand from hand Pulls toy by string Gross pincer grasp Some fine pincer grasp	Rings a bell Uncovers hidden toy [shown] Manipulates two objects, i.e. one in each hand
12/12	Furniture walk or hand held Attains sitting Has trunk rotation Crawls on hands and knees Equilibrium in sit	Waves bye-bye 'Give me' games Sociable to people Plays with self in mirror	Initiates vocalization Babbled monologue when alone Uses three words appropriately Can chew solid food Follows unseen sound	Fine pincer approach Index finger point Opposition grasp Sees and picks up tiny things off floor	Finds a hidden toy Accept three cubes Takes object out of container Tries to copy with pencil
18/12	Walks well: wide base-gait, flat feet; centre of gravity between feet Equilibrium in stand Squats, stoops, trots Throw, hits, kicks ball	Looks at book and enjoys it Feeds self with cup; uses spoon	Uses five words appropriately Names a picture — dog, cat, horse, ball, book, cup	Holds several blocks in one hand Puts three bricks in tower Places pegs in a board	Recognizes a circle; puts two circles in a board Puts cubes back in box Points to body parts
24/12	Walks up and down stairs with rail Jumps off step Seats self in chair Throws ball into basket Reaches outside base Forward weight shift in walking	Helps with drawing Asks for things Will cooperate on command Very mother-dependent Often emotionally labile Plays beside rather than with others	Four syllable/phrases 4—8 common objects identified Names four pictures	Can open screw top Builds tower, five bricks Scribbles Draws strokes with a pencil Pincer grasp of pencil	Screws open a toy. Puts circle, square and triangle in board

Table 1
Continued

Age	Postural/motor	Social/emotional/behavioural	Hearing/vocalization/speech/language	Visual/eye—hand manipulative	Performance
36/12	Walks up and down stairs one foot per step. Walks on tip toes Copies cross leg sit	Gives name Knows sex and age Cooperative Loves to play Imitates. Likes to succeed	Six syllable sentences, two adjectives, 12—20 pictures Some immature consonants	Builds tower of eight bricks Threads 6—12 beads	Copies circle and a cross Cuts with scissors Knows big and little Knows money Repeats three number sequence
48/12	Hops three steps Walks line for 4 feet Marches to music Runs fast on flat surface — no falls	Very changeable Often aggressive — 'know all' Can undress Plays with older children	Six colours Comprehends two items and tells use of and uses personal pronouns	Cuts paper Draws a man Early tripod grasp Definite hand preferred	Height, weight, length comparisons, e.g. which is tallest Counts to 4 Matches by colour and size
60/12 [5 years]	Runs up steps Jumps rope 15 cm [2 feet together] Running kick	Cooperative Performs all sensory motor tests [tactile and kinaesthetic]	Names opposites Ten syllable sentence Shows 12 different aspects of a picture	Draws △ Has good dynamic tripod grasp	Counts 10—15 Can name which goes faster Builds model gates
72/12 [6 years]	Jumps three steps Throws and catches a ball in hands Runs very fast outside — no falls	Knows full address Can go on errands Has play-mates and names them	Names letters of alphabet Numbers, shapes and sizes	Writes name [prints] Draws triangle and three letters without copy	Knows opposite to high is low, also right and left Can repeat five digit sequence.

picture appears to be clearer and it is possible to identify more accurately infants in whom development is normal, delayed or definitely abnormal (Burns *et al.* 1989).

Theoretical Basis of Movement

There are differing schools of thought about development of motor performance. The more long-standing approach follows a theory of maturation based on the early work of Gesell (1954) and later Wyke (1975) who generally describes early development in terms of neural maturation. This theory supports the view that the integrity of the basic structure of the brain and the timing of the processes of cell division and proliferation, neuronal migration, differentiation and maturation, glial cell expansion, dendrite elaboration, neural myelination and process formation are important precursors of normal development (Volpe 1981).

Another view considers the development of con-

trolled movement as a self-organizing process whereby there is a close interactive and dynamic link between the infant's level of skills, the intrinsic properties of movement and the demand of the task (Corbetta and Thelen 1994). This dynamic systems approach tends to link biomechanical and behavioural variables. Thelen and Ulrich (1991) observed that 'the motivational aspect of locomoting towards a desired goal is independent of the means of achieving that goal. Infants will scoot, roll, shuffle, creep, crawl or use a wheeled device to reach a desired object often 6 months or more before they can walk. It is not the translation of intention into motor action that limits locomotion, but the developmental readiness of the sensory and neuromotor elements needed for particular postures and actions' (pp. 40—41).

It is most likely that maturation, learning, perception, practice and emotional factors all contribute. When there is a problem of development it is important to recognize that there are a number of ways of approaching intervention, remediation and opening opportunities for further development. From the maturational perspective, movement begins in utero and increases as the brain and nervous system mature. Even in utero there exist fairly elaborate facilitatory and inhibitory reflexogenic feedback systems to motoneuronal pools from the mechanoreceptors. Progressive sophistication of the neuromuscular control systems involves the development of cortical projection systems, enabling the acquisition of feedback and servocontrol systems affecting movement. In these systems, response can be modulated up or down from either peripheral or central regulatory mechanisms. Furthermore, inhibition as well as excitation appears to play an important role in the control and differentiation of movement. In 1975 Wyke stated that 'although movements of parts of the body are effected by the synchronously coordinated contraction and relaxation of striated muscles operating, for the most part, over joints — the stimulus to produce such movements and the control mechanisms that regulate their execution and bring them to an appropriate stop, are neurological' (p. 19). Despite this it is still not clear how and where the appropriate motor commands that are sent to the muscles are tailored in accordance with the mechanical requirements of the task (Paillard 1988). See Figure 1.

Motor Control

In the development of motor control during the first 2 years there is evidence of both increasing maturation of the nervous system and learning through experience. Studies have shown that soon after birth

Figure 1   Fun Activities Require Muscle Control

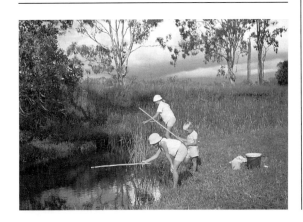

the newborn infant can orient towards a visual stimulus and has a variety of movements some of which are fairly stereotypical patterns, called primitive or infant (reflex) patterns of movement while others follow no consistent pattern. Within a few months, the child can reach and grasp an object, but the biomechanical characteristics of this reaching vary considerably between infants (Corbetta and Thelen 1994). In the early months, background postural control is inconsistent and unreliable. Through feedback from sensory receptors various postural and movement adjustments are established and successful outcome of goal-orientated movement occurs more consistently. After further experience, anticipatory or feedforward postural control occurs. According to Haas and Diener (1988) this preparatory activation is essential for effective and economic motor performance. In fact, Woollacott et al. (1989) studied the activation of postural muscles in very young children and found that feedforward activation to stabilize the trunk can occur in advance of a reaching movement of the arm in infants under 12 months.

Functional or Voluntary Movement

Functional or voluntary movement is composed of two interactive components: (1) a stable support which includes postural adjustment to preserve orientation of the body in the field of gravitational forces, and (2) a displacement or movement towards a goal (Figure 2). The stabilizing action normally precedes the second component which is concerned with the voluntary action. These components, however, are intertwined in variable synergies. Three characteristic

Figure 2   Stable Postural Control by 12 Months

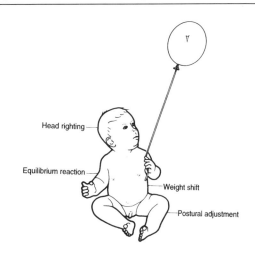

features of synergies underlying postural adjustment associated with goal-directed segmental movement have been outlined by Massion (1984). These are:

(1) their anticipatory nature which minimizes the extent of disturbance to posture and equilibrium caused by movement; (2) their ability to adapt efficiently to the conditions under which the movement is performed; and (3) the influence of instruction which modifies the pattern as a function of the task. In addition, Paillard (1988) drew attention to the importance of the context in which the movement was occurring. Changing postural constraints, different motivations and emotions and concurrent tactile, visual and proprioceptive inputs have a marked influence on the type of motor response used. The nervous system obviously has an incredibly adaptive capacity and a wide range of performance strategies. A strategy for postural control and movement on a stable (ground) base will be different from postural adjustment and control of movement in an unstable situation or in a moving environment. Furthermore, individual strategies will vary considerably. A child with poor feedforward or feedback mechanisms will require different strategies to a child with postural mechanisms that are both efficient and effective.

Development of Movement: Basis for Effective Performance

The building blocks for later effective and efficient motor performance which are laid down in the first 2 years after birth include an ability to sustain a stable postural background, perform volitional movement and maintain equilibrium as well as to plan and carry out the desired action in a coordinated controlled manner. Over a number of years the child will build on this base by using movement to perform and repeat a large variety of activities in a range of postures and situations, will develop an efficient interplay of muscle action, strength, flexibility and endurance, a range of joint movement and a level of coordination and control that enables performance of highly skilled activities.

Posture and Movement in the First 12 Months

The overall postural presentation of the newborn is one of flexion, but within a couple of weeks the baby starts to stretch out into more extended postures. Flexion may be accentuated in the prone position due to the influence of the tonic labyrinthine reflex (TLR) while in supine an increase in trunkal extensor tone due to the influence of the same reflex can be noted. The knees and elbows remain flexed, but, the hips tend to abduction and the shoulders mildly retract. The influence of these early TLR patterns of movement may be assessed by supporting the child upright in sitting, holding around the chest and gradually lowering backwards (or forwards). Presence is indicated by a positive arching into extension as the head (labyrinth) moves 45 degrees or more towards the supine (or trunk flexion as the head is moved forward) as illustrated in Figure 3. This method of testing overcomes the problem of differentiating between muscle weakness (the head only drops but no trunk arching), behavioural resistance to pull to sit and the TLR. Similarly, the flexor response can be seen as the head and trunk is moved forward.

As the infant attains more extension when supine, an asymmetrical posturing of the arms is frequently noted. This asymmetrical tonic neck reflex (ATNR) may be stimulated by the turning of the head. Neck rotation results in the facial limbs extending and the occipital limbs flexing. In the infant about 4–6 weeks post-term, the influence of ATNR is marked and sometimes quite strong in the upper limbs. Lacey *et al.* (1987) observed a dominant ATNR pattern of movement, particularly in the lower limbs in very premature infants, who later demonstrated abnormal motor development. Other reproducible fairly stereotyped patterns of movement which can be elicited during the first few weeks after birth include the grasp reflexes in both feet and hands in response to touch on the palmar or plantar surfaces, the placing response to touch on the dorsum of the foot or hand, the Moro reflex in response to sudden movement of the head, primary standing stimulated by weight through the feet, and the walking reflex when weight and centre of gravity is moved forward. For the

Figure 3   Testing for Evidence of Tonic Labyrinthine Reflex (TLR)

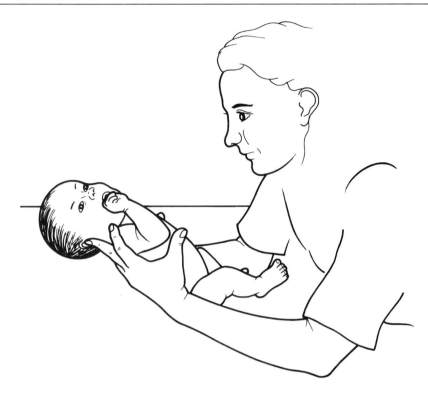

assessment of these and any other infant/primitive (reflex) reproducible patterns of movement it is important to follow specific testing procedures.

During these first few weeks the infant is starting to follow visually a small object or face moved horizontally and then vertically, and by about 6 weeks the infant will smile in response to appropriate input. Feeding is important for both mother and baby. Success in feeding provides the mother with positive feelings about herself and her baby. Early oral intake is in the form of repeated bursts of primitive sucking where the tongue presses the nipple/teat against the hard palate and gradually changes over the first 2 months into a stronger suck pattern where the tongue moves down behind the lower gum and the intraoral pressure is reduced to stimulate the flow of fluid. Control of head position plays an important role in the development of both eye follow and feeding.

The control of the head position while being picked up and held in sitting at first is intermittent and bobbing, but soon becomes stable while at the same time social interaction and interest in immediate surroundings motivates a desire to keep the head erect (Figure 4). Stability of head control when prone is usually associated with stability of the shoulder girdle during support on elbows or hands appearing usually by about the fourth month. About the same time, when supine, the head can be maintained centrally and hands brought to the midline (Figure 5).

Playing with hands or feet is frequently noted over the next month or two. Head control in all positions and throughout movement is largely dependent on the development of head righting to gravity.

Figure 4   Early Head Control in Supported Sitting

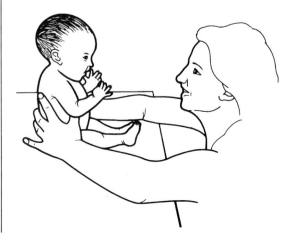

Figure 5 Centralizing to the Midline. Baby centralizing upper and lower limbs, eyes focusing centrally on mother

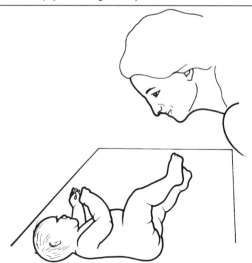

As the infant enters the third month after term early signs of head righting to gravity may be observed. Gradually over the next 3 months an immediate and automatic adjustment of the head to gravity in supported vertical (forward, back and sides) and horizontal (ventral, side and dorsal) positions will develop (Figure 6). Other automatic postural righting reactions collectively called 'body righting' include the response of the body and limbs to turning the head, the realignment of the head to a changed position of the body and the segmental alignment of the body to itself as observed when the upper or lower trunk is rotated around the central body axis (Peiper 1963, Bobath and Bobath 1972).

Figure 6 Testing Head Righting (Lateral) in Horizontal Support

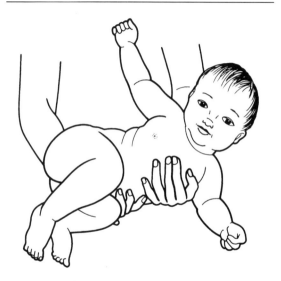

By the sixth month or soon after, a positive Landau reaction (head, trunk and hip extension in ventral suspension) will usually be present (Figure 7). These automatic postural reactions are associated with the maintenance of posture against gravity and subtle postural realignment during changes of position. The Landau reaction appears to be important in the development of upright posture.

Basic postural stability using the trunk flexors, extensors and rotators needs to be established as the base on which a plethora of motor abilities can be built. A number of supporting and weight-shift reactions occur during the activities of prone elbow support, creeping, crawling on hands and knees as well as in standing. It is important to recognize the difference between infant primary standing reflex and the positive supporting reaction observed in supported standing from about 6–9 months onwards (Touwen 1976). A positive support reaction is indicated by co-contraction of muscles around a joint providing a firm but dynamic pillar of support. This is often preceded by a shift of weight on to the particular limb or joints.

Achievement of control in and out of positions is facilitated by the ability to shift weight to one side, to support or stabilize the joints of the weight-bearing limb and thus allow the non-supporting limb to move freely. (See Figure 8).

Lateral and then diagonal weight shift may be observed also as the infant starts creeping, crawling on hands and knees and achieving standing (Figures 9 and 10). Raising the centre of gravity, as in sitting, crawling, standing and walking, places a demand for equilibrium not previously required. At first, displacement will cause a protective response of the limbs in the direction to which the body is falling, but an antidisplacement response or equilibrium reaction is soon noted.

Figure 7 The Landau Reaction

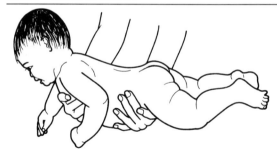

Figure 8   Lateral Weight Shift to Right Shoulder

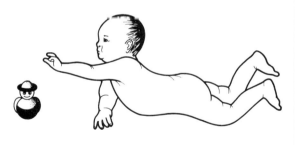

Figure 9   Diagonal Weight Shift – Shoulder to Opposite Hip

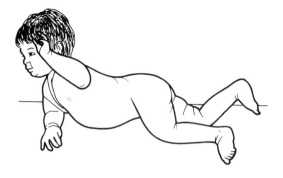

The more unstable and complex the position, the more need there is to learn new strategies of equilibrium and thus balance to maintain the desired position.

Balance is the functional expression of the interplay of all reactions to maintain a steady state. Control of weight shift, stability and equilibrium are particularly evident as the centre of gravity is raised in standing and the child starts to step out independently. Early walking is basically a side-to-side motion on a relatively wide base with the centre of gravity maintained within that base. Taking a step forward narrows the base and requires a weight shift to the supporting leg to free the stepping leg for movement as well as good dynamic muscular control around the hip and pelvis of the supporting leg (Figure 10). This is usually achieved 4–6 months after first independent steps. Throughout the second 12 months the development of motor control, independent bipedal locomotion, coordinated grasp and release, constructive play and verbal communication and independence in basic activities, continue.

The Hand in Infant Development

The hands play a very important role in motor development and develop unique skills. In addition to the

Figure 10   Weight Shift to Left Hip to Allow Right Leg Free to Place Forward

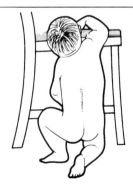

important grasp and manipulation of objects, the hands hold, support, protect, assist in balance, and provide an important avenue for learning, communication and social interaction. The hand is tactilely sensitive and from the outset a grasp response can be stimulated by touch. This grasp reflex can be often observed while the baby is feeding and grasping the mother's finger. This palmar reflex is stimulated by touch to the palm. At the same time the hand will open reflexly in response to touch or pressure on the back of the hand. This placing reflex is often demonstrated by touching the back of the hand on the edge of a table and the infant will extend the wrist and fingers and 'place' the heel on the table. Gradually the stereotyped flexion of the fingers into the palm is replaced by a 'seeking' action in response to touch to the lateral border of the hand (Twitchell 1970) (Figure 11).

By 10–12 weeks the infant will often turn the hand and follow a touch to the ulnar side before grasping the object. Frequently the infant will then turn to look at the hand and object. Sometimes the infant will

Figure 11   Tactile or Seeking Grasp

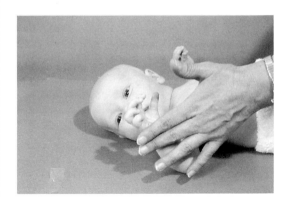

Figure 12   Clutching — Plucking Using Ulnar Fingers

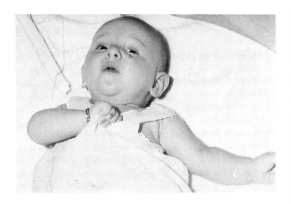

attempt to repeat the activity with a rather uncoordinated grasp. By about the third month the infant plucks the clothing with the lateral (ulnar) three fingers and soon clasps the hands in the midline (Figure 12). At first this appears to be unintentional.

By the fourth month, holding objects or clothing for a short period is frequently observed and the infant may reach to grasp a ring or other suitable object held in an appropriate position (i.e. to the side of midline). The infant, at first, may or may not visually direct the intention to grasp. The patterns, use and control of hand movements continue through palmar approach and grasp using fingers and palm (Figure 13) and then, gross pincer between base of thumb and index finger.

At first an infant will place both hands on to a toy in the midline, but later when given two objects to hold will drop one. While holding one object they may take it from the holding hand with the free hand. This action, called transference, normally occurs after 6 months of age and appears to precede being aware of

Figure 13   Palmar Approach

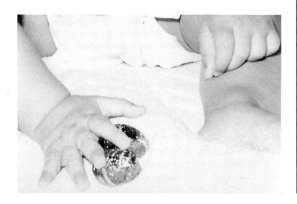

Figure 14   Take from — Transfer

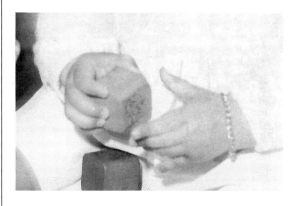

holding one object in each hand and banging one object with or on to another. See Figure 14.

Between 9 and 12 months, fine pincer, index pointing and poking and thumb—index opposition become more and more part of everyday play (Figures 15 and 16). The hands by this time are used to feeling different textured surfaces, finding and picking up tiny things, feeding food to the mouth, expressing and communicating wants and providing social interaction in the form of waving and clapping. It appears that children who perform more object-exploring activities, both manipulative and oral, are more coordinated than infants who do not (Kopp 1974).

Once opposition has been achieved, the tips of the thumb, index and middle finger tend to be used to hold an object and in initial controlled release (Figure 17). This type of grasp gives little control, so for scribbling with a pencil the cross palmar (supinator) pattern provides the child with a more satisfying outcome and tends to replace the immature tripod finger hold. Over the next 12 months the infant moves around the environment more freely and hands are used to poke, explore, play and attempt basic tasks. Coordination is poor and the outcome variable. A summary of infant prehension is provided in Table 2. The development of manipulative and fine motor skills forms an important part of early childhood development and is addressed in the next chapter.

Role of Sensation in Infant Development

Sensory input and feedback is very important in the development and control of posture, movement,

Figure 15   Fine Pincer – Thumb to Side of Index Finger

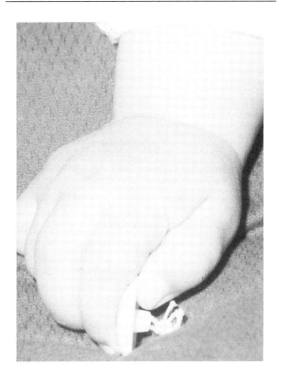

Figure 16   Opposition – Tips of Thumb and Index Finger Opposed

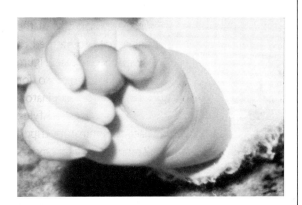

Figure 17   Placing of Object – Use of Tripod Fingers

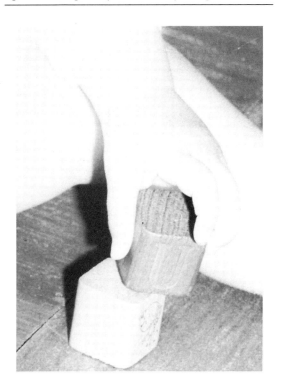

pressure or body movement. Six successive stages in the emergence of sensory awareness have been identified by Holt (1977, p. 229). Initially the infant shows a preoccupation with one input at a time. This stage is followed by an increasing flexibility and ability to switch from one channel to another. Subsequently there is a level of comprehension of the tactile, visual and auditory nature of an object. It is noticeable how

Table 2
Sequence of Infant Prehension

- grasp reflex
- tactile/seeking grasp
- ulnar plucking/clutching
- palmar grasp
- gross pincer
- transference
- hold two objects
- fine pincer
- index pointing
- opposition
- placing object
- finger tripod
- cross palmar

balance, coordination and in the learning of skills. It is important also in social/emotional interaction, learning about the environment in which one lives and moves and in cognitive development. The major sensory systems involved in motor development are the tactile, proprioceptive, vestibular, visual and auditory systems.

In the newborn, a number of infant patterns of movement or responses can be elicited by sensory input such as touch (face or hand), light, sound, joint

an infant of 8–9 months explores the different 'feels' of objects and surfaces. The fourth stage described is the ability to associate consecutively different sensory impressions about the same object followed by a capacity to associate simultaneously the different sensory impressions. The final stage described involves the ability to receive simultaneous sensory impressions from different objects and select or attend to the important and ignore or inhibit the unimportant.

An important aspect of development is integration, that is, the multiple links between receptive and expressive systems and channels. A difficulty or dysfunction in any aspect of integration is likely to have multiple effects on performance or in some instances provide an avenue for compensation. Perception, which is the conscious awareness and interpretation of sensory information, is an important element, together with decision-making and organization, in motor-skill learning. Perception and motor-skill learning form an important part of early childhood development.

REFERENCES

Ausubel, DP, Sullivan, EV (1970) *Theory and Problems of Child Development*, 849 pp., 2nd edn. Grune and Stratton: New York.

Ayres, AJ (1972) *Sensory Integration and Learning Disorders*, 294 pp. Los Angeles: Western Psychological Services.

Bobath, K, Bobath, B (1972) Diagnosis and assessment of cerebral palsy. In: Pearson, PH, Williams, CE (eds) *Physical Therapy Services in the Developmental Disabilities*, pp. 31–35. Springfield: Charles C. Thomas.

Burns, YR, O'Callaghan, M, Tudehope, DI (1989) Early identification of cerebral palsy in high risk infants. *Australian Paediatric Journal* 25: 215–219.

Burns, YR, Souvlis, T, Bullock, MI (1984) The first five years of development of children born pre-term. *Australian Journal of Physiotherapy* 30: 192–202.

Corbetta, D, Thelen, E (1994) Interlimb coordination in the development of reaching. In: van Rossum, JHA, Laszlo, JI (eds) *Motor Development: Aspects of Normal and Delayed Development*, pp. 11–24. Amsterdam: VU Uitgevverij.

Drillien, CM, Thomson, AJM, Burgoyne, K (1980) Low-birthweight children at early school age: a longitudinal study. *Developmental Medicine and Child Neurology* 11: 26–47.

Drillien, CM, Pickering, RM, Drummond, MB (1988) Predictive value of screening for different areas of development. *Developmental Medicine and Child Neurology* 30: 294–305.

Flehmig, I (1992) *Normal Infant Development and Borderline Deviations*, 279 pp. New York: Thieme.

Gesell, A (1954) The ontogenesis of infant behaviour. In: Carmichael, L (ed.) *Manual of Child Psychology*, 2nd edn. New York: John Wiley.

Hass, G, Diener, H-C (1988) Development of stance control in children. In: Amblard, B, Berthoz, A, Clarac, F (eds) Posture and Gait: Development, Adaptation and Modulation. *Proceedings of the Ninth International Symposium on Postural and Gait Research*, Marseille, pp. 49–58.

Holt, KS (1977) *Developmental Paediatrics Perspectives and Practice*, 311 pp. London: Butterworths.

Kopp, CB (1974) Fine motor abilities of infants. *Developmental Medicine and Child Neurology* 16: 629–636.

Lacey, J, Henderson-Smart, D, Edwards, E *et al.* (1987) Can preterm neurological assessment predict motor outcome at 1 year? *Proceedings of the Tenth International Congress of the World Confederation for Physical Therapy*, Sydney, pp. 263–266.

MacDonald, JA, Burns, YR, Mohay, HA (1991) Characteristics of neurosensorimotor performance of very low birthweight and high risk infants at six years of age. *New Zealand Journal of Physiotherapy* Dec.: 17–20.

Mandich, M, Simons, CJR, Ritchie, S *et al.* (1994) Motor development, infantile reactions and postural responses of pre-term and at risk infants. *Developmental Medicine and Child Neurology* 36: 397–405.

Martenuik, RG (1979) Motor skill performance and learning: considerations for rehabilitation. *Physiotherapy Canada* 31: 187–202.

Massion, J (1984) Postural changes accompanying voluntary movements. Normal and pathological aspects. *Human Neurobiology* 2: 261–267.

Paillard, J (1988) Posture and locomotion: old problems and new concepts. In: Amblard, B, Berthoz, A, Clarac, F (eds) Posture and Gait: Development, Adaptation and Modulation. *Proceedings of the Ninth International Symposium on Postural and Gait Research*, Marseille, pp. viii.

Peiper, A (1963) *Cerebral Function in Infancy and Childhood*, 693 pp. International Behavioural Science Series. New York: Consultants Bureau.

Sameroff, AJ (1980) Social and environmental influences on the developing nervous system. In: Sameroff, AJ (ed.) Neonatal Neurological Assessment and Outcome: Influences on Development. *Ross Conferences on Pediatric Research*, Columbus, Ohio.

Sinclair, D (1989) *Human Growth After Birth*, 259 pp., 5th edn. Oxford: Oxford University Press.

Smyth, MM, Wing, AM (1984) *The Psychology of Human Movement*, 339 pp. London: Academic Press.

Thelen, E, Ulrich, BD (1991) Hidden skills. *Monographs of the Society for Research in Child Development* 56: 1–98.

Touwen, BCL (1976) Neurological development in infancy. *Clinics of Developmental Medicine* 58. Spastics International Medical Publications. London: Heinemann.

Twitchell, TE (1970) Reflex mechanisms and the development of prehension. In: Connolly, K (ed.) *Mechanisms of Motor Skill Development*, pp. 25–45. London: Academic Press.

Volpe, JJ (1981) *Neurology of the Newborn*, 648 pp. Philadelphia: WB Saunders.

Williams, HG, Fisher, JM, Tritschler, KA (1983) Descriptive analysis of static postural control in 4, 6, and 8 year old normal and motorically awkward children. *American Journal of Physical Medicine* 62: 12–26.

Woollacott, MH, Shumway-Cook, A, Williams, H (1989) The development of posture and balance control in children. In: Woollacott, MH, Shumway-Cook, A (eds) *Development of Posture and Gait Across the Life Span*, pp. 77–96. Columbia: University of Southern California Press.

Wyke, B (1975) The neurological basis of movement: a developmental review. In: Holt, K (ed.) Movement and Child Development. *Clinics in Developmental Medicine* 55: 19–29. Spastics International Medical Publications. London: Heinemann.

3

Motor Development – 2 to 6 Years

YVONNE BURNS

Selectivity of Movement and Gaining Control
•
Sensory Awareness and Perception
•
Motor Planning (Praxis)
•
Hand Preference
•
Motor Skill Acquisition

The period from 2 to 6 years is often regarded as early childhood. At no time in the developmental continuum is there any particular change in growth or development that indicates a division between one period and another, but an arbitrary division into periods of infancy, early childhood or preschool period, school-age or prepubertal period and adolescence can be helpful in identifying important aspects of growth, maturation and development. At all ages all aspects of development such as cognition, speech and language, social and emotional changes as well as posture and movement must be considered together with the physical changes of body structures.

The 2-year-old is energetic and self-focused. The basic motor abilities of head control, sitting, crawling, walking, squatting and climbing have been achieved and allow exploration of the environment providing experiences of space. Manipulative abilities are sufficient to allow some investigation of objects and test 'what happens when' (cause and effect). The knowledge base is expanding – many words are understood and the use of speech for communication is beginning.

During the period from 2 to 6 years the child will acquire motor and sensory motor abilities and skills which are necessary for effective and efficient performance in daily functional activities, schoolwork and learning, and sport and recreation. They will progress from individual play to group participation. As the child moves into school and the peer group challenge emerging skills and abilities, these will be modified, adapted and perfected to meet the demands of an increasing variety of situations. In the previous chapter attention was drawn to the basis of motor control and voluntary movement. During early childhood an increasing ability to coordinate components of movement and to use patterns of movement more appropriate to the task is observed.

Selectivity of Movement and Gaining Control

The achievement of motor skills and abilities not only involves increasing control of balance, muscle strength, coordination in terms of timing, effort and direction, the number of possible repetitions and the speed at which they are performed, but also the changing patterns of control. The 2-year-old has basic abilities and motor independence but little skill. Over the next 3 to 4 years the child develops a more consistent and stable postural background, more rhythmical patterns of movement, less overflow in terms of associated movement and synkinesis, an increasing ability to select and isolate the sequence of movement most appropriate to the task and an improving ability to modify or adapt movement to changing needs. An understanding of these changes may be gained through following the development of a number of well-known activities.

Gross Motor Abilities

WALKING AND RUNNING

While the basic pattern of mature gait in terms of heel strike, mid-stance knee flexion and ankle–knee mechanism is usually present within 40 weeks of initial independent walking, at about 2 years of age (Burnett and Johnstone 1971), considerable variability and change occurs during the period of early childhood (Rose-Jacobs 1983). A visit to a preschool or kindergarten playground to observe children of various ages walking and running will clearly illustrate a number of differences between the younger 2-year-olds and the 5–6-year-old children. When walking and running the child of 2 years shows a considerable amount of extraneous movement and expends a great deal more energy than the 5- or 6-year-old. The 2-year-old displays a degree of toeing-out and variance in speed, stride and rhythm.

By 3 years, improved pelvic–hip muscle control and balance throughout the stance and step-forward phase allows more uniformity of length, height and step width and heel–toe weight transfer, but variability and an increased energy expenditure persist. The 4-year-old has often achieved an easy, smooth, swinging, rhythmical, energy cost-effective style of walking pattern (Espenschade and Eckert 1980), but some variability and immaturity persists to school age.

Running involves push-off and strength to propel the body forward. Inefficiencies in patterns of locomotion are often emphasized when the child runs, but walking at slow speeds is more likely to identify problems of hip–pelvic stability.

Control of balance is maturing and changing during this 2–6 year period with some studies reporting that mature patterns of control are not evident until about 7 years of age (Woollacott et al. 1987, Riach and Starkes 1993).

CLIMBING

Climbing is a fun challenge to most children (Figure 1). Many children start to climb on to a low step or furniture about the same time as walking alone, but considerable variability with age exists especially in relation to stairs. Children who have stairs in the home may start to crawl up stairs a little before those who do not have the opportunity. The ability to ascend precedes the ability to descend. When walking, the placement of both feet on the same step precedes the ability to alternate step placement (one foot per step).

Figure 1   Climbing at 12 Months

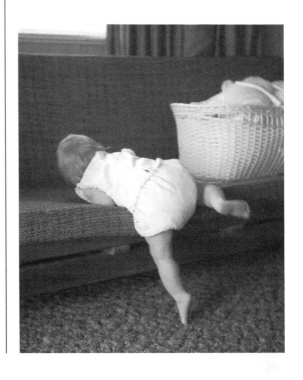

With help many children will ascend stairs by 2 years, but may crawl down backwards. When starting to walk upstairs by themselves, the second foot is placed on the same step beside the first. Alternate feet per step going up may begin even before the child can manage coming down in the upright position. Normally going up with alternate feet is achieved by 2.5 to 3 years and coming down within the next 6 months.

JUMP, HOP, GALLOP AND SKIP

The first attempts to jump involve a one-foot-off-the-ground action, but by 2 years some children may be starting to lift both feet together. By 3 years progressing forward jumping two feet together is usually possible and the ability to hop on one foot may be starting.

By 5 years most children can broad jump 60 cm (Figure 2), jump two feet together over a rope held 15 cm from ground, and hop up to 10 hops on one foot. The ability to gallop putting the body weight on to the forward foot precedes the ability to skip the legs alternately. The latter may not be achieved until about the sixth year (Espenschade and Eckert 1980). Immaturities or delays in regard to these motor skills may be due to a number of factors and in themselves give limited information about the development of movement. If a child is failing to achieve expected levels of gross motor ability it is important to consider all neurological, musculoskeletal and sensorimotor aspects of the background to the activity as well as the components of the performance itself.

Figure 2   Broad Jump at 5 Years

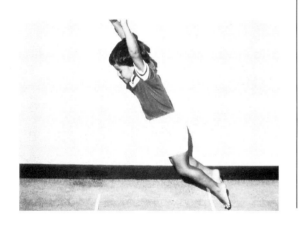

BALL CATCHING

The changes in movement pattern observed in catching a ball illustrate increasing control and dissociation of movement as well as improving ability to judge velocity and direction of an approaching ball. Between the ages of about 2 and 3 years children tend to hold their arms straight out in front of the shoulders, elbows straight and palms facing up and wait for a relatively large ball to lob into their arms. Then they start to bend the elbows and supinate the forearms to 'catch' the ball in the elbow angles, but shoulder movement continues to provide the main adjustment. Gradually a more relaxed posture and improved sense of timing allow the child to drop the elbows to the side of the body, but nevertheless they continue to catch the ball within the forearms. By about 5 years the shoulders and elbows are more relaxed, the child adjusts the body more appropriately to the direction of the incoming ball and the ball is caught in the two hands. Through the more relaxed arm position the child is able to absorb the force of the caught ball. Even at 6 years not all children can catch a small ball in either two or one hand. A pattern of increasing control and ability to adjust force and direction can be observed also in the lower limb during the process of learning to kick a stationary then a moving ball. Children with a normal postural and sensory motor background improve ball skills with practice.

Fine Motor Abilities

The importance to the child of fine motor and manipulative ability in this age group is reflected in their desire to build constructively and with imagination using blocks or other such materials, to copy or mimic adult activities, to play with balls, to thread, draw, cut with scissors and to write. Many of these activities performed by 4- to 5-year-olds require considerable proximal or shoulder–elbow stability as well as small muscle strength and kinaesthetic awareness (see Figure 3).

To illustrate the main points, the changes which occur through this period in several fine motor and upper limb activities will be followed.

Figure 3   Accessory Stabilization During Fine Motor Activity (4 Years)

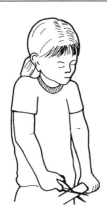

Figure 4   Dynamic Tripod

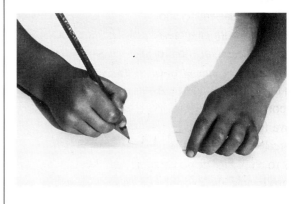

PENCIL GRIP: FROM MAKING A MARK TO WRITING

The first grip of a pencil and attempt to make a mark may be seen soon after 12 months of age. The pencil is held at the end with the distal part of the thumb, index and middle fingers. There is no control and the pencil usually falls or slips from the fingers. Over the next few months the child finds that a firmer grip on the pencil can be achieved through use of cross palmar (cylindrical) grasp and forceful scribbling may be the result. Soon after 2 years, ability to imitate a vertical and then a horizontal stroke may be noted. As described by Rosenbloom and Horton (1971) and Holle (1976) in the early stages of pencil use, the hand grasps the pencil, but the movement is performed by the shoulder. Control of the movement gradually moves more distally with less shoulder and more elbow movement while the pencil is now held between the thumb and index finger. At first the fingers hold the pencil stiffly and there is a degree of wrist flexion. Between the fourth and sixth years the child moves towards the development of a more mature dynamic tripod grasp (Figure 4). This involves resting the lateral or ulnar border of the hand and semiextended wrist on the supporting surface while the middle finger which supports the pencil is stabilized on the ring and little fingers, the index finger guides the fine, precise movements and the thumb provides the pressure. Efficient and effective control of the pencil mark is produced by minute degrees of finger and wrist flexion.

GRASP FOR FEEDING

The grips used to hold a spoon or fork for feeding follow a similar pattern to that described in pencil control. To take food to the mouth without spilling also requires control over forearm pronation/supination. In the early stages when a cross palmar grip is used the food is scooped on to the spoon using pronation. To keep the food in the bowl of the spoon while moving it to the mouth requires supination. The ability to unscrew and screw-on the top of a jar or toy also requires control of forearm rotation. These activities are often achieved soon after 2 years of age although it may take up to 4 years for the child to use eating utensils in an adult fashion.

CUTTING WITH SCISSORS

This is a difficult task for the preschool child, requiring the ability to isolate thumb and index finger abduction, eye–hand coordination, small muscle strength and discrete timing of the actions of both hands. Sensation and feedback play an important role in the development of all these manipulative and fine motor skills.

Sensory Awareness and Perception

An aspect of particular importance and change during this period is the increasing awareness and interpretation of sensory information. Globally referred to as sensorimotor perception, it is often further divided into more specialized areas such as visual, auditory, kinaesthetic, motor or spatial perception, or a combination of these. Kinaesthesis is of particular importance for the monitoring of movement, detection of errors and error-corrective changes (Laszlo and Sainsbury 1994). Although Lefford (1970) reports that over 90% of children aged 4 years have fully differentiated hand–finger discrimination perceived visually or tactual-kinaesthetically, the ability to reproduce demonstrated finger and hand positions is only just beginning at this age (Lynch *et al.* 1992). There is evidence to suggest that in terms of memory, it is not the motor programme that is remembered, but the kinaesthetic information generated during the movement (Laszlo and Sainsbury 1994). This has important implications for remediation programmes involving problems of kinaesthesia. Tactility and vision also play an important role in motor control, perceptual development and the concepts of space and spatial relationships.

Motor Planning (Praxis)

The ability to deduce purposefully a solution to a problem involves planning. When it involves selection of appropriate movement it is called motor planning. The child who goes behind the piece of furniture to retrieve a ball which rolled underneath or pulls a chair to the door to reach the handle displays an ability to motor plan. It may be said that planning is first seen in the child who wriggles and rolls across a space to reach a toy or pulls the cloth on which it is placed. Cratty (1979) indicated that the most marked changes in this regard were seen between 2 and 4 years of age. Assessment of motor planning may involve the ability to undertake a task not previously experienced, to copy correctly a visually demonstrated limb posture or action and to plan a motor response to a verbally described task. A child with a problem in this area may have all of the components of normal movement, but be unable to select or sequence the appropriate action and as a result be seriously disadvantaged.

Hand Preference

This title is used rather than 'handedness' or 'dominance' for a definite reason. Children tend to show a preference to use one hand more than the other any time from 12 months onwards. In some children this is marked and consistent, while in others it is less consistent and either hand may be used for the same or different tasks. There is some evidence that hand preference may be task related and that consistency of hand use for a task may be as important as total preference for one side. Denkla (1974) found evidence indicating motor skills involving strength, repetitive speed, use of tools and sequencing tended to be performed better with the right hand while motor tasks involving spatially accurate tactual and visual placements tended to be performed equally or better by the left hand of right-handed subjects.

Great care should be taken before attributing problems of learning or motor performance to handedness. Although mixed or undecided hand preference is sometimes found among children who have motor coordination or learning problems it is most important to identify the underlying reason. A child with a strong or marked preference for one hand should be assessed also to ensure that there is no deficit or dysfunction of the other side.

Task-related preference may be noted also in the lower limbs where stability may be better on the non-skilled preferred leg. The significance of laterality and crossed laterality is complex and as yet unresolved.

Motor Skill Acquisition

Skill is the highest level of motor functioning. A number of theoretical models have been and continue to be proposed because the actual process is as yet unclear. These models include a process of 'trial and error', a selected learning hypothesis and an information processing model as suggested by Martenuik (1979). For further information regarding various learning models refer to the psychology literature. From the physiotherapists' perspective it is clear that in addition to normal neurosensorimotor integrity, task orientation and motor planning, motivation and effort, memory of previous experience and practice, all play an important role in skill acquisition. It is likely that genetic inheritance also contributes to the selection, motivation and special attributes of specific skills. To date, physiotherapists have been inclined to place considerable emphasis on understanding the development of the infant and child under 2 years of age. The tendency to consider the preschool child who is running around playing energetic games and asking endless questions as perfectly normal should be avoided. The developmental changes which occur during this preschool period are important and any aspects of concern should be addressed by relevant investigation and assessment.

REFERENCES

Burnett, CN, Johnson, EW (1971) Development of gait in childhood: Part II. *Developmental Medicine and Child Neurology* 13: 207–215.

Cratty, BJ (1979) *Perceptual and Motor Development in Infants and Children*, 310 pp., 2nd edn. New Jersey: Prentice-Hall.

Denkla, MB (1974) Development of motor coordination in normal children. *Developmental Medicine and Child Neurology* 16: 729–741.

Espenschade, AS, Eckert, HM (1980) *Motor Development*, 360 pp., 2nd edn. Columbus: Merrill.

Holle, B (1976) *Motor Development in Children: Normal and Retarded*, 218 pp. Copenhagen: Munksgaard.

Laszlo and Sainsbury (1994) Adequate kinaesthetic development: prevention of perceptual–motor dysfunction or clumsiness. In: van Rossum, JHA, Laszlo, JI (eds) *Motor Development: Aspects of Normal and Delayed Development*, pp. 71–88. Amsterdam: Uitgeverij.

Lefford, A (1970) Sensory, perceptual and cognitive factors in the development of voluntary actions. In: Connolly, K (ed.) *Mechanisms of Motor Skill Development*, pp. 207–224. London: Academic Press.

Lynch, MR, Raymer, ME, Elvery, JH *et al.* (1992) The development of hand position sense. *New Zealand Journal of Physiotherapy* April: 15–20.

Martenuik, RG (1979) Motor skill performance and learning: considerations for rehabilitation. *Physiotherapy Canada* 31: 187–202.

Riach, CL, Starkes, JL (1993) Stability limits of quiet standing postural control in children and adults. *Gait and Posture* 1: 105–111.

Rose-Jacobs, R (1983) Development of gait at slow, free and fast speeds in 3 and 5 year-old children. *Physical Therapy* 63: 1251–1258.

Rosenbloom, L, Horton, ME (1971) The maturation of fine prehension in young children. *Developmental Medicine and Child Neurology* 13: 3–8

Woollacott, M, Debu, B, Mowatt, M (1987) Neuromuscular control of posture in the infant and child: is vision dominant? *Journal of Motor Behaviour* 19: 167–186.

4

Motor Development – Primary School Child to Adolescence

PAULINE WATTER

Progression of Physical Status: Primary School to Adolescence
•
Developmental Trends in Sensorimotor Responses

Reflecting on the continuous nature of development it is evident that there are no clear-cut steps in abilities from preschool to primary school age, but rather a smooth transition based on increasing maturity of perception, responses and control. The child beginning school needs to be socialized, vocal, independent for activities of daily living and ready for formal learning. These skills are developed progressively through play and meaningful interaction with other children and adults.

Physically, the preschool child develops control over movements such as climbing, jumping, hopping, galloping and sometimes skipping, as well as over fine finger movements. The asymmetrical movements like galloping and hopping tend to emerge on the preferred side first, and only some time later on the non-preferred side. There is usually a marked reduction in this asymmetry between the fifth and sixth year. This produces a more even stride which in turn affects the quality of running, for example. It is interesting to watch small children when a particular skill is developing, for their play often focuses on activities that

use the new pattern of movement. This provides the practice necessary to perfect control of the emerging pattern, and lays the foundation for the development of further more complicated patterns.

While modern school entry classes are not as rigid as in the past, the demands on the children are still quite different from those for preschoolers in terms of limiting movement and behaviour. That children may begin school from just 5 years of age to more than 6 years has marked implications for both the child and teacher, since the change in maturity and control between 5 and 6 years is considerable.

Between 5 and 6 years of age much maturation will occur in all of the areas described earlier, and the main issue is that the development of the individual child needs to be at a school appropriate level for the child to have satisfactory experiences. The child's 'readiness' reflects the developmental status of that individual within the general framework of expected skill acquisition for the age.

It is important to consider what the specific demands of acceptable school behaviour imply with respect to the neurodevelopment of the child. The child must have enough motor coordination to stand in line, walk into class, and negotiate the desks, chairs and stairs. They must have adequate postural control and equilibrium reactions to sit on a chair even when turning the head to look at someone or reaching to the floor, and sufficient muscle tone to maintain positions at the desk without undue fatigue. The child needs to be able to concentrate, listen, follow instructions and remember information being learned. Hand sensation and motor control must be adequate for efficient manipulation of the pencil and scissors, while the child must also plan or organize appropriate responses such as formation of letter shapes or positioning of the letter on the page. Short-term memory will be developing rapidly so information can be stored and retrieved as necessary.

Neurosensorimotor skills are used to allow participation in group play requiring running, skipping, ball skills and balancing, all now within a framework of formal games, rules and taking turns. In addition to these issues, others of emotional development and control, attitude and behaviour have to be considered. There is increasing socialization of emotional responses, cooperation, and ability to operate independent of external controls and to plan work independently. Such maturation continues throughout the primary school years and beyond.

Other important changes occur in cognitive functions, largely relating to the level of operation, such as moving from concrete to conceptual levels of reasoning. This underpins the changes in teaching strategies which mirror maturational changes, and the introduction of increasingly difficult concepts such as in mathematics.

It is easy to understand how difficulties in any of the areas described can contribute to poor adjustment to school life. The child's successes or failures in the class and playground affect attitudes, behaviours and self-esteem, and may set the pattern for later adolescent experiences.

Progression of Physical Status: Primary School to Adolescence

Maturation is generally reflected in increased physical size, strength and speed. While following general trends, the rate of maturation is highly individual and may be affected by familial patterns and diet. Normal movements become increasingly controlled, smoother and faster, as well as easier and more automatic in their execution. They also become more complex in their combinations and sequences. It is these combinations which provide the skills necessary to carry out particular sports activities which emerge strongly during middle primary school years (8–9 years onwards). An example of this is seen when ball-throwing skills are refined to bowling a cricket ball, or when running and hopping are refined to gymnastics.

As with the earlier skills such as hopping or jumping, the more complex patterns at first require concentration, planning and effort. As they improve with practice, the child's focus shifts to forward planning the next play of the ball, or anticipating the next position, rather than centring on how the child is carrying out the current task.

It is largely accepted that in early primary children there are minimal differences on most parameters between boys and girls (Thomas and French 1985, Gallahue 1989), and that the minor differences that are seen are largely due to the effects of environmental pressures. This changes in late primary children and with the onset of puberty.

Physical Skills

Children are acquiring mature control over the fundamental patterns of movement by about 6 years of age. Once this stage has been reached, they begin the transition to the development of more specialized movement patterns (Gallahue 1989). According to Gallahue, there appear to be some exceptions to the early control over fundamental patterns, such as the ability to strike the ball and to volley, both of which require sophisticated visual skills and develop later than other lower-level skills. Perhaps these two skills are not fundamental at all, hence their later acquisition.

Changes in strategies for postural control are also documented around this period in children's development. Studies by Woollacott and Shumway-Cook (1989) and Riach and Starkes (1994) suggest that postural control in children over 7 years of age is similar to that of adults. Riach and Starkes (1994) conclude that 4- to 7-year-olds use ballistic (fast open-loop) methods of control, while from 8 years on they use sensory guided (closed-loop) methods. According to Riach and Starkes (1994) both open and closed loops are dependent on feedback or sensory information. The difference between these two methods is that the corrective movement in open-loop control is ballistic and its effectiveness is not known until after the movement, while in closed-loop control the corrective movement itself is monitored by sensory feedback.

As children get older they have more adaptable long latency postural responses, which become progressively more refined and effective (Woollacott and Shumway-Cook 1989). Further, by the age of 7, a child's stability limits approach those of an adult's, and are largely predicted by physical factors related to growth, including height, weight and foot length (Riach and Starkes 1993).

As well as having efficient control of fundamental motor patterns, the young primary school child has a fully developed dynamic tripod grip with good postural control at the desk. Fine motor skills improve on the same parameters as gross motor skills discussed earlier (faster, smoother, easier). Such changes mirror the physiological changes occurring. For example, improved pencil control, in part, reflects refinements in kinaesthesis, feedforward and planning of the movements required, while increased speeds of finger tapping reflect, in part, improved reciprocal inhibition and dissociation of movements.

Sugden (1980) notes that the child at 6 years of age has slower performance speed than an adult, and that the speed of performance decreases as information load increases. There is also a negative correlation between speed and accuracy (Livesey and Laszlo 1979). Keele (1973) and Megaw (1975) argue that in serial move-

ments, the amount of slowing is due to the processing of feedback associated with the previous movement, and that this increased with the accuracy demanded by the previous movement. Interestingly, Sugden (1980) demonstrates a progressive and significant decrease in reaction times in children from age 6 through to 12 years, with each group significantly different from the others. Once the child was older than 6 years, the information load did not affect the reaction time, reinforcing the notion that it is the forward planning or processing related to the information load which produces the decrease in performance speed as tasks become more complex. There is continuing debate in this area, however, typified by the suggestion of Wade and Whiting (1986) that time required for feedback processing decreases with increasing age. It seems, however, that a major limiting factor on speed of performance is the processing speed (Laszlo and Bairstow 1985). Another issue disregarded by many is the diadochokinetic nature of the test movements used in the studies reported earlier, and that factors that affect rapid alternating movement could have a direct effect on performance. Arnheim and Sinclair (1979) present performance scores for children aged 4 to 12 years on a range of motor tasks. On all these timed measures, they demonstrate a steady improvement with increasing age, but fail to consider adequately the quality of performance. In any physiotherapy assessment this is an issue of primary importance and physiotherapists need normal values for motor tasks that reflect quality as well as speed.

Hand Skills

By 5 years of age most children have acquired a dynamic tripod grip, and are physically ready for more controlled use of the pencil, usually in the form of prewriting activity. Cognitive readiness and teaching alone are not sufficient for acquisition of hand skills such as writing. The tactile, proprioceptive and visual systems provide feedback (separately and together) which contributes to the development of appropriate fine motor skills, and their importance must not be overlooked.

Certain hand movements have been the subject of investigation, including finger drumming, finger tapping and sequential finger thumb opposition. All improve with respect to smooth flow of movement, improved diadochokinesia, and increasing number of repetitions as has been described for the gross motor abilities. Similarly, the improving ease of execution and automaticity of control are also features of advancing maturity. By adding the pressure of speed to movement execution, subtle differences in motor control may be exhibited (Denckla 1974). In her article, Denckla reports gains in the number of possible repetitive and successive finger movements between 5-, 6- and 7-year-olds, but no significant differences between 8-, 9- and 10-year-olds. No gender-based differences are reported for this study, although some studies do show gender differences. Unfortunately, inadequate reporting and differences in techniques affect the usefulness of the data.

Comparing performance of preferred and non-preferred hands also highlights particular differences in response and control which will follow normal patterns, and therefore allow comparison in suspect populations. For example, Denckla (1974) reports excessive asymmetries in function favouring the right hand in right-preferring children who are very young or brain damaged.

Ball Skills

The acquisition of ball-handling skills is one of those areas that are particularly affected by the amount of practice, attention and level of frustration. It is common for normal children inexperienced in such tasks to perform poorly, but they will improve given practice. In comparison, children with problems may not improve with practice, but need special input or assistance. Consequently there will be a large variation in skill within the normal community, depending upon the activity and interest of the family and the individual, as well as what opportunities are available at school through the physical education programme, and during play.

CATCHING

There is a normal sequence through which most children will progress when learning ball skills. As described in the previous chapter, the preschooler goes from a chest receive to catching between the forearms using a large ball. The child moves on to catching between parallel hands, and the 5-year-old child will often achieve this at least with a 20 cm ball.

The 6-year-old is beginning to catch a tennis ball within the hands, and the hands can be held away from the body. Thus a 5-year-old at school may not catch a tennis ball whereas many 6-year-olds may be able to do so. Both are normal, and all children cannot be expected to perform similarly.

The next stage, being able to drop and catch a ball using two hands, often appears between 6 years and 6 years 6 months. Dropping the ball and using one hand to catch it with the hand under the ball like a cup comes next. By 7 years most children can drop the ball and catch it with the hand on top of the ball (spider catch) while at the same time they are starting to pat-bounce a tennis ball. These 7-year-old skills coincide with the improvement in wrist control and isolated movement of fingers needed for cursive writing. Further improvement occurs with the child being able to stay on one spot and control the ball rather than having to chase it, as well as being able to do tricky games. Such games include being able to drop–clap the hands and catch the ball, or throw the ball in the air–clap–catch. Increasing the number of claps before catching, or introducing body turns (for example) all serve to increase the difficulty of the task, and are enjoyable challenges for children over 8 years. At this stage, if not earlier, games such as hand ball become popular, utilizing combinations of developing skills. Further development occurs if the child becomes involved in sport-specific training.

THROWING

Noticeable changes can be seen between the throwing styles of younger and older children. The actual timing of the progression of these skills is largely dependent on opportunity and practice, and later perhaps on gender-based expectations.

When a young child begins to throw the ball, the movement tends to be a push produced by shoulder and elbow action. The ball often remains in front of the shoulder before release, and the release tends to be downwards with the fingers spreading. There is very little rotation involved and little organized foot placement. See Figure 1.

Figure 1   Throwing Action of a 2-Year-Old: (A) Preparation (B) Following Release

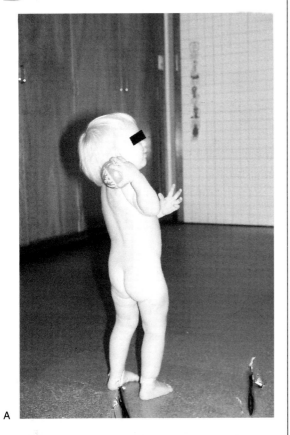

A

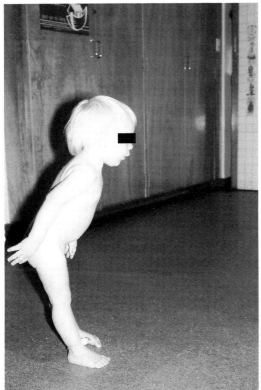

B

In the early school years the child swings the throwing arm up sideways and back with elbow flexion, until the ball rests near or behind the head. The arm swings forwards high over the shoulder, and the trunk flexes as the arm moves forward. There is some associated trunk and shoulder rotation, while the leg on the throwing side steps forward.

The mature pattern is seen when the arm is lifted back with more shoulder abduction than previously, and the opposite arm or elbow is elevated for balance during the swing-back phase. There is good rotation throughout the body while the throwing arm moves horizontally forward, with the forearm rotating until the thumb points down. The opposite foot is placed forward during the throw (Gallahue 1989).

As children mature, differences in throwing styles may become apparent between boys and girls, but these are mainly acquired and social differences, not being based on superior strength or other physical factors. Some authors, however, believe that boys are biologically advantaged to some degree in this area (see later). Once increasing upper torso strength appears in pubescent boys, then differences in strength of throw and the use of shoulder action gives boys an advantage over girls, and this difference is then maintained.

Issues of Gender and Performance: Does Sex Affect Skill?

Boys and girls of young primary school age are similar with respect to body composition, having equal ratios of fat to muscle (Malina 1984), as well as being comparable in terms of body type, strength and limb length. Puberty lasts for about 4.5 years, with girls entering puberty an average of 2.5 years earlier than boys (Gallahue 1989). Girls experience their peak growth spurt on average 2 years earlier than boys (Thomas and French 1985) which results in the earlier termination of their long bone growth and subsequent lesser height (Espenchade and Eckert 1980).

During and after puberty, boys produce increased levels of testosterone which is related to their increase in muscle tissue. This in turn gives them an advantage in any activity that requires strength or endurance. Boys become heavier and taller than girls with the effects of puberty (Thomas and French 1985), with more lean body mass (Burmeister 1975) as well as broader shoulders and narrower hips (Roche and Maliner 1983). Boys also develop greater arm and calf circumferences than girls (Roche and Malina 1983), and have smaller triceps skinfolds (Frisancho 1981).

Reviewing the literature it seems that most of the differences in performances of young boys and girls are small and can be explained in terms of cultural and social pressures, in that they are reduced to insignificance by added exposure and training, and changed attitudes in the adults dealing with young children. There appear to be true differences which could be ascribed to biology in throwing distance and velocity of throw between young primary school boys and girls (Thomas and French 1985). In these activities boys are marginally advantaged at 3 to 4 years of age, and this increases as they mature. In other tasks, such as balance and tapping, it appears that boys and girls perform equally well until puberty, after which boys do better. On tasks such as the dash, sit-ups or runs, boys are slightly advantaged in early childhood and prepuberty, but after puberty their advantage is much more marked. This is due to larger muscles and longer limbs as a result of pubertal development in boys (Thomas and French 1985). As with many aspects of life, the motor outcomes reflect a combination of biological and environmental influences.

By the age of 17 years, there is little overlap in performance of boys and girls in skills that reflect strength, power, endurance or speed (Thomas and French 1985). Girls tend to level off in many skills after puberty, while boys continue to improve in most areas (Gallahue 1989). As a general rule, boys increase in power and endurance after puberty, but lose flexibility. Girls on the other hand tend to plateau on measures of speed and strength at the onset of puberty, but maintain flexibility.

On the issue of flexibility, it is interesting to note that it decreases in both boys and girls during the pre-pubescent growth spurt, probably because long bone growth precedes the muscle and tendinous extension (Micheli and Micheli 1985). This produces tight musculotendinous units which may resolve as the child moves on through puberty. Beyond this point, changes in flexibility are more likely to reflect changes in activity levels rather than true biological factors (Gallahue 1989), and girls tend to outperform boys at all ages.

Aerobic Endurance

Circulatory changes which occur in children as a function of maturation include a decline in the resting heart rate in both boys and girls from age 6 years to approximately 12 to 14 years of age, with girls having a slightly higher rate than boys at all ages (Thomas 1984) as well as having slightly lower diastolic and systolic blood pressure (Shaver 1981). Maximal rate also declines for both sexes with increasing age (Thomas 1984). In general, there is a gradual increase in both maximum cardiac output and maximum stroke volume as children age, and this accounts for part of the gains in absolute maximum oxygen uptake seen in growing children (Thomas 1984). Maximum oxygen consumption increases as a function of age until 18 to 20 years of age, and may be further improved by training (Gallahue 1989). Thomas also notes that the sex, age and size of a child affects his or her absolute values for heart rate, stroke volume and cardiac output during exercise, and that these are also affected by the degree of training.

Preadolescent children demonstrate less improvement with training than adults. They have a lower level of haemoglobin in the blood compared with adults or post-pubertal teens (13 g/100 ml blood compared with 14–15 g/100 ml blood) which limits oxygen uptake and in turn limits training effects. Review of the literature by Thomas (1984) suggests that improvement with training in preadolescents is mainly due to improved cardiac output, while in adults this is augmented by increased oxygen-carrying capacity of the blood due to higher haemoglobin concentration.

Adenosine triphosphate (ATP) is used to produce muscular contraction during both aerobic and anaerobic metabolism. Activities that depend on strength bursts or short-term speed use anaerobic metabolism to deliver the essential oxygen. Once the work extends from 21 to 120 seconds, anaerobic glycolysis is responsible for the increase in ATP production. Children exhibit low levels of the enzyme phosphofructokinase (PFK) compared with adults (approximately 40% adult values) which limits the rate of glycolysis and hence the amount of oxygen available for work. The post-pubertal increase in the levels of PFK relates to biological factors and perhaps to the physical effect of training (Thomas 1984) and may explain the improved work tolerance in this age group.

Postural Changes

Changes in the postures adopted by young children have been dealt with earlier. The preschool and perhaps early school-age child often appears in standing to have a protruding abdomen, with a lumbar lordosis and extended knees. This is frequently attributed to inadequate space for the abdominal organs in a child ready to grow rapidly.

As the growth spurt occurs, the posture alters, assuming a more adult alignment. At various times through the primary school years children may present with tightness in particular muscle groups as a direct result of growth-related factors. The most common pattern noted is the development of tight hamstrings, probably in conjunction with rapid long bone growth (7–10 years). In normal children this is a temporary condition, alleviated by catch-up lengthening in the affected muscle groups.

It is interesting to speculate further as to the effect of increasingly sedentary lifestyles of children, and indeed adults, on the development of tight muscles, and the secondary effects of this in terms of limiting functional movement, the use of inefficient resting postures and predisposition to injury. Other issues that need to be considered include the possible development of scoliosis in girls during late primary school, and the adjustments made by the body to accommodate the changing shape, particularly of the pubescent girl due to redistribution of body tissue.

Developmental Trends in Sensorimotor Responses

Proprioception

Proprioception throughout the body progressively matures during early childhood. By 6 years of age kinaesthesis is well developed, and the child can recognize and accurately copy arm and body position in space without visual cueing. The hands, however, appear to increase in their proprioceptive accuracy at least until age 8 years (Lynch et al. 1992) and probably until age 10 or 12 years (research in progress). The improvement in the child's ability to appreciate and copy difficult hand, finger and wrist positions relates not only to an ability to feel the position but also to forward plan the copying required by the other hand. Without visual cueing, the confirmation that the result is correct depends upon proprioceptive feedback from the copying hand.

One aspect of developing proprioception is seen in the child's ability to produce specific hand positions relating to the emergence of writing skills. From about 4 years, the child progressively develops the ability to produce isolated lumbrical activation with the wrist in extension (Ireland 1991, Ireland and Watter 1995). This produces the 'tent' position where the child can keep the wrist on the table and the metacarpophalangeal joints flexed, while the interphalangeal joints remain extended. This is the position required for the static tripod grip; to progress on to the dynamic tripod, the child needs to be able to isolate distal finger movements against the background 'tent' position. This control develops progressively between 4 and 6 years of age, mirroring the changes that occur in the young school age child in pencil grip and pencil manipulation. Both will depend upon the progressive maturation of the proprioceptive system in conjunction with cortical control.

Although social trends will often influence some aspects of the angle and pencil hold, proprioception provides the feedback for final adjustment of pencil angle and direction, as well as the physical pressure required. Rapidly executed movements are the hallmarks of increasing maturation and produce mature manipulative skills. Bairstow and Laszlo (1981) have found a strong correlation between kinaesthetic ability and both writing and drawing.

Some authors support the progressive maturation of the proprioceptive system at least up to 7 years of age (Laszlo and Bairstow 1985, Crowe et al. 1987), while others refer to a decline in acuity in older adults (Barrack et al. 1983, Skinner et al. 1984). Although many authors have studied proprioceptive function in the hand and arms, it also plays an important role in postural setting in preparation for activity. The child has to be aware of and monitor the relative positions of body parts throughout movement in order to provide a stable background for movement.

Synkinesis

Synkinesis refers to mirror movements which occur in the upper limbs, usually involving 'symmetrical homologous muscles on the contralateral side' (Lazarus and Todor, 1987). They are a subgroup of the more general associated reactions, and are noticeable in young children but should gradually fade as the child ages. They can be seen in normal individuals during tasks that require considerable effort, and in some children with minor motor problems or cerebral palsy during easy activity. When young children are developing control over emerging skills, it is common to see strong synkinesis in the contralateral limb. With maturation, movement becomes more easily controlled and elicitation of synkinesis is less likely. When synkinesis remains strong under normal conditions, it implies poor dissociation or inhibition of overflow activity or an immature degree of inhibition.

In general, the intensity and frequency of synkinesis increases as task difficulty increases (Wolff et al. 1983, Todor and Lazarus 1986). Fog and Fog (1963) report that synkinesis is apparent from 2 years of age and can remain until 14 or 16 years of age, especially when movements require effort. Other authors have demonstrated periods of marked decline in the frequency and strength of synkinesis during the middle primary school years, particularly between 6 and 10 years of age (Lazarus and Todor 1987, Fog and Fog 1963).

Nass (1985) claimed that if other factors such as strength of voluntary contraction remain constant, then the level of synkinesis decreases as age rises. It also appears that synkinesis is more marked when the non-preferred hand is the working hand (Cohen et al. 1967, Ashton 1973, Todor and Lazarus 1986), but the reasons remain unclear. One final point is that synkinesis can be readily inhibited by voluntary control or merely by directing attention to its occurrence (Cohen et al. 1967, Lazarus and Todor 1991). This has implications for care during testing.

Diadochokinesis

This ability to alternate action of an agonist and antagonist rapidly, often tested as rapid pronation/supination of the forearm, is supposedly a reflection of the level of central nervous system maturity. The primary concern is that through reciprocal inhibition, excessive antagonist co-contraction is prevented, thereby allowing smooth coordinated movement to occur. That part of the inhibition occurring after the onset of agonist activity (E.M.G. recorded), depends to a large degree on sensory feedback from the contracting muscle (Leonard et al. 1990), and as such may depend in part on maturity of the child for its integrity. According to Smyth and Wing (1984), poor ability to perform diadochokinetic movements relates to deficits in the relative timing of components of the motor control programme.

A secondary factor which becomes apparent when young children perform such tasks is that they rapidly lose the ability to limit movement to the one joint being tested. Thus, if the diadochokinetic movement being tested is pronation/supination of the forearm, in younger children there is often progressive loss of control of the elbow and shoulder positions. As children mature, rapidly alternating movements become faster and more easily controlled, continue for longer before control is compromised, and are more isolated to the desired movement.

The importance of the integrity of such aspects of movement control becomes clear if particular examples are considered. The rapid up/down strokes of initial writing can be considered a diadochokinetic movement which is stressed more by cursive writing than by printing. Later, the flexor movements are considered to be the major component of rapid writing. Stable background postural setting and dissociation of the distal finger movements is required, as well as alternation of direction of finger movements. These physical factors must operate efficiently in conjunction with planning the movement to make the letter shape and calculating the amount of effort needed. If the alternation fails, a vital link in the complex chain of requirements for writing is missing, compromising the eventual quality and speed of the output.

The improvement in diadochokinetic control with increasing age is implied in studies such as those of Denckla (1973, 1974) who investigated finger tapping and drumming. There is little information documenting changes in this feature other than the qualitative aspects noted earlier. Since it plays such an important role in the production and maintenance of smooth coordinated movement, further studies would be valuable.

Short-term Memory

The psychological and educational literature demonstrates that there is a continuous improvement in the ability of normal children to remember sequences or strings of information, whether in the verbal, visual or motor domains. Remembering given instructions (verbal, or parts of a motor sequence or a visual pattern) in order to plan a response before initiating one is an important aspect of short-term memory, and the sequential component is an essential element of the spatiotemporal ordering of both the command and the response.

Various neurodevelopmental physiotherapy assessments use a modified verbal short-term sequential memory test which is not loaded for language, and which is the subject of ongoing clarification as to its reliability in adults and children, and to changes related to maturation. It has been customary not to use this test before 5 years of age, but most 5-year-olds can be expected to repeat simple rhythmic sequences of up to 5-beats which they hear (but do

not see), being clapped. It appears that the number of claps recalled rises systematically at least for 5-, 7- and 9-year-olds (Alderson 1994). If the patterns used are open or non-rhythmic, are language-loaded or require reversal of order on responding, the task is much harder. Memory for arhythmic patterns is consistently below that for rhythmic patterns with the same number of beats. There are differences in adult's level of function related to the amount of musical training.

Memory for movements will be affected by the number of items to be retained as well as the precision requirements of the task (Wilberg 1991). Long-term memory for motor skills is said to be highly resistant to forgetting once the skill has been learned, even after extended periods of time (months or years) (Rosenbaum 1991). Short-term or working memory for movements is better when the movement to be recalled or reproduced has been actively generated, rather than passively positioned (Rosenbaum 1991). This suggests that active involvement aids memory for task requirements. Kelso and Stelmach (1976) make similar claims with respect to the accuracy of memory for positioning movements, an important consideration for physiotherapists who may be evaluating kinaesthesia in the hands or arms.

Summary

It is evident that development is an ongoing process which follows a general pattern but proceeds at an individual rate for every child. Children will have transition periods when they move from one stage or level to the next, when new skills are emerging or being learned. Certainly, child development is not a simple linear process, and the unique combination of ability, experience, maturation and environmental pressures needs to be considered for each child. It is also important to learn from the range of professionals who contribute to knowledge about the many facets of child development.

REFERENCES

Alderson, L (1994) An investigation of developmental trends in auditory clap patterns. Honours Thesis, Department of Physiotherapy, University of Queensland.

Arnheim, DD, Sinclair, WA (1979) The Clumsy Child, 319 pp. St. Louis: CV Mosby.

Ashton, R (1973) Associated movements in Yoruba school-children. *Developmental Medicine and Child Neurology* 15: 3–7.

Bairstow, PJ, Laszlo, JI (1981) Kinaesthetic sensitivity to passive movements in children and adults, its relationship to motor development and motor control. *Developmental Medicine and Child Neurology* 23: 606–616.

Barrack, RL, Skinner, HB, Cook, SD et al. (1983) Effects of articular disease and total knee arthroplasty on knee joint-position sense. *Journal of Neurophysiology* 50(3): 684–687.

Burmeister, W (1975) In: Thomas, JR (1984) *Motor Development During Childhood and Adolescence*, 294 pp. Minneapolis: Burgess.

Cohen, HJ, Taft, LT, Mahadeviah, MS et al. (1967) Developmental changes in overflow in normal and aberrantly functioning children. *Journal of Paediatrics* 71(1): 39–47.

Crowe, A, Keessen, W, Kuus, W et al. (1987) Proprioceptive accuracy in two dimensions. *Perceptual and Motor Skills* 64: 831–846.

Denckla, MB (1973) Development of speed in repetitive and successive finger movements in normal children. *Developmental Medicine and Child Neurology* 15: 635–645.

Denckla, MB (1974) Development of motor co-ordination in normal children. *Developmental Medicine and Child Neurology* 16: 729–741.

Espenschade, AS, Eckert, HM (1980) *Motor Development*, 360 pp., 2nd edn. Columbus: Merrill.

Fog, E, Fog, M (1963) Cerebral inhibition examined by associated movements. In: Bax, M, MacKieth, R (eds) *Minimal Cerebral Dysfunction*, 104 pp. National Spastics Society Medical Education and Information Unit. London: Heinemann

Frisancho, AR (1981) New norms of upper limb fat and muscle areas for assessment of nutritional status. *American Journal of Clinical Nutrition* 34: 2540–2545.

Gallahue, DL (1989) *Understanding Motor Development: Infants, Children, Adolescents*, 563 pp., 2nd edn. Indiana: Benchmark Press.

Ireland, P (1991) An analysis of the development of the lumbrical finger pattern in combination with wrist extension in normal four, five and six year old children. Honours Thesis, Department of Physiotherapy, University of Queensland.

Ireland, P, Watter, P (1995) The development of lumbrical control in children aged four to six years. *Australian Journal of Physiotherapy* 41(1): 13–18.

Keele, SW (1973) *Attention and Human Performance*, 360 pp. Pacific Palisades: Goodyear

Kelso, JAS, Stelmach, GE (1976) Central and peripheral mechanisms in motor control. In: Stelmach, GE (ed.) *Motor Control: Issues and Trends*, pp. 1–40. New York: Academic Press.

Laszlo, JI, Bairstow, PJ (1985) *Perceptual–Motor Behaviour. Developmental Assessment and Therapy*, 207 pp. New York: Praeger Scientific.

Lazarus, JC, Todor, JI (1987) Age differences in the magnitude of associated movements. *Developmental Medicine and Child Neurology* 29: 726–733.

Lazarus, JC, Todor, JI (1991) The role of attention in the regulation of associated movement in children. *Developmental Medicine and Child Neurology* 33: 32–39.

Leonard, CT, Moritani, T, Hirschfeld, H et al. (1990) Deficits in reciprocal inhibition of children with cerebral palsy as revealed by H reflex testing. *Developmental Medicine and Child Neurology* 32: 974–984.

Livesey, JP, Laszlo, JI (1979) Effect of task similarity on transfer of performance. *Journal of Motor Behaviour* 11: 11–21.

Lynch, RM, Raymer, ME, Elvery, JH et al. (1992) The development of hand position sense. *New Zealand Journal of Physiotherapy* April: 15–20.

Malina, RM (1984) Human growth, maturation and regular physical activity. In: Boileau, RA (ed.), *Advances in Pediatric Sport Sciences*, pp. 59–84. Champaign, IL: Human Kinetics.

Megaw, ED (1975) Fitts tapping revisited. *Journal of Human Movement Studies* 1: 163–172.

Micheli, LJ, Micheli, ER (1985). Children's running: special risks? *Annals of Sports Medicine* 2: 61–63.

Nass, R (1985) Mirror movement asymmetries in congenital hemiparesis: the inhibition hypothesis revisited. *Neurology* 35: 1059–1062.

Riach, CL, Starkes, JL (1993) Stability limits of quiet standing postural control in children and adults. *Gait and Posture* 1: 105–111.

Riach, CL, Starkes, JL (1994) Velocity of centre of pressure excursions as an indicator of postural control systems in children. *Gait and Posture* 2(3): 167–172.

Roche, AF, Malina, RM (1983) In: Thomas JR (1984) *Motor Development During Childhood and Adolescence*, 294 pp. Minneapolis: Burgess.

Rosenbaum, DA (1991) *Human Motor Control*, 411 pp. New York: Academic Press.

Shaver, LG (1981) *Essentials of Exercise Physiology*, 310 pp. Minneapolis: Burgess.

Skinner, HB, Barrack, RL, Cook, SD (1984) Age related decline in proprioception. *Clinical Orthopaedics and Related Research* 184: 208–211.

Smyth, MM, Wing, AM (1984) *The Psychology of Human Movement*, 339 pp. New York: Academic Press.

Sugden, DA (1980) Movement speed in children. *Journal of Motor Behaviour* 12: 125–132.

Thomas, JR (1984) *Motor Development During Childhood and Adolescence*, 294 pp. Minneapolis: Burgess.

Thomas, JR, French, KE (1985) Gender differences across age in motor performance: a meta analysis. *Psychological Bulletin* 98(2): 260–282.

Todor, JI, Lazarus, JC (1986) Exertion levels and the intensity of associated movement. *Developmental Medicine and Child Neurology* 28: 205–212.

Wade, MG, Whiting, HTA (1986) *Themes in Motor Development*, 371 pp. Dordrecht: Nijhoff.

Wilberg, RB (1991) *The Learning, Memory and Perception of Perceptual–Motor Skills*, 350 pp. New York: North-Holland.

Wolff, PH, Gunnoe, CE, Cohen, HJ (1983) Associated movements as a measure of developmental age. *Developmental Medicine and Child Neurology* 25: 417–429.

Woollacott, M, Shumway-Cook, A (1989) *Development of Posture and Gait Across the Life Span*, 319 pp. South Carolina: University of South Carolina Press.

5

Intrauterine Differentiation and Growth of the Neuromusculoskeletal System

JOAN COLE

Somite Development
•
Development of the Neural Tube
•
Folding of the Embryo
•
Skeletal Development
•
Development of Muscle
•
Neuromotor Control System

The period of intrauterine life in humans is one of sequential, orderly development of a variety of interdependent functional systems. These processes equip the newborn infant with basic survival functions and the capacity to continue to develop in strength and ability in a suitably conducive environment.

While an understanding of all aspects of embryological and fetal development is relevant to physiotherapists, the development of the neuromusculoskeletal system is of particular importance to those concerned with the management of children who demonstrate developmental delay. While a wide range of information is available describing skeletal and neural development, the contribution of muscle development and its association with the emergence of the normal motor competencies has aroused little research interest.

This chapter examines the available descriptions of the intrauterine evolution of the neuromusculoskeletal system and the relevance of this information to sensory motor development in infants whose intra-uterine movement experiences have been severely curtailed. The contribution of intrauterine movement to emerging sensory motor competencies in the early months of extrauterine life is central to the present discussion. The relationship of each area of development to the others and their participation in the development of movement during fetal and early post-natal life is addressed.

The embryo develops from the cluster of 16–32 cells known as the morula which enters the uterus via the fallopian tube at about the sixth day after conception. The cells which make up the morula have the capacity to form both the embryo and all those other components necessary to support the embryo as it implants into the uterus and connects with the maternal support systems arising in response to the fertilization of the ovum.

The first stage of cell differentiation in the morula occurs when space begins to appear between the cells such that a cavity is formed and the structure becomes known as the blastocyst (that is a number of cells with pluripotent capacity formed around a fluid-filled cavity). As the cavity becomes more definitive, one end emerges as the embryonic pole or the location at which those cells from which the embryo develops first appear. This concentration of cells is known as the embryoblast. It is surrounded by cells which make up the external covering of the embryoblast, known as the trophoblast. In turn, the trophoblast has two components: the syncytiotrophoblast which lies at the embryonic pole and is involved in invading the uterine wall during implantation and the formation of the placenta; and the cytotrophoblast which continues as the external enclosure of the developing embryo and its membranes.

At the beginning of the second week after conception, the cells of the embryonic pole are sorted into two layers to form the germinal disc. The layer which lies in apposition to the invading syncytiotrophoblast is known as the epiblast or primary ectoderm and that which relates directly to the cystic cavity of the blastocyst is known as the hypoblast or the primary endoderm. The epiblast rapidly develops its own cavity, the amnion, and produces cells which surround it and form the amniotic membrane. By the eighth week of life the amniotic cavity will completely surround the developing embryo.

The hypoblast produces cells which move out to line the inner wall of the blastocyst forming two separate cavitites which replace the blastocyst with its surrounding layer of cytotrophoblasts. The primary yolk sac is the first of these and is a cavity directly related to the emerging embryo. Once it is formed, the space between the primary yolk sac and the cells of the cytotrophoblast enlarges and is filled with extraembryonic reticulum (connective tissue) produced by the cells of both the cytotrophoblast and those of the primary yolk sac. Extraembryonic mesoderm, which arises from the proliferation of cells of the epiblast, then forms a lining for both the interior wall of the cytotrophoblast and the exterior wall of the primary yolk sac with a space developing between the two layers. This space, the chorionic cavity, gradually enlarges so that by the 13th day, the embryonic disc with its dorsal amnion and ventral yolk sac lies encased in the chorionic cavity to which it is connected by a thick band of mesoderm known as the connecting stalk. Within the same time-frame, the primary yolk sac becomes detached from the embryo and is replaced, through a further outgrowth of hypoblastic cells, by a secondary or definitive yolk sac which appears to play a major role in haemopoiesis (the development of blood cells). The sequence of events described so far is outlined in Figure 1.

Figure 1   The transformation from blastocyst (A) to embryo from the time of implantation into the uterine wall at day 7 to day 14 when the embryo floats in the chorionic cavity attached to the uterine wall by the connecting stalk (C). From Moore and Persaud (1993).

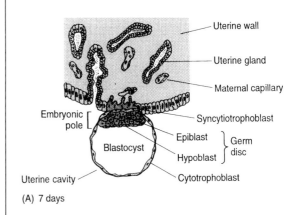

(A) 7 days

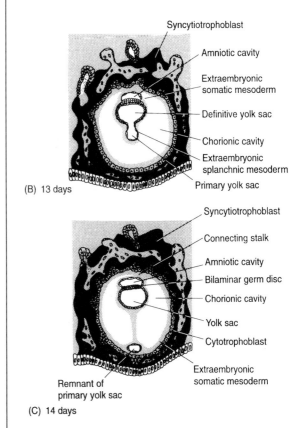

(B) 13 days

(C) 14 days

Gastrulation (the process of formation of the trilaminar embryo) and neurulation (the emergence of the neural tube, the precursor of the central nervous system) follow on through the third week of development. At the beginning of the third week, the primitive streak appears. This is a midline structure which emerges at the caudal end of the epiblast and grows to about the centre of the disc where it develops a depression, the primitive pit, surrounded by some cell overgrowth, the primitive node. Because the primitive streak identifies the midline and the dorsal surface of the germinal disc and the location of the primitive pit indicates the end at which the head will form, anterior and posterior aspects and the right and left sides of the body together with its general orientation are defined by the appearance of these two structures (Figure 2).

Cells from the epiblast (the dorsal cell layer in which the primitive streak and pit appear) migrate through the primitive pit, inducing changes in the hypoblast which then forms the secondary or definitive endoderm. At the same time a third layer, known as the mesoderm, is formed. The mesoderm can be thought of as forming the filling in a three-layered sandwich with the definitive endoderm and the ectoderm as the encasing layers. The superior and inferior ends of the gut tube are identified at this stage as two areas where the endoderm and ectoderm fuse without an intervening layer of mesoderm. The buccopharyngeal membrane at the rostral end identifies the location of the mouth and the cloacal membrane at the caudal end indicates the location of the anus. The relevant structural changes occurring at this stage are shown in Figure 2.

Thus, at the end of the third week of gestation the principal building blocks for subsequent differentiation and growth are in place and the orientation in space of the emerging embryo is readily identifiable. Any teratogenic influence (for example a viral infection which can cross the placenta), obviously has the potential to disrupt this finely balanced process of differentiation. That potential remains a threat throughout the first 16 weeks as the trilaminar disc is gradually transformed into the embryo and fetus. Moore (1988, p. 61) identifies the critical periods in development for those who are interested in further reading.

Somite Development

The cells of the mesodermal layer spread out on either side of the midline defining structure, the notochord. The formation of the notochord is induced by the migration of cells from the primitive streak through the primitive pit. The vertebral column forms around the notochord which persists after birth in a much-modified form, contributing to the annulus pulposus of the intervertebral discs. On either side of the notochord, the lateral plate mesoderm, as it is known, divides into three distinct compartments (Moore and Persaud 1993), the paraxial, the intermediate and lateral cell aggregations.

As the name suggests, the paraxial component of the lateral plate mesoderm occupies the area immediately lateral to the notochord. Initially a continuous cell mass, this portion of the mesoderm divides first into separate whirls of cells called somitomeres (Larsen 1993). The seven most cranial of these remain as somitomeres and contribute to the muscles of the face, jaw and throat as the face develops between weeks 4 and 10 (Larsen 1993). The remainder subsequently form discrete segmented blocks known as

Figure 2 Dorsal surface of the bilaminar germ disc showing the primitive streak which marks the dorsal surface and the buccopharyngeal and cloacal membranes which indicate the rostral and caudal ends of the developing embryo. A is provided for orientation. Arrows shown in B indicate migration of cells to form the emerging mesoderm. From Moore and Persaud (1993).

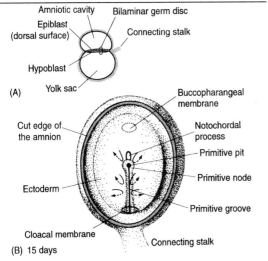

Figure 3   Identification of the three columns of mesoderm. Paraxial forming somites and their derivatives; intermediate mesoderm forming the urogenital system; lateral plate mesoderm forming the connective tissue and muscle of viscera and limbs, serous membranes of pleura, pericardium and peritoneum, blood and lymph cells, cardiovascular and lymphatic systems, spleen and adrenal cortex. The level of the cross-section is indicated by the dotted line. From Moore and Persaud (1993).

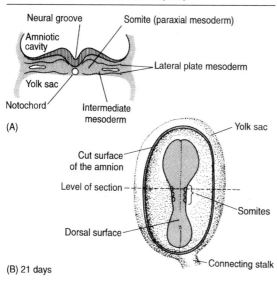

(A)

(B) 21 days

somites. The divisions of the mesoderm and the formation of the somites are shown in Figure 3.

Bilateral somite formation begins in the third week of gestation and continues in a craniocaudal direction to the 30th day of gestation when 42 to 44 somitic pairs can be identified in a dorsal view of the embryo (Larsen 1993). Some of these disappear, leaving a total of 37 somites which contribute to the formation of the musculoskeletal system. The somites provide those structures of the trunk devoted to support, protection and movement. Support and protection are provided by the bony, cartilaginous and fibrous structures, movement is provided by the voluntary musculature and the peripheral nerves. The contribution that each group of somites makes to the development of the infant is shown in Figure 4.

The compacted mass of cells which constitute the somites gradually separate (Larsen 1993) to form blocks of cells which fulfil specific roles. The more superficial cells from the medial, cranial and caudal

Figure 4   Structures formed by the surviving somitomeres and the 37 pairs of somites.

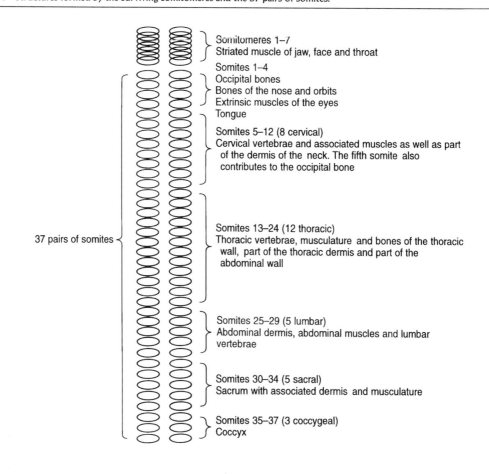

surfaces of the somite migrate to encompass the notochord and form the sclerotome from which is derived the vertebrae, their ligamentous attachments and the dura mater (Mastaglia 1981). Dermatomes, which form the corium of the skin, are constituted by the migration of the cells of the lateral superficial layers of the somite. The remaining portion makes up the myotome which moves dorsally to form a flat muscle plate (Mastaglia 1981). This differentiation occurs at each somite, producing a repeating developmental sequence, a process known as metamerization. Figure 5 shows how the somite at one level differentiates.

Development of the Neural Tube

The nervous system begins to develop with the appearance of the neural plate on the dorsal surface of the trilaminar embryo. The neuroectodermal cells differentiate from those of the surrounding ectoderm as a result of an induction process triggered by the notochordal process and the influence of the underlying mesoderm. This phase of neural induction marks the first stage of the development of the neural control system (Cowan 1982).

At approximately the beginning of the third week of gestation the cells of the neural plate begin to proliferate on either side of the midline, forming the neural folds (see Figure 3). Overgrowth of these neural folds causes the two separate sides of the structure to meet in the midline, transforming the flat plate of emerging neural tissue into a tube. The neuroectodermal cells separate from the remainder of the ectodermal layer. The rest of the ectodermal cells later differentiate to form the skin and cover over the mesodermal (bone, muscle) and neuroectodermal (neural tissue) components. From this tubular structure, the central nervous system develops. Neuroectodermal cells from the neural folds, which are isolated by the closure of the neural tube, collect on either side of the neural tube, forming the basis of the autonomic nervous system. The steps in neural tube formation are shown in Figure 6. The neural tube closes from the centre, zipping up in both caudal and rostral directions. It remains open at the cranial end (rostral neuropore) and caudal end (caudal neuropore), finally closing at these points on days 24 and 26 respectively.

The closed neural tube ends at somite 31 and an alternative form of development is required to provide the sacral and coccygeal components of the emerging spinal cord. These are provided by secondary neurulation in which, as the primitive streak regresses, it forms the mesodermal caudal eminence, a solid neural core which then cavitates longitudinally and unites with the neural tube. Secondary neurulation is complete by the end of the sixth week of gestation (Larsen 1993). The process of secondary neurulation is shown in Figure 7.

Figure 5   Differentiation of the somite into its sclerotome, myotome and dermatome components and migration of the sclerotome to form the vertebral body and arch. From Moore and Persaud (1993).

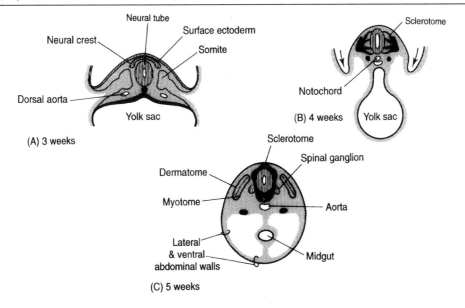

Figure 6   Overgrowth of the neural groove (A) causing closure of the neural tube and isolation of the cells from the crest of the groove (neural crest cells, B). The isolated cells contribute to the ganglia of the peripheral and autonomic nervous systems (C). The neural tube closes from the centre towards the rostral and caudal neuropores (D). From Moore and Persaud (1993).

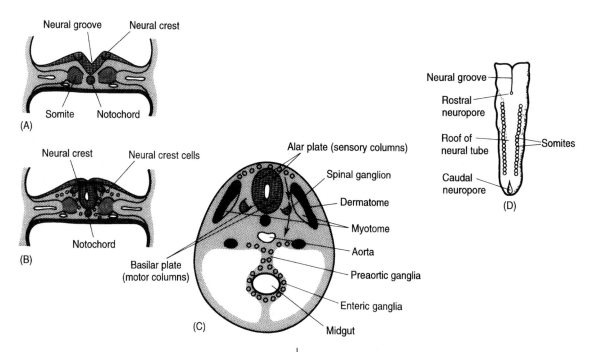

Failure of closure is associated with most of the common abnormalities of the neural tube ranging from spina bifida occulta (failure of formation of one or more vertebral arches) to spina bifida cystica with meroanencephaly (failure of closure of the rostral neuropore with consequent failure of formation of the telencephalon). Such major defects are also usually accompanied by rachischisis or failure of fusion of the vertebral arches (Moore and Persaud 1993).

From the beginning of the formation of the neural tube, the three primary vesicles of the brain (prosen-cephalon, mesencephalon and rhombencephalon) are apparent as wider areas of the neural plate. During week five of embryonic life, the primary vesicles further divide to form five secondary vesicles (the prosencephalon forms the telencephalon and diencephalon; the mesencephalon forms the metencephalon and the myelencephalon).

A period of cell proliferation follows formation of the neural tube in which the various populations of neuronal and glial cells are formed. The cells of the neuroepithelium lining of the central canal of the

Figure 7   Secondary neurulation, the process by which the lower end of the neural tube is formed from the remnants of the primitive streak. From Moore and Persaud (1993).

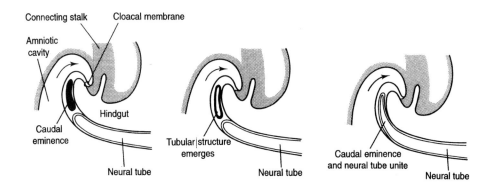

neural tube are the centre of this proliferation and the area in which they are found is known as the germinal matrix or ventricular layer of the developing neural tube. The extent of cell proliferation varies in different parts of the central nervous system, being greatest in the telencephalon and diencephalon with least activity occurring in the brainstem and spinal cord.

A most striking feature of the period of cell proliferation is the way in which particular populations of cells are always developed in the same sequence. For example, the cells of the deepest lamina of the cerebral cortex (lamina VI) appear first and the most superficial layer (lamina I) develops last. In general, it can be said that the larger neurones form first, and large populations of neurones usually develop over a prolonged period of time (Cowan 1982). Thus it has been suggested that the spatial and temporal aspects of this process of formation follow a specific pattern (Cowan 1982).

Neuronal migration is the next stage of neural development (Cowan 1982); on withdrawal from the proliferating cycle of cell development, the majority of neurones migrate to their functional location. Most neuronal aggregation occurs in the mantle layer which forms the grey matter. The mantle layer of the brainstem and spinal cord is arranged in two sets of paired columns, the alar plates which lie on the dorsal region and give rise to sensory cells and the basilar plates which lie ventral to the alar plates and give rise to motor cells. From these cells the peripheral nerves and many of the cranial nerves develop (see Figure 6).

Similar migrating cells which have a common destination and function group together in a process known as cell aggregation, the next step in central nervous

Figure 8 The process of folding which transforms the embryo from a flat plate to a tubular structure seen in longitudinal section (A and B) and in cross-section (C and D). From Moore and Persaud (1993).

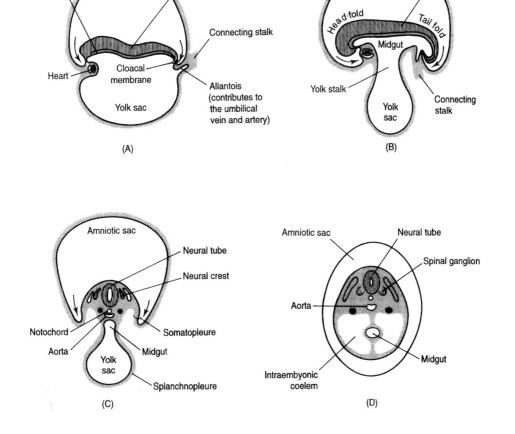

system development. While it is apparent that neural cells undergo differentiation primarily at the time of formation of the neural plate, complete cytodifferentiation does not occur until the cell is ready for migration and aggregation.

Cytodifferentiation is the next stage of neural development and is characterized in neurones by the formation of specific dendritic and axonal processes and neurotransmitter precursors which are known to distinguish differing populations of these cells. The cell processes form the marginal (or outer) layer which will eventually become the white matter of the nervous system as the process of myelination starts in the late fetal period. The myelin-producing oligodendrocytes are neuroglial cells which originate from the germinal matrix after the formation of neuronal cells ceases. Myelination in the peripheral nervous system is produced by Schwann cells which are derivatives of neural crest cells.

With the appearance and differentiation of the various cell groupings, the need for communication amongst cells of any one population and between different populations emerges. This represents the phase of the formation of synaptic connections (Cowan 1982). It would appear that, early on, neurones acquire the necessary positional information with respect to the population of other neurones to which they belong and axons travel to their destinations through the locomotor property of their growth cones (Larsen 1993). Chemotactic cues or molecular markers facilitate this pathfinding ability of the growth cones. Preferential secretion of trophic substances may assist the axon and its growth cone (Larsen 1993).

Folding of the Embryo

The embryo is transformed from a two-dimensional, three-layered flat structure to a three-dimensional series of parallel tubes by the process of embryonic folding which begins on the 22nd day of gestation. Folding is brought about by the differential rates of growth of the ectodermal and mesodermal layers which overgrow and surround the endodermal layer attached to the non-growing yolk sac. Folding occurs

around the longitudinal axis as shown in cross-section in Figure 8. Longitudinal folding causes the lateral edges of the ectodermal and mesodermal layers to come together in the ventral midline. As this occurs the endoderm, which is continuous with the yolk sac, grows much less rapidly and both structures are gradually surrounded by the enfolding ectodermal and mesodermal layers. Failure of midline closure can result in gastroschisis which is a protrusion of the viscera into the amniotic cavity. It differs from omphalocele which is a herniation of the abdominal contents into the umbilical cord rather than a failure of midline closure (Moore and Persaud 1993).

By the end of the fourth week of gestation, the flat embryonic disc has become a series of tubes. The endoderm, with the remains of the yolk sac, forms the gut tube. The gut tube is completely surrounded by the mesoderm (forming the walls of the trunk) which is in turn covered by the ectoderm, providing the skin covering for the total structure. On the dorsal surface of the ectoderm, the neural tube has already formed and is surrounded by the components of the differentiating somites which form the vertebral column, the muscles of the vertebral column and the dermis of the skin overlying the posterior aspect of the emerging embryo. Since the amnion is attached to the ectodermal layer, the amniotic cavity comes to surround the embryo as it is swept ventrally by its attachment to the folding ectoderm.

Coinciding with the folding around the longitudinal axis, the rapidly growing rostral (or head end) of the embryo also begins to fold. The tubular structure which forms the neural tube folds twice anteriorly (the cervical and mesencephalic flexures) and subsequently once posteriorly (the pontine flexure) in the region of the pons and fourth ventricle (Figure 9A), aligning the telencephalon on the diencephalon and brainstem (Figure 9B).

Skeletal Development

The elements of the bony skeleton begin to differentiate from the time of the appearance of the somites (Moore and Persaud 1993), that is, around the 20th day of gestation. Skeletal development

Figure 9   Appearance of the flexures at the rostral end of the neural tube and the formation of the primary vesicles of the brain. From Moore and Persaud (1993).

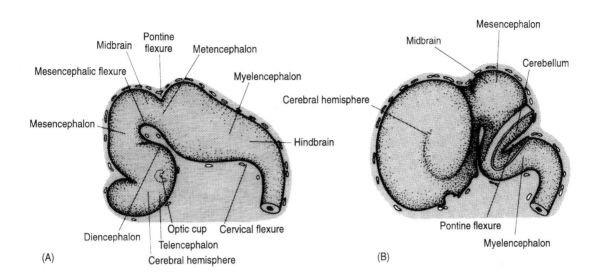

emanates from the mesenchyme (a loosely organized material which forms embryonic connective tissue) of the paraxial mesoderm. It is a pluripotent tissue in that it has the capacity to develop into fibroblasts, chondroblasts or osteoblasts. In addition to the mesodermal cells of the somites, it is derived also from splanchnic mesoderm and a further small proportion arises from the neuroectodermal neural crest cells (Williams et al. 1989) which contribute to the bones of branchial arch origin such as the mandible, maxilla, the malleus and the incus. The bones of the skull are derived from the lateral plate mesoderm.

Bone originates in one of two ways. Membranous bones develop directly from mesenchymal cells by periosteal or endosteal ossification. Long bones undergo enchondral ossification, that is they are derived from a cartilaginous model. Both types of bone formation start with mesenchymal condensation following which there is cellular differentiation. In membranous bone, induction starts rapidly following the original condensation. A matrix of prebone is laid down in which calcium phosphate is deposited, trapping the osteoblasts (Moore and Persaud 1993), which subsequently become osteocytes. Initially disorganized, the spicules of new bone arrange themselves into layers around emerging blood vessels forming the system of Haversian canals. Membra-

nous bone derives its outer layers of compact bone as a result of the action of peripheral osteoblasts which continue to form new plates of prebone in the superficial layers. The central layer is less well organized and is also subjected to resorption as a result of osteoclastic activity. It is in this spongy centre that the mesenchymal cells also demonstrate their haemopoietic potential as bone marrow develops in the interstices. The skull and the axial skeleton are formed from membranous bone, the appendicular skeleton is formed by enchondral ossification.

Around the 30th day of embryonic life the limb buds appear in the lateral plate mesoderm, the emergence of the upper extremity preceding that of the lower extremity by 2 days (Moore and Persaud 1993). The condensed mesenchyme which forms the limb buds is overlayed by the apical ectodermal ridge, and the process of induction of limb growth is interdependently related to limb bud formation and appearance of the apical ectodermal ridge. Damage to or failure of the apical ectodermal ridge can result in limb deficiencies such as phocomelia (partially formed limb) or amelia (absence of the limb).

By the sixth embryonic week, the segments which represent the articular components of the limbs appear, and hyaline cartilage models of the bones can be seen; Figure 10 shows this sequence of events. Since they emerge first, skeletal elements act as the primary determinants of soft tissue organization. The limbs gradually rotate medially through the sixth to eighth weeks, the lower limbs to a greater extent than the upper limbs. This rotation causes the arms to come to a position in which the elbows point posteriorly and the hands come together in the midline. In the lower extremities the rotation allows the legs to assume a position in which the knees point towards the head and the feet take on a plantigrade orientation. The rotation causes the dermatomes to spiral around the limb providing the apparently complex pattern of neural supply to the skin and muscles of the limbs.

Ossification occurs initially in the diaphysis or shaft of the long bones at the primary ossification centres and has begun in all such bones by the end of the embryonic period (Moore and Persaud 1993). Secondary ossification centres at the ends or epiphyses of these bones do not begin to appear until the end of the fetal period, and most emerge during infancy. Fusion between the bone formations of the primary and secondary ossification centres does not occur until the full adult dimensions of the limb have been achieved.

Bone continues to develop in post-natal life; the tissue grows in length, volume and weight until each segmental component, at an appropriate time in the individual's development, reaches skeletal maturity. Skeletal maturation is marked by the consolidation of bone in its adult dimensions and the disappearance of the centres of ossification. In addition, bony tissue is subjected to constant remodelling all through life. There is a delicate interplay between continuous osteogenesis and the two processes of bone destruction, osteolysis by osteocytes and resorption by osteoclastic cells.

Figure 10 Formation of the upper limb from development of the limb bud with its apical ectodermal ridge at 4 weeks to the emergence of the phalanges at the end of the sixth week. From Moore (1988). By permission of Mosby-Year Book, Inc.

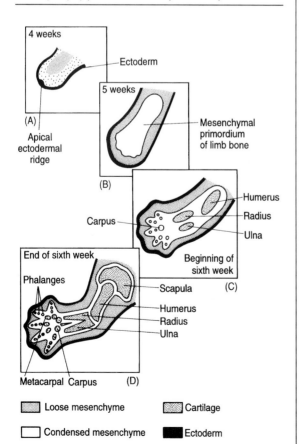

Factors Affecting Bone Formation

While the control of the rate and extent of bone growth is genetically determined, it is a multifactorial characteristic influenced by such factors as social class, number of siblings, quality of diet and illness. Tanner (1986) suggests that the severity of a growth-retarding influence depends upon how early in life it is encountered and the duration of time over which it acts. He states that: '. . . [these] two influences can be combined into the simple statement that the further an animal is below its [own] growth curve at the start of rehabilitation the worse the ultimate deficit' Tanner (1986, p. 176).

Although Tanner is concerned with nutritional rehabilitation, the statement has relevance for physiotherapists since bone formation is also shaped by weight-bearing and the pull of actively contracting skeletal muscle. For an infant showing developmental delay affecting the ability to produce smooth coordinated activity at will, the influence of movement limitation on the shaping of bone may be almost as significant as the effect of poor nutrition. The child's muscular system may be forced to compensate for mechanical disadvantage as a result of the limitation of appropriate growth and shaping of the skeleton which has occurred with the failure of the movement stimulus to bone growth. Add to this the feeding difficulties frequently encountered in infants who demonstrate abnormal motor development and the problem movement limitation presents for such children is clear.

Development of Muscle

All human behaviour, apart from glandular secretion, is the result of activation of contractile proteins in muscle (Wyke 1975). Muscle can be considered the principal effector organ for observable behaviour. The voluntary musculature of the body develops from three principal cell lines in the embryo, the paraxial and lateral plate mesoderm and the branchial arches. The origin of the rectus muscles of the eye is uncertain (Moore and Persaud 1993), but it is suggested that they are derived either from the occipital somites (somitomeres) or some elements of the paraxial mesoderm (Larsen 1993).

Each myotome divides to form hypaxial and epaxial components (Moore and Persaud 1993). From the epaxial cells the dorsal musculature of the trunk is derived. The hypaxial cells produce the prevertebral muscles and those of the abdominal wall (Figure 11). The somatopleuric part of the lateral plate mesoderm provides the genesis of the limb musculature. The contribution of the myotomes to the muscles of the extremities remains a subject of much discussion (Mastaglia 1981, Williams et al. 1989, McLennan 1990).

As metermerization continues, splitting, realigning and fusion of muscle plates occurs (Mastaglia 1981) so that most muscles develop as a combination of mesodermal cells of differing segmental origin. The origins, however, can be detected readily in the mature organism as the innervation of the muscle retains its association with the segmental level of the developing neural tube. Most muscles demonstrate multisegmental nerve supply.

Figure 11 Formation of trunk and limb muscles. The myotome of each somite divides into epaxial and hypaxial components to form the trunk musculature. The muscles of the limbs arise from the lateral plate mesoderm. From Moore (1988). By permission of Mosby-Year Book, Inc.

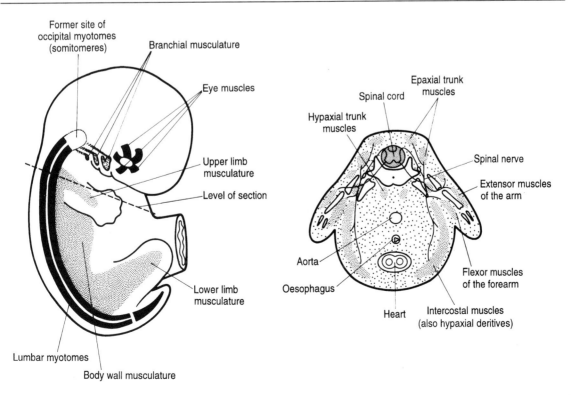

Muscle originates as mononucleated cells capable of mitotic division. Two forms of the cells have been identified by electron microscopy in a study of human fetal tissue (Webb 1972). Presumptive myoblasts are identifiable by gradual elongation of form, markedly granulated, large nuclei and the bulge imparted to the cell by the large nucleus. The more mature stage of development is represented by the myoblast according to Webb (1972). The myoblast is recognizable by its fusiform shape and the presence of actin and myosin filaments in the cytoplasm. The myoblasts are intimately associated with the syncytial structure which develops as a result of the fusion of the first generation of primitive myoblasts and is known as the primary myotube (Landon 1992, McLennan 1990).

The primary myotubes have a centrally located nuclear core, peripheral myofilaments and appear around the fifth week of human development (Webb 1972). The peripheral structures consist of contractile proteins arranged into isotropic and anisotropic bands to produce the typical cross-striated appearance in the 9–12-week fetal specimen (Webb 1972). These primary structures tend to be collected together with the cell membranes in apposition. Associated with them are undifferentiated cells which are considered to be the precursors of subsequent generations of myotubes (Kelly and Zacks 1969). With continued maturation, the primary myotubes give way to myotubes which are distinguishable by the relocation of the nuclei of the cells to the periphery as a result of the large increase in contractile protein which invades the central cytoplasm and forces the nuclei to vacate the previous position. The primary myotubes in the process of enlarging and becoming identifiable as myotubes, separate from the original cluster. Subsequent generations of stem cells, some of which contain myofilaments, surround the maturing primary myotubes in their newly developed isolation (Kelly and Zacks 1969). By the 20th week of gestation few myotubes remain (Mastaglia 1981) as this precursor of the muscle cell takes on the characteristics of a muscle fibre. Subsequent generations of myotubes, known as secondary myotubes (McLennan 1990) are responsible for the increase in muscle fibre numbers during the period

of late fetal development. These arise by fusion of stem cells that are continually dividing and remain in close association with the developing primary myotubes.

Mastaglia (1981) has indicated that the fascicular pattern observed in skeletal muscle is probably a result of subsequent generations of myotubes developing from these satellite stem cells around the original primary myotube. Webb (1972) proposed that the proliferation of fibroblasts occurring from 12 to 14 weeks of gestation forms the myotubes into bundles which can be seen to be surrounded by endomysium and perimysium. Following the development of muscle fibres, their differentiation into functionally separate types can be demonstrated. It is now commonly accepted that muscle can be classified histochemically into two basic categories of fibre. The classification is based upon the work of Dubowitz (1966) and Brooke and Kaiser (1970).

Dubowitz (1966) identified muscle fibres as type I which he described as rich in nicotinamide adenine dinucleotide diaphorase (NADH) and poor in phosphorylase, and type II which demostrate the opposite characteristics. Based on a selection of autopsy material taken within 48 hours of birth from 12 full-term and 21 preterm born infants and 17 fetuses, Dubowitz divided the differentiation of muscle fibres in intrauterine life into three phases.

Phase I   no obvious division into fibre types (12–18 weeks gestation)
Phase II   the appearance of both type I and type II fibres but with a preponderance of type II fibres (20–26 weeks)
Phase III relatively equal proportions of both types (30 weeks gestation onwards)

Dubowitz did not identify subgroups of fibres; however, later workers have done so. Brooke and Kaiser (1970) distinguished three different subgroups of the type II fibre, based upon the myosin ATPase staining characteristics of this group of fibres after preincubation in media of differing pH. These they named types IIA, IIB and IIC.

Subsequently, Collin-Saltin (1978) reproduced the Dubowitz (1966) study using techniques as described by Brooke and Kaiser (1970), to identify the timing of the appearance of the differing subgroups of type II muscle fibres in the fetus and infant. Her sample consisted of 68 abortuses, 13 preterm and 5 full term delivered subjects. The results demonstrated agreement with the Dubowitz (1966) finding with respect to the numbers of type II fibres present, but showed that the type II fibres are initially of the undifferentiated type IIC group. A few differentiated type IIA and type IIB fibres begin to appear between 31 and 37 weeks of gestation. Collin-Saltin (1978) reported that it was not until 38 to 40 weeks of gestation that the relative proportions of type I and differentiated type II fibres approached the distribution found in adults which was described by Dubowitz (1966) as occurring from the 30th gestational week onwards. The sequence of differentiation in the third trimester of development is shown in Figure 12.

Research now needs to look at the timing of the differentiation of the myotubes into types I, IIA, IIB and IIC. Until recently opinion has been divided over whether fibre differentiation is a product of neural innervation or occurs independently before innervation takes place. The current view (Landon 1992) is that the primary myotubes form the type II fibres and subsequent generations of myotubes make up the type I fibre population.

Several authors such as Goldspink (1980), Moore and Goldspink (1985) and Salmons and Vrbová (1969) have suggested that activity is important in muscle fibre differentiation and subsequent hypertrophy, at least in animal models. Bowden and Goyer (1960) reported

Figure 12   Percentages of type I and type IIA, B and C muscle fibres present at different stages of normal gestation. Graph drawn using data from Collin-Saltin (1978).

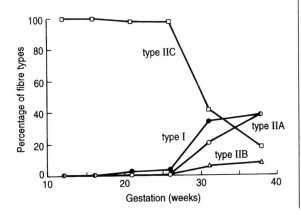

that the most rapid growth in muscle development in human infants can be seen in the diaphragm, a muscle in constant use. At birth the mean diameter of muscle fibres taken from the diaphragm is twice that of the mean diameter of limb muscles (Bowden and Goyer 1960). In addition to the importance of activity in the development of muscle, thyroid hormone activity has been shown to be an essential element in the transition from fetal to adult myosin synthesis (Rubenstein et al. 1988). These findings suggest that the inactivity, feeding difficulties and hormonal imbalance that are characteristic of very premature infants and those showing developmental delay, may have detrimental effects on the continued development of the muscular apparatus.

The lack of movement may have other outcomes. Crawford (1973) and Ziv et al. (1984) have shown persistent muscle shortening in immature animals as a result of the imposition of constant postures. The shortening was due to disruption of the balance between the contractile protein developed and the length of the muscle tendon. With stretching of the shortened muscles as a consequence of normal activities, the muscles showed growth of the tendon rather than an increase in sarcomere formation to accommodate the demands of the new situation. In mature muscle, fixation in the shortened position does not produce this effect. Instead, loss of muscle protein occurs as sarcomeres are absorbed but tendon length is not necessarily altered. With the resumption of normal activity, lengthening after immobilization takes place as a result of sarcomere replacement so that the muscle belly-to-tendon length ratio is restored (Goldspink 1980).

While muscle is known to be particularly adaptable tissue (Lieber 1986b), reports have indicated that the mechanical properties of muscle are altered in young animals subjected to persistent muscle shortening during development. The animals produce peak torque values at a point in the range of movement that differs markedly from the values recorded for control animals of the same age or for mature subjects whose muscles have been treated in the same manner (Goldspink 1980, Williams and Goldspink 1978). Lieber (1986a) has provided the explanation for this alteration in muscle mechanics. He pointed out that the number of sarcomeres in parallel within the muscle belly is proportional to the force the muscle can develop while the number of sarcomeres in series is proportional to the velocity of contraction of the whole muscle. Reduction of sarcomeres therefore will decrease the capacity of the muscle to produce the required force at an appropriate velocity. Maintenance of the normal resting length of muscle seems to be critical in infants and young children if the mechanical properties of muscle are to develop normally (Crawford 1973, Williams and Goldspink 1978, Gossman et al. 1982, Ziv et al. 1984).

Sarnet (1992) gives two examples of the effect of changes in the normal resting length. Infants with phocomelia develop small muscles in their phocomelic limb. These muscles are made up of fewer sarcomeres which are shorter in length than they would be in a normal limb. If the phocomelic limb has reduced range of motion, disuse atrophy involving type II fibres will subsequently occur. The second example relates to tenotomized muscle in which, as a result of reduction in the tension-developing capacity of the muscle, the sarcomeres shorten as does the whole muscle belly. The muscle fibres may subsequently develop central core lesions. Equally, the persistent postures forced upon infants who have limited capacity for voluntary movement (for example, very preterm infants, infants with cerebral palsy) may contribute to the development of altered muscle mechanics as muscle and bone fail to develop optimally, consequently reducing the infants' potential for motor skill development.

Neuromotor Control System

Over twenty years ago Humphrey (1964) demonstrated in aborted human fetuses that movement could be elicited in response to stimulation by the middle of the eighth week of embryonic life. Recent ultrasound examination of early fetal movement has confirmed that this finding is consistent with the emergence of movement in utero in the human fetus (Birnholz et al. 1978, Ianniruburto and Tajani 1981, de Vries 1987). For movement to occur the afferent and efferent connections of the neural control system must be functional to produce this reaction to stimulation.

The initial phases of neural development were outlined earlier. The two final phases involve cell death during development and the elimination of unwanted synapses and neural processes. All but a few cell populations exhibit a high proportion of cell death, which can result in the loss of more than half the cells originally occurring in some groupings. Cell death coincides with the formation of synapses on to neighbouring neurones, is generally linearly related to the size of the neural field to which the projection is being made, and it is impossible to distinguish in advance those neurones which will survive and those which will not (Cowan 1982). Presumably, initial overproduction ensures that the cell population is sufficient to establish the connections necessary to make the unit functional. Subsequent cell elimination may be designed to structure the system in the most efficient manner and remove redundancy.

The elimination of synapes and cell processes is unrelated to the phase of cell death and usually occurs at a later stage in neural development. There is some suggestion that the phenomena observed in this phase of development are related to trophic influences associated with the degree of synaptic activity generated by successful processes and synapses. For example, a lack of stimulation associated with absence or reduction in normal intra-uterine movement may have a detrimental effect because the necessary trophic influences are not provided to some neurones which are essential to normal movement development.

The most frequently studied model of the phase of elimination is that associated with the connection between the neuromuscular junction of skeletal muscle and the anterior horn cells of the spinal cord. Neuromuscular junctions can be identified in the human embryo by the 10th week of gestation (Landon 1992). The nerve fibres spread out among the middle of the developing myotubes forming simple knob-like endings. Initially unmyelinated, myelination commences in the peripheral nervous system at about 16 weeks gestation. While the motor endplates gradually become more organized, they do not reach a fully developed state until several months after birth. Originally, more than one nerve axon may make contact with the single end-plate of a group of myotubes; however, following birth these extra axonal connections are withdrawn so that each end-plate receives innervation from only one axon of a motor neurone. There appears to be an upper limit to the number of myotubes a single axon can innervate, producing a motor unit of finite size (Landon 1992). Vrbovà et al. (1988) have reported that this reorganization of synaptic inputs to skeletal muscle end-plates in the early postnatal stage of development is dependent on activity.

The sensory innervation of the muscle sensory organs (muscle spindle and golgi tendon organs) are among the first axons to make contact with developing muscles occurring at about the 18th day (muscle spindle) and the 21st day (golgi tendon organs) of gestation. The muscle spindle initially only contains one or two intrafusal muscle fibres with up to four or five being present at one week post-natally. As is the case for the emerging muscle spindles, the golgi tendon organ does not reach its mature form until 2–3 weeks after birth (Landon 1992). Thus control of tension development and the capacity to sustain that tension are not well developed in infants born before term.

Summary

While much is known about the development of the human embryo and fetus, attention is usually focused on the development of systems which facilitate survival, particularly for those infants born before the full 40 weeks of gestation. Thus the respiratory, alimentary and neural systems have been extensively examined, but the musculoskeletal system and its interaction with the central nervous system has been less well described.

To understand the interactions of the neural, muscular and skeletal systems which enable the individual to produce smooth, coordinated, voluntary movement it is essential to know the origins of each of the separate cell lines which are the foundations of the mature systems. An understanding of the contribution of the ectodermal and mesodermal layers of the trilaminar embryo to the development of the neuromusculoskeletal system enables the physiotherapist to identify more readily the origin of abnormalities in the development of the system. Equally, knowledge of the factors which influence differentiation and growth of bone, muscle and neural tissue will provide a basis for evaluation of the possible relationships between prenatal development, and delay in the emergence of motor skills or the continuing limited mastery of motor skills in some children.

Physiotherapists have long been acquainted with the limitation imposed on movement by disruption of the central nervous system through failure during development or subsequent damage. However, insufficient attention has been given to the consequences for the musculoskeletal system associated with any event which limits movement, be it birth before 32 weeks of gestation when the immature organism is unable to cope with the overpowering influence of gravity, damage to the neural control system or other movement-limiting conditions.

In dealing with infants and young children who have limited motor abilities, and where damage to the central nervous system has occurred (as in cerebral palsy) the physiotherapist must pay careful attention to secondary limitations placed on the emerging musculoskeletal system. Unless due care is exercised, the neural damage will be compounded by lack of muscular and skeletal development. This could lead to alteration in the biomechanics of movement and consequent loss of motor skill and efficiency.

For infants who demonstrate delayed motor development (for whatever reason), early intervention to promote optimal development in the musculoskeletal system could counterbalance other limitations of the contributing systems. Unless such intervention occurs early and in line with normal continuing postnatal development of muscle and its neural interactions, the original neural damage or failure of development is likely to be compounded by failure of muscle and its attachments and innervation to keep pace with the demands placed upon it as the infant grows.

REFERENCES

Birnholz, JC, Stephens, JC, Faria, M (1978) Foetal movement patterns: a possible means of defining neurological developmental milestones in utero. *American Journal of Roentgenology* 130: 537–540.

Bowden, DH, Goyer, RA (1960) The size of muscle fibres in infants and children. *Archives of Pathology* 69: 188.

Brooke, MH, Kaiser, KK (1970) Muscle fibre types: How many and what kind? *Archives of Neurology* 23: 369–379.

Collin-Saltin, A-S (1978) Enzyme histochemistry of skeletal muscle of the human foetus. *Journal of Neurological Sciences* 39: 169–185.

Cowan, WM (1982) A synoptic view of the development of the central nervous system. In: Nicholls, JG (ed.) *Repair and Regeneration of the Nervous System*, pp. 7–24. New York: Springer-Verlag.

Crawford, GNC (1973) The growth of striated muscle immobilised in extension. *Journal of Anatomy* 114: 165–183.

de Vries, JIP (1987) *Development of Specific Movement Patterns in the Human Foetus*. Groningen: Drukkerij van Denderen BV.

Dubowitz, V (1966). Enzyme histochemistry of developing human muscle. *Nature* 211: 884–885.

Goldspink, G (1980) Growth of muscle. In: Goldspink, G (ed.) *Development and Specialization of Skeletal Muscle*, pp. 19–35. Cambridge: Cambridge University Press.

Gossman, MR, Sahrmann, SA, Rose, SJ (1982) Review of length-associated changes in muscle. *Physical Therapy* 62 (12): 1799–1808.

Humphrey, T (1964) Some correlations between the appearance of human foetal reflexes and the development of the nervous system. *Progress in Brain Research* 4: 93–135.

Ianniruberto, A, Tajani, E (1981) Ultrasonographic study of foetal movements. *Seminars in Perinatology* 5: 175–181.

Kelly, AM, Zacks, SI (1969) The histogenesis of rat intercostal muscles. *Journal of Cell Biology* 42: 135.

Landon, DN (1992) Skeletal muscle — normal morphology, development and innervation. In: Mastaglia, F, Lord Walton of Detchant (eds) *Skeletal Muscle Pathology*, pp. 1–87. Edinburgh: Churchill Livingstone.

Larsen, WJ (1993) *Human Embryology*. New York: Churchill Livingstone.

Lieber, RL (1986a) Skeletal muscle adaptability. I: Review of basic properties. *Developmental Medicine and Child Neurology* 28: 390–397.

Lieber, RL (1986b) Skeletal muscle adaptability. II: Muscle properties following spinal-cord injury. *Developmental Medicine and Child Neurology* 28: 533–542.

McLennan, IS (1990) Early development and fusion of muscle cells. In: Meisami, E, and Timiras, PS (eds) *Handbook of Human Growth & Development Biology.* Vol II Developmental Biology of Organ Systems Part A: Muscle, Blood and Immunity, pp. 3–23. Ann Arbor: CRC Press.

Mastaglia, F (1981) Growth and development of the skeletal muscles. In: Davis, JA, Dobbing, J (eds) *Scientific Foundations of Paediatrics*, pp. 590–620. London: William Heinemann Medical.

Moore, KL (1988) *Essentials of Human Embryology*, 4th edn. Philadelphia: BC Decker.

Moore, GE, Goldspink, G. (1985) The effect of reduced activity on the enzymatic development of phasic and tonic muscles in the chicken. *Journal of Developmental Physiology* 7: 381–386.

Moore, KL, Persaud, TVN (1993) *The Developing Human*, 5th edn. Philadelphia: WB Saunders.

Rubenstein, NA, Lyons, GE, Kelly, AM (1988) Hormonal control of myosin heavy chain genes during development of skeletal muscles. In: *Plasticity of the Neuromuscular System*, Ciba Foundation Symposium 138, pp. 35–51. Chichester: John Wiley.

Salmons, S, Vrbová, G (1969) The influence of activity on some contractile characteristics of mammalian fast and slow muscles. *Journal of Physiology* 201: 535–549.

Sarnet, H (1992) Developmental disorders of muscle. In: Mastaglia, FL, Lord Walton of Detchant (eds) *Skeletal Muscle Pathology*, pp. 211–236. Edinburgh: Churchill Livingstone.

Tanner, JM (1986) Growth as a target-seeking function. In: Falkner, F, Tanner, JM (eds) *Human Growth.* Vol I Developmental Biology and Prenatal Growth, (2nd edn) New York: Plenum Press, pp. 167–179

Vrbová, G, Lowrie, MB, Evers, J (1988) Reorganization of synaptic inputs to developing skeletal muscle fibres. In: *Plasticity of the Neuromuscular System*, Ciba Foundation Symposium 138, pp. 131–151. Chichester: John Wiley.

Webb, JN (1972) The development of human skeletal muscle with particular reference to muscle cell death. *Journal of Pathology* 106: 221–228.

Williams, PE, Goldspink, G (1978) Changes in sarcomere length and physiological properties in immobilized muscle. *Journal of Anatomy* 127: 459–468.

Williams, PL, Warwick, R, Dyson, M, Bannister, LH (1989) *Gray's Anatomy*, 37th edn. Edinburgh: Churchill Livingstone.

Wyke, B (1975) The neurological basis of movement — a developmental review. In: Holt KS (ed.) *Movement and Child Development*, pp. 19–33. Clinics in Developmental Medicine 55. London: William Heinemann Medical Books.

Ziv, I, Blackburn, N, Rang, M, Koreska, J (1984) Muscle growth in normal and spastic mice. *Developmental Medicine and Child Neurology* 26: 94–99.

Developmental Anomalies

DAVID TUDEHOPE

Fetal Brain Development
•
Timing of Events Which Cause Neurological Deficit
•
Prenatal Factors Causing Neurological Deficit
•
Perinatal Factors Causing Neurological Deficit

Fetal Brain Development

There is a continuum of brain development from the time of conception right through gestation and until the end of the first decade of life (Dobbing 1981). The pattern of brain growth and development consists of neurogenesis, neuronal regression, neuronal migration, glial development and myelination (see Figure 1).

The first evidence of neural tissue is present from about 18 days after conception when the neural crest develops which subsequently forms the neural tube. The stages in formation of the human central nervous system are best dated from the time of fertilization (Table 1).

During the embryonic period (4–13 weeks) there is a phase of rapid neuroblast multiplication. There is massive overdevelopment of neurones, 80% of which regress leaving the adult number by 18 weeks after conception. Neurones are produced deep in the brain and migrate to the cortex and other sites up until 25 weeks of gestation. During the rapid growth phase from 24 weeks until the end of the second year

of post-natal life, glial cells are produced and migrate to their final sites. This process is associated with myelination which continues to 12 years of age. Functional integrity depends on dendritic arborization whereby each neurone is in contact with approximately 10 000 other neurones. These connections

Figure 1   The Pattern of Brain Growth and Development

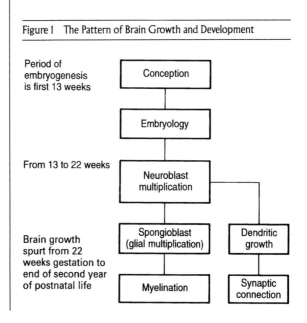

Table 1

Stages in Formation of the Human Central Nervous System

Time	Developmental event
0	Fertilization
1 week	Implantation
2 weeks	Formation of the primitive streak and notochord
18 days	Formation of the neural plate
23 days	Formation of the rostral and caudal neuropores
25 days	Closure of the rostral neuropore
27 days	Closure of the caudal neuropore; formation of a blood supply for the neural tube
4th week	Formation of the three primary brain vesicles
5th week	Beginning of formation of embryonic cerebrospinal fluid; division of primary brain vesicles into five secondary brain vesicles

between neurones are called synapses and establishing new synaptic contact is part of the learning process. The brain is not an homogeneous organ and different areas of the brain grow at different times and rates. Thus, growth restriction at one time, for example with malnutrition, may distort the general growth pattern of the brain or act specifically on certain brain structures (e.g. cerebellum 16–25 weeks).

Timing of Events Which Cause Neurological Deficit

Factors adversely influencing brain growth and development may operate at different times. Community-

Table 2

Causes of Neurological and Neurosensory Handicaps in Childhood Related to the Onset of Insult

Prenatal	Perinatal	Postnatal
Downs' syndrome	Perinatal asphyxia	Hypothyroidism
Other chromosomal disorders	Intracranial haemorrhage	Inborn errors of metabolism
Syndromes	Periventricular	
Viral infection	Leukomalacia	
Neural tube defects		Meningitis
	Hypoxia, acidosis, hypotension	
Intrauterine growth retardation	Oxotoxic drugs	Trauma
	Kernicterus	Apparent life threatening event (ALTE)
Toxins and drugs	Hypoglycaemia	
Alcohol	Apnoea	

based studies on the timing of events which cause neurological handicap in children suggest that prenatal insults account for 70–75% of cases, perinatal insults 20% (half in preterm and half in term infants) and postnatal events 5–10%. The more common causes of neurological handicap are listed according to the time of insult in Table 2. Unlike general body growth the brain has only one opportunity of optimal development and thus any distortion of growth at a particular time may be irreversible.

Prenatal Factors Causing Neurological Deficit

Prevention of Neurological Deficit

Health care workers are in a unique position to reduce childhood neurological deficit. Periconceptual counselling of diabetic women and tight control of diabetes will minimize the incidence and severity of birth defects. Periconceptual dietary supplementation with folic acid has been shown to reduce dramatically, although not abolish, the recurrence of spina bifida. Genetic counselling provides facts about genetic conditions and reproductive risks so that couples may make informed decisions about their reproductive future. Situations where it is appropriate to offer genetic counselling to couples include previous birth defect, family history of a genetic condition, and a pregnancy in women of over 35 years. Prenatal diagnosis is a rapidly growing area of obstetrics and many couples are prepared to take the risk of a birth defect provided the condition can be detected during the pregnancy. Relatively few conditions can be treated in utero once a diagnosis is made. Prenatal fetal diagnosis gives the couple the opportunity of termination of pregnancy or psychological preparation for the birth of a defective child. Prenatal diagnosis is usually by analysis of fetal tissues obtained by either chorionic villous sampling at 10–12 weeks or amniocentesis at 16–18 weeks gestation. Structural defects can be detected by ultrasound with good definition of most structures by 18 weeks gestation. Techniques for obtaining fetal tissue are cordocentesis and fetal skin biopsy. Antenatal screening programmes with testing of maternal blood for α-fetoprotein, βHCG and oestriol can reduce the rate of live births with neural tube defects and Down's syndrome.

The routine neonatal physical examination at birth is designed to detect occult anomalies such as congenital heart disease, congenital dislocation of the hip, cataracts and undescended testes, thereby providing the potential for optimal management. Auditory brainstem-evoked response and otoacoustic emission hearing tests should be performed in newborn infants considered to have an increased risk (usually 2–5%) of sensorineural hearing loss (see Table 3).

Nutritional advice on the desirability of breast-feeding and nutrient supplementation with iron or vitamins may minimize subsequent deficits. Neonatal biochemical screening programmes for inborn errors of metabolism such as phenylketonuria, cystic fibrosis, galactosaemia and hypothyroidism enable diagnosis in a presymptomatic phase so that appropriate treatment will prevent or minimize subsequent handicap. Childhood immunization programmes against hepatitis B, poliomyelitis, tetanus, diphtheria, whooping cough, haemophilus influenza B, measles, mumps and rubella are designed to eradicate these diseases and their devastating sequelae.

Table 3

Indications for Routine Auditory Assessment of the Newborn

Family history of hearing impairment
Congenital perinatal infection, particularly rubella, cytomegalovirus, syphilis
Anatomical malformations:
cleft palate
ear anomalies
syndromes (e.g. Down's, Treacher-Collins')
Hyperbilirubinaemia:
> 425 μmol/l for full-term infants
> 255 μmol/l for infants < 1500 g
Bacterial meningitis
Severe perinatal asphyxia
High aminoglycoside serum levels
Extreme prematurity
< 30 weeks gestation
< 1250 g birth weight

Congenital Abnormalities, Malformations and Deformations

Registers of birth defects generally report incidences of 2–3% of all births having major congenital abnormalities and about 7% for minor imperfections if all skin haemangiomas, preauricular skin tags, etc. are included. The incidence of congenital abnormalities is highest in preterm and small-for-gestational-age (SGA) infants.

A major birth defect is one that interferes with the function of all or part of the body or is severely disfiguring whereas a minor birth defect has little or no interference with function and is not severely disfiguring. Congenital abnormalities are disturbances of morphogenesis and are usually classified into malformations and deformations (Figure 2).

Malformations result from a disturbance of growth during embryogenesis, for example congenital heart disease. Deformations result from later changes in previously normal structures by destructive pathological processes or intrauterine forces, for example talipes, bowel atresia, aqueduct stenosis. Deformations may be multiple or single and frequently have common aetiological factors which include primigravidity, oligohydramnios, abnormal presentation (e.g. breech), multiple pregnancy, uterine abnormality (e.g. fibroids), septate uterus and growth retardation. Intrinsic forces may cause a localized deformation, for example talipes equinovarus or a deformation sequence. A deformation sequence refers to the moulding effects of an intrauterine constraint, examples are the oligohydramnios sequence with contrac-

Figure 2   Problems of Morphogenesis Resulting in a Sequence of Defects

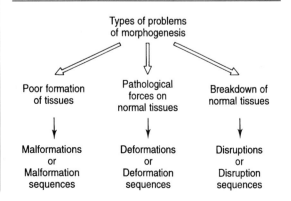

77

tures, facial dysmorphism, pulmonary hypoplasia or breech deformation sequence (oblique head deformation) with plagiocephaly and torticollis. Intrauterine contractures (known as arthrogryposis) occur as a result of limitation of fetal joint mobility from such factors as fetal crowding, intrinsic neuromuscular deficit, connective tissue and skeletal defects and extrinsic constraint.

The frequency, expected incidence and recurrence risk for selected major congenital malformations are included in Table 4. Causes of congenital malformation are genetic (Mendelian mode of inheritance) in 20%, chromosomal 10%, environmental 6–9% (includes infection, drugs, chemicals, radiation, maternal metabolic disease), unknown 35–40% and polygenic inheritance 25–30%. Many birth defects including most cleft lips and/or palates, cardiac defects, talipes, dislocation of hip, Hirschsprungs disease and neural tube defects are inherited as polygenic or multifactoral disorders. This implies that the recurrence risk for the next offspring varies from 2 to 5% when there is one affected first-degree relative. Thus, there is a genetic predisposition and frequently also an environmental trigger.

TERATOLOGY
Teratology is the study of the causation of birth defects and particularly focuses on identifying any environmental triggers for the disorders of polygenic inheritance or unknown aetiology. A teratogen is an agent (chemical, drug, virus or radiation) that produces physical defects in the offspring. A fetotoxin is an agent causing damage of any kind to the fetus. A mutagen is an agent that causes a permanent transmissible change in the genetic material. The critical periods in embryogenic development for the deleterious effects of teratogens have been extrapolated from the rubella experience. Different organ systems are affected at different times and examples of critical periods are: brain 15–25 days, eye 25–40 days, heart 20–40 days, limbs 24–36 days and ear 40–60 days after conception. The history of perinatal medicine has been punctuated with teratogenic disasters from a variety of drugs including hormones (diethyl stilboestrol), antipsychotics (thalidomide), anticonvulsants (valproate), antimicrobials (chloramphenicol), antineoplastics (aminopterin), anticoagulants (warfarin) and most recently vitamin A analogues or oral retinoids for treatment of severe acne and psoriasis.

ALCOHOL EMBRYOPATHY
Excessive alcohol intake in early pregnancy during the period of fetal organogenesis can result in a specific syndrome of growth failure, facial abnormalities, microcephaly, skeletal and visceral abnormalities (Jones, 1988). Subsequently, there is usually delayed psychomotor development. Approximately one-third of infants born to chronic alcoholic women develop the fetal alcohol syndrome whilst others have less obvious manifestations such as growth failure, mild intellectual deficit, hyperactivity and specific learning difficulties.

SMOKING IN PREGNANCY
Maternal smoking has a dose-dependent effect on decreasing fetal weight due to impaired uterine perfusion with structural placental changes, and increases in fetal carboxyhaemoglobin and fetal erythropoiesis. Complications in smokers compared with non-smokers include infertility, spontaneous abortion, impaired fetal well-being, placenta praevia, abruptio placenta, amniotic fluid infection and premature rupture of membranes. Longitudinal evaluation of infants

Table 4
Observed Rate, Expected Incidence and Recurrence Rate for Selected Major Congenital Malformations

	Rate per 1000 births*	Expected incidence†	Recurrence risk
Total malformations	19.7	1:30	
Central nervous system	1.0	1:375	4%
Eye	0.15	1:3000	
Ear	1.0	1:600	
Cleft lip and/or cleft palate	1.3	1:400	2–6%
Intestinal	0.3	1:900	
Cardiovascular system	1.3	1:400	3%
External genitalia	1.6	1:300	
Limbs	7.6	1:75	
Chromosomal	1.0	1:600	1.5%

* Rates for Mater Mothers' Hospital 1990–1993
† Expected incidence obtained from AIHW National Perinatal Statistics Unit March 1993

born to maternal smokers and subsequently reared in a smoke-filled environment demonstrate increased rates of hyperactivity at 4 years, growth failure, impaired intellectual performance and increased risk of sudden infant death syndrome (SIDS).

SUBSTANCE ABUSE IN PREGNANCY

A wide variety of drugs such as alcohol, amphetamines, barbiturates, codeine, heroin, methadone, benzodiazepams and cocaine are abused in pregnancy. Cocaine is the most frequently abused drug in pregnancy in the USA but in the UK and Australia heroin and methadone are the most common. The illicit use of these drugs is associated with increased fetal and neonatal deaths, intrauterine growth retardation and prematurity. Perinatal intoxication with cocaine is associated with major behavioural and psychomotor problems as well as increasing likelihood of birth defects and SIDS. Long term follow-up studies of infants born to narcotic-addicted mothers are showing little if any fetal imprinting effect on cerebral development.

PRENATAL MATERNAL INFECTIONS

Several infectious agents have minimal or no maternal effects, but represent major threats to the fetus and neonate. Some infectious agents, such as rubella, cytomegalovirus and toxoplasmosis, cross the placenta in utero (vertical transmission) whilst other infectious agents (herpes simplex, human immunodeficiency virus (HIV), varicella, hepatitis B) are acquired around the time of birth (perinatal acquisition). Maternal infections which may cause congenital abnormality (see Figure 3) include rubella, toxoplasmosis, syphilis, cytomegalovirus and parvovirus B19 whilst others may only set up a state of chronic infection (e.g. hepatitis B, HIV, hepatitis C).

OTHER TERATOGENS

Chemical agents such as pesticides and waste products have not been subjected to rigorous teratogenic studies in man. Recent experience with dioxin contamination in the insecticide 2,4,5T and its possible association with spina bifida and renal agenesis (Potter's syndrome), however, suggests that much more rigorous surveillance of chemicals is necessary

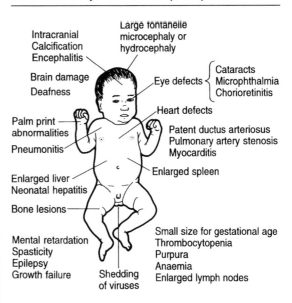

Figure 3   Schematic Representation of the Clinical Features of Prenatal Infections (Levene and Tudehope 1993)

in the future. Several studies have suggested that a high fever (>39°C) irrespective of whether it is associated with viral infection, sauna bath or faulty electric blanket may be teratogenic at critical periods of embryogenesis. Maternal diseases such as diabetes mellitus, maternal hyperthyroidism (Graves disease), maternal phenylketonuria and idiopathic thrombocytopenic purpura predispose the fetus and neonate to increased risk of congenital malformation. Antenatal evidence of polyhydramnios (amniotic fluid volume >2 litres) is frequently a sign of an underlying birth defect such as oesophageal atresia, bowel atresia, chromosomal anomaly or neural tube defect. Chronic polyhydramnios may also be associated with multiple gestation and maternal diabetes.

Intrauterine Growth Retardation and the Small-for-Gestational-Age Infant

The growth-retarded fetus is susceptible to intrauterine death, perinatal asphyxia and subsequently neonatal morbidity. Small-for-gestational-age (SGA) infants are a heterogeneous group at risk of perinatal morbidity and mortality. Their long-term morbidity depends on the cause and severity of the growth retardation and appropriate management of presenting problems. Of those SGA infants in whom the cause remains undetermined, 40% are constitutionally small and have a good long-term outcome. Determinants of birth weight may be operative before conception, at conception or between conception and birth. The incidence of SGA varies between countries and depends on definition, but is usually 2–3% of all births in industrialized countries. Socioeconomic and ethnic factors will influence this incidence. Subdividing the heterogeneous SGA population into more homogeneous groups offers the potential of establishing a better understanding of the underlying cause of the problem and therefore more accurate prognoses and more appropriate plans for post-natal management.

The classification of growth retardation as intrinsic implies an abnormality at the time of conception or within the first trimester and includes chromosomal anomalies, fetal infection, primordial dwarfism, the effects of maternal drugs such as alcohol and constitutional factors. Generally these babies have equal growth retardation of weight, length and head. Extrinsic implies a later onset of growth retardation and is usually associated with impaired uteroplacental perfusion and an inadequate supply line of nutrients and/or oxygen. Maternal factors include hypertension, diabetes mellitus with vascular complications, renal disease, cardiac disease, sickle cell disease and collagen disorders.

Neonatal risks for the SGA infant include perinatal asphyxia, hypoglycaemia, infection and congenital malformations. The ultimate outcome is dependent on the cause of aberrant growth, timing and duration of the insult, the severity of the growth retardation, the degree of intrauterine or post-natal asphyxia, the post-natal course and the socioeconomic status of the family. SGA infants born at term are prone to more developmental, behavioural and learning problems than appropriately grown infants born either at term or preterm. Babies who are both SGA and preterm have a greater risk of serious neurological handicap than SGA babies born at term or appropriately grown preterm infants. If catch-up growth occurs, especially with head circumference, the eventual IQ score is higher than in those infants whose head remains small.

Perinatal Factors Causing Neurological Deficit

Approximately 20% of neurological handicaps in a paediatric community can be attributed to perinatal factors with equal but quite different contributions from term and preterm infants.

Term Infants

Perinatal insults causing neurodevelopmental disability include perinatal asphyxia, birth trauma and intracranial haemorrhage.

PERINATAL ASPHYXIA

The term 'asphyxia' is widely misused in medicine. Asphyxia is a condition of impaired gas exchange leading, if it persists, to progressive hypoxaemia and hypercapnia. Perinatal asphyxia is used to indicate an impairment of gas exchange during or soon after labour and hypoxic ischaemic encephalopathy is used to describe the illness thought to stem from such impairment. There is a widespread belief that asphyxia and cerebral palsy follow adverse intrapartum events and that they can be prevented by optimal obstetric care. Although this belief has fostered litigation against obstetricians, there is little scientific evidence to support it. It was hoped that routine fetal heart rate monitoring would prevent fetal asphyxia and cerebral palsy, but this has not occurred because perinatal asphyxia is an uncommon cause of cerebral palsy and routine intrapartum fetal heart rate monitoring and acid–base status do not prevent asphyxia or cerebral palsy. Blair and Stanley (1988) estimated that only 8% of cerebral palsy can be attributed to perinatal asphyxia.

The clinical severity of hypoxic ischaemic encephalopathy is graded as mild (irritability, hyperalert, hypotonia), moderate (lethargy, seizures, marked abnormalities of tone, gavage feeding) or severe (coma, prolonged seizures, severe hypotonia, prolonged apnoea). The severity of hypoxic ischaemic encephalopathy is a useful guide to long-term prognosis. Babies exhibiting mild encephalopathy have an excellent prognosis, those with moderate encephalopathy have a 25% risk of serious sequelae including cerebral palsy and mental retardation, and those with severe encephalopathy have an 80% chance of dying or surviving with severe handicap. Although 3% of all babies born have a 1 minute Apgar score of 0–3 and 2% have a 5 minute Apgar score of 0–6, only 6 babies per 1000 show clinical features of hypoxic ischaemic encephalopathy. Other predictors of long-term outcome in infants with features suggestive of perinatal asphyxia are cord blood pH, cranial ultrasound, cerebral blood flow velocity, intracranial pressure and computerized tomography and nuclear magnetic resonant imaging and spectroscopy.

BIRTH TRAUMA

Birth trauma injuries may be sustained either during labour or at delivery and may occur despite skilled obstetric care. The decreased incidence in birth trauma over recent years has been attributed to changing trends in obstetric management such as caesarean section instead of difficult vaginal delivery. It is estimated that significant birth injury (excluding asphyxia) occurs in 0.2/1000 live births and is more likely in breech and preterm deliveries. Significant birth injuries leading to developmental anomalies include injuries to the head such as subaponeurotic haemorrhage, skull fracture, nerve injuries and intracranial haemorrhage.

Nerve injuries in the newborn may be due to stretching, compression, twisting, hyperextension or separation of nervous tissue. The nerve injuries are classified as neuropraxia, axontomesis or neurotomesis. Nerve injuries in the newborn include facial nerve palsy (usually lower motor neurone), brachial plexus palsy (Erb's or upper brachial plexus palsy, Klumpke's or lower brachial plexus palsy and total paralysis of the arm), recurrent laryngeal nerve palsy and spinal cord injuries.

INTRACRANIAL HAEMORRHAGE

Intracranial haemorrhage in the term infant is usually related to birth trauma and less often to asphyxia. Subarachnoid haemorrhage is usually associated with a good prognosis, if there are minimal neurological signs in the newborn period, even when neonatal convulsions occur. Subdural haematomas fortunately have become rare and are predominantly related to

cephalo–pelvic disproportion, abnormal presentation and excessive moulding of the head. There are three basic types of subdural haemorrhage – tentorial laceration, falx cerebri laceration and rupture of superficial cerebral veins. Infants with a tentorial or falx cerebri laceration exhibit a catastrophic collapse after birth and die suddenly, whereas those with the milder type have bleeding over the temporal cerebral lobe and present with focal convulsions or a chronic subdural effusion with subsequent hydrocephalus. Intracerebral haemorrhage is relatively rare in term infants and frequently relates to the battered fetus, coagulation disturbance, cerebral artery occlusion, thrombocytopenia or arteriovenous malformation.

Hypoglycaemia

Glucose, like oxygen, is essential for normal brain function both as the major metabolic fuel and as a precursor of essential macromolecules during the rapid phase of brain growth in the baby. It cannot now be disputed that hypoglycaemia causes brain damage, nor that effective management of hypoglycaemia protects from this neural damage. What is in dispute is the definition of hypoglycaemia. Previously, Cornblath and Schwartz (1976) defined hypoglycaemia in the term infant as blood glucose <1.7 mmoll^{-1} and in the preterm infant as <1.1 mmoll^{-1}. Recent physiological evidence suggests that the blood glucose should be maintained at 2.6 mmoll^{-1} in both term and preterm infants and that the previous classification of asymptomatic or symptomatic hypoglycaemia be abandoned. A series of case reports from 1959 to 1975 revealed 79 of 158 (50%) of babies with symptomatic hypoglycaemia impaired at follow-up. Koivisto et al. (1972) reported 13 of 85 (15.2%) of babies with symptomatic hypoglycaemia being impaired at follow-up compared with 3 of 56 (5.4%) control infants. In this study the incidence of impairment of asymptomatic infants of 4 of 66 (6.1%) was similar to that of control infants. Lucas et al. (1988) confirmed neurodevelopmental disability in infants with moderate asymptomatic hypoglycaemia (blood glucose <2.6 mmoll^{-1}) in infants of birthweight <1850 g.

Hyperbilirubinaemia

The classic presentation of kernicterus in the newborn is progressive development of lethargy, rigidity, opisthotonos, high-pitch cry, fever and convulsions over a period of 24 hours. This is followed by death in 50% of cases. At autopsy there is bilirubin staining and necrosis of neurones, especially in basal ganglia, hippocampus and subthalamic nuclei. Survivors of kernicterus often demonstrate choreoathetoid cerebral palsy, high-frequency deafness, mental retardation and paralysis of upward gaze (Parinaud's sign). Preterm infants rarely manifest the previous features, but may manifest more subtle bilirubin brain damage consisting of mild disorders of both motor function and cognitive function (minimal cerebral dysfunction). High-frequency hearing loss is the commonest feature of the bilirubin encephalopathy syndrome and is most commonly seen in preterm infants. The levels of unconjugated bilirubin which cause brain damage are not known, but it is probably only free non-protein bound bilirubin that is dangerous. Acidosis, asphyxia, prematurity and drugs that compete for bilirubin binding sites, predispose infants to kernicterus possibly by opening the blood–brain barrier to bilirubin molecules. There is considerable disagreement as to what constitutes a critical level of unconjugated hyperbilirubinaemia for both term and preterm infants. The management nomograms for term and preterm infants clearly differentiate between haemolytic and non-haemolytic disease.

Preterm Infant

Although the low-birth-weight (LBW) infant may be either preterm or SGA or both, the problems faced by the LBW infant in the neonatal period and subsequently, depend on whether the infant is born too early or is growth retarded. See Table 5 for a classification of newborn infants according to birth weight, gestational age or size for gestational age.

Preterm birth is the foremost problem in obstetric practice today. Where possible, the woman in preterm labour should be transferred to a very specialized perinatal unit. Survival rates for preterm infants vary considerably from one centre to another depending on whether quoted figures are corrected for labour

Table 5

Classification of Newborn Infants According to Birth Weight, Gestational Age or Size for Gestational Age

	Incidence in Australia
Birth weight	
< 2500 g – low birth weight (LBW)	6.5%
< 1500 g – very low birth weight (VLBW)	1.3%
< 1000 g – extremely low birth weight (ELBW)	0.6%
Gestational age [completed weeks after last normal menstrual period]	
< 37 weeks – preterm	7%
> 42 weeks – post-term	6%
Size for gestational age	
weight between +2 SD* and −2 SD from mean – appropriate for gestational age (AGA)	95%
weight < −2 SD from mean – small for gestational age (SGA)	2.5%
weight > +2 SD from mean – large for gestational age (LGA)	2.5%

* Standard deviation

Table 6

Survival Rates to Hospital Discharge for LBW and Preterm Infants analysed by birth weight and gestation age at Mater Mother's Hospital (Tudehope, Gray, Steer 1990–1993)

Birth weight [g]	Survival rate
500–999 g	78%
1000–1499 g	90%
1500–1999 g	95%
2000–2499 g	98%
Gestational age [weeks]	
24–25	62%
26–27	84%
28–29	89%
30–31	99%

ward deaths, lethal malformations and outborn infants. Survival rates for LBW and preterm infants at a major maternity hospital, the Mater Mothers' Hospital 1990–1993, are shown in Table 6.

CLINICAL PROBLEMS FOR THE PRETERM INFANT

Most organ systems are undergoing continued structural and functional development during the last 3 months of intrauterine life. Premature birth requires adaptation to extrauterine life before these organ systems are adequately developed.

ing into a primary ischaemic area of brain or as result of a venous infarct.

Post-haemorrhagic ventricular dilatation occurs in up to 40% of infants with periventricular haemorrhage. Measurements of the lateral ventricles are usually taken on coronal section of ultrasound examination at the level of the foramen of Munro. Normal ventricular size is ≤ 3 mm, mild ventricular dilatation 4–7 mm, moderate 8–12 mm and severe >12 mm. Severe ventricular dilatation is associated with symptoms of raised intracranial pressure including apnoea, poor feeding, irritability, sutural separation and 'setting sun' appearance of eyes. Treatment consisting of acetazolomide (Diamox), serial lumbar punctures and a ventriculo–peritoneal shunt is frequently required for severe ventricular dilatation.

Porencephaly refers to the cystic cavities in one or both cerebral hemispheres following an intraparenchymal haemorrhage.

PERIVENTRICULAR LEUKOMALACIA (PVL)

PVL literally means softening of the white matter around the ventricles and is now recognized as a major risk factor for the subsequent development of cerebral palsy. The lesion is due to underperfusion in the watershed region of the periventricular white matter. The region is particularly vulnerable to ischaemic insults between 27 and 33 weeks gestation. The diagnosis is made by real-time ultrasound and multiple cystic cavities develop which later fill with glial tissue. A magnetic resonance image scan at 12 months of age in an ex-preterm child who has spastic diplegia will usually show altered myelination.

RETINOPATHY OF PREMATURITY (ROP)

This condition was formerly known as retrolental fibroplasia and is a common condition affecting the most immature infants. Studies in the 1950s demonstrating a direct association between oxygen dosage and the development of retrolental fibroplasia resulted in tightly controlled use of oxygen with a decline in incidence of ROP. Currently it occurs predominantly in extremely low-birth-weight (ELBW) infants and the relationship between oxygen and ROP is much more complex than originally thought. An Australian study reported an incidence

Main Problems of Prematurity

- birth asphyxia
- thermal instability
- lack of the primitive survival reflexes of suck, swallow, cough and gag, with high incidence of milk aspiration
- jaundice
- pulmonary diseases
- metabolic disturbances
- patent ductus arteriosus – congestive heart failure
- intracranial lesions – periventricular haemorrhage, periventricular leukomalacia
- infection – perinatal and nosocomial
- gastrointestinal intolerance and necrotizing enterocolitis
- ophthalmic lesions – retinopathy of prematurity
- surgical lesions
- haematological disorders
- renal immaturity

PERIVENTRICULAR HAEMORRHAGE (PVH)

The incidence of PVH is 40% for infants of birth weight less than 1000 g and 30% for those of 1000–1500 g. The bleeding occurs in the germinal matrix (or subependymal plate) which lies over the head of the caudate nucleus. Rupture into the ventricle occurs in 70% of cases of PVH. The germinal matrix is present between 24 and 34 weeks of gestation and rapidly involutes after this time. Bleeding is due to rupture of fragile capillaries within the germinal matrix and is associated with respiratory distress syndrome (RDS), mechanical ventilation, metabolic acidosis and coagulation disturbances. The extent of PVH is graded 1–4 (Tudehope et al. 1989):

Grade 1: subependymal haemorrhage
Grade 2: intraventricular haemorrhage filling
          < 50% of ventricle
Grade 3: intraventricular haemorrhage filling
          > 50% of ventricle
Grade 4: intraparenchymal haemorrhage

Intraparenchymal haemorrhage may be due to bleed-

of 13% for ROP developing in infants admitted to a neonatal intensive care unit (Yu *et al.* 1982). The incidence is almost 80% in babies of less than 1000 g birth weight. Approximately 80% of infants with acute proliferative ROP showed complete regression of retinal changes.

The diagnosis of ROP is made clinically by indirect ophthalmoscopy after prior pupillary dilatation and examination by a paediatric ophthalmologist. ROP is staged according to the international classification (Committee for the Classification of ROP 1984).

Stage 1: a thin line of demarcation in the periphery of the retina separating the avascular retina anteriorly from the vascularized retina posteriorly

Stage 2: the line is more extensive and forms a ridge

Stage 3: vascular proliferation immediately posterior to the ridge

Stage 4: retinal detachment – subtotal

Stage 5: Retinal detachment – total

Stages 1 and 2 usually regress completely to normal and it is only stage 3 that may require treatment.

Plus disease   Plus is added to any stage of ROP if the following signs of activity are seen:

- tortuosity and engorgement of retinal vessels
- vascular engorgement and rigidity of the iris
- vitreous haze

There is now effective treatment for severe acute ROP and screening is a necessary clinical procedure in all at-risk infants. All infants less than 1500 g or less than 32 weeks gestation should be screened, with the first examination at about 32 weeks post-menstrual age. Infants with ROP of Stage 3, zone 2 are said to reach threshold and probably will benefit from cryotherapy or laser therapy. Cryotherapy in infants with threshold ROP improves outcome by about 50% compared with non-treated infants (Cryotherapy for ROP Cooperative Group 1988).

HEARING IMPAIRMENT

Profound hearing and visual impairments are major causes of severe handicap arising from the neonatal period. Assessment of hearing in high-risk infants is

Table 7

Complications in the First Year of Life of Preterm Infants

Medical	
Respiratory	nasal congestion, exacerbation of bronchopulmonary, dysplasia, recurrent wheezing, sudden infant death syndrome (SIDS)
Cardiac	patent ductus arteriosus, ventricular septal defect
Ophthalmic	retinopathy of prematurity, strabismus, myopia
Auditory	sensorineural hearing loss, conductive dysfunction
Surgical	inguinal hernia, umbilical hernia, undescended testes, hydrocoele
Gastrointestinal	vomiting, gastro-oesophageal reflux, constipation, colic
Neurological	
Major	spastic diplegia, hypotonia, hemiplegia, quadriplegia, hydrocephalus, microcephaly, mental retardation
Minor	ataxia, incoordination, specific learning difficulties, minimal cerebral dysfunction, attention deficit disorders
Miscellaneous	
	child abuse, neglect, deprivation, behavioural disturbances, emotional disturbances, failure to thrive

possible before the child leaves the neonatal unit and early diagnosis is essential for optimal management. Hearing impairment is either conductive, sensorineural or mixed. Sensorineural deafness requires hearing aids and occurs in about 3% of graduates from a neonatal intensive care unit, whereas conductive deafness has been reported in 58% for infants under 1500 g (Tudehope *et al.* 1992). Infants with a significant risk for hearing loss should be screened before discharge from the neonatal intensive care unit with auditory brainstem-evoked response or otoacoustic emission studies (see Table 3).

FOLLOW-UP OF PRETERM INFANTS

The healthy preterm infant whose weight is appropriate for gestational age (AGA) should grow at the same rate as a term infant of the same post-conceptual age. Common complications in infants in the first year of life to preterm infants are listed in Table 7.

The World Health Organization has provided definitions for the commonly misused terms, impairment, disability and handicap.

Impairment — Any loss or abnormality of psychological, physiological or anatomical structure or function

Disability — any restriction or lack of ability (resulting from an impairment) to perform an activity in the manner or within the range considered to be normal

Handicap — a disadvantage for an individual that limits or prevents the fulfilment of a role that should be normal for that individual

The various handicaps, disabilities and impairments sustained by preterm infants manifest at different times through the first and subsequent years of life (see Figure 4).

SPECIALIZED FOLLOW-UP CLINICS

Infants who are at risk of chronic handicapping conditions should be followed up in special multidisciplinary clinics, or by their paediatricians. Infants requiring specialized follow-up would include very low-birth-weight (VLBW) infants, and those with severe perinatal asphyxia, intracranial haemorrhage, neonatal convulsions and abnormal neurological examination at discharge and those requiring mechanical ventilation. Frequently, preterm infants suffer from iatrogenic diseases due to neonatal care in hospital; these include oxygen toxicity as well as hearing deficits, rickets and a wide range of deformities.

Summary

The knowledge obtained by the physiotherapist on the prenatal and perinatal causes of developmental anomalies is not only intellectually satisfying, but also assists in treatment of the child and family. Many of the aetiological factors causing neurological deficit result in specific neurosensory problems. The aware physiotherapist is able to design a more appropriate treatment programme. An understanding of the causation of a child's disability is likely to improve rapport with parents and can lead to better counselling and handling of parents. Aetiological factors such

Figure 4 Handicaps in Very Low Birth Weight (VLBW) Infants Related to Corrected Ages (Adapted from Desmond et al. 1980)

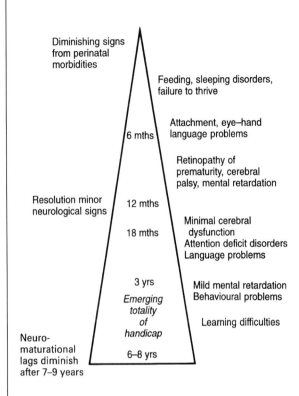

as extreme prematurity contributing to extensor patterns or the 'dystonia' syndrome (Drillien 1972, Tudehope et al. 1981, Burns et al. 1984) might well influence the introduction of developmental handling programmes and subsequent prognostic counselling. The physiotherapist might recognize specific developmental patterns which may be attributable to aetiological factors not previously identified.

REFERENCES

Blair, E, Stanley, F (1988) Intrapartum asphyxia: a rare cause of cerebral palsy. *Journal of Pediatrics* 112: 515–519.

Burns, Y, Fitzpatrick, MP, Mohay, H (1984) A four year follow-up of infants with signs of neuro-developmental deviation. *Australian Journal of Physiotherapy* 30: 75–80.

Committee for the Classification of Retinopathy of Prematurity (1984) The international classification of retinopathy of prematurity. *Pediatrics* 74: 127–133.

Cornblath, M, Schwartz, R (1976) *Disorders of Carbohydrate Metabolism in Infancy,* 501 pp. Philadelphia: Saunders.

Cryotherapy for Retinopathy of Prematurity Cooperative Group (1988) Multicenter trial of cryotherapy for retinopathy of prematurity: preliminary results. *Pediatrics* 81: 692–706.

Desmond, MM et al. (1980) The very low birthweight infant after discharge from intensive care: anticipatory health care and development course. *Current Problems in Pediatrics* 6: 5–59.

Dobbing, J (1981) The later development of the brain and its vulnerability. In:

Davis, JA, Dobbing, J (eds) *Scientific Foundation of Paediatrics*, pp. 742–759, 2nd edn. London: Heinemann.

Drillien, CM (1972) Abnormal neurological signs in the first year of life in low birth weight infants. Possible prognostic significance. *Developmental Medicine and Child Neurology* **14**: 575–584.

Jones, KL (1988) In: *Smith's Recognizable Patterns of Human Malformation*, pp. 491–494, 4th edn. Philadelphia: Saunders.

Koivisto, M, Blanco-Sequerios, M, Krause, U (1972) Neonatal symptomatic and asymptomatic hypoglycaemai: a follow-up study of 151 children. *Developmental Medicine and Child Neurology* **14**: 603–614.

Levene, MI, Tudehope, D (1993) *Essentials of Neonatal Medicine*, 438 pp., 2nd edn. Oxford: Blackwell Scientific.

Lucas, A, Morley, R, Cole, TG (1988) Adverse neurodevelopmental outcome of moderate neonatal hypoglycaemia. *British Medical Journal* **297**: 1304–1308.

Tudehope, D (1992) The low birth weight infant. In: Clements, A (ed.) *Infant and Family Health in Australia*, pp. 69–77, 2nd edn. Melbourne: Churchill Livingstone.

Tudehope, D *et al.* (1981) Minor neurological abnormalities during the first year of life of infants of birth weight <1500 gm. *Australian Paediatric Journal* **17**: 265–268.

Tudehope, D *et al.* (1989) Neonatal cranial ultrasonography as predictor of 2 year outcome of very low birthweight infants. *Australian Paediatric Journal* **25**: 66–71.

Tudehope, D, Gray, P, Steer, P (1990–1993) *Annual Reports of Department of Neonatology*, Mater Mothers' Hospital.

Tudehope, D *et al.* (1992) Audiological evaluation of very low birth weight infants. *Journal of Pediatrics and Child Health* **28**: 172–175.

Yu, VHY, Hookham, DM, Navej, RM (1982) Retrolental fibroplasia — controlled study of four years experience in a neonatal intensive care unit. *Archives of Disease in Childhood* **57**: 247–252.

Section C:

Assessment and Evaluation of Outcome

PROLOGUE: YVONNE BURNS

Prologue

YVONNE BURNS

Assessment provides the basis for clinical problem-solving, decision-making, selection and modification of intervention techniques or approaches to management and evaluation of outcome. The changing and complex nature of development means that one of the first tasks facing the physiotherapist is to determine what aspects of the child need to be assessed. It is important to choose the most appropriate tests or measures which will ensure meaningful results, give a balanced profile of the child's abilities, and identify potential difficulties. The most suitable context in which to undertake the assessment should be considered.

No one test or type of assessment is suitable for all purposes. While a standardized test will be used to provide the initial baseline and problem identification, another type of assessment may be more helpful for the measurement of small clinical change during or after an intervention. Furthermore, an assessment of function/performance within the child's usual environment may be most appropriate for the child with a moderate to severe physical disability at home, at school or within a vocational setting.

Whatever type of assessment or test is used, it is important to ensure that standardized procedures and techniques are followed and outcomes and results are recorded. The physiotherapist's knowledge, experience and understanding of motor and psychosocial development as well as movement analysis is crucial for good clinical decision-making regarding intervention.

Section C considers paediatric physiotherapy assessment in terms of the principles and purposes of assessment, the aspects to be considered (such as different presentations, age, background, environment or context), and whether as a team or individual assessment. The assessment process is presented, including preparation, history, observation, testing, recording reporting and planning intervention. In addition, the types of assessment available and some of those currently being used by practising physiotherapists are outlined.

Yvonne Burns

Throughout the world, health costs are rising rapidly and there is increasing pressure on health care professionals to demonstrate the effectiveness of treatments or interventions. It is essential that clinical and research physiotherapists face the issue and determine ways of effectively evaluating outcome. Chapter 8 looks closely at the complex issue of 'outcome' measurement. Patient outcome is determined by a number of inter-linking factors, including the status of the child before intervention, the environment in which the child functions and subtle or indirect influences. Despite the complex nature of the problem all physiotherapists can and should become involved in developing improved measures of patient 'outcome'. Single or small group study design may be useful to clinical physiotherapists for evaluating intervention.

7

The Process of Physiotherapy Assessment for Children

YVONNE BURNS AND CATHERINE HIGGINS

Physiotherapy Paediatric Assessment
•
Administration of an Assessment
•
Type of Assessments

Assessment of movement is an essential component of the repertoire of skills of a physiotherapist. In paediatrics, the physiotherapist requires special knowledge and skills. Assessment of motor development, posture, sensory responses, movement and particular functions must take into account the ongoing changes associated with growth and system maturation, inherited characteristics, individual variations and the constant transactions occurring between the child and the environment. The preceding chapters have set the scene in respect to child, family and therapist interactions and aspects of normal and abnormal development.

This chapter presents the general principles of physiotherapy assessment in paediatrics, the reasons for assessment, the process and special features, selection of appropriate tests or evaluations and the range of assessments currently being used by physiotherapists. Developmental neurosensorimotor assessments will be addressed in some detail. Assessments specific to other conditions will be discussed in relevant sections of later chapters.

Physiotherapy Paediatric Assessment

Physiotherapy paediatric assessment is the process of gathering information about an infant or child to determine their level of physical well-being and functional ability. The problems which may interfere with movement must be determined through the evaluation of motor development and postural control and the neurological, musculoskeletal, cardiorespiratory and other systems likely to influence the quality of motor performance. Function should be evaluated in the context of the child's usual environment and personal needs. Accurate interpretation of assessed information must be based on a thorough knowledge of normal development of the respective body systems and developmental performance as well as the presenting signs of dysfunction or abnormality. Assessment can be considered as the initial phase of, or precursor to, intervention, as it provides a baseline and focus for treatment and programme implementation. Assessment not only identifies the problems to be addressed but also recognizes what is normal.

Principles of Assessment

Assessment involves the following:

Information	this includes reason for referral, relevant history and results of other tests/investigations, age of the child, any known growth or developmental factors, special social or family factors
Observation	an essential first step during which presenting abilities, problems and specific characteristics can be noted before entering into the child's personal space to administer specific tests
Administration	tests may involve palpation, measurement, specific positions, movement or inputs. It is important to ensure that these tests are age-appropriate, as well as condition- and aspect-specific; it is essential that intervention during an initial or baseline assessment is avoided
Recording	accurate recording of measurements, responses, scores or grades, or description of performance is crucial
Interpretation	in the light of knowledge of normal development, reason for referral and results of the current assessment, a decision regarding the need for and type of physiotherapy intervention should be determined. If the condition is known, care is required to ensure that diagnosis bias (i.e. finding symptoms to support diagnosis) does not

influence interpretation. In research, assessors should be 'blind' to diagnosis/history or previous results which may bias results

Any major or long-term illness is likely to have an adverse affect upon aspects of the child's motor, intellectual or social development. Therefore, an assessment/examination of any sick child should include at least a brief evaluation of their development. A physiotherapy developmental assessment should check:

- age-appropriateness of gross and fine motor functions
- neurological status
- musculoskeletal status
- developmental postural and balance reactions
- sensorimotor responses and/or perception
- motor skill ability and coordination

Identification of developmental delay or dysfunction should lead to appropriate action. It may be that a more detailed developmental assessment is indicated, referral for other investigations or the inclusion of appropriate developmental interventions into the child's overall programme.

The Context of Assessment

Development is a continuing, complex, interrelated process of change. During development considerable variability as well as general conformity occurs within the context of a broad but recognized sequence of events. Different levels of maturation, ability and experience in all of these aspects are likely to lead to considerable variation not only between children but in the same child in different settings. Furthermore, a child's performance often depends upon a number of events occurring simultaneously. Before starting, it is important therefore to address the assessment setting or environment, the approach of the assessor, the timing and sequence of presentation of the test or assessment procedures, the child in terms of coping, self-esteem and respect, as well as the involvement of parents or carers. The assessment setting may be a hospital, special centre, nursery, preschool or school or the child's own home. Whatever the setting, the organization of the room and the attitude of all those present should provide a suitable environment. The assessor should have knowledge and training in understanding children and use an approach suitable to the age and special needs of the child and family.

There are a number of different types of assessment and approach. These include developmental, functional and disability- or condition-specific assessments. Other assessments are designed to consider specifically the child's interactions within a familiar environment.

Ecological Assessment

Ecological assessment is a structured process of gathering formal and informal information about the child within their usual environment. Although mainly used by school psychologists to examine the child's usual behaviour, the environment surrounding the behaviour and the individual–environment link (Carlson et al. 1980), it offers a useful model for assessment of motor function and performance. This approach of regarding the child and the environment as a single unit involves assimilation of information from widespread sources such as parent and teacher interviews, check-lists and observations as well as formal standardized testing (Milliken and Buckley 1983). The ecological assessment process is particularly suitable for the preschool and school-age child as it incorporates a broad perspective of the child and will often identify issues that may be detrimental; for example a negative attitude that is adversely affecting the child's self esteem, or an aspect of the environment that is inhibiting progress, e.g. lack of access and need for a ramp or personal equipment.

Why Assess?

The type of physiotherapy assessment undertaken will vary according to the ultimate purpose and use of the information. The aim of the assessment may be to:

- contribute to the diagnostic process by identifying aspects of concern and ascertain why the child is not reaching expected or age-appropriate levels of motor performance.

- screen a population of children to identify those who may require more specific assessment and possible intervention
- set a baseline for intervention by identifying current strengths or normal functioning as well as primary and secondary abnormalities and potential problems
- follow-up children considered to be 'at risk' for problems of motor development
- determine the effectiveness and efficacy of an intervention programme
- evaluate the results of the application of a specific technique, equipment, orthoses or treatment
- identify access or other functional needs

Through assessment, interpretation of results and comparison with normal standards and/or specific criteria, physiotherapists can decide whether a child's performance is within the expected normal range, requires physiotherapy intervention or needs further investigation. Treatment and intervention programme planning based on accurate and detailed assessment is more likely to address the specific needs of the child and avoid inopportune treatment than a cursory or inappropriate assessment.

To meet the changing needs of an infant or child, reassessment and clinical problem-solving are an integral part of on-going developmental intervention programmes. It is essential in cases of long-term intervention that from time to time, perhaps every 3, 6 or 12 months depending on age and condition, a formal review assessment be undertaken to compare with the initial or baseline assessment. For longitudinal follow-up the same assessment or similar testing process should be used to allow valid comparison.

Cautions

Instigating the process of assessment carries enormous professional responsibility (Derstine 1989). The act of undergoing assessment may place a 'label' upon the child that is inaccurate or unwarranted, causing concern for the child and the child's family or caregivers. Furthermore, the act of administering an assessment may give parents and caregivers expectations of service delivery, which on interpretation of assessment results may not be warranted (King-

Thomas and Hacker 1987). Assessment does not necessarily mean that physiotherapy intervention is required or advisable. In some cases, monitoring the child's process may be more appropriate or referral to another professional may be required. In conditions where there is deterioration, repeated failure or loss of previously acquired abilities can lead to strong negative emotional responses and diminished self-esteem. Inaccurate, inadequate or inappropriate assessment can also result in an outcome that may be detrimental to the future of the child and/or family.

Which Assessment Tool?

Selection of the most appropriate test or assessment process will depend upon:

- the purpose of the assessment
- the condition and severity of presentation of the infant's/child's problem
- the child's age
- the approach of the physiotherapist
- the environment and background of the infant or child to be assessed
- the availability of the test proforma

These factors will now be looked at in more detail.

PURPOSE OF THE ASSESSMENT

The purpose of the test may be guided by the origin of the referral for physiotherapy assessment. The infant or child could be referred by a doctor within the medical system, by a concerned parent, or by a teacher at a school. The information required to provide input to a medical diagnosis will have a different emphasis and focus to that of a parent or school. Although specific information about the underlying components of the child's motor abilities provides an important background for the formulation of an individualized physiotherapy treatment plan, an educational team would require information that is heavily biased towards function. If the purpose is to screen a population of children, for example at a preschool, a test which identifies that a child is not reaching the standard of their peers may be all that is needed to indicate that further investigation or detailed assessment is warranted.

For the purpose of research the researcher must find a test which definitely meets the requirements of reliability and validity. The use of poorly designed or inappropriate measures or assessments could be detrimental to the outcome of the research and may mean many hours of wasted work. Research undertaken by physiotherapists may use instrumentation (such as goniometers and angle finders to assess joint range or spirometers to assess respiratory function), timed or measured tasks, written tests, evaluative and predictive measures or inventories (Bailey 1991). Developmental tests may be standardized or non-standardized. A standardized test is accompanied by a manual which will provide the researcher with background information on the test such as the procedure used for obtaining the norms, the population chosen as the normative group and the degree of validity and reliability obtained for that test. Information relating to trials performed should also be included.

The researcher must use the chosen tool only in the manner dictated in the test manual and administer it only to the population described therein under preset conditions, otherwise the results of the test cannot be ensured to be valid or reliable. Observer bias is another major factor which may disrupt the internal validity of a study (Bailey 1991).

CHILD-SPECIFIC ASSESSMENT

History/Diagnosis Some tests are originally designed to be administered to children with certain disabilities. For example, the *Gross Motor Function Measure* (Russell *et al.* 1993) is designed for assessment of children whose disability is cerebral palsy. The *Visual Assessment and Programming* and *Capacity Attention and Processing* (VAP CAP) provide an assessment and programming package for children with visual impairment (Blanksby 1992).

Physiological status If a child is hungry, fearful, not well and/or in pain, performance and response to tests can obviously be affected. Tired or hungry infants and young children do not perform well so assessments should be timed to coincide with awake or play periods.

Physical impairment The degree of physical impairment will influence the choice of assessment tools.

A child with severe physical disability would not be able to achieve even basic motor milestones so an assessment involving advanced gross motor activities (run, jump) would be inappropriate. In this situation a basic neurodevelopmental assessment could be performed to look at qualitative aspects of the child's movements, balance, postural reactions and responses to sensory input and quantitative aspects such as joint range and muscle strength. A functional assessment may give further helpful information.

Sensory Disabilities Sometimes the nature of the child's disability may actually limit the performance of the 'hands on' phase of assessment as a child who is tactile defensive or has vestibular dysfunction may not like to be handled. In this case, an assessment tool which contains large observational components may be most useful in gaining an assessment of the child's abilities. Other children such as those with hearing impairments, may be unable to follow assessment instructions without the assistance of signing or demonstration of the tasks. Children with visual impairments may hesitate to perform some tasks due to fear of movement or unfamiliarity with the environment. If specific sensory-adapted tests are not available or suitable, normal tests/procedures may need to be modified.

Intellectual Abilities An intellectual impairment may limit the administration of particular assessments because of the child's difficulty in comprehending instructions. The presence of parents or use of motivational toys or music may gain the child's attention and cooperation in specific tasks. Consistency and patience are important in the development of trust.

Communication Abilities The child's communication abilities may also influence the type of testing performed. A child with receptive language problems will not cope easily with complex commands during the assessment. Any device the child needs for communication should be present at the assessment and the use of signing may be necessary for a child with a hearing impairment.

Sociocultural Aspects It is important to avoid assessments containing any items of cultural or social bias that would compromise a child's performance.

AGE OF THE CHILD

Most tests are designed for certain age groups. The choice of an assessment may be influenced by the age of the child. For example, a developmentally based assessment may be of more value in the evaluation of infants and young children when developmental status is most relevant, or when the degree of dysfunction is relatively mild. In the case of older children, especially those with a more moderate or severe disability, the clinician may choose an assessment that focuses on testing a child's functional abilities. In all situations it is important that the test items and the way they are administered are age-appropriate. Use of age-inappropriate equipment or approach can adversely affect the level of cooperation and even undermine the child's self-esteem.

APPROACH OF THE PHYSIOTHERAPIST

The personal attributes of physiotherapists can also influence the choice of assessment. This choice will depend on the content and extent of a physiotherapist's experience and the circumstances and areas of practice in which they currently work or have worked in the past. The physiotherapist who adopts a flexible approach to assessment will attempt to use different assessment tools as warranted or try new tools as they become available.

ENVIRONMENTAL FACTORS

The setting in which assessment is carried out may depend on the preliminary choice of assessments. Some assessments are carried out in a quiet area, perhaps away from the child's usual environment. Others are administered in a more ecological setting such as in the area of function under assessment, for example in the classroom or at home, and incorporate information from others to whom the child is well known. However, environmental factors pertain not only to the setting in which a physiotherapist would administer an assessment, but also to the human and physical resources available such as persons present (parents, psychologist, other therapists) and assessment equipment.

DISCIPLINE-SPECIFIC OR TEAM ASSESSMENT

Whether a discipline-specific assessment is performed and/or team assessment depends on the team dynamics and the information needed. If detailed gait analysis is required, then the physiotherapist would probably perform a discipline-specific assessment to determine a child's functional ability in this area. However, if a broad idea of a child's mobility is required, then a team assessment which covers mobility in one of its domains could be administered by a selected member of the team, not necessarily the physiotherapist.

USER FRIENDLINESS OF THE ASSESSMENT

Overall design features and cost of the assessment tool also need to be considered. The test may have to be relatively portable for ease of administration in different settings. The test should be of suitable duration and of sufficient interest, and if possible fun, to hold the attention of the child and the examiner. Time available is also a consideration when choosing how long to devote to a certain assessment procedure and whether the information gained is worth the time invested.

Choosing a suitable tool to use to perform an assessment requires the physiotherapist to consider all options, become familiar with various assessment tools and adopt a flexible approach to this important stage of intervention. If one tool is insufficient to give comprehensive information then a combination of tests should be used. Additionally, many physiotherapists work in team settings, so the baseline data gathered by each team member using discipline-specific assessments, can be amalgamated. Each team member can interpret their findings and share the implications of it. This will provide a more comprehensive picture of the child's abilities.

The value of the assessment depends not only on the selection of an appropriate tool but also on the way in which it is administered.

Administration of an Assessment

Figure 1 depicts the process of assessment and the steps undertaken to compile a comprehensive profile of the child. The following section will explore the components of the process in more detail.

Preparation

FAMILIARIZATION WITH THE ASSESSMENT TOOL

Once an assessment protocol or tool is chosen, the physiotherapist will need to practise the format and procedure of the test. Any equipment required to administer the test will need to be collected, but usually the test kit will provide the items or they can be easily obtained in most paediatric settings. Often the administration time will be suggested in the manual. Some authors recommend specialized training before administration but Rogers (1987) states that the need for special training may reduce the usability of the test. As training may not be easily accessed, the test procedure outlined in the manual should be clear and concise and the test procedures easy to learn. This will encourage physiotherapists to use the tool and assist in the 'demystification' of a new assessment tool.

ASSESSMENT TIME

A suitable time for the parents or caregivers to attend the assessment must be made. Whenever possible avoid meal and sleep times, as a hungry or sleepy child does not perform well. The assessment protocol should be outlined before the assessment and the parents or caregivers reminded about the purpose of the assessment and how the information will be used, for example to plan treatment. Allow sufficient time for the assessment to be carried out in a relaxed manner in appropriate surroundings. Sometimes it is helpful to have both parents present, especially in the case of a young child. Other times or with older children, the child may cooperate better in the absence of the parents or caregivers.

Depending on the assessment tool chosen, the test may need to be administered at the one appointment,

Figure 1   The Assessment Process

Purpose	Diagnostic	Screening	Intervention
	Professional responsibility		Research
Context	Movement focused	Collaborative	Ecological/clinical
Selection	Test specific to purpose of assessment		

Undertaking the assessment

Preparation – testing, environment, equipment
History/background – obtain and read reports, interview, network
Observation
Testing
Recording
Interpretation
Report – numerical (computer), written and/or videotape
Amalgamate the information of other assessments/investigations

Child's abilities/disabilities known
‖
Formulate physiotherapy goals
‖
Collaborate with team

Monitor / Intervene

Reassess to establish
if intervention
now required

Treatment provision
Design physiotherapy
programme

Reassess to establish
efficacy of intervention

especially if it is a standardized test. A standardized test should also be administered in the manner described in the test manual. Sometimes detailed assessment for planning intervention may require more than one appointment. Baseline assessments should be completed before intervention begins.

To obtain an accurate picture of the child's abilities/disabilities, the child should feel comfortable and at ease with the assessment throughout the duration of the test. Some children are wary of a test situation due to past experiences and the physiotherapist may need to create an atmosphere that feels less imposing to the child. The physiotherapist should develop good verbal and non-verbal communication skills. If the child does not perform a test item well or continues to have difficulty performing or repeating a task, it may be best to move on to something else or try to test the task in a different way at another time (if it is not a standardized test item). Avoid creating a negative situation by prolonging or persisting with an assessment item the child has failed, as a loss of

confidence or cooperation can adversely affect performance in following test items. Some children have challenging behaviour so the physiotherapist may need to ascertain first if any behaviour management strategies have been instigated and should use these consistently throughout the assessment process.

VENUE

The environment should be warm and safe. Privacy may need to be considered as the child may have to be suitably undressed. Infants over 3 months old may be best assessed on a large clean padded area on the floor. Age-appropriate toys should be available. Avoid small objects which can be accidently swallowed. Observing children in a familiar environment will provide the best setting for observation of functional abilities, but this may not be possible. If a test is designed to be administered in a group situation, an educational setting such as a school can be ideal. Some assessments can be undertaken while the child participates in the school programme or a group.

TEAM

Parents, care-givers and/or other professionals (therapists, psychologists, doctors, teachers or nurses) may be involved in the assessment of the child. In this case it may be advantageous to undertake assessments concurrently with other members of the team. It is important that the primary assessor for each aspect of the assessment be prearranged to avoid confusing either the child or the parent during the assessment.

EQUIPMENT

The assessment procedure will flow more smoothly if all the necessary test items are readily available. Neurodevelopmental assessment normally requires very little specialized equipment. The equipment needed will depend on the age and disability of the child being tested.

Equipment ideas

Room equipment and furniture
Suitable floor coverings — carpets, mats
A chair and table with perhaps an option of adaptive seating
Stairs/parallel bars
Pillows
Bean bags
Padded plinth

Equipment for testing age-appropriate tasks and fine motor skills
Puzzles
Books
Jump rope
Pencils, crayons and paper
Different sized balls/bat
Toys — noisy, visually interesting (keep small toys away from infants and young children)
Threading beads
Screw toys

Equipment for testing neurological, musculo-skeletal, sensorimotor and physical status
Tendon hammer
Blindfold
Small torch
Stop watch
Optokinetic strip of fabric
Music cassettes — rhythm
Goniometer/angle finder
Small items for stereognosis
Cotton wool, pin, paper clip
Tactile toys — different textures
Tape measure
Vibrator
Bell or noisy toy
Finger puppet
Blowing toys

Other equipment for testing sensorimotor areas, balance and postural reactions and equipment for positioning
Large therapy balls
Balance beam
Scooter board
Wedges — cutout
Balance board
Spinning box
Steps
Roll

Background Information

The first step in the assessment process is usually to assimilate background information and generate a history of the child's condition and progress. Obtaining a history will provide insight into which assessment path to follow, the child's prognosis and any precautions or contraindications of which to be mindful while handling the child. Aspects of the child's history that may need to be obtained are:

- medical history, e.g. diagnosis, surgery, investigations, medication
- familial history, e.g. incidence of disabilities, developmental problems
- birth history, e.g. pregnancy, duration of labour, instrumentation used
- developmental history, e.g. achievement of milestones, regression
- psychological history, e.g. behaviour, likes/dislikes, interests

- educational history, e.g. school attendance, alternative settings
- service delivery history, e.g. provision of therapy services, agencies involved

Methods of obtaining this information may involve some or all of the following:

- interviews with the parents or caregivers
- written check-lists for the parents or caregivers to complete detailing the child's attainment of developmental milestones and their impression of the child's current abilities
- with the permission of the parents and caregivers, using reports from other professional service providers involved with the child

Information may be gained while observing the child in various situations. During this part of the proceedings it is important to establish rapport with the child, family and caregivers. A good history will facilitate the choice of a suitable formal assessment tool and will avoid duplication of service delivery or inappropriate intervention.

Sensitivity is required when asking parents and caregivers about the history of the child's condition and obtaining personal information about the family and family dynamics. If this history-taking is done early in the assessment process, rapport may not be fully established and it can take time for the parents and caregivers to reveal personal details. Sensitivity is particularly important when obtaining the family history to determine the incidence of a special disability or condition. Sometimes the parents and caregivers are still 'grieving'; questioning may upset them or they may be grateful for the opportunity to talk about it. Much information can be gained from previous records, so discretion is required in choosing the appropriate time and questions to be asked. Questions should be kept relevant and concise. Avoid jargon to ensure that the child, family or caregivers understand what is being asked of them.

Observation

Physiotherapists can perform part of their assessment through informal observation, perhaps during the initial meetings with the child's family. An overall idea of the child's basic physical status and abilities can often be gained by observing the child at play. For example, observe: patterns of movement, posture of the head, trunk and limbs, spontaneous voluntary or involuntary movement; purpose and planning; eye contact; verbalization; alertness and social responsiveness. The effect of any specialized equipment that is being used by the child can also be observed.

Observation can be formalized through the use of recording methods, for example:

- rate of behaviour in which frequency of the target behaviour is recorded
- check-lists of behaviours performed by children with certain disabilities against which a parent or caregiver can mark off the occurrences of the particular negative or positive behaviours, for example rocking, self-stimulation or self-initiated rolling
- rating scales which assign a numerical value to rate the frequency, quality or amount of a behaviour, for example 1 'never occurs' to 5 'always occurs' (Huber and King-Thomas 1987, p. 5).

These methods can assist in formulating a basic profile of the behaviours of the child and provide valuable insight into the areas that require more detailed objective assessment. For example, the child avoiding being touched or different textures or surfaces may indicate to the physiotherapist that the child has problems processing tactile input. Therefore, assessment of the tactile system should be targeted as a vital area for testing.

Preliminary movement analysis and observation of aspects of abnormal patterns of movement can occur while observing the child at play, eating and interacting with others. This is also a suitable time for the examiner to discover some of the child's interests and preferences in regards to activities, toys and distractions, in preparation for more direct handling of the child by the physiotherapist. Once a rapport with the child has been established, the child will usually be more cooperative and this should expedite the remainder of the assessment process. Only then should the examiner proceed with the next step in the assessment process, that of more in-depth hands-on assessment which requires the examiner to enter the child's space.

Physiotherapy Neurodevelopmental Checklist

GENERAL ABILITIES	Primitive reflexes (contd) R L
Gross Motor	— withdrawal
head control	— stepping
roll over	— Moro
crawl	— Galant
sit	— abdominal
stand	— tonic labyrinthine reflex
walk	— asymmetrical tonic neck reflex
ability to change position	— symmetrical tonic neck reflex
run	Pathological movement patterns
stairs	— adducted thumbs
jump	— scissored legs
hop	— internal rotation with extension
kick	— external rotation with abduction
catch	— upper limb synergies
walk straight line	Abnormal eye movement or position
stand on one leg	(nystagmus, squint)
other	

Fine Motor

MUSCULOSKELETAL

	UL LL Trunk
grasp — maturity	Muscle power / imbalance
— quality and / or efficiency	Contractures
intrinsic action	Fasciculation
coordination	Atrophy
wrist and finger movement	Gower's sign
finger dexterity	Joint range of movement
isolated finger movement	Joint deformities
threading	Structural problems
writing	e.g. scoliosis
drawing	congenital dislocation of the hip
hand preference	Orthopaedic surgery

NEUROLOGICAL SIGNS R L	Comments
Basic tone — upper limbs	
— lower limbs	
Active tone — upper limbs	
— lower limbs	
Deep tendon reflexes — knees	
— elbows	
Clonus	
Tremor — type	
— amplitude	
Involuntary movements	
Associated reactions	
Primitive reflexes	
— mouthing, rooting	
— suck and swallow	
— gag	
— hand grasp	
— foot grasp	
— extensor thrust	
— crossed extension	
— hip adductor reflex	

POSTURE AND BALANCE R L

Postural stability during activities
— gross motor
— fine motor
(e.g. lying, sitting, standing)
Placing
Positive support — upper
             — lower
Weight shift — upper (lateral/diagonal)
             — lower
Head righting — forward (optical)
     Vertical — back
            — side
     Horizontal — prone
            — supine
            — side
Body on body righting
Landau
Protective reactions
Parachute — arms
         — legs
Equilibrium — sitting
            — standing
Posture and balance relative to position

SENSORY MOTOR

Tactile R L
General localization of touch
Double simultaneous
Specific tactile localization on fingers
Graphaesthesia
Stereognosis
Reaction to pain

Proprioception
Finger position awareness
Limb position awareness — upper
                     — lower
Automatic position adjustment
Synkinesis
Static hold — with vision
          — vision occluded
Arm extension test
— arm position
— hand position
— loss of position
— excessive stabilization

Vestibular R L
Vest. head righting
Post-rotatory response
— oculomotor nystagmus
— postural reaction

Ocular Motor R L
— eye follow
— fix and release
— dissociation of head
   and eye movements
— convergence
— fast follow
— optokinetic nystagmus
— eye—hand coordination

Auditory motor
— localization of direction
— following of unseen sound
— listening to sound

Motor Planning (Praxis)
Organization of body
— visual copy
— verbal instruction
Cross midline
Skills
— ability to learn new skills
— diadochokinesia
— thumb to alternate fingers
— auditory tap pattern
— rhythm and timing

Perceptual Motor (necessary if no occupational therapist is available)
Visual motor
— drawing, copy simple shapes, mazes, mannequin, form board, joining dots, draw a man (house), assembling barrels (by shape, size), sequencing, figure-ground

BEHAVIOURAL RESPONSES
To — examiner
     — individual tests
     — environment
     — parents
Consistency of response
General coping ability

Comments

Testing

Physiotherapy assessment involves tests which require handling, palpation, passive movement of limbs and other contact techniques so it is advisable to start with the least-threatening tests. The child should be positioned to provide the most appropriate support or, in the case of a standardized test, according to the positions described in the test manual. With a non-standardized tool, the test positions used during assessment should be recorded so that a subsequent examiner will be able to replicate the procedure. In this way, the child's optimal performance will be observed and interpretation of comparisons between performances can be made. It is often advisable to avoid lying the child down until their confidence has been gained. Some infants are fearful in prone position while others dislike being supine. It is advisable to plan which tests you will need to perform in each position, e.g. sitting, kneeling, prone, supine, to avoid unnecessary handling and changes of position. See the neurodevelopmental check-list for aspects which may need to be tested.

Recording the Assessment and Outcome

Record-keeping is a vital component of the assessment process and such records can:

- create a legal record to justify the outcome of the assessment such as the decision to provide a particular physiotherapy programme
- be referred to at a later date to allow comparison of the child's abilities and to show change in the child's function
- supply the foundation for ongoing intervention and programme re-evaluation.
- provide a means to share information with other team members
- promote continuity of service provision; information on assessment and intervention previously implemented will be accessible and useful for subsequent providers of a physiotherapy service to that child and prevent excessive duplication of service

Recording anecdotal information, such as a child's incidental displays of function, likes/dislikes, or adverse responses, can also be helpful to a physiotherapist new to the child. When there is a change of staff this can assist in easing both child and physiotherapist through the transition process of getting to know each other.

Paul-Brown (1994) states that clinical record-keeping should comply with federal and state laws and meet the standards and regulations of the facility for whom the professional works. Assessment records should include:

- the child's personal identification details, such as name, age, address
- date of the assessment
- referral source and other service-providers involved
- client diagnosis and comprehensive history as outlined previously
- assessments undertaken and results
- interpretation of assessment results and implications of results
- statement of prognosis if relevant
- recommendations based on client's functional needs
- signature and professional title of the examiner and/or documenter

The rationale for choosing various assessment tools and the recommendations made on the basis of assessment, such as intervention, referring on to another or seeking another investigation, should all be documented. Records should be checked for accuracy, contain common terminology and be written legibly in ink or typed so that they can be used and understood by potential users at a later date (Paul-Brown 1994).

Many physiotherapists take an objective but qualitative approach to assessment and its recording. They often record the presence, and categorize the type of muscle tone and the abnormal reflex activity or movement. They also describe observed movement patterns, balance and postural reactions and motor responses to sensory input. However, this qualitative reporting of assessment may require standardization since the results of research into these assessment techniques often indicate poor reliability. Kathrein (1990) reported on the inter-rater reliability of the assessment of muscle tone. Her research showed low inter-rater reliability in the clinical setting. She found that the results reflected factors such as:

- lack of standardization of the technique used to assess the tone
- lack of consistent terminology to describe tone and the degree of tone present
- lack of a category to describe abnormal fluctuating or variable tone

Recording Format

Some formalized tests provide assessment logs or forms to be completed which can save time provide a profile of the child's abilities and can be kept as a record of the assessment. A number of these forms are designed to allow recording of subsequent assessment results on the same page for easy comparison, but this practice tends to bias subsequent assessment results. The following authors allow some of the record forms published in their tests to be photocopied for the clinicians use, according to copyright specifications:

- Department of Education, Queensland (1994) – neurodevelopmental assessment format, joint range procedure, manual muscle testing forms, wheelchair and adaptive seating assessment forms and preoperative check-list forms
- Blossom and Ford (1991) – joint range procedure, posture assessment, wheelchair posture assessment and general record-keeping ideas
- Cusick (1990) – biomechanical and joint motion record-keeping forms

It may be helpful to videotape a child's performance, especially from a different visual angle to that of the examiner. This can allow later observation of the videotape to gain a different perspective and provide a permanent record of the child's movements for later comparison.

Confidentiality is extremely important and the distribution of information should only be allowed if written permission has been given by the parents or legal caregivers on behalf of the child. Records should be kept in a safe and secure storage area to maintain this confidentiality. It is also important to use discretion as to what is recorded. Value judgements based on a physiotherapist's personal value system should be omitted.

Scoring the Test and Interpreting the Assessment Results

If using a standardized test, the assessment tool will usually explain the method of scoring. Some tools have a computer program to assist in scoring. Rogers (1987), noted that a manual should also explain to the tester how to deal with test items that were not completed or were performed incorrectly by the child. Raw scores in themselves are not significant until they are compared to the test standard.

The interpretation of results is an important phase of the assessment process and carries with it much responsibility. It is from assessment information that treatment is indicated and programmes are developed. The appropriateness of the assessment to meet these needs has far-reaching consequences for the child, as programmes that are not appropriately directed may be wasting valuable intervention time. In the growing child, there are often critical ages when well-directed treatment may prevent life-time complications, deformity or disability. For example, a young child who, on assessment, is not reaching age-appropriate motor milestones may not be moving sufficiently to provide the necessary formative sensory experiences and correct skeletal modelling and alignment to prevent pathological contractures of muscles and joint structures.

Reassessment Schedule

Reassessment, which is a process of revisiting the assessment arena after a period of time, is integral to providing a physiotherapy service to a child as they grow and respond to intervention. Change may be demonstrated by reassessment results indicating the efficacy of the physiotherapy programme or it may be shown that the expected outcome is not being achieved. The frequency of reassessment will depend on the child's disability, age, the rate of progress and the nature of intervention undertaken since the last assessment.

It is at this time that we see that the assessment process is actually part of the continuum of intervention. As reassessment becomes intermingled with episodes of treatment and programme implementation, the outcome of each reassessment helps the physiotherapist to become vigilant and dynamic in response to the changing needs of the growing child.

Type of Assessments

Standardized Tests

Standardized tests are structured and have a fixed content, a prescribed method of administration, a fixed scoring system and should be administered to the specified population as outlined in the test manual (Bailey 1991). They may be norm or criterion referenced. Standardization refers to the procedure of administering the test to subjects under consistent conditions (Montgomery and Connolly 1987) and taking the test through a 'normalizing' process, which establishes a level of validity and reliability in regard to the 'normal' population (Bailey 1991). According to Jacobs and Logigian (1989), in the case of non-standardized tests, a uniform procedure in administering the test may be prescribed, but normative data, reliability and validity have not been established and it is therefore difficult to compare results of subsequent tests. After reviewing much of the accompanying literature to assessment tools which claim to be standardized, it is apparent that some authors have become more flexible in their interpretation of the term 'standardized', especially in regard to the order of presentation of test items to the child.

Norm-referenced Tests

Norm-referenced tests allow comparison of a child's test score to that of scores already obtained from an assessment of a large, representative reference group of peers, i.e. the child's performance is compared to the performance of other children. A reference group could be either a group of children without a disability or a group of children with a similar condition to the child being tested, for which norms have been obtained (Haley *et al.* 1989). These tests use norma-

tive values to interpret an individual's performance and can therefore establish developmental age levels and differences among individuals. They must be administered in a standard manner as specified in the test manual and should demonstrate reliability and validity. Tests are not necessarily linked to intervention, as items included in the test are not based on task analysis and may not be sensitive to, or directly related to, interventional objectives. Care should be taken in using norm-referenced tests to gauge the effects of instruction or intervention. They are more suitable for diagnostic or school placement purposes (Montgomery and Connolly 1987) and can indicate the need for further specific assessment.

Examples of norm-referenced tests are:

- *Peabody Developmental Motor Scales and Activity Cards* (Folio and Fewell 1983) which is a standardized screening or formal assessment tool used to measure gross and fine motor skills in children from birth to 6 years and 11 months in a check-list format.
- *Movement Assessment Battery for Children* or Movement ABC (Henderson and Sugden 1992), is developed from the Test of Motor Impairment (TOMI) by Stott *et al.* (1984) which can be used as a screen (check-list format) or as a more formal restandardized edition of the TOMI to provide both qualitative and normative measures of a child's motor competency in the areas of manual dexterity, ball skills and static and dynamic balance. The test targets the age group 4 to 12 years.

Criterion-referenced Tests

Criterion-referenced tests examine the performance of a child against a set of predetermined criteria which are designed to assess quality of age-appropriate responses (Burns 1992). It provides an index of competence independent of the performance of others and depicts a continuum of ability ranging from lack of proficiency to an expected level of performance of a set task (Rogers 1987).

In some criterion-referenced tests, items of the test are developed from task analysis and are sensitive to the effects of instruction and can therefore be used to measure the effects of such instructions by recording change in the child's subsequent performances [Montgomery and Connolly 1987]. Information from criterion-referenced tests may therefore be used for programme planning and evaluation of intervention.

Examples of criterion-referenced tests are:

- *Gross Motor Function Measure* (GMFM) (Russell *et al.* 1993) which was developed to be administered to children with cerebral palsy. It is used to measure a change in a child's gross motor function over a period of time using a pool of 88 items across various dimensions such as lying and rolling, sitting, through to walking and running. The scoring system takes into account the effect of aids or orthoses on performance and allows later recording and comparison of performance with such aids.
- *Developmental Programming for Infants and Young Children* (Schafer and Moersch 1981) which assesses areas of development such as gross motor, perceptual/fine motor, cognition, language, social and self-care for the age groups, birth to 35 months and 3 to 6 years. By systematic evaluation of the child's development, an individualized curriculum can be designed.

Norm-referenced and criterion-referenced tests can be further subdivided into developmental and functional assessments. Some criterion-referenced tests have an element of each focus, i.e. they may primarily be functionally focused but will also provide normative data, depending on how they are used and what age groups they are used to assess. The manual accompanying the test will outline the intention of the authors. Norm-referenced tests usually provide a broad overview of the age-related cognitive, language, social and motor performance of an infant or child.

A number of these tests are designed for use by other professionals such as psychologists or speech pathologists. Physiotherapists should be aware of their professional boundaries as some of these tests are restricted to a particular professional group and accreditation may be required before use is permitted.

Developmental Tests

The *Griffiths Abilities of Children* (Griffiths 1970) and the *Bayley* (Bayley 1969) are two well-known norm-referenced tests of overall development of infants and young children. General developmental tests usually contain items of gross and fine motor performance, but the pass/fail scoring format provides little qualitative information. Technically, the child may pass the set task but the quality of movement used may not be normal. Although a general developmental test will provide a broad profile of the child, the physiotherapist usually requires more specific information about the quality of the child's movement patterns. Developmental criterion-referenced tests therefore play an important role in providing more qualitative information about a child's motor and neurological development.

The *Neuro-Sensory and Motor Developmental Assessment for Infants and Young Children* (NSMDA), evaluates gross and fine motor performance, neurological status and primitive reflexes, posture and balance reactions and motor responses to sensory input at specified ages from 1 month to 6 years (Burns 1992). Its purpose is to identify problems and strengths of motor performance at certain ages and it is suitable for longitudinal follow-up of infants and children at risk of later problems. The test has been used successfully in identifying infants with cerebral palsy as well as less obvious motor dysfunction (Burns *et al.* 1989, Macdonald *et al.* 1990).

The *Motor Assessment of Infants* (MAI) useful to the age of 12 months (Chandler *et al.* 1980) evaluates a child's muscle tone, primitive reflexes, automatic reactions and volitional movement in the first year of life and targets children who have been treated in a neonatal intensive care unit. According to Derstine (1989), the authors state that the purpose of the test is to identify motor problems in infants up to the age of 12 months; provide grounds for early intervention; monitor the effects of physical therapy for the stated age group; assist research; and enhance the observational skills of the examiner through evaluation of children with and without disabilities.

Early identification of a child's problems in these areas allows discussion with the parents about the implications of the child's diagnosis, implementation of early intervention programmes and subsequently the prevention of perhaps a more severe level of disability for that child (Derstine 1989). The NSMDA and MAI are both useful for identifying infants who may have motor difficulties.

An example of a developmental test for the school-aged child is the *Battelle Developmental Inventory* (Newborg *et al.* 1984) which can be used in school or clinical settings. Its domains are personal, social, adaptive, motor, communication and cognitive.

Screening Tests

Stowers and Huber (1987) suggest that developmental tests can be divided into two groups, screening tests and those that provide a more detailed profile of a child's abilities and problems. Screening tests aim to detect the possible or definite presence of deviations from the norm and are used to indicate if further assessment or intervention is required by comparing children's abilities to those of their peers. An example of a screening test is the *Miller Assessment for Preschoolers* (also known as the MAP) developed by Miller (1988). This test was designed to identify students with pre-academic problems which may affect the child's abilities to progress developmentally at the same rate as their peers. It covers the areas of sensory and motor abilities, cognitive abilities and combined abilities which involve complex tasks. It is norm-referenced, standardized and individually administered.

Functional Assessments

Fraser *et al.* (1990) state that for some clinicians, assessments with a more functional focus will yield more valuable data as they determine an individual's abilities to perform certain everyday functional tasks or skills in their usual environment whereas a developmental assessment determines an individual's maturation and how the individual functions compared to normative data. Tests with a more functional focus are particularly useful in the case of the older child whose physical disability is of a significant degree. Children with a moderate to severe motor disability may attain basic milestones but the quality and efficiency of their movement patterns may never reach a level that can be considered within normal limits.

These types of tests contain domains such as mobility, self-care and social cognition and place an emphasis on:

- determining the child's level of functional competence in key daily activities in their everyday environments, usually school or home
- considering the effect of an assistant or equipment on progress
- measuring the child's independence rather than normality

It is the more relevant content validity that distinguishes functional tests from the more traditional developmental assessment approaches as only a limited amount of appropriate functional content is sampled in the traditional developmental tools (Haley *et al.* 1989, 1991). For example, for an 8-year-old child with cerebral palsy of the severe spastic quadriplegia type, the fact that the child is 'developmentally functioning' at a 9-month-old level is irrelevant. It is more important for this child to ascertain the potential to transfer independently from chair to toilet or to achieve independent mobility. An example of such a tool is The *Pediatric Evaluation of Disability Inventory* (PEDI) (Haley *et al.* 1992) designed to assess young children with physical disabilities with or without an associated cognitive disability. It has three functionally oriented domains of self-care, mobility and social function. It rates the child's capability and performance of functional tasks using:

- a Functional Skills Scale which rates functional skills for which the child has shown a level of mastery
- a Caregiver's Assistance Scale which measures the level of assistance the child requires from the caregiver to perform a functional activity
- a Modifications Scale which takes into account the environmental adaptive equipment used by the child to perform functional daily activities

Clinical uses of the PEDI include the ability to detect a functional deficit or delay, to evaluate an individual or group's progress over time, and as an outcome measure for programme evaluation.

Team Assessments

Other test instruments are designed for team use such as the *Carolina Curriculum for Preschoolers with Special Needs* by Johnson-Martin *et al.* (1990) and the *HELP for Special Preschoolers* (Santa Cruz County 1987) which can be used by teams operating at home, preschool or daycare settings and requires little training to administer. The *Functional Skills Screening Inventory* by Becker *et al.* (1986) includes a behavioural check-list for assessing children with moderate to severe disability, from 6-years-old through to adulthood, in domains based on life skills such as personal care, communication and community living. These tests are intended to be administered and interpreted by the team which includes parents and caregivers. Often teachers, psychologists, occupational therapists, physiotherapists and speech therapists have been involved in the development of an assessment. All or only some of the team may be involved in the actual administration of the assessment and assessment may occur in a variety of settings using a more ecological approach as described earlier.

So it can be seen that a test may be described in a number of ways. A type of continuum can be said to exist with some tests not absolutely at either end of the scale. The following grouping of movement tests is not meant to be definitive but merely illustrative of the types of descriptors used when discussing different assessments. The features of these assessments have been described already, under these descriptors.

In summary, the physiotherapist must be aware of the range of types of tests, their characteristics and the uses of each, to make informed and effective choices. Some more recent tests are listed in Table 1.

Types of Assessments Available

Norm-referenced
- Peabody Developmental Motor Scales and Activity Cards
- Movement ABC

Developmental
- Miller Assessment for Preschoolers
- Developmental Programming for Infants and Young Children
- Batelle Developmental Inventory
- Neuro-Sensory and Motor Development Assessment

Therapy-specific
- Gross Motor Function Measure
- Gross Motor Performance Measure (to be published)
- Motor Assessment of Infants

Criterion-referenced
- Gross Motor Function Measure (1993)
- Motor Assessment of Infants
- Developmental Programming for Infants and Young Children

Functional
- Pediatric Evaluation of Disability Inventory

Team
- Carolina Curriculum for Preschoolers
- HELP for Special Preschoolers
- Functional Screening Skills Inventory

Table 1
Some Recent Assessment Tools Used by Physiotherapists

Name	Purpose	Target population	Domains	Test descriptors
NSMDA Neuro-sensory and Motor Developmental Assessment (Burns 1992)	Physiotherapy. To evaluate neurosensory motor development for clinical/research purposes. Useful for predicting motor development outcome. Assessor: physiotherapist	Children at the ages: 1, 4, 8, 12, 18 months and 2, 3, 4 and 6 years	Gross and fine motor, neurological, primitive reflexes, postural reactions and sensory motor areas. Uses scales for 1–4 for item scores and 1–5 for functional grades of the domains	Standardized criterion-referenced. Testing time: varies according to age/cooperation
Movement ABC Revised TOMI by FA Moyes and SE Henderson (Henderson and Sugden 1992)	To identify and evaluate the movement problems that can determine a pupil's participation and social adjustment at school and to plan programmes for remediation and management. Assessors: teachers or health professionals	To address level of child's motor competence in the age range of 4–12 years for children with mild to moderate disabilities	Manual dexterity, ball skills, static and dynamic balance. Check-list considers child task performance within environment	Standardized norm-referenced test and check-list (2 components). Testing time: 20–30 mins (individual)
Gross Motor Performance Measure (Boyce et al. 1993; companion to GMFM below	To measure clinically important change in motor performance, or quality of movement of children with cerebral palsy	Cerebral palsy	Five performance attributes: weight shift, alignment, coordination, dissociated movement, stability using 20 gross motor function measure items	
Gross Motor Function Measure 2nd edn. (Russell et al. 1993)	To measure gross motor function over time in clinical and research settings. Can retest a dimension and score performance with use of aids or orthoses	Cerebral palsy. Validity and reliability study specific to those with head injury is required. Feedback from therapists indicates generally suitable for this population	88 test items: lying and rolling, sitting, crawling and kneeling, standing, walking, running and jumping	Standardized criterion-referenced observational. Testing time: 45–60 mins (individual)

PEDI Pediatric Evaluation of Disability Inventory [Haley et al. 1992]	Validation studies underway. Uses include: ● detect functional deficit ● evaluative measurement of individual group progress in programmes ● outcome measure for programme evaluation of pediatric rehabilitation or education programmes For use by physiotherapist, occupational therapist, nurse, speech language pathologist, educator, psychologist and other professionals	Children with physical disabilities with or without cognitive disabilities. Normative data available between 6 months and 7.5 years. Scaled data available for children of all ages. Not intended as a developmental assessment for babies and older children with minimal disabilities	Measures capability and performance of functional activities of 3 domains: ● self-care ● mobility, including basic transfer skills, indoor and outdoor locomotion, stairs and parameters of speed, distance and safety ● social function	Functional, ecological criterion-referenced but normative standard scores available based on sample of children without disability Testing time: 30 mins. Parent interview: 45–60 mins.
Infanib [Ellison 1994]	Quick and simple screen for infants at risk of neuromotor dysfunction.	Birth to 12 months.	Twenty items grouped into five subclasses: primitive reflexes, righting reactions, postural and vestibular responses, proximal and distal tone.	Screening tool Testing time: 15 mins.
TIME The Toddler and Infant Motor Evaluation [Miller and Roid, 1994]	Diagnostic assessment to evaluate motor abilities of young children	Birth to 3.5 years	Quality of movement and its relationship to function is evaluated. Subtests include: mobility, stability, motor organization, social/emotional abilities and functional performance	Standardized, developmental and diagnostic. Can be used as a screen. Observational with parent elicited responses. Diagrammatic record forms.

Thought Provokers

- A 2-year-old with development delay was not responding to attempts to encourage walking. Assessment by a physiotherapist revealed leg length difference, limitation of hip abduction, persistent posturing of the hip into flexion and reluctance to weight bear. The child was referred for orthopaedic assessment and dislocation of the hip was confirmed. This child had been assessed previously by several health professionals but because her physical features indicated she had a well-known syndrome which was confirmed by chromosomal screening she had never been undressed and fully assessed. What are the indications of hip dislocation?

- Foot orthotics were prescribed for a 3-year-old child who presented with marked pronation of the feet. After a short time, the parents noted the child was falling more frequently and a deterioration in gait had occurred so they requested a second opinion. Assessment revealed muscle weakness, particularly of his extensors and abductors and asymmetrical limitation of movement in the lower trunk. A rare syndrome was later diagnosed. What explanation can you give for the adverse effect of the orthotics?

- An infant of 4 months presented with persisting extension of the trunk and increased muscle tone was thought to be the cause. When positioning and handling to inhibit overuse of trunk extensors failed to help, a more experienced physiotherapist was asked for advice. Assessment revealed extreme weakness of neck and trunk flexor muscles (perhaps due to prolonged abnormal positioning in utero). A programme to stimulate and facilitate trunk and neck flexor muscles to encourage normal developmental activities led to a positive outcome. Think of other situations where different causes can lead to similar presentation.

- Children with Down's syndrome have joint laxity and a few children have malformation of atlanto – occipital or atlanto – axial joints which can result in subluxation. Consider the implications of omitting to check if the child has had this aspect investigated and how it could affect programme planning, particularly as the child started to participate in rigorous activities.

REFERENCES

Bailey, DM (1991) *Research for the Health Professional: A Practical Guide*, 226 pp. Philadelphia: FA Davis.

Bayley, N (1969) *Bayley Scales of Infant Development*. New York: The Psychological Corporation.

Becker, H, Schur, S, Paoletti-Schelp, M et al. (1986) *Functional Skills Screening Inventory (FSSI): An Instrument to Assess Critical Living Skills*. Austin, Texas: Functional Resources Enterprises Inc.

Blanksby, D (1992) *VAP CAP – The VAP CAP Handbook* (Visual assessment and programming and capacity attention and processing). Royal Victorian Institute for the Blind Education Centre, Australia.

Blossom, B, Ford, F (1991) *Physical Therapy in Public Schools – A Related Service*, Vol. 1. Rothwell, GA: Rehabilitation Publications and Therapies Inc.

Boyce, W, Gowland, C, Russell, D et al. (1993) Consensus methodology in the development and content validation of a gross motor performance measure. *Physiotherapy Canada* **45**: 94–100.

Burns, YR (1992) *N.S.M.D.A. Physiotherapy Assessment for Infants and Young Children*, 48 pp. Brisbane: CopyRight Publishing.

Burns, YR, O'Callaghan, M, Tudehope, DI (1989) Early identification of cerebral palsy in high risk infants. *Australian Paediatric Journal* **25**: 215–219.

Carlson, CI, Scott, M, Eklund, SJ (1980) Ecological theory and method for behavioural assessment. *School Psychology Review* **9**: 75–82.

Chandler, LS, Andrews, MS, Swanson, MW (1980) *Movement Assessment of Infants: A Manual*. Rolling Bay: Chandler, Andrews and Swanson.

Cusick, B (1990) *Progressive Casting and Splinting for Lower Extremity Deformities in Children with Neuromotor Dysfunction*, 401 pp. Tucson: Therapy Skill Builders.

Department of Education, Queensland, Australia (1994) Therapy assessment in an educational setting. In: *Assessment Resource Folder for Physiotherapists*, Brisbane Australia, Low Incidence Support Centre, Therapy Services, Department of Education Queensland.

Derstine, S (1989) Tests of infant and child development. In: Tecklin JS (ed). *Pediatric Physical Therapy*, pp. 16–39. Philadelphia: JB Lippincott.

Ellison, P (1994) *The Infanib*. Tucson: Therapy Skill Builders.

Folio, MR, Fewell, RR (1983) *Peabody Developmental Motor Scales and Activity Cards*. Allen, Texas: DLM Teaching Resources.

Fraser, BA, Hensiger, RN, Phelps, JA (1990) *Physical Management of Multiple Handicaps: A Professional's Guide*, pp. 41. London: Paul H Brookes.

Griffiths, R (1970) *The Abilities of Young Children*. London: Child Development Research Centre.

Haley, SM, Hallenborg, SC, Gans, BM (1989) Functional assessment in young children with neurological impairments. *Topics in Early Childhood Special Education* **9**: 106–127.

Haley, SM, Coster, WJ, Faas, RM (1991) A content validity study of the pediatric evaluation of disability inventory. *Pediatric Physical Therapy* **3**: 177–184.

Haley, SM, Coster, WJ, Ludlow, LH et al. (PEDI Research Group) (1992) *Pediatric Evaluation of Disability Inventory*. Boston: New England Medical Centre Hospital.

Henderson, SE, Sugden, DA (eds) (1992) *Movement Assessment Battery for Children*, 240 pp. UK: The Psychological Corporation.

Huber, CJ, King-Thomas, L (1987) The assessment process. In: King-Thomas, L, Hacker, BJ (eds) *A Therapist's Guide to Pediatric Assessment*, pp. 3–10. Boston: Little, Brown and Co.

Jacobs, K, Logigian, MK (1989) Learning disabilities. In: Logigian, MK, Ward, JD (eds) *A Team Approach for Therapists Pediatric Rehabilitation*, pp. 95–153. Boston, MA: Little, Brown and Co.

Johnson-Martin, NM, Attermeier, SM, Hacker, B (1990) *Carolina Curriculum for Preschoolers with Special Needs*, pp. 334. Baltimore: Paul H Brookes.

Kathrein, JE (1990) Interrater reliability in the assessment of muscle tone of infants and children. *Physical and Occupational Therapy in Paediatrics* 10: 27–41.

King-Thomas, L, Hacker, BJ (eds) (1987) *A Therapist's Guide to Pediatric Assessment*. Boston: Little, Brown and Co.

Macdonald, JA, Burns, YR, Mohay, HA (1990) Characteristics of neuro-sensori-motor performance of very low birthweight and high risk infants at six years of age. *New Zealand Journal of Physiotherapy* 19: 17–20 (corrected reprint).

Miller, LJ (1988) *Miller Assessment for Preschoolers Manual*, 1988 Revision, 160 pp. San Antonio: The Psychological Corporation/Harcourt Brace Jovanovich.

Miller, LJ, Roid, GL (1994) *The TIME Toddler and Infant Motor Evaluation*, 296 pp. Tucson: Therapy Skill Builders.

Milliken, RK, Buckley, JJ (1983) *Assessment of Multihandicapped and Developmentally Disabled Children*, pp. 45–62. Rockville, MD: Aspen Systems.

Montgomery, PC, Connolly, BH (1987) Norm-referenced and criterion-referenced test: use in pediatrics and application to task analysis of motor skill. *Physical Therapy* 67: 1873–1876.

Newborg, J, Stock, JR, Wnek L, Guidubaldi, J, Svinicki, J (1984) *Battelle Developmental Inventory.* Allen: DLM Teaching Resources.

Paul-Brown, D (1994) Clinical record keeping in audiology and speech-language pathology. *American Speech–Language–Hearing Association* May : 39–42.

Rogers, JC (1987) Selection of evaluation measurements. In: King-Thomas, L, Hacker, BJ (eds) *A Therapist's Guide to Pediatric Assessment*, pp. 19–33. Boston: Little, Brown and Co.

Russell, D, Rosenbaum, P, Gowland, C *et al.* (1993) Gross Motor Function Measure, pp. 112. McMaster University, Children's Developmental Rehabilitation Programme, Chedoke-McMaster Hospitals and Hugh MacMillan Rehabilitation Centre, Ontario, Canada.

Santa Cruz County Office of Education (1987) *HELP for Special Preschoolers Ages 3 to 6: Assessment Checklist and Activities Binder.* Palo Alto: Vort Corporation.

Schafer, DS, Moersch (eds) (1981) *Developmentl Programming for Infants and Young Children*, 5 vols. Ann Arbor: University of Michigan Press.

Stott, DH, Moyes, FA, Henderson, SE (1984) *Test of Motor Impairment: Henderson Revision.* Guelph, Ontario: Brook Educational.

Stowers, S, Huber, CJ (1987) Developmental and screening tests. In: King-Thomas L and Hacker BJ (eds) *A Therapist's Guide to Pediatric Assessment*, pp. 43–142. Boston, MA: Little, Brown and Co.

8

Evaluating Outcomes

PRUE GALLEY

Outcome Measurement
•
Single-subject Experimental Design

Each paediatric physiotherapist aims to provide appropriate and effective care. The desirable goal of physiotherapy intervention is that the end results or 'outcomes' are both useful and beneficial to the child and his or her family.

Patient 'outcome' is one of three categories used to define quality of care: structure, process and outcome (Donabedian 1988). 'Structure' covers those attributes which describe the material and human resources as well as the organizational structures of the settings in which physiotherapy occurs. 'Process' of physiotherapy care includes concepts such as the technical competence of the therapist and the quality of the therapist/child and parent/therapist relationships.

The concept of 'outcome' focuses on the physical, psychological and social well-being of the child and stands for the effects of physiotherapy care on the child's health. It also includes ideas such as improvements in knowledge and behaviour that impact on health; patient satisfaction with care (Cleary and McNeil 1988) and overall life satisfaction. The term

'health-related quality of life' has been suggested to represent this multidimensional concept (Jette 1993).

Knowledge about the links between process and outcome is unclear in many areas of rehabilitation (Lohr 1988). This problem is not unique to physiotherapy (Johnston and Granger 1994, Rogers and Holm 1994) but, like other health professionals, physiotherapists need to ask hard questions relating to the outcomes they actually obtain and the real costs involved in achieving them.

Very little has appeared in the physiotherapy literature focusing on these issues so far although there is some evidence of attempts by paediatric physiotherapists and others to address this, particularly in the area of cerebral palsy management. To date, results have been unclear and inconclusive which is partly due to the limitations in methodology used (Royeen and DeGangi 1992) and the lack of appropriate measures which reflect change in functional status (Boyce et al. 1991a). This situation presents an exciting challenge to all physiotherapists.

The concept of outcome is patient-centred as ultimately the true test of the effectiveness of physiotherapy intervention is whether the child can function in his or her natural environment as a result of such intervention. It focuses on the individual. This means that many variables need to be considered: hence making the study of outcomes very complex.

Kane (1994) has proposed a generic equation to summarize this complexity:

$$\text{Outcomes} = f \text{ (baseline, patient factors, environment, treatment)}$$

Outcomes are the results which reflect some change in health status over a period of time; therefore it is necessary when considering 'outcomes' to include 'baseline' measures. This allows for later comparisons to be made.

The issue of individual differences is also embedded in this equation as 'patient factors' and 'environment'. Clinical variables such as whether a child has cerebral palsy, spina bifida, juvenile rheumatoid arthritis or cystic fibrosis of a particular severity interact with demographic variables such as age, sex, socioeconomic status and educational support. The physical and psychosocial environment in which the child lives also impacts on outcome. These are factors over which the physiotherapist has little control.

'Treatment' is also a difficult issue to address, for although the physiotherapy treatment may be specific for a particular child, other professionals are also contributing to the treatment component. Isolating the unique contribution made by physiotherapy intervention when so many interventions and other life events, including maturation, have been occurring in parallel appears overwhelming, but it is a necessary task to undertake.

Central to achieving progress with this task is a commitment by paediatric physiotherapists to developing and validating outcome measures which can be used by clinicians, researchers, administrators and educators to show what physiotherapy really does. Relying on tests generated by other disciplines such as psychology and special education does not fully serve the child because the physiotherapy dimension is not fully expressed.

A key concept in the measurement of physiotherapy outcomes is the importance given to the involvement of the patient in their evaluation. Self-report measures feature in any complete consideration of outcome measurement (Jette 1993, Fuhrer 1994).

More needs to be done in developing and validating tests for particular paediatric groups and subgroups, particularly in relation to the evaluation of functional abilities (Mitchell 1992) and other health-related measures of quality of life (Jette 1993). Research and development of test instruments is very time-consuming which may explain in part why there are so few available, but there is evidence that physiotherapists and others are beginning to address this issue (Russell *et al.* 1989, 1994, Boyce *et al.* 1991b).

Outcome Measurement

Measurement is central to the concept of outcomes in order to demonstrate the effectiveness of what has been done in a statistically appropriate way. The difficulty is that at the present time many important factors cannot be readily measured except in crude terms. An example of this is the difficulty presented when trying to quantify relationships or 'quality of life'. The tendency to consider that only those things that are measurable using today's techniques are all that matters is to be avoided, but at the same time there is a pressing need for paediatric physiotherapists to attempt to improve the quality of their measurement tools. This activity needs to be done within the framework of adherence to those standards now specified for test developers and end users (Task Force on Standards for Measurement in Physical Therapy 1991).

In recent years, physiotherapists have shown increasing interest in measuring outcome. The next few years should see much more attention being paid to the use of standard outcome measures.

An outcome measure is defined as:

'a measurement tool (instrument, questionnaire, rating form, etc.) used to document change in one or more patient characteristics over time' (Cole *et al.* 1994). These changes can range from the area of physical functioning (such as in basic activities of daily living) to changes in the perception of the child and its family as to the child's overall sense of well-being.

The process of developing such measures is in its infancy in physiotherapy but all physiotherapists can become involved. Therein lies the challenge. Some of the tasks to be done by physiotherapists as a professional group include:

- identifying those patient characteristics that are influenced by physiotherapy; it is here that the single-subject experimental design with its patient-centred focus (Gonella 1989) could prove a useful first step
- developing valid and reliable instruments that are sensitive to changes in these characteristics over time (Johnston et al. 1991)
- adopting key physiotherapy outcome measures as 'gold-standards' and encouraging their universal use (Cole et al. 1994)
- providing feedback from users to those involved in developing instruments to enable refinements to be made

Choosing the appropriate outcome to measure will depend on the merits of each case. Ashburn et al. (1993) after reviewing research into the effectiveness of physiotherapy in the rehabilitation of stroke have emphasized the need for the aims of physiotherapy to be clear so appropriate outcome measures are selected. For example, there is an important difference between measuring performance of movement and performance of function as the more global scales of independence do not measure patterns of movement and how they change over time.

In paediatric physiotherapy improvement of the quality of movement is an important goal. The assumption is that this will lead to improved function but this is not always the case. Both types of measure may be necessary to obtain a more accurate picture of the effectiveness of physiotherapy intervention, although overloading the child with too much testing is to be avoided.

A key issue is that ideally only those instruments that are standardized are used. This means that information

as to the purpose, target group, instructions as to how and when the instrument is to be administered and scored, interpretation of scores and evidence of the instrument's validity and reliability are available to all users. Unfortunately, few instruments in physiotherapy reach this standard at present but it is important that physiotherapists are aware of these demands to enable them to be more discriminating when choosing instruments that are currently available and interpreting the physiotherapy literature on outcomes.

One advantage of using standardized outcome measures is that scores obtained may be pooled for use in epidemiological databases. Scores so obtained in different settings for groups of children with similar disabilities can be aggregated to obtain an overall more powerful measure of outcomes of physiotherapy that are more universal and not dependent on the treatment setting.

A causal link between process and outcome, however, cannot be unequivocally established by these means. Rather it requires the use of randomized controlled trials which tend to be expensive but by measuring outcome it is more likely that problems warranting the expense of such research can be more systematically identified. Unfortunately, large-scale outcome studies are also expensive.

Single-subject Experimental Design

One method that is becoming increasingly used by physiotherapists in their attempt to link the process of physiotherapy intervention to patient outcomes is the single-subject experimental design (Gonella 1989, Riddoch and Lennon 1994). This approach which focuses intensively on a small number of subjects is more manageable in terms of numbers and expense. Its attractiveness is that it has the potential to enable all clinicians to function productively as clinical scientists.

Although results cannot be generalized from a single-subject study, a physiotherapy intervention if replicated over a series of patients, strengthens the case for its potential generalizability (Evans 1994). A randomized controlled trial conducted as a follow-up to these strong preliminary investigations would be more likely to produce significant results which in turn could be used to enhance the physiotherapy knowledge base. The attractiveness of this systematic approach to monitoring what is done is that it enables clinicians to function as clinical scientists in their daily work (Mitchell 1992, Sim 1994) as they seek answers to the question 'Does this treatment (or treatments) work with this particular patient (or patients)?' (Evans 1994).

There are many single-case experimental designs that can be used but they are all characterized by the following:

(i) the sequential introduction and withdrawal or variation of the treatment intervention; and

(ii) the use of frequent and repeated outcome measures (Ottenbacher 1986).

A baseline is first established using repeated measures to provide a standard for later comparisons.

The most basic method is the AB design where A represents the 'no treatment' baseline phase and B, the treatment phase (see Figure 1).

This design can be extended to create, ABA, ABAB and other designs. The studies by Bower and McLellan (1992, 1994) into the effects of physiotherapy intervention for children with cerebral palsy illustrate the potential as well as some of the problems of this method in what is a most complex treatment area. Goal-setting in the precise terms necessary for use of a single experimental design approach can be a difficult exercise for physiotherapists who are used to setting more general treatment aims (Bower and McLellan 1994) but this is a challenge that clinicians will need to accept if they are to participate fully in evaluating treatment outcomes. It cannot be avoided.

It is also possible to use a BAB design in situations when a particular treatment is already in place. Repeated measures of the target behaviour are made during the treatment (B) phase and continued when the treatment is withdrawn (A) and then reintroduced (B).

Withdrawing treatment once it has been introduced may not be a realistic or ethical option for some patients so the use of multiple baseline designs is

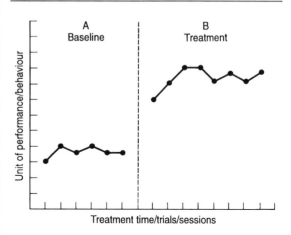

Figure 1   Graph illustrating the Basic AB Single-case Experimental Design

advocated (Evans 1994, Sim 1994). Here the treatment intervention is introduced at staggered times across separate baselines (Ottenbacher 1986). It is possible for the physiotherapist to examine: (i) one target outcome across multiple subjects (see Figure 2); (ii) multiple target outcomes in one subject; or (iii) one target outcome in one subject across multiple settings. Whatever design is chosen, measurements must be kept consistent across phases. The measures should achieve a level of stability before a new phase is introduced. Ideally 6 to 8 data points in each phase is considered the minimum (Kazdin 1982).

Systematic measurement and recording procedures are central to the application of single-subject experimental designs. The behaviour to be modified needs to be defined, for example, a specific motor response or a functional outcome. Decisions relating to the setting, data collection method and the time period for collecting data need to be made in advance. Data are systematically recorded and plotted initially in graph form and measurement is continued until the requirements of the chosen design are satisfied (Ottenbacher 1986).

The patterns created by plotting the repeated measures over time can be analysed visually to detect changes between phases in level, variability, trend and slope. Sometimes differences are obvious but in most situations this is not the case so more rigorous statistical analysis is required. Use of statistical procedures specially developed for single-subject experimental design studies is highly desirable if this

Figure 2 Graph Illustrating a Multiple Baseline Design. A target outcome across four children is shown; note the staggered introduction of the treatment/intervention phase as represented by the broken line

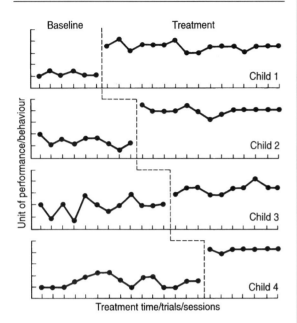

method is to be more widely accepted by the scientific community (Riddoch and Lennon 1991). Some statistical methods that have been used include: (i) the split-middle method of trend estimation ('celeration line' approach); (ii) two standard deviation band method; and (iii) the C statistic (Nourbakhsh and Ottenbacher 1994).

Relating outcomes to the process of physiotherapy presents a demanding task to all physiotherapists. Evaluating treatment outcomes is part of that work. Fortunately, there are now an increasing number of methods that can be used although much more research and development by physiotherapists is necessary to do this well. Therein lies the challenge.

REFERENCES

Ashburn, A, Partridge, C, De Souza, L (1993) Physiotherapy in the rehabilitation of stroke: a review. *Clinical Rehabilitation* 7: 337–345.

Bower, E, McLellan, E (1992) Effect of increased exposure to physiotherapy on skill acquisition of children with cerebral palsy. *Developmental Medicine and Child Neurology* 34: 25–39.

Bower, E, McLellan, E (1994) Measuring motor goals in children with cerebral palsy. *Clinical Rehabilitation* 8: 198–206.

Boyce, WF, Gowland, C, Rosenbaum, PL et al. (1991a) Measuring quality of movement in cerebral palsy: a review of instruments. *Physical Therapy* 71: 813–819.

Boyce, WF, Gowland, C, Hardy, S et al. (1991b) Development of a quality-of-movement measure for children with cerebral palsy. *Physical Therapy* 71: 820–832.

Cleary, PD, McNeil, BJ (1988) Patient satisfaction as an indicator of quality care. *Inquiry* 25: 25–36.

Cole, B, Finch, E, Gowland, C et al. (1994) *Physical Rehabilitation Outcome Measures*, 222 pp. Toronto: Canadian Physiotherapy Association.

Donabedian, A (1988) The quality of care. How can it be measured? *Journal of the American Medical Association* 260: 1743–1748.

Evans, J (1994) Physiotherapy as a clinical science: the role of single case research designs. *Physiotherapy Theory and Practice* 10: 65–68.

Fuhrer, MJ (1994) Subjective well being: implications for medical rehabilitation outcomes and models of disablement. *American Journal of Physical Medicine and Rehabilitation* 73: 358–364.

Gonella, C (1989) Single-subject experimental paradigm as a clinical decision tool. *Physical Therapy* 69: 601–609.

Jette, AM (1993) Using health-related quality of life measures in physical therapy outcomes research. *Physical Therapy* 73: 528–537.

Johnston, MV, Granger, CV (1994) Outcomes research in medical rehabilitation. *American Journal of Physical Medicine and Rehabilitation* 73: 296–303.

Johnston, MV, Findley, TW, DeLuca, J et al. (1991) Research in physical medicine and rehabilitation. XII. Measurement tools with application to brain injury. *American Journal of Physical Medicine and Rehabilitation* 70: 40–56.

Kane, RL (1994) Looking for physical therapy outcomes. *Physical Therapy* 74: 425–429.

Kazdin, AE (1982) *Single-case Research Designs*, 368 pp. New York: Oxford University Press.

Lohr, KN (1988) Outcome measurement: concepts and questions. *Inquiry* 25: 37–50.

Mitchell, RU (1992) The quality of evaluation in physical therapy. *Critical Reviews in Physical and Rehabilitation Medicine* 4: 61–77.

Nourbakhsh, M, Ottenbacher, KJ (1994) The statistical analysis of single subject data: a comparative examination. *Physical Therapy* 74: 768–776.

Ottenbacher, KJ (1986) *Evaluating Clinical Change*, 243 pp. Baltimore: Williams & Wilkins.

Riddoch, J, Lennon, S (1991) Evaluation of practice: the single case study approach. *Physiotherapy Theory and Practice* 7: 3–11.

Riddoch, J, Lennon, S (1994) Single subject experimental design: one way forward? *Physiotherapy* 80: 215–218.

Rogers, JC, Holm, MB (1994) Accepting the challenge of outcome research: examining the effectiveness of occupational therapy practice. *American Journal of Occupational Therapy* 48: 871–876.

Royeen, CB, DeGangi, GA (1992) Use of neurodevelopmental treatment as an intervention: annotated listing of studies 1980–1990. *Perceptual and Motor Skills* 75: 175–194.

Russell, DJ, Rosenbaum, PL, Cadman, DT et al. (1989) The Gross Motor Function Measure: a means to evaluate the effects of physical therapy. *Developmental Medicine and Child Neurology* 31: 341–352.

Russell, DJ, Rosenbaum, PL, Lane, M et al. (1994) Training users in the Gross Motor Function Measure: methodological and practical issues. *Physical Therapy* 74: 630–636.

Sim, J (1994) The ethics of single-system (n+1) research. *Physiotherapy Theory and Practice* 10: 211–222.

Task Force on Standards for Measurement in Physical Therapy (1991) Standards for tests and measurements in physical therapy practice. *Physical Therapy* 71: 589–622.

Section D:

Preparing for Management

PROLOGUE: YVONNE BURNS AND JULIE MACDONALD

Prologue

YVONNE BURNS AND JULIE MACDONALD

Physiotherapists work in a wide variety of contexts and with a complex range of conditions affecting a broad age group from those born some weeks before their expected birth date through the preschool and school years into the teenage and possible post-school years. It is imperative therefore that the physiotherapist has some understanding of the special attributes and needs of various age groups, cultures, families and themselves, as well as the knowledge of the assessment and treatment principles of the presenting problems.

The opening chapter of Section D provides a broad overview of the principles of management addressing aspects of clinical reasoning, home programmes and various techniques often found within the repertoire of skills of a physiotherapist. The next chapter looks at a number of different contexts in which a physiotherapist may be working with preschool and school-aged children and draws particular attention to the importance of communication and interaction between various services, professional colleagues, the child and the family.

Equipment, aids and orthotics frequently form an important or an essential role in the management or treatment of a range of conditions. It is pertinent therefore that, while addressing different management approaches and service delivery contexts, the following chapter presents an overview of a range of apparatus, discussing prescription and use. Considerable practical detail is included.

Evaluation of any form of intervention is essential. Computerized gait analysis and its use in the evaluation of gait with and without orthotics (as described in Chapter 12) can assist in clinical decision-making and provide objective measurement of outcomes of intervention.

9

Principles of Physiotherapy Management

YVONNE BURNS

Clinical Reasoning and Problem-Solving
•
Basic Principles of Management
•
Home Programmes
•
Physiotherapy Intervention

Physiotherapists working in paediatrics meet infants, children and adolescents with a wide range and degree of impairment, disability, illness, dysfunction and problems of movement. Underlying any condition of childhood even of relatively short duration are the ongoing changes of growth, maturation and development. Nelson *et al.* (1969) point out that any examination of a child or programme of management which does not assess developmental status and evaluate how the illness or treatment may affect growth or development, is incomplete.

Children are neither miniature adults nor lesser beings but unique individuals with their own set of inherited biological and personality characteristics which are constantly impinged upon and shaped by a variety of environmental factors including parental, cultural and societal attitudes (Ausabel and Sullivan 1970). Assessment and treatment must recognize that the significance of age-related physiological, anatomical, developmental and emotional aspects of the individual are as important as knowledge of the condition, its presenting signs, symptoms and likely outcome.

Some conditions adversely affect a number of body systems or aspects of growth and development while in other conditions the primary pathology may be confined to one system but the secondary effects could be more widespread. The emotional implications of illness and disability on the child and family must not be downgraded or overlooked. The practise of encouraging parents to stay with their child while in hospital and of discharging them home as soon as feasible, reflects awareness of the emotional stress that separation or hospitalization can cause a child.

Any assessment and treatment plan of an infant or child for any condition should consider all aspects of growth and development, including those specific to the condition. For example, after surgery, the need for a child to be nursed for prolonged periods in a particular posture or position may result in a delay in some aspects of development and must be addressed as part of the rehabilitation.

The physiotherapist in paediatrics is frequently a first-contact practitioner and sometimes, for example in schools, may be the only health professional within the team. The responsibility for well-substantiated advice and programme planning in these situations can be even greater than when the referral has come from within the health care system. Clinical reasoning and problem-solving are important physiotherapy skills.

Clinical Reasoning and Problem-Solving

According to Terry and Higgs (1993) 'clinical reasoning can be broadly interpreted as the thinking and decision-making processes associated with clinical practice' (p. 47). It has been described as a hypothetico-deductive reasoning process which involves the development of a clinical hypothesis from data collected and then the testing of this hypothesis as the basis for diagnostic and treatment decisions (Dennis and May 1987). Grant and Marsden (1987), however, place emphasis on the clinician's knowledge base. Dennis and May (1987) found that, although physiotherapy clinicians prefer a systematic style of decision-making, in practise they tend to blend the gathering of data and decision-making in a spiral process with each piece of new information being related to previous knowledge and past experiences to modify or refine the initial decisions. Although the complex relationship between knowledge and reasoning is not yet fully understood, it is apparent that a sound, well-organized knowledge base greatly enhances effective clinical reasoning. A number of personal factors such as individual preferences and values, style of thinking and critical reflection, motivation as well as extrinsic factors such as learning, prior experience, current clinical trends and observation of colleagues can have considerable impact on clinical reasoning and decision-making.

Owing to the individual set of attributes, problems and needs of each child, the physiotherapist must use knowledge, experience and clinical reasoning to determine the problems and priorities needing attention in designing a suitable treatment programme. Previous experience can bring considerable advantage to the situation (watch an experienced clinician at work and note how they quickly integrate an array of information and come to a clinical decision with ease and efficiency). On the other hand, over-reliance on experience can be a disadvantage if there is a tendency to draw conclusions without substantive evidence to back the decision. There is never room for complacency — the best therapists are always learning.

The beginning practitioner may find it useful to consider what is known about the child and the presenting condition, the perceptions and assumptions gained about the situation, what knowledge and experience the physiotherapist can contribute and to recognize what is not known at the time.

WHAT IS USUALLY KNOWN

- Information regarding the child and possibly family history
- reason for referral (parent, doctor or teacher concerns) and possibly a diagnosis
- any previous investigations and results
- results of the current assessment

WHAT IS PERCEIVED

- potential problems
- the attitude of child and family
- the impact and influence of past experience on the child/family

WHAT IS NOT USUALLY KNOWN

- the effect of the condition on ongoing growth and development
- the potential abilities of the individual child
- the compounding and interactive effects of the original illness/impairment and ongoing changes

WHAT THE PHYSIOTHERAPIST BRINGS TO THE SITUATION

- knowledge of motor development and general development of infants/children
- knowledge of the clinical presentation of a number of conditions likely to be pertinent to the child in question
- skills in physiotherapy assessment and treatment
- an ability to interpret clinical assessment findings

and a knowledge of contraindications and precautions

- personal attributes and abilities particularly relevant to the approach to and management of children

Basic Principles of Management

Whatever the presenting condition, age, race or background of the child the following basic principles apply (see also Figure 1).

- respect the infant/child as an individual as well as showing respect for the family
- establish appropriate communication with child and parents/carers
- gain pertinent information and history about the child and relevant family background
- ensure confidentiality of all information and no transmission without parent and/or child permission
- demonstrate readiness to seek all available knowledge about the condition and results of other tests/assessments
- undertake a thorough physiotherapy assessment (structured observation and specific tests) relevant to the condition, identifying

those factors that are normal as well as problems and aspects of concern

- interpret findings in the light of total assessment(s) and other knowledge about the child
- screen for developmental problems, particularly those relevant to posture and movement
- ascertain the situation in which treatment is likely to occur; if the condition is likely to involve the family in long-term management then determine the home situation, parental abilities and those of back-up personal and physical resources
- establish with parents/carers and other professionals involved a plan of management, the aims and type of treatment(s) to be implemented by whom, when, where and how and the expected results
- determine the time of review/reassessment and outline a likely future plan of management

Management of Infant and Young Child

Parents play the crucial role in the care and treatment of most infants and young children. The exception is in the case of some acute illnesses where highly

Figure 1   Basic Principles of Management

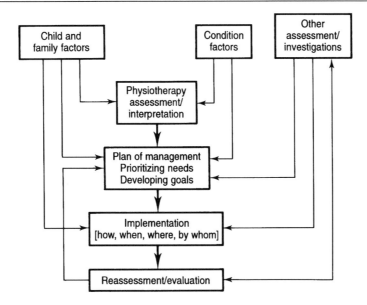

specialized care is required. To ensure they can undertake this role to the best of their ability, parents require a clear understanding of the features and problems associated with the condition, the aims of the care procedures and treatment techniques as relevant to their child and the expected response to each aspect of treatment. When appropriate, this should be provided in writing. Parental involvement sometimes occurs in hospital where they complement the care provided by the hospital team, but in most conditions the parents must continue all or some of the treatment at home. This is usually referred to as a 'home programme'.

Home Programmes

Home programmes must be tailored to the individual needs of the child as well as his or her family. This may present a challenge due to the life style or type of dwelling of the particular family. In multicultural countries such as Australia it is of importance also to recognize and respect different cultural and racial child-raising practices. As pointed out by Scherzer and Tscharnuter (1982) while an infant's behaviour is affected by the family, the family's responses are affected by those of the infant. An infant who is unresponsive or irritable due to a brain lesion is likely to initiate in the family less responsiveness, interaction and even handling than a normally responsive infant thus diminishing the quality and quantity of important social, emotional and physical interaction. The role of the family and parents in the care and rearing of their child must not be usurped but rather developed and supported. Parents often need to become an advocate for their child but to do this they need confidence in their own abilities. It is important therefore to recognize when parents need confirmation of their abilities.

Physiotherapists involved in planning, teaching and reviewing home programmes must have an understanding of the needs of parents as well as those of the infant/child (as explained in the opening section of this book). Parents have many roles to play as parent to other children, partner to each other, son/daughter to own parents, and as neighbour and

workmate within a community and cultural group. Communication at all levels is of primary importance. Mutual respect and trust enable parents, child and physiotherapist to work together in harmonious partnership. Avoid anxiety or animosity which can be easily conveyed to the infant or child.

Normally home programmes start on an informal level when the children are very young, but as they reach kindergarten and preschool age programmes in these group settings tend to become more structured and formal. At school age, children may attend the regular school with their peers. In some countries attendance may be determined by their physical and or intellectual capabilities while in others all children are eligible to attend government schools.

When devising a home programme, remember all the activities in the life of the infant or child: bathing, dressing, nappy change or toilet, eating, being lifted, nursed and carried, playing, interacting and communicating with others and sleeping. Life involves visits to friends, shopping, holidays and some times of hardship, grief and anxiety. All need to be considered.

The first step in helping parents to understand their child's needs is to include them in the assessment explaining the reason for each test and whether the outcome is normal or outside the expected range for age. They are then in a better position to discuss their own areas of concern and indicate their priorities for intervention. It is important to set the aims of each technique/activity in the home programme and to ensure that the parents/carers understand these aims and the expected responses or outcomes. They are then in a better position to initiate their own ideas. It is best to agree upon a small number of clear aims (about three), especially in the early stages. There may be several ideas or options involved in achieving each aim.

Record the programme with or for the parents in a way that they can understand. Never assume a parent can read or read your writing. A home programme book is a good idea with use of diagrams and stick figures or even photographs to show what you mean. Video is increasingly used, particularly if the family cannot visit the therapist regularly.

Throughout the following chapters a number of

different treatment approaches and techniques will be described either specifically or as part of a case story. These case scenarios are fictitious, but typical of clinical presentations experienced in paediatric physiotherapy practices. Physiotherapists have a broad range of skills and specific techniques from which to select the most appropriate for a particular child. It is often difficult for the beginning practitioner to bear in mind a whole spectrum of possible interventions and to take on board new techniques or approaches. It is important to ascertain what these new approaches have to offer, how they compare with those already in use, and how they can be evaluated. Using the example of approaches to treatment of neurological and developmental conditions, a way of categorizing commonly used interventions into major groupings is presented next in an attempt to aid the selection of the most appropriate interventions.

Physiotherapy Intervention

Physiotherapy interventions can be considered to fall into a number of different categories, from those that involve little participation or action from the child and are therefore therapist- or adult-dependent through to those that rely on self (child) initiative and problem-solving. These approaches must not be considered in isolation as many are complementary and a number can be integrated concurrently into a treatment programme. As a child develops and matures there can be a trend to move from less reactive approaches to more of those that involve the child to a greater degree in the control of their own movement and decision-making. The importance of having clear aims and expectations of any intervention cannot be overstressed. Here we consider some of the techniques, from least to most child involvement.

TECHNIQUES THAT DO NOT ELICIT A SPECIFIC RESPONSE

These include use of **equipment** designed to support not facilitate and to lift, to carry or for transport.

SPECIFIC INPUT TO ELICIT OR FACILITATE AN AUTOMATIC RESPONSE

Specific sensory input may be given to elicit a desirable response or prior to other techniques. Sensory input may be useful in activating an improved muscular response (Rood 1962) or making the child more aware of the part to be moved. General or specific tactile, proprioceptive, vibratory or vestibular stimulation may be useful in some settings while in others the use of vision or hearing may be helpful in providing input specific to the improvement of balance, coordination, rhythm and perceptual motor development. Use of these techniques will be elaborated in chapters discussing severe and multiple disability and motor coordination difficulties.

The use of specific **handling techniques** will facilitate postural, equilibrium and other automatic reactions while at the same time inhibiting less-desirable primitive and tonic reflex patterns of movement. This technique, often called neurodevelopmental facilitation, was developed by Bobath and Bobath (1964). It aims to provide a more normal sensorimotor background of postural tone and movement and is useful in the treatment of developmentally delayed infants and in infants and children with normal or increased muscle tone associated with cerebral palsy. It is also a useful early-stage technique following traumatic brain damage. It is well-described by Scherzer and Tscharnuter (ch. 8, 1982). Handling, facilitation and positioning by parents and carers during day-to-day activities is an important element of this approach (Finnie 1974). One should recognize the limitation of facilitation in most infants and children with very low muscle tone.

Positioning during other activities can be helpful in eliciting more sustained or dynamic desirable postures. Dynamic equipment used for standing or seating (Pope et al. 1994). In the child with low tone, ensure that dynamic postures are used and that the time spent in positions that may cause overstretching around joints is minimized.

DIRECTED TASKS

Encouragement to perform desirable activities through the use of **goal-directed play** is an extremely useful strategy when dealing with children who have generalized motor developmental delay. Play is the natural learning experience of childhood and should be fully utilized in any intervention strategy.

Task activities are also useful in developing movement strategies, an ability to motor plan and a sense of achievement which will in turn often motivate the child to try again or venture into new territory. The Conductive Education approach uses task series aimed specifically at teaching the children to gain basic control over their movement for the achievement of function (Hari and Tillemans 1984).

It is often necessary to include specific **exercises** designed to strengthen, lengthen or develop a desired movement pattern. Compliance, however, can be a problem at any age and motivators may be necessary to achieve the desired number of repetitions.

MOTOR LEARNING

It is fascinating to watch how a developmentally normal child learns by doing and how many times they repeat an activity. The ways children learn have been studied for many years by psychologists. Baddeley (1984) draws attention to what physiotherapists can learn from these studies and how it may affect programme planning. The contributions of what is inborn and therefore due to maturation and what is subsequently learned are not yet clear but it is known that the two are interwoven in the pattern of ongoing development of structure and function.

Learning involves repetition which may be gained through play, daily routines, group activities such as action songs (visual / verbal instruction), movement to music or repeating prescribed movements or exercises. In the last, compliance may be poor unless there is a specific child-selected / accepted goal or encouragement through peer group participation.

Conditioning involves rewarding a desirable response. As mentioned later in Chapter 23, it is desirable to identify the most appropriate reward system. This often involves a process of controlling the environment to provide selected feedback. Baddeley (1984) describes 'open-loop' control as 'those sequences of movements, or motor programmes which can be selected from a store of programmes held in motor memory and used in response to some environmental demand' (p. 37).

Visual or auditory input in the form of **biofeedback** may be used through the strategic placement of 'switches' or pressure-sensitive devices to reward desired responses or remove reward when undesirable response is made by the child.

Relationship play involves the child interacting with a paired adult, another child or a small group of children. It aims to build up self-awareness and self-confidence through 'doing' with another, various activities which usually involve a considerable amount of body contact, through for example, touching or supporting, while at the same time developing improved coordination, sequencing and rhythm of movement. This type of programme developed by Sherbourne (1990) is suitable for a group of ambulatory children with intellectual impairment.

Skill acquisition involves learning and practice. For effective and efficient functioning, skills should not be learnt in isolation (splinter skills) but should form part of an integrated whole in the context of day-to-day living. Unfortunately, sometimes children have difficulty transferring skills learnt in a formal 'therapy' situation to the 'real' world.

PROBLEM-SOLVING

It is preferable for children with a movement disability to gain an ability to plan and execute solutions to their own movement problems. Motivation to try, confidence in themselves as individuals, an understanding of their own abilities and difficulties and a repertoire of basic plans of action are all desirable attributes. Comprehension of language forms an important basis for problem-orientated approaches of management but children with limitations in this area can also achieve a useful level of independent problem-solving ability through the provision of opportunities to take responsibility for achieving a goal.

CHALLENGE TO SUCCEED

There is nothing like a challenge to motivate a mentally active child or adult into action. Successful achievement has a very positive effect on self-esteem and confidence. Most challenges mean some degree of initial failure, but once the goal is in sight the drive to achieve becomes even greater. On the other hand, repeated failure and repetitive negative feedback will discourage, leading to loss of confidence and self-esteem. One of the most important skills of intervention is the ability to set goals that are achievable and meaningful but that will also challenge, and to give feedback that encourages but is realistic. It is important to allow a degree of failure as well as success. The ability to enable a young infant or child with severe or multiple sensory and physical impairments to achieve, with minimal assistance, a self-initiated goal is probably one of the most important skills of the physiotherapist.

INDEPENDENCE

Independence in mobility, function, communication and decision-making are medium- to long-term goals for most young people with chronic disabilities. It is never too soon or the child too disabled to start providing opportunities for responsibility and independence.

Physiotherapists have a broad repertoire of skills and use a wide range of techniques in the treatment of children. The most important skills are the ability to communicate effectively with and without words, to develop a sense of trust and to respect each child and adult as an important individual person. Some techniques frequently used by physiotherapists are summarized in the list below and discussed in later chapters. The list does not include all techniques, but will serve as a useful reference.

Techniques used by Physiotherapists

Positioning

- the infant for development of postural reactions
- the child for function
- to encourage best-possible response and inhibit the abnormal

Facilitation

- for infant handling
- in the presence of increased tone

- to increase strength and sequencing of reactions/movement patterns

Sensorimotor

- sensory input to elicit specific reflex response then integrate into function
- to stimulate a desired motor response, particularly in a child with severe neurological disorder
- to increase general sensory input

Exercises

- to increase muscle strength, control or patterns of movement
- to prevent or control dysfunction, weakness or deformity which are specific to the condition being treated

Postural stability

- specific exercises to facilitate or activities to control dynamic central (trunk) and proximal joint stability
- provide background control during phasic activity. This is especially important in the presence of low muscle tone, muscle weakness or postural instability

Ranging

- active or supported active movement to maintain or increase range of movement
- passive movement in the absence of active movement. Extreme care is necessary when passively ranging any immature joints. In the presence of hyperactive stretch reflex (spasticity) passive stretching is likely to aggravate the condition.

Plasters/Casting

- use of plaster-casting in weight-bearing is useful for gaining joint range (Ricks and Eilert 1993)
- allows/encourages more normal patterns of weight-bearing in children with cerebral palsy or after head injury (Sussman 1983, Watt et al. 1986)
- a special exercise programme is essential during and after plasters

Specialized techniques

- physiotherapists use a number of specialized techniques to gain a desired response (for example, respiratory techniques to clear airways)

Orthotics, splints

- physiotherapists make, use and prescribe a wide range of aids and equipment specific to the needs of the individual child and condition being treated

Electrotherapeutic techniques

- biofeedback has been found to be useful
- Functional Electrical Stimulation (FES) has been used with children (Carmick 1993a,b; Hazelwood et al. 1994)

Care should be taken with any electrotherapeutic agents, as children are not reliable reporters of what they feel. Ultrasound should be avoided near to or over joints and growth plates.

Hydrotherapy

- provides a useful medium for exercise, gaining strength and movement control, balance and confidence

Hippotherapy and Riding Therapy

- useful for improving balance and postural control

REFERENCES

Ausabel, DP, Sullivan, EV (1970) *Theory and Problems of Child Development*, pp. 849, 2nd edn. New York: Grune and Stratton.

Baddeley, H (1984) Motor Learning. In: Levitt, S (ed.) *Paediatric Developmental Therapy*, pp. 34–43. Oxford: Blackwell Scientific.

Bobath, B, Bobath, K (1964) The facilitation of normal postural reactions and movements in the treatment of cerebral palsy. *Physiotherapy* 54: 3–19.

Carmick, J (1993a) Clinical use of neuromuscular electrical stimulation for children with cerebral palsy, Part 1: Lower extremity. *Physical Therapy* 73 (8): 505–513.

Carmick, J (1993b) Clinical use of neuromuscular electrical stimulation for children with cerebral palsy, Part 2: Upper extremity. *Physical Therapy* 73 (8): 514–525.

Dennis, JK, May, GM (1987) Practice in the year 2000: expert decision making in physical therapy. *Proceedings of the 10th International Congress of the World Confederation of Physical Therapists*, Sydney, pp. 543–551.

Finnie, N (1974) *Handling the Young Cerebral Palsy Child at Home*, 306 pp. London: Heinemann.

Grant, J, Marsden, P (1987) The structure of memorized knowledge in students and clinicians: an explanation for diagnostic expertise. *Medical Education* 21: 92–98.

Hari, M, Tillemans, T (1984) Conductive Education. In: Scrutton, D (ed.) *Management of the Motor Disorders of Children with Cerebral Palsy*, pp. 19–32. London: Heinemann.

Hazelwood, ME, Brown, JK, Rowe, PJ et al. (1994) The use of therapeutic electrical stimulation in the treatment of hemiplegic cerebral palsy. *Developmental Medicine and Child Neurology* 36: 661–673.

Nelson, WE, Vaughan, VC, McKay, RJ (eds) (1969) Prologue to developmental pediatrics, *Textbook of Pediatrics*, 1589 pp, 9th edn. Philadelphia: Saunders.

Pope, PM, Bowes, CE, Booth, E (1994) Postural control in sitting. The SAM system: evaluation of use over three years. *Developmental Medicine and Child Neurology* 36: 241–252.

Ricks, NR, Eilert, RE (1993) Effects of inhibitory casts and orthoses on bony alignment of foot and ankle during weight bearing in children with spasticity. *Developmental Medicine and Child Neurology* 35: 11–16.

Rood, MS (1962) The use of sensory receptors to activate, facilitate and inhibit motor response, autonomic and somatic developmental sequence. In: Sattely, C (ed.) *Approaches to Treatment of Patients with Neuromuscular Dysfunction*. Third International Congress — World Federation of Occupational Therapists, Iowa, pp. 26–37.

Scherzer, AL, Tscharnuter, I (1982) *Early Diagnosis and Therapy in Cerebral Palsy*, 289 pp. New York: Dekker.

Sherbourne, V (1990) *Developmental Movement for Children*, 121 pp. Cambridge: Cambridge University Press.

Sussman, MD (1983) Casting as an adjunct to neurodevelopmental therapy for cerebral palsy. *Developmental Medicine and Child Neurology* 25: 804–805.

Terry, W, Higgs, J (1993) Educational programmes to develop clinical reasoning skills. *Australian Journal of Physiotherapy* 39: 47–51.

Watt J, Sims D, Harkham, F et al. (1986) A prospective study of inhibitive casting as an adjunct to physiotherapy for cerebral palsied children. *Developmental Medicine and Child Neurology* 28: 480–488.

10

Physiotherapy Services for Preschool and School-aged Children

AMANDA CROKER AND MEGAN KENTISH

The Disability Movement – A Brief History
•
The Transition from Infancy
•
Early Intervention
•
Parents Views and the Family
•
Critical Periods for Physiotherapy Intervention
•
Models of Service Delivery
•
Team Approaches
•
The Provision of Physiotherapy Services

As children reach preschool and school age they experience an increasing number of environments and contexts. This can pose challenges as well as expanding opportunities for the development of skills, and achievement of functional goals. Physiotherapy intervention must take into account these changing environments and contexts.

Physiotherapy services for children may be available through health systems (hospital or community based), government departments providing disability services, educational agencies, non-government specialized agencies and private practitioners. The way in which these services are made available and delivered to children is influenced by the political, cultural, economic and legislative forces existing in the particular location. In countries struggling to provide basic health and education services, the prevalence of children with disabilities is higher than it would otherwise be, and infrastructure may be poorly developed.

Elkins (1993) suggests that lower prevalence of disability, and well-developed services for children with disabilities are indicators of the economic well-being of a society.

In this chapter the principles of physiotherapy management for preschoolers and school-aged children are discussed taking into account their health and educational needs. It is important for the physiotherapist to have some awareness and understanding of the changes that have occurred (and will continue to occur) in the delivery of services to people with disabilities over the recent decades. A brief history of the disability movement is given. The influence of the setting and the coordination of physiotherapy services across settings and agencies is also explored. Early intervention provision is discussed with particular emphasis on family issues. Finally, the requirements for physiotherapy intervention during the school years are also addressed.

The Disability Movement – A Brief History

Historically, societies have tended to organize services to children with more significant disabilities through institutions and often with funding from non-government agencies. Children were sometimes separated from their families and lived in residential settings. Throughout the 1970s, the Disability Rights Movements gained strength, especially in the USA and pressure came to bear on governments to enact legislation and provide services that would facilitate more equitable participation in community life for people with disabilities.

The philosophy of normalization originated in Scandinavia, but was developed further by Wolfensberger (1972) in the USA. He described normalization as the provision of as normal or typical a situation for persons with disabilities as can be achieved, using methods that are also normative in a particular society. Deinstitutionalization of people with disabilities, and 'mainstreaming' of children with disabilities from segregated to regular schools have been features of this process.

During the 1970s the federal government of the USA passed legislation (Education for all Handicapped Children Act of 1975) which has had a significant effect on the development of services to children with disabilities both in that country and subsequently in other countries such as Australia. In the USA, Acts mandated that educationally related services such as physical therapy be provided by education authorities. Further legislation in 1986 (Education of the Handicapped Act Amendments) extended the mandate to include early intervention services.

Some of the principles underpinning this legislation included:

- Individualized Education Plans (IEP) which required annual written goal statements, outcome measures, and the services necessary for implementation to be documented
- least-restrictive environment which required docu-

mented services to be delivered as close as possible to the regular classroom
- Due Process which gave parents the right to challenge decisions of education systems
- parental participation would be assured in all the processes

Other countries have not legislated so specifically regarding services to children with disabilities. In Australia, for example, a Disability Services Act was passed in 1986 and a Disability Discrimination Act in 1992, but there has been no specific Act mandating what services children require in order to benefit from their education. The education acts in the various states of Australia have been amended during the 1980s, to extend the right to a free public education to all children (including those who had previously been considered ineducable).

At the international level the United Nations (UN) developed Standard Rules on the *Equalization of Opportunities for Persons with Disabilities* which were adopted by the General Assembly in late 1993. The International Year of Disabled Persons (1981) and the subsequent World Program of Action concerning Disabled Persons had provided a strong impetus for progress towards these internationally agreed to UN Standard Rules. The spirit and intent of all the disability legislation when applied to the provision of special education for children with disabilities, should mean that they can be enrolled at their local community school and receive an appropriate educational programme which is adequately resourced, if this is deemed by all concerned to be the least restrictive environment.

For children with physical or multiple disabilities the provision of physiotherapy services is often a vital factor in their successful access to, and participation in, an educational programme. The integration of these children into their local school instead of being clustered in a segregated setting requires increased resourcing for physiotherapy services.

Policies and legislation can enforce the enrolment practices of schools, and redirect resources, but changes in attitude cannot be affected so directly. The child with multiple disabilities may attend a local school, but it is the positive attitudes of the school staff, the degree of teamwork, and the quality of the programmes that contribute significantly to the outcomes.

The Transition from Infancy

As children grow and develop from infancy to early childhood, there is a transition from a family-orientated environment to a broader, more challenging environment. This environment may include play group, child care, kindergarten, preschool, school and a variety of community settings. The growth and development of the child normally leads to increasing independence in these various settings and establishes links with the community.

Early intervention programmes and play groups are community settings commonly used for ongoing physiotherapy management. Generally, they provide services to children with a variety of needs but in some instances programmes have been established to cater for children with the same or similar conditions, for example, intellectual difficulties or neurological problems.

Physiotherapy services must adapt to meet the needs of children as they move from the home, to the preschool, hospital and community during their preschool years. The transition from one agency to another may potentially be difficult for parents and children. This transition may be from a home-based programme or specialized hospital-based service to a preschool educationally based programme with parents less involved in the actual intervention programme. Separating from a child and needing to acknowledge the child's new level of independence or lack of independence at a time when other children are achieving this poses its own challenges to the parents. Coordinated planning and preparation by all agencies involved is required.

Early Intervention

Early intervention in the first five years of life may be described as a systematic and planned effort to promote development through creating an appropriate environment and the opportunity for beneficial experiences. Focus, rationale, timing, duration, intensity and location are important dimensions of early intervention programmes. Furthermore, facilitating the child's development and supporting the family are the primary objectives.

Most early intervention programmes are designed to ensure that the developmental process, experiences and relationships closely approximate those compatible with the principles of normal child development. They should also foster the development of the child and strengthen family/child relationships (Guralnick and Bennett 1987). Strategies should be included to help parents recognize some of the unique aspects of their child. Preventative strategies to minimize the occurrence of secondary complications while providing a developmentally appropriate environment are important dimensions of early intervention.

The rationale of early intervention stresses the importance of early years for developing children and the role environment plays in that development. Research indicates that environmental events can substantially alter the course of development during early years (Guralnick and Bennett 1987).

Moore (1990) describes the aims of early intervention as follows:

- promotion of the social, emotional, intellectual and physical growth of young children with developmental problems to take maximum advantage of their potential for learning
- prevention of the development of secondary disabilities in young children with developmental problems
- support of the families of young developmentally disabled children so as to enable them to meet the needs of children as effectively as possible

Guralnick and Bennett (1987) suggest that the following three broad target populations can be identified as benefiting from early intervention:

1. infants and children at increased environmental risk (poverty, adolescent mothers)
2. infants and children at increased biological risk (prematurity, very low birth weight, birth trauma/asphyxia, syndromes)

3. infants and children with established developmental delays or disability

The services may be home- or centre-based or a combination of these, and may be provided by a range of agencies. Home-based services focus on assisting parents or caregivers to acquire effective intervention skills.

As a child reaches the preschool years, services are more likely to become centre-based where the child attends a particular setting on a regular basis. This setting may be in a classroom, hospital or community. The focus is usually more child-orientated but parental involvement remains vital.

Parents Views and the Family

For their services to be most effective, physiotherapists should:

- assist parents to see their child as a child first, not as a problem to be fixed by the experts
- collaborate with others, using the key person in the child's life, for example the parent, the child-care worker or teacher, and sharing knowledge and skills
- never assess for assessment's sake; make any assessment relevant to real life
- use the appropriate natural times and settings which encourage the postures, movements, skills and tasks that you are attempting to achieve with the child
(Queensland Parents of People with Disability, 1993)

The family plays a critical role in nurturing the young child and not only provides for the child's physical needs but also fosters the development of the child (Case-Smith 1991). Children with special needs are best served by meeting the needs of the family. Therefore, when considering management of the preschool and school-age child it is essential that the physiotherapist recognize not only the individual differences of the child but also the characteristics of the family and the close interlinking between them.

Physiotherapists have long recognized the need to consider each person as unique and to assess and treat accordingly, taking into account factors such as age, expectations and personality type. The char-

acteristics of the family, including their cultural background, the diversity of individuals' characteristics, and their resources and ability to cope, should influence the way in which the physiotherapist interacts and works with the family to provide appropriate treatment for the child.

A key element in individualizing programmes is the involvement of the family working with professionals to set goals for the child that will guide the development of appropriate intervention strategies.

Baxter (1989) noted that parents expected professionals to be helpful and forthcoming with information and practical advice, to be interested and to treat them with consideration and respect. Indeed, service delivery is much more likely to be effective if professionals show support for parents while helping to facilitate access to the type of assistance that parents require (Baxter 1989).

Case Study 1

Sam is a 6-year-old boy who sustained a significant head injury and a spinal cord injury which resulted in (R) hemiplegia and T6 paraplegia respectively. He also suffered residual short-term memory loss and language difficulties. After the initial management in intensive care, Sam was managed by the rehabilitation team at the paediatric hospital. Planning for discharge to a small country town began early and eventually Sam's rehabilitation was transferred to the local hospital therapists.

Because the therapists who were to see Sam had limited paediatric experience, support and liaison were planned to include a video of individual and combined therapy sessions with written reports. These were sent to the country therapists before Sam's discharge. An outreach visit by the paediatric team was then planned for shortly after the discharge to meet and discuss problems with the physiotherapist who was to see Sam at the local school, to visit Sam's old grade one class to assist in planning for early integration back into school, and to visit the family at home.

It is important to recognize that discharge from hospital represented a time of stress and anxiety for Sam's family. This family not only had the stress of the recent accident and the consequences of Sam's injuries, which caused considerable grief, but they also had the challenge of coping with Sam in a home environment which was not yet suitable for wheelchair access. The physiotherapist's sensitivity and understanding is important during this stage to help reinforce the family's ability to adapt, cope and meet each problem as it arises.

The physiotherapist and other team members form a collaborative partnership with the family, and this partnership recognizes the family's role in deciding what is important for the family unit. Understanding the family's concerns and needs is integral to effective rehabilitation.

A combined programme that is meaningful and beneficial must meet the priorities of the family and fit in with their daily routine as well as meeting Sam's daily life needs. Effective team work, good interagency communication and close collaboration with the family are essential.

The physiotherapist must recognize that families at various stages may explore alternative therapies and treatments. Physiotherapy service providers should respect families' rights, as well as fulfilling professional responsibilities by providing any available information to assist families in their decision-making. It is in the best interests of the child for the family to be reassured that if they choose to leave they can return at any stage to the physiotherapy service.

The different cultural backgrounds of families should be considered by the physiotherapist in service delivery. When working with children with special needs and their families there is no single correct way to achieve a desired outcome, but rather many possible alternatives.

Inclusion of siblings in management may be beneficial for all family members and will allow siblings to obtain accurate information about the nature of the disability and the opportunity to develop their own coping strategies within a supportive, informed environment.

Professionals must be aware of the increased potential for stress in families with a child with a disability. Cavangh and Ashman (1985) identify a number of potentially stressful issues for these families, including difficulties in marital and family relationships, greater feelings of social isolation and more difficult socioeconomic circumstances. Physiotherapists may need to provide practical suggestions about how to access information regarding the availability and type of supports, respite services and financial assistance schemes.

The physiotherapist has a role in adapting home programmes to take into account the physical capacity of the carers, as well as educating them in manual handling techniques and back care.

Critical Periods for Physiotherapy Intervention

All children have a potential requirement for physiotherapy during their childhood or adolescence. They may be hospitalized and need respiratory management or mobilization following orthopaedic procedures, or sustain a sporting injury requiring outpatient treatment. Other children may present with acquired brain injury requiring rehabilitation, both in hospital and for some time afterwards, depending on the extent of the lesion and subsequent disability.

Children with disabilities (both congenital and acquired) tend to have critical periods when the requirement for physiotherapy intervention is greatest. These critical periods include:

- rapid developmental change (young children)
- growth spurts which can affect muscle balance, posture and balance
- access to and appropriateness of new environments, for example
  - classroom furniture and playground equipment

- mobility requirements (rails, ramps, lifts, etc.)
- education of new staff about the child's physical abilities and needs
- deterioration of function (as in progressive neuro-muscular conditions)
- conditions that flare up (as in juvenile chronic arthritis)
- physical preparation for a particular vocation or leisure activity

Models of Service Delivery

At different times and stages, different agencies may be used to provide necessary support and treatment. The choice of agency will be influenced by location, required intensity, availability or critical periods in the child's development.

Service provision can be described by direct, monitoring or consultation models. Direct therapy or 'hands on' intervention refers to assessment of the child followed by treatment that is delivered on a one-to-one basis or in a small group setting by the physiotherapist. Monitoring requires the physiotherapist to assess the child and plan the intervention, with programme delivery by other team members. There would be ongoing contact to review and update the programme. Consultation refers to the physiotherapist assisting with problem-solving on the basis of need and ongoing contact may not be necessary.

In hospital the direct therapy model may be the most appropriate. Within the context of school it may be more appropriate for physiotherapy strategies to be included in the overall classroom programme and to be carried out by other team members with appropriate monitoring by the physiotherapist. In both situations success is largely dependent on the accuracy of assessment, the appropriateness of programme development and the skill of the person carrying out the programme.

As a child's needs change, the method of service delivery may also change. The continuum of services remains the issue for the child and family, but appropriate consultation, planning and communication should facilitate continuity of services.

Team Approaches

A multiprofessional team can provide comprehensive assessment information which allows for effective team planning and decision-making. Effective team decision-making has been recognized as important in the design of quality programmes for children and their families (Flemming and Flemming 1983). Consistency between home, therapy and educational programmes is facilitated when team members work together with the family.

Team members are determined by the child's needs and by the resources within the appropriate agencies. In rural areas, geography and human resources within the region may influence the team's composition. Involvement of parents or immediate carers in the team is always vital and the concerns, goals and resources of families are critical in the planning and implementation of an intervention programme. Physiotherapists should collaborate with family and professional team members to determine the overall focus of services and to select the approaches that will be most effective for the child.

Several types of team are discussed in the literature and these are categorized according to the way in which team members are coordinated, how children are assessed and how programmes are planned and implemented.

MULTIDISCIPLINARY TEAM

In this case, each professional assesses the child and determines priorities, goals and intervention strategies (Muhlenhaupt 1991). However, interventions may be implemented in isolation from each other (Bailey 1984). Services are often provided through a specialized centre such as a hospital, but may also be home-based (Muhlenhaupt 1991). Parents may have the responsibility of coordinating the different services participating in their child's intervention programme.

INTERDISCIPLINARY TEAM

Here, each professional evaluates the child independently. However, the interdisciplinary team members review the assessment results together and collaborate to decide on priorities and goals and to plan and coordinate the intervention programme. Achievement of goals requires ongoing planning and communication between team members working together in an interactive and coordinated manner (Bailey 1984).

TRANSDISCIPLINARY TEAM

Sometimes professionals work together throughout the assessment, planning and implementation of the intervention programme. The sharing of both information and skills is the basis for this approach and involves a much greater degree of collaboration than other practices (Rainforth *et al.* 1992), resulting in fewer persons involved in direct programme implementation with the child and family (Sparling 1980).

Giangreco *et al.* (1989) suggest that these team models are interrelated and represent an historical evolution of teamwork. The isolation of the disciplines from each other in the multidisciplinary model often leads to unmet needs for children with more complex problems. The lack of collaboration in actual assessment and intervention in the interdisciplinary model can also limit team effectiveness. The transdisciplinary team model depends heavily on positive team interaction. Each of these models may be appropriate in certain settings and address specific therapy needs. It is the needs of the child that should determine the model guiding the service delivery, not those of the team. The processes of teaming rather than the characteristics attributed to one particular team model have been the focus of more recent literature. The processes of collaboration and consultation have been highlighted as being critical to effective team functioning (Swan and Morgan 1993).

Professionals involved in the provision of intervention programmes go through a cycle of assessment, planning, implementing, evaluating progress, modifying the plan along the way, evaluating outcomes and organizing follow-up, referring elsewhere or discontinuing the service as appropriate. How this occurs and the selection of a particular team approach depends on the requirements of the service, the philosophy underlying the programme, tradition and the experience and preference of the staff.

The Provision of Physiotherapy Services

A variety of agencies provide physiotherapy services for preschool and school-age children with special needs. These include: health-care agencies with services provided through specialized paediatric hospitals, general hospitals both in urban and rural settings and community centres; education systems providing services in both mainstream and special schools, as well as a variety of early intervention programmes for children under school age; independent agencies which may be disability specific and provide a variety of services in a variety of settings; and the private practitioner.

Interagency collaboration often becomes necessary so that available resources are pooled to meet the needs of the children and their families. Collaborative efforts between family members and professionals from all agencies with appropriate communication results in coordination and continuity of care. This becomes particularly important as children transfer between programmes, or as families access consultative services from one agency while their child attends another. A case manager may be appointed to facilitate the transfer of information from one agency to another, coordinate potential areas of overlap and prevent duplication of services. In some situations parents assume this role.

Case Study 2

Tanya is an 11-year-old girl who has cerebral palsy (spastic quadriplegia). She has been attending a special school in a large city which employs physiotherapists on staff. Tanya and her family, together with members of her educational team have agreed that Tanya's educational needs would best be met in her local community school where her brother and sister are enrolled. They agree that the necessary supports would need to be made available such as teacher aide time, specialized equipment, therapy, and training for school staff.

> *Tanya is mobile on flat surfaces using a walking frame, but her tendoachilles are shortening with her current growth spurt, and walking is becoming more difficult. Everyone agrees that it would be ideal for Tanya to be as mobile and independent as possible before her change of school.*
>
> *The family made an appointment to see Tanya's orthopaedic surgeon at the children's hospital and the special school physiotherapist sent a report to the hospital physiotherapist who will be attending the clinic. Although Tanya has responded well to serial casting in the past, it was decided that surgical releases would be more beneficial at this stage.*
>
> *The special school and hospital physiotherapists liaised to ensure the following:*
>
> - *that the hospital staff were informed of Tanya's handling and positioning requirements and how to use her equipment (including her communication device)*
> - *the family were provided with support at home (domiciliary nursing and physiotherapy were organized)*
> - *the hospital physiotherapist and the orthopaedic surgeon organized with the orthotist for bilateral hinged ankle foot orthoses to follow removal of the cast; the school physiotherapist was to monitor their use during mobility training sessions at school*
>
> *Three months after surgery Tanya's mobility goals were achieved and the process of transition to the local community school began.*

School Services

Physiotherapists are increasingly involved in supporting children's access to, and participation in, their school programmes. Blossom and Ford (1991) discuss the need for the physiotherapist to have a good understanding of the child's condition and how this affects their movement ability. In addition, the physiotherapist should identify the barriers faced in the school setting as well as the expectations and requirements for functioning in that environment. The demands placed upon the child regarding endurance, mobility, strength and dexterity should be identified. The child with subtle problems of motor control or sensorimotor perception often needs as much or more assistance than one who has a more obvious physical disability.

The focus of physiotherapy in the school setting is to contribute to the learning outcomes of the child with special needs. Physical access and participation in appropriate classroom programmes are primary goals. This may include advice regarding environmental alterations and the provision of appropriate equipment as well as programme planning and implementation as part of the educational team. At critical periods in the child's development it may be necessary for the child to access physiotherapy from other agencies. Effective communication and close liaison between therapists is essential. To work effectively in the school setting, the physiotherapist should be familiar with the influence of factors such as school culture, the school community expectations, the policies and procedures of the local and broader educational administration, and working as an educational team member.

The benefits of integrated therapy in educational settings are highlighted by Rainforth and York (1987). Indeed, integrated therapy is an essential feature of the transdisciplinary approach and enables the child to be provided with more consistent, comprehensive programming and more meaningful outcomes (Giangreco *et al.* 1989).

Hospital Services

Physiotherapy services for children with acute or ongoing conditions are often provided in the hospital setting where physiotherapy assists in their recovery. Those children who have ongoing medical conditions or disabilities may require intermittent involvement or blocks of treatment at critical periods throughout childhood and adolescence.

In the hospital setting, the doctor and consulting specialist largely determine the overall management plan into which other services such as nursing and therapies are interwoven. The parents normally stay close by or visit regularly and play an important role. Many large children's hospitals also have a school on site and children attend or continue school from their beds.

Specialized paediatric hospitals cater for children with more complex needs by the provision of multidisciplinary clinical teams. Outpatient clinics provide the opportunity for review by team members who have particular expertise in various conditions such as cystic fibrosis, burns management and spinal disabilities. Other specialized services such as orthotics and prosthetics and provision of customized seating and mobility aids are usually linked to the paediatric hospital. Physiotherapists who work within these services and specialized clinics have usually developed a high level of knowledge, expertise and clinical judgement and are a valuable resource to other physiotherapists. They have an important role in providing information and support to the transferring child's local service provider. This may include verbal, written and visual communication (such as video) to local hospital physiotherapists, private practitioners and physiotherapists from other agencies.

Community Services

The movement towards inclusion of children with disabilities within their local community has been accompanied by increasing demands for locally based services. Agencies have responded to this demand by moving away from centre-based services and towards the development of outreach services to local communities.

Rural Services

Services in rural areas present more of a challenge to the physiotherapist providing intervention programmes for children with special needs. Geographical considerations and lack of human resources in the local area influence the model of service delivery available. Assessment and programme planning may occur either through visits to a metropolitan centre or via an outreach service to the child's local commu-

nity. The programme may then be implemented by local personnel including family members and school staff. Regular monitoring by the physiotherapist is necessary. It is important that the programme be both practical and realistic for the child, family and school staff, as well as appropriate to their environment.

Case Study 3

Peter is a 7-year-old boy with spina bifida who lives on a large farming property and attends the local one-teacher country school. He attends a specialized paediatric hospital in a large metropolitan centre for specialized clinics, periodic physiotherapy and provision of equipment. There is no local physiotherapy service. A community agency has just started providing outreach programmes to the area once every 2 months and this includes physiotherapy services. Peter's family were keen to access this new service when told about it. The hospital physiotherapist referred Peter to this service and liaised directly with the physiotherapist who would provide the outreach service.

In the past, information to the school was conveyed by video to educate the school staff. Peter's parents also passed on relevant information. A number of key issues relating to day-to-day management had previously been identified and other concerns were noted during a school and home visit. These included setting out a timetable for ambulation, assisting with sporting programmes and managing a number of safety and access issues in the playground. The physiotherapist, together with the parents and school staff, identified the development of independence in mobility and living skills as a primary goal, and various strategies for encouraging this were discussed.

Both the hospital and outreach physiotherapists continue to liaise closely with each other and Peter's family. Benefits of the outreach service have included increased confidence for all concerned and improved compliance at school. The parents report feeling more supported and relieved of much of the responsibility of having to manage Peter's physiotherapy programme on their own.

REFERENCES

Bailey, D (1984) A triaxial model of the interdisciplinary team and group process. *Exceptional Children* 51(1): 17–25.

Baxter, C (1989) Parent perceived attitudes of professionals: implications for service providers. *Disability, Handicap and Society* 4(3): 259–269.

Blossom, B, Ford, F (1991) *Physical Therapy in Public Schools – A Related Service*, Vol. I. Roswell, GA: Rehabilitation Publications and Therapies Inc.

Case-Smith, J (1991) The family perspective. In: Dunn W (ed). *Paediatric Occupational Therapy*, pp. 319–331. Thorofare, NJ: SLACK Inc.

Cavangh, J, Ashman, AF (1985) Stress in families with handicapped children. *Australia and New Zealand Journal of Developmental Disabilities* 11(3): 151–156.

Education for all Handicapped Children Act. Public Law 94-142. US Congress Senate, 94th Congress, 1975.

Education of the Handicapped Act Amendments of 1986. Public Law 99-457. US Congress Senate, 99th Congress, 1986.

Elkins, J (1993) Review of the Queensland school curriculum special education: issues and comparative analysis. *Shaping the Future* 3: 160–204.

Flemming, DC, Flemming, ER (1983) Consultation with multidisciplinary teams: a program of development and improvement of team function. *Journal of School Psychology* 21: 367–376.

Giangreco, MF, York, J, Rainworth, B (1989) Providing related services to learners with severe handicaps in educational settings: pursuing the least restrictive option. *Paediatric Physical Therapy* 1: 55–62.

Guralnick, MJ, Bennett, FC (1987) A framework for early intervention In: Guralnick, MJ, Bennett, FC (eds) *The Effectiveness of Early Intervention for At-Risk and Handicapped Children*, pp. 3–29. Orlando: Academic Press.

Moore, TJ (1990) Helping young children with developmental problems: an overview of current early intervention aims and practices. *Australian Journal of Early Childhood* 15: 3–8.

Muhlenhaupt, M (1991) Components of the program planning process. In: Dunn, W (ed) *Paediatric Occupational Therapy*, pp. 125–136. Thorofare, NJ: SLACK Inc.

Queensland Parents of People with a Disability Inc. (1993) *Statement on Therapy with Children.*

Rainforth, B, York, J (1987) Integrating related services into community instruction. *Journal of the Association of Persons with Severe Handicaps* 12(3): 188–198.

Rainforth, B, York, J, MacDonald, J (1992) *Collaborative Teams for Students with Severe Disabilities, Integrating Therapy and Educational Services*, 284pp. Baltimore: Paul Brookes Publishing.

Sparling, JW (1980) The transdisciplinary approach with the developmentally delayed child. *Physical and Occupational Therapy in Pediatrics* 1(2): 3–16.

Swan, WW, Morgan, JL (1993) *Collaborating for Comprehensive Services for Young Children and their Families: The Local Interagency Coordinating Council*, 249 pp. Baltimore: Paul H Brookes.

Wolfensberger, W (1972) *The Principle of Normalisation in Human Services*, 258 pp. Toronto: National Institute on Mental Retardation.

11

Aids and Orthotics

JOHN GILMOUR AND MEGAN KENTISH

Wheelchairs
•
Lower Limb Orthoses
•
Initial Use of Orthoses
•
Aids to Assist Mobilizing

The child whose mobility or normal function is reduced may be unable to explore or fully discover and interact with their environment. As a result emotional, intellectual and physical development may suffer. A child with a disability needs the stimulus of movement so that they not only experience different surroundings but also experience movement itself.

The use of aids and orthoses can be an important factor in the management of disability in children. Aids and orthoses discussed in this chapter will include orthotic devices for the lower limb, standing and walking aids, as well as various wheelchairs and other mobility devices. These items are often given the generic term of 'equipment'. Some equipment may be specific, highly technical and at times expensive in order to be successful; however, there are many everyday items that can be used by the clinician and carers that may assist in meeting the needs of the child.

Equipment is used as a part of a total patient management programme and, as such, should augment other components such as therapy and home programmes, school and life style needs of the family. The provision of equipment is a dynamic process of constant change and requires regular monitoring as the child grows and develops to ensure best-possible outcomes.

Wheelchairs

Wheelchairs can be used to assist in meeting the mobility and positioning needs of the child with disability. By appropriately addressing these needs, the development, function and quality of life of the child can be enhanced.

The major groups of children who may require a wheelchair and positioning through adaptive seating systems include those with the following:

- muscle weakness such as muscular dystrophies and spinal muscular atrophies
- muscle paralysis such as spina bifida and spinal cord injury
- abnormal muscle tone such as cerebral palsy,

acquired brain injury and various syndrome presentations

- orthopaedic conditions such as juvenile chronic arthritis, osteogenesis imperfecta, arthrogryposis and congenital limb deficiencies

There are two basic factors to consider in the provision of wheeled devices for the child with disability: (1) mobility; (2) positioning. Most wheeled devices will have a dual role, meeting both mobility and positioning needs.

Mobility

Wheelchairs and other wheeled devices allow for, or enhance, mobility for children with special needs. The benefits of improved mobility include:

- greater exploration of the environment
- increased independence
- improved function
- increased peer group interaction
- greater access to education and the community
- improved family mobility allowing greater community access

Movement allows interaction with the environment, and is considered to be crucial to the development of the child. Wheeled mobility, therefore, may be provided at a very young age for some children (Trefler *et al.* 1993). Early mobility aids may include scooter boards, castor carts, modified trikes and bikes, powered toy cars and a variety of strollers and wheelchairs. Children progress according to age, needs, abilities and the availability of equipment.

Some children will be completely dependent on the wheelchair and accompanying adaptive seating system in order to meet their mobility needs and also allow for positioning that will improve function. Other children may not rely exclusively on a wheelchair as they have some ambulatory skills; however, safety, endurance, energy expenditure or speed requirements do not allow them to keep up with family or peers. School work or fine motor function may be compromised by fatigue or abnormal tone in these children. The use of a wheelchair for some or all of their mobility may address these issues.

To prescribe the most appropriate mobility aid for the child and family, the team needs to consider the physical, sensory and cognitive abilities of the child, the nature and prognosis of the disability and the environments in which the child will function.

For children whose physical, sensory or cognitive disability precludes self-propulsion or the use of powered chairs, attendant-propelled mobility is necessary. Upper limb function will help to determine the ability of the child to self-propel. If self-propelling is so slow and difficult so as to be non-functional and cause frustration to the child, or causes excessive fatigue or unacceptable changes in tone, powered mobility may be considered.

It is important to note for what activities and in which environments the child and family propose to use the chair — home, school, recreation or community. Terrains of these various environments and methods of transporting family members and the chair are also important factors to consider. Knowledge of safety guidelines and regulations regarding transportation of wheelchairs and their occupants should be accessed by health professionals.

Wheeled mobility devices fall into three broad categories: self-propelled; attendant-propelled; and power-driven.

Self-propelled Mobility Equipment

Young children may have a castor cart or scooter board as their first method of wheeled mobility and as a way to introduce them to self-propulsion. Modified bikes and trikes may be suitable mobility devices for some children; however, most children with disability who are able to self-propel rely on manual wheelchairs for mobility. See Figure 1.

While a small proportion of children with disabilities may use their lower limbs to propel and steer the wheelchair, by far the majority will use their upper limbs to propel the chair.

LIGHTWEIGHT MANUAL WHEELCHAIRS
All self-propelling wheelchairs should be lightweight and of an appropriate size and design to promote optimal mobility and function (Figure 2). This ensures protection of upper limb joints and low energy expenditure during propulsion. Successful

Figure 1   Early Mobility Equipment. A, Castor cart; B, motorized car; C, customized tricycle

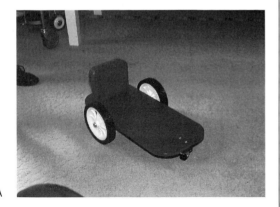

A

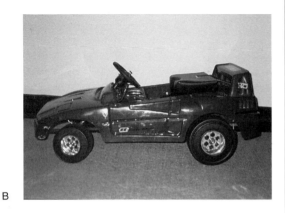

B

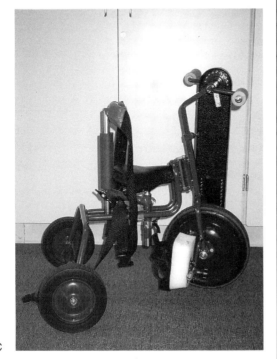

C

Figure 2   Lightweight Manual Wheelchair, providing optimal mobility, function and recreation

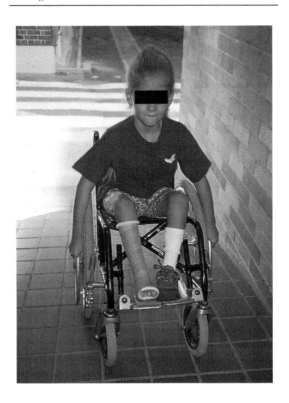

wheelchair propulsion relates to the user's ability, the design characteristics of the wheelchair, and the suitability of the wheelchair (Hughes *et al.* 1992).

Lightweight wheelchairs may be commercially available or may be custom-made depending upon the individual needs of the child. Understanding the options and various components available in lightweight wheelchairs is necessary for sound decision-making during the prescription process. Figure 3 shows the components of a manual wheelchair.

A lightweight wheelchair that features 'adjustability' allows for individual set up of the chair and ensures the user is able to achieve maximum performance in the chair (Figure 4). Appropriate individualized adjustments to the chair result in:

- improved posture, stability and comfort
- improved manoeuvrability
- reduced energy expenditure for propulsion
- improved suitability for specific activities

Figure 3   Manual Wheelchair Components

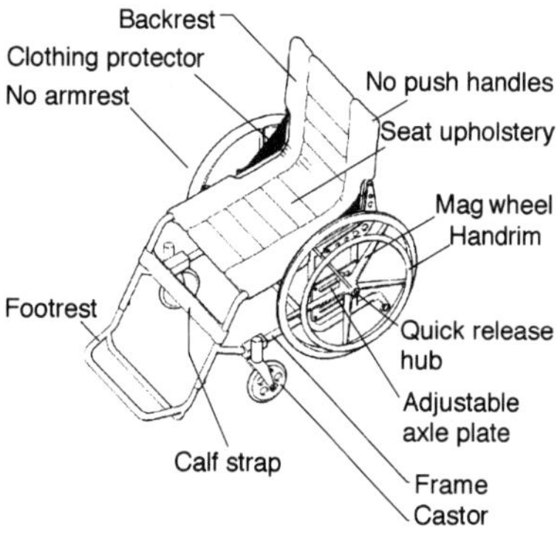

Backrest Clothing protector No armrest No push handles Seat upholstery Mag wheel Handrim Footrest Quick release hub Adjustable axle plate Calf strap Frame Castor Lightweight manual wheelchair	**FRAMES**	*Folding frames* ● easy storage ● transport in vehicle or roof hoist ● warp, play and lack of rigidity can be problematic ● less adjustable than rigid frames *Rigid Frames* ● generally lighter in weight ● no play therefore more manoeuvrable/responsive/less energy to propel ● greater strength and stability therefore more tolerant of heavy use ● usually the choice for sports use ● transport may be difficult unless wheels are removable ● fold-down back is a useful option
	TYRES	*Pneumatic* ● provide cushioned ride (shock absorbing) ● better traction in wet ● easily repaired if punctured ● cheap and readily available *High pressure* ● less resistance ● easier to push and manoeuvre ● more suitable for sports use ● lighter in weight ● less cushioned ride outdoors ● less traction in wet
	WHEELS	*Spoked wheels* ● stronger and more shock absorbing ● slightly lighter weight ● higher maintenance due to spokes ● spoke hub arrangements can be arranged to increase performance *Mag wheels* ● more durable ● lower maintenance ● less shock absorbing ● heavier
	CASTORS	*8" or 6" Pneumatic* ● shock absorbing, therefore, smoother ride ● good for travel over rough terrain ● higher maintenance ● less clearance for footplate adjustment *5" Urethane* ● increased manoeuvrability of chair ● less rolling resistance ● less shock absorption ● often chosen for sports use ● low maintenance ● good foot clearance *3" Urethane* ● similar to roller blade wheel ● usually sports use only ● minimal rolling resistance ● difficult to use outdoors unless skilled

Figure 3   Continued

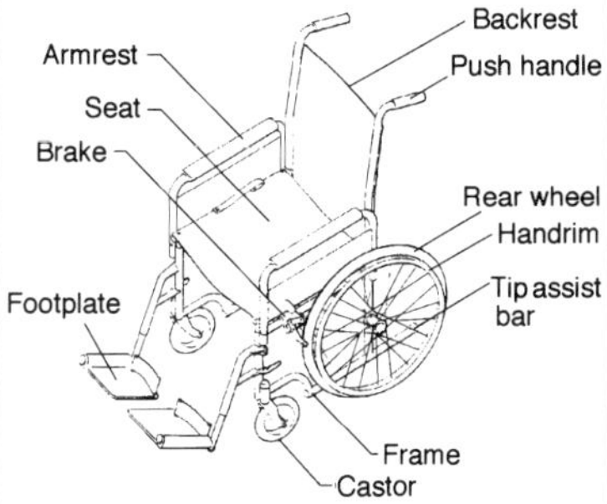

Armrest —
Seat —
Brake —
Footplate —

Backrest
Push handle

Rear wheel
Handrim

Tip assist
bar

Frame
Castor | BRAKES | *Toggle*
• most common style
• push or pull to apply
• high or low mounting
• consider reach and ease to engage
• consider position for transfers
• consider position for stroking of the wheels to propel

Extended handles
• longer lever arm makes brakes easier to apply
• within closer reach for small children
• allows for poor sitting balance

Scissor
• fold completely out of the way
• good clearance for transfers
• good for sports chairs
• maybe expensive option
• difficult to engage |
| | ARMRESTS | *Armrest*
• useful for weight shifting and propping to maintain position
• allow for easy mounting of tray
• desk style allows closer access to table top
• increase the width and weight of the chair
• may interfere with stroking when self-propelling
• removable or swing away for ease of transfer
• protective of clothing |
| | FOOTPLATES | *Footplate*
• adjustability important to allow for growth
• consider suitability for standing transfers
• fixed, fold-up, swingaway, removable footplate or tube options
• tube type footrests less likely to cause skin breakdown
• angle important in control of tone or spasm (often 90°–100°)
• feet tuck decreases length of chair / increases manoeuvrability |
| | ACCESSORIES | *Handrims*
• plastic-coated provide more traction for weak grip
• capstans — projections from handrims — may be useful if grasp is limited
• capstans positioned vertical, oblique, horizontal
• number of capstans can be varied

Anti-tip bars
• prevents backwards tipping
• important safety feature for less-skilled users
• must be turned up for curbs

Calf straps
• prevents feet from slipping backwards or hitting castors
• useful for spasm
• heel loops may be an alternative

Spoke protectors
• protects hands and fingers from spokes

Clothing or thigh protectors
• prevent skin rub from wheels on soft tissue of thighs
• usually not necessary if armrests used
• may be solid or cloth
• cloth – less risk of scrapes / skin breakdown during sideways transfers
• cloth may stretch out of shape more readily

Push handles
• allows carer to push the chair therefore height important
• may assist with functions such as reaching to floor or repositioning |

Figure 4   Wheelchair Adjustment Parameters

Camber 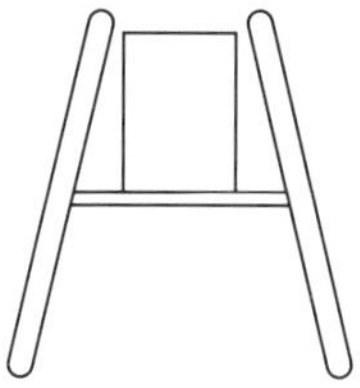	• more natural pushing action (easier to push down and out) • increased turning ability • increased side-to-side stability due to increased width of wheelchair base • increased space for fingers at top of wheel so good for sports • sporty look • wider chair — may affect doorway access • reduced area for sitting — watch for rubbing • preset angle of 0, 3, 6, 9 or 12° in some chairs • achieved by placing washers between axle block and frame in some chairs
Wheel toe-in/toe-out 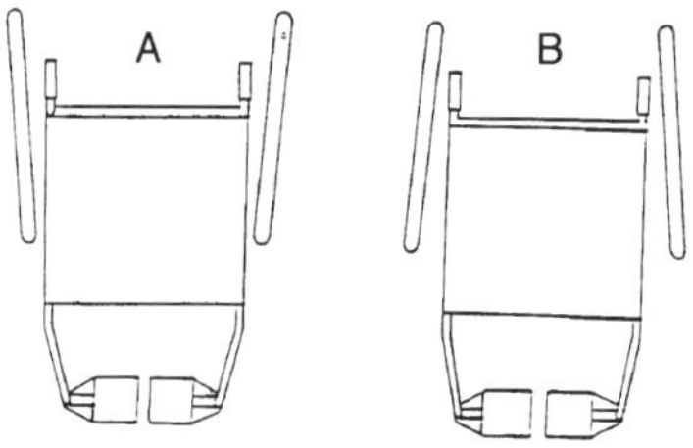 A B	• refers to rear wheel alignment (should be set in neutral) • must be adjusted for when seat angle changed and in a wheelchair with camber • if incorrectly aligned, wheelchair may veer in one direction or have greater resistance to rolling • measure distance between wheel rims front and back to check alignment • adjust by using washers to space axle block or through rotation of axle bar

Back axle position (up/down) 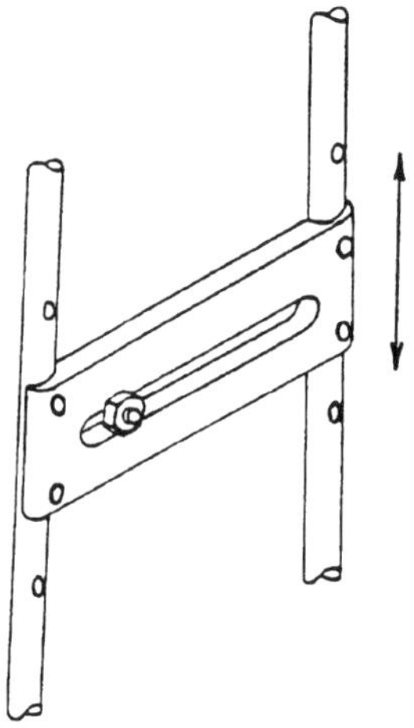	• adjustment of back axle position may require:
	  – realignment of front castor angle to maintain these perpendicular to the ground, otherwise the front of the chair rises and falls as the chair moves along
	  – possible repositioning of brake blocks
	  – adjustment of backrest to maintain upright position
	• affects the rear height of chair to floor
	• if height is lowered:
	  – increased performance in turning/manoeuvring
	  – the chair is more stable
	• may change seat/backrest angle
	• changes degree of elbow flexion during pushing

Back axle position (forward/back) 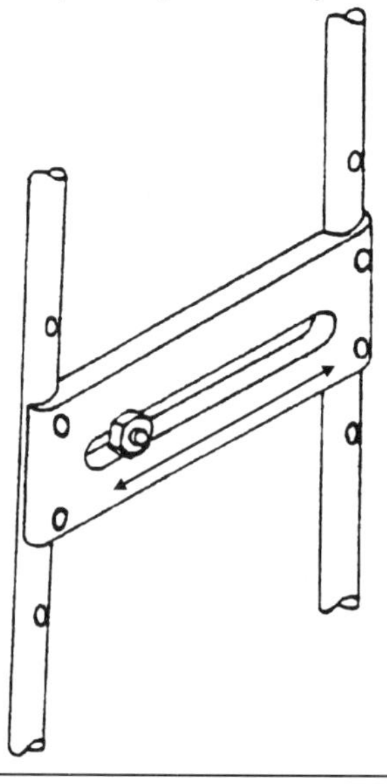	• back axle forward brings the user closer over the centre of gravity
	  – chair becomes more 'tippy', greater weight at rear of chair
	  – easier to do 'wheelies'
	  – easier to propel forward/energy efficient
	  – use anti-tip bars where the increased 'tippiness' is problematic
	• back axle back results in greater stability, however reduces performance

Figure 4   Continued

Back angle 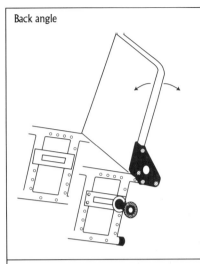	• assists with positioning of child for improved stability/function/comfort • folding frame chairs usually do not allow for adjustment • rigid frame often allows adjustment of back rest

Seat height to floor 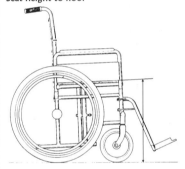	• affects accessibility to tables
	• affects transfers
	• height altered by:
	  — changing rearwheel size and castor fork length
	  — moving back axle up or down and adjust castor fork length

Wedge 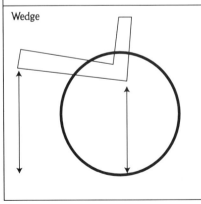	• wedge achieved by adjusting back axle/back angle • usually not possible with folding frame • may improve posture and stability in sitting • backrest height may be reduced • transfers may be more difficult • wedge may be built in to frame design

Consultation with appropriate agencies or physiotherapists with expertise in this area may assist with these adjustments. However, it is important to note that this 'adjusting' of the chair is an ongoing process as the child grows and develops, and function and skill change. The child and parents should be encouraged to take an active role during the adjusting of the chair, just as they do in the selection of a wheelchair.

Attendant-propelled Mobility Equipment

For infants and young children, prams and strollers provide appropriate mobility. Large collapsible strollers with a nylon slung seat/backrest are available for the older child who is reliant upon a parent or carer for propulsion. These strollers are usually easy to manoeuvre and push; however, they may require modification to assist with appropriate positioning of the child. They are generally considered to be unsuitable for the school-aged child. Other mobility devices such as beach buggies, rickshaws or running buggies may be chosen or used for specific activities, depending on the needs of the family and child and the availability of resources. In general, however, wheelchairs are the most commonly used mobility device for children with a level of disability that dictates attendant propulsion.

WHEELCHAIRS

The components of attendant-propelled wheelchairs may be similar to those of self-propulsion chairs, but it is not necessary for these chairs to have large rear wheels or the same performance features as self-propelled wheelchairs. Important features are those that meet both positioning needs of the child and the needs of the attendant who pushes the chair.

Positioning needs of the child include:

- safety features such as seat belts, arm-rests and spoke protectors
- features to address both comfort and function, as dictated by the level of disability and the needs of the child – adaptive seating systems and frames to allow mounting of such systems may be required. Adaptive seating systems are discussed later in the chapter.

Features to consider that assist in meeting the needs of the attendant who pushes the chair include:

- access allowing ease of transfers and positioning of the child
- effective braking system for the attendant
- appropriate handle height
- tilt-bar to assist with gutters and steps
- light in weight to allow for ease of pushing and transportation (in and out of cars or public transport)
- manoeuvrability with stability for ease of pushing

As with all equipment, durability, reliability and cosmesis must be considered.

TILT IN SPACE AND RECLINE WHEELCHAIRS

Children with severe physical disability, such as marked spastic quadriplegia or marked hypotonia,

may present with an inability to maintain an upright posture in a standard fixed-angle wheelchair. Neurological influences and poor postural abilities combined with the effect of gravity may result in a situation that requires a seating system which allows for variation of the total patient position in space. These children may also have significant pelvic and spinal deformities. The child can be positioned upright, semireclined, reclined or in some chairs tilted forward to allow for various daily activities. The 'tilt in space' and 'reclining' wheelchairs offer some of these variations (see Figure 5).

'Tilt in space' allows for the normal seated angle relationship of the hips, knees and ankles to be retained whilst altering the orientation of the person in space. These relationships may be vital in the management of tonal influences or to the muscular and functional abilities of the child. Armrest angle adjustment may be required to allow a tray surface to remain in a horizontal position. There may be a

Figure 5   Tilt-in-space and Recline Wheelchairs. A, Wheelchair with adaptive seating in backward tilt; B, recline wheelchair – note elevated legs

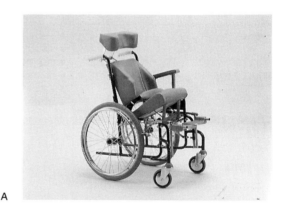

A

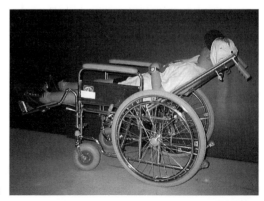

B

requirement to forward tilt the seating unit to improve postural abilities and muscle activation in response to gravity and in turn improve function of the child. It is not possible to maintain this position for prolonged periods and a programme using this position should be graded to suit individual children.

'Reclining' wheelchairs offer a reclined or semireclined position for the child with corresponding changes of hip, knee and ankle angles. This is achieved by rearward recline of the backrest and elevation of the legrests. This position may be useful for children with degenerative neuromuscular conditions, severe hypotonia, ventilated patients or those with insufficient range of movement in the hips. Patients with strong primitive reflexes and extensor tone, or those with hamstring contracture may be disadvantaged by or not tolerate recliner positioning. This emphasizes the importance of trialling the chair.

Appropriate support of the lower limbs must be considered as seat and leg length relationships vary as recline is introduced. If this is not achieved, discomfort and pressure problems may result. Children who sit in reclined positions may require specialized cushions for pressure relief. Headrest support should always be provided with recline chairs. Many children may benefit from a slight backrest recline (10–15°) as this may place less demands on head and trunk control and result in a more relaxed position and reduced tone (Bergen and Colangelo 1985).

Powerdrive Mobility Equipment

Electric toy cars, scooters and other powered mobility devices are available, are often cheaper than conventional powerdrive wheelchairs and may also have more cosmetic appeal to some users. Scooters offer similar outdoor mobility to some powerdrive wheelchairs; however, it is important for prescribers and users to be cognizant of the differences in performance and use. Scooter features include:

- increased turning circle
- decreased manoeuvrability
- seating support usually limited and modification difficult
- reasonable sitting balance required to operate tiller
- functional use of both hands usually required

POWERDRIVE WHEELCHAIRS

Powerdrive chairs are generally prescribed if a person is unable to be functionally independent in a manual wheelchair or the effort of manual propulsion is detrimental to other daily functions. The major advantage of powerdrive wheelchairs is that they allow independent indoor and outdoor mobility over significant distances with minimal physical demands on the user. Improved access, function and independence result.

Many powerdrive wheelchair users have significant physical deformities requiring adaptive seating and various control options for operating the chair. Powerdrive wheelchairs incorporate a number of options including variable height function. The control device can be mounted for hand, foot, chin, crown control and sip-puff. Figure 6 shows some of these options.

There have also been significant advances in the technology involved with the electronics and motor systems of these chairs. Most control boxes are computer programmable and have variable speed settings. Safety and reliability have been increased with the introduction of electromechanical braking and the use of gel batteries. Advances in frame design provide floating and variable suspension to improve rough surface driving and in turn, increased safety and community access for the user.

Recent research notes that children as young as 2 years of age, and persons previously thought to be intellectually unsuitable, have been successfully tested for powerdrive mobility (Trefler et al. 1993). Prescribers are therefore encouraged to keep an open mind when considering potential users of this form of mobility equipment. It is important to provide adequate trialling time to allow opportunity for learning necessary skills. The early use of switch-operated toys may help develop the concepts necessary to use a powerdrive wheelchair successfully. These considerations are particularly important for those children with neurological disorders who have multiple impairments.

A number of skills should be considered important for operation of a powerdrive wheelchair. These include:

- adequate motor planning skills
- spatial awareness

Figure 6   Powerdrive Wheelchair. A, Chin control; B, manual control; C, variable height option allowing independent transfers and improved function

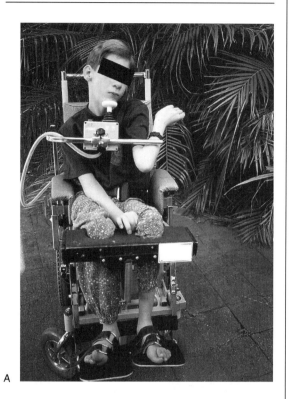

A

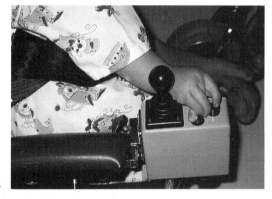

B

- adequate visual abilities
- a form of motor control which allows for consistent operation of the control device

These factors should be assessed functionally in the chair.

The child should demonstrate the potential to, or show the ability to:

- turn the chair on and off
- stop and start on command or at set points
- negotiate obstacles including doorways and paths
- avoid steps, gutter edges

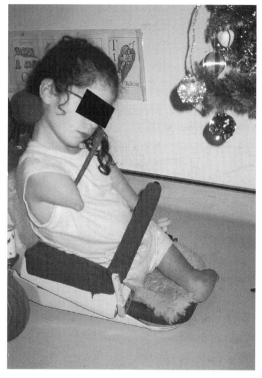

C

- show directional control
- develop safety awareness of themselves, others and environmental setting

These skills may take time to develop depending on age, ability and opportunity to use a powerdrive wheelchair. It is vital to trial the accessibility of the environments in which the chair is to be used as well as to ascertain the family's ability to transport and maintain the chair. A back-up manual chair or manual base may be required when the powerdrive chair is being serviced and when transportation or terrain limit the use of the power component of the chair.

The disadvantages of powerdrive wheelchairs must be considered during the prescription process. They include:

- the expense of initial purchase and ongoing maintenance
- the need for regular maintenance
- larger size and reduced turning circle when compared with manual chairs — components are up to 20 kg in weight which influences transportation of the chair
- the operator is sedentary which may result in

reduced physical fitness, increased potential for obesity, and less opportunity to maintain weakened muscles.

Positioning

There has been considerable literature discussing both 'normal' seating and seating for the disabled population. Factors such as comfort and function with energy efficiency are prominent in these discussions.

'Normal' sitting has been classified as a dynamic posture of the body (Andersson and Ortengren 1974, Andersson *et al.* 1975, Basmajian 1985.) This functional posturing involves regular shifts of one's centre of gravity and shifting from side to side to relieve soft tissues from pressure, and vary muscle activity, thus reducing fatigue. Sitting is used for a wide variety of functions and postures and activity levels vary from relaxing in a recline to leaning forward in an alert position. A child with disability may not be able to move and change position readily, making pressure, discomfort and fatigue all important issues to consider when addressing seating for these children.

PRINCIPLES OF SEATED POSITIONING

The pelvis as the starting point. The pelvis is the key point of sitting posture (Zacharchow 1988). A stable midline position of the pelvis, i.e. avoiding rotation and tilt with equal weight-bearing on the ischial tuberosities provides the base from which movement of the head, trunk and limbs can occur or develop (Waksvik and Levy 1979). Hip flexion, abduction and external rotation enhances pelvic stability.

Symmetry. Symmetrical midline orientation of the trunk, head and limbs is important for function (Bergen and Colangelo 1985). Head position will also have a major influence on the total seated posture for children with increased tone and abnormal reflex activity. Asymmetry of position is accepted when deformities are fixed, or when abnormal tone is so great that to achieve symmetrical posture the child would be subjected to undue forces. See Figure 7.

Stability. Stability in sitting is enhanced when a

Figure 7 Child with Cerebral Palsy with extremely high tone. A, Marked pelvic asymmetry and scoliosis — posterior view; B, adaptive seating to accommodate high tone and fixed deformity

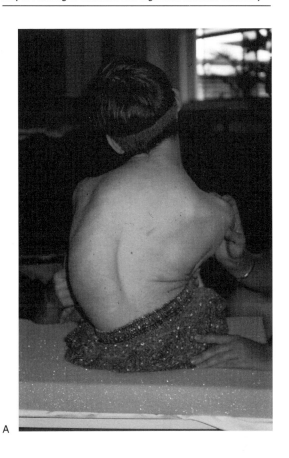

A

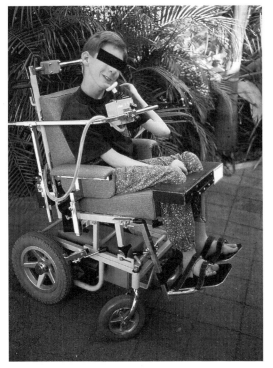

B

Figure 8 Child with Neurological Impairment. A, Poor position in stroller; B, width of wheelchair and slung upholstery offering little stability; C, child symmetrical and stable in adaptive seating.

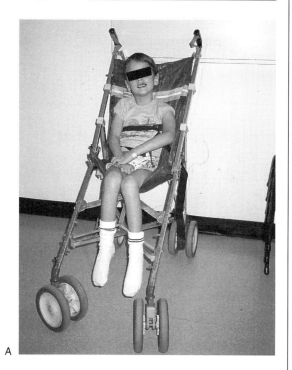

A

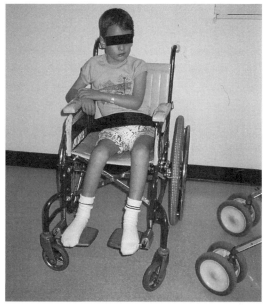

B

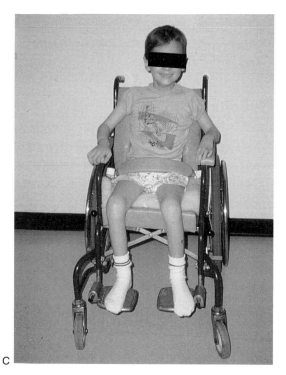

C

saggy seat which may cause pelvic obliquity, adducting hips, sacral sitting and other deviations. See Figure 8.

Backrest and armrests provide assistance to stability of sitting (Zacharchow 1988). Appropriately positioned footplates ensure adequate pressure distribution to the thighs, feet and buttocks (Waksvik and Levy 1979), and will add to the stability of the child. Care should be taken not to provide so much support to the child that seating becomes a 'passive' position. If dynamic seating can be encouraged, improvements in function and postural responses can occur. Seating can therefore be used as an adjunct to the therapy programme.

ADAPTIVE SEATING SYSTEMS

Seat support alone may not provide adequate support for children with significant physical disability or asymmetry. Use of adaptive seating may be necessary to assist in addressing common goals — improvement in the child's position, function and comfort. Various wheelchair frame types (adjustable frames, tilt in space and recliner) as well as postural supports will assist in meeting the positioning needs of the child. Postural supports used in adaptive seating may be commercially available or manufactured to meet the individual needs of the child. The use of the more common components are outlined in Figure 9.

stable base of support is achieved. Various components of the chair assist in positioning the pelvis and providing appropriate stability. The use of a firm seat rather than a slung seat will enhance stability and position (Bergen and Colangelo 1985). If a slung seat is chosen for reasons of convenience, it is important that the child and parents know the importance of having taut upholstery, rather than a stretched

Figure 9   Common Components Used in Adaptive Seating

Seats	Solid flat	Anterior wedged	Posterior wedge	Contoured	Asymmetrical
	• often foam on ply • provides firm base of support • prevents poor leg position due to seat sag	• wedge usually half depth of seat • assists in maintaining hip flex • limits sacral sitting; extensor tonus	• may reduce 'C' curve and sacral sitting • promotes active postural extension • grade time on this seat as endurance may be poor	• buttock area sculpted • ischial shelf limits forward slide • leg troughs • slight adductor pommel • foam density variations may be used in different sections	• allows for marked unilateral femoral length difference • allows for fixed deformity • usually incorporates other seat additions

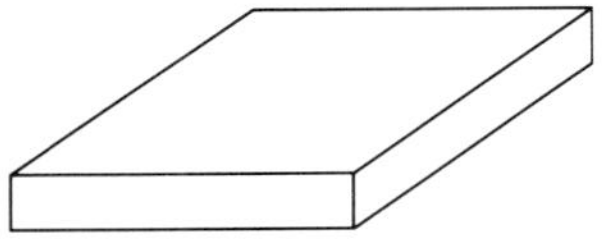

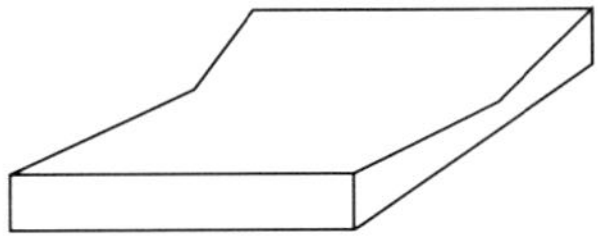

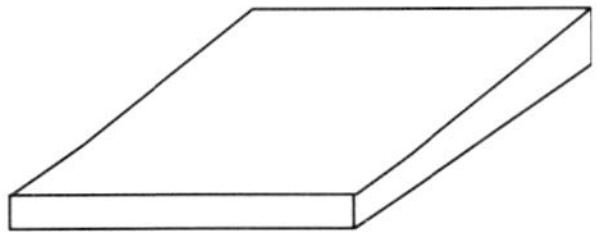

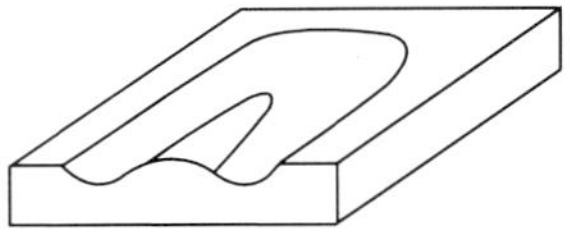

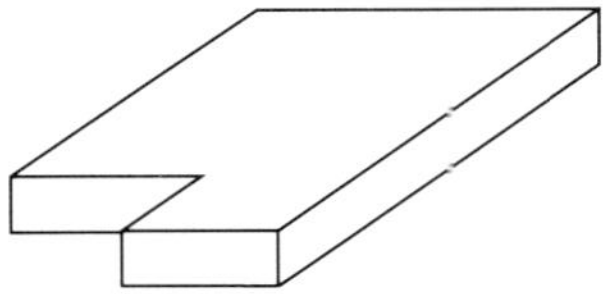

Seat additions	Adductor pommel	Abductor blocks	Hip blocks	Knee blocks	
	• located anteriorly and centrally on seat • generally removable mounting for ease of client transfer • length important to not contact adductor muscles	• located anterolateral edge of seat • usually fixed to frame or incorporated in seat • used on any seat style • length variable according to control needed • limits excessive abduction position of lower limb	• located to rear of seat • used to assist in control of pelvic position • often angled out • deep curved backrest if low may provide some control of pelvis	• located on to anterior edge of seat • must be removable • assists in location of femurs • control is via tibial tuberosities • assists in limiting forward slip of patient • position should be pain free	

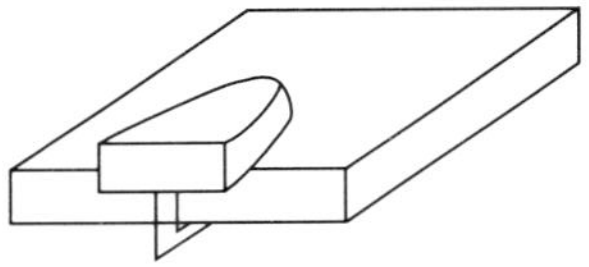

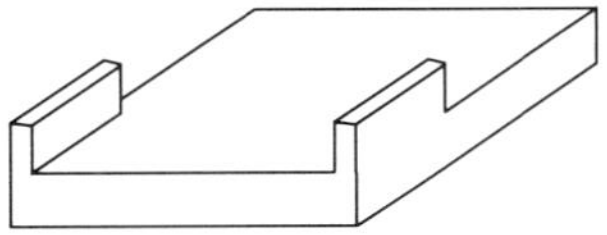

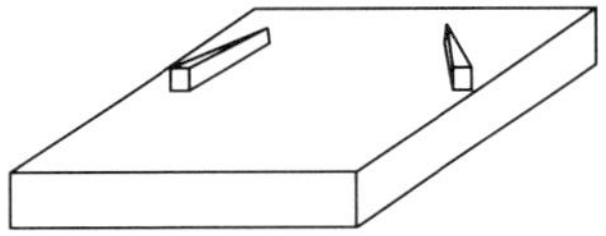

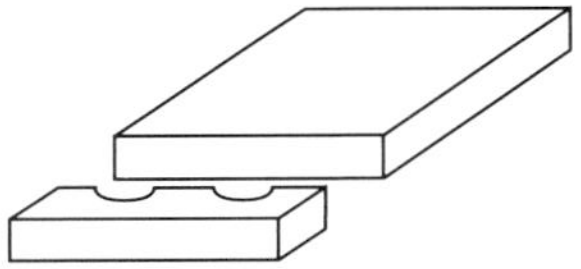

Figure 9   Continued

Backrests	Flat	Curved	Deep curved	Removable lateral supports	Asymmetrical

	• provides firm support
	• can be mounted anteriorly or posteriorly to uprights
	• position influences seat depth
	• limits kyphotic posture due to elimination of sling sag
	• height of backrest above seat can to allow for gluteal bulk
	  – provides lumbar support
	  – allows for observation of pelvic position in chair
		• as for flat backrest, plus
		• mild contour provides awareness of centralized upright sitting posture
		• encourages active correction
			• as for flat backrest, plus
			• provides postural support laterally of trunk and pelvis
			• depth of curve determined by the amount of support needed
			• shaped to allow upper limb positioning and function
				• used in conjunction with flat backrest
				• provided in various shapes and sizes
				• usually bilateral but may be unilateral
				• generally removable mountings and may be multiadjustable
				• forces required may limit corrective abilities
				• often used in conjunction with hip block for three-point fixation
					• designed to accommodate complex fixed spinal/pelvic deformity
					• specialized manufacture
					• position in relation to frame uprights variable

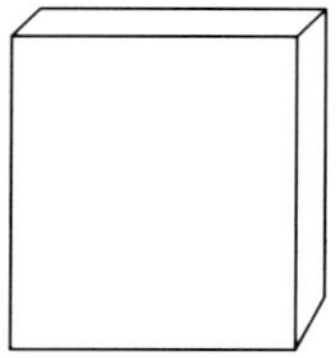

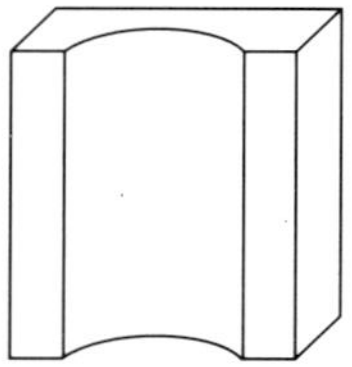

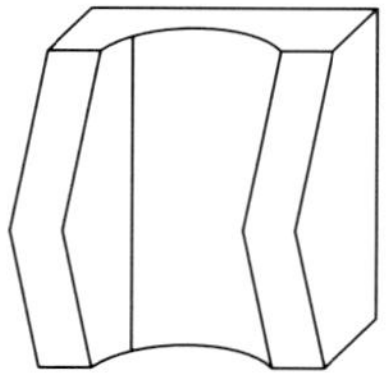

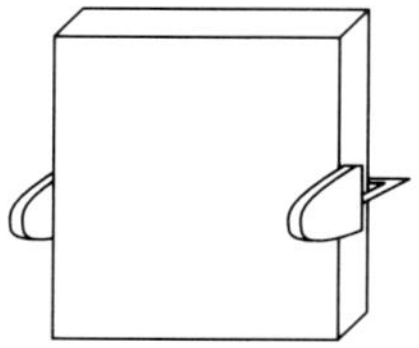

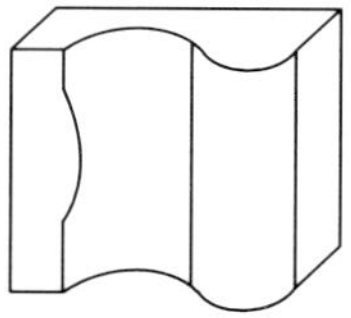

Headrests	Flat	Contoured
	• height and width variable • removable or fixed mounting • can be offset or in line with backrest • important safety feature if child transported in chair in vehicle	• assists in maintaining centralized head position • often multiadjustable mounting • support under occiput to limit abnormal extension

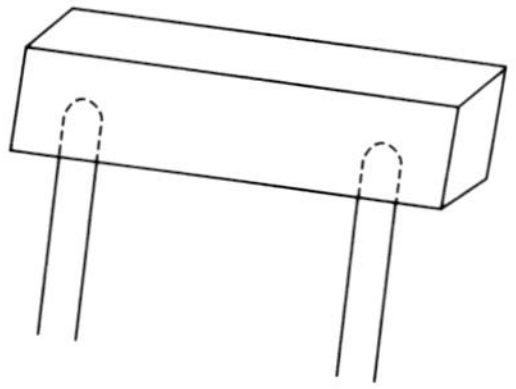

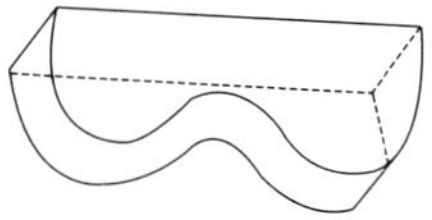

Figure 9   Continued

Straps	Pelvic	H harness/Vest	Chest strap	Calf strap
	• various materials – leather, padded leather, nylon webbing • width variable • various fixing mechanisms and positions • important in maintaining pelvic position • angle of attachment may vary 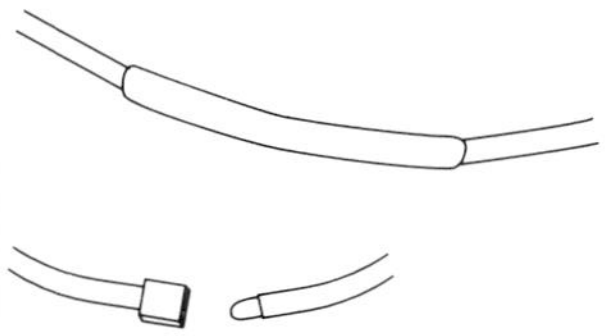	• can be continuous with pelvic strap • can be removable from pelvic strap • attaches to headrest or over higher backrest for correct line of pull • assists in limiting flexed trunk posture • useful when transporting occupant • chin poke posture should be avoided 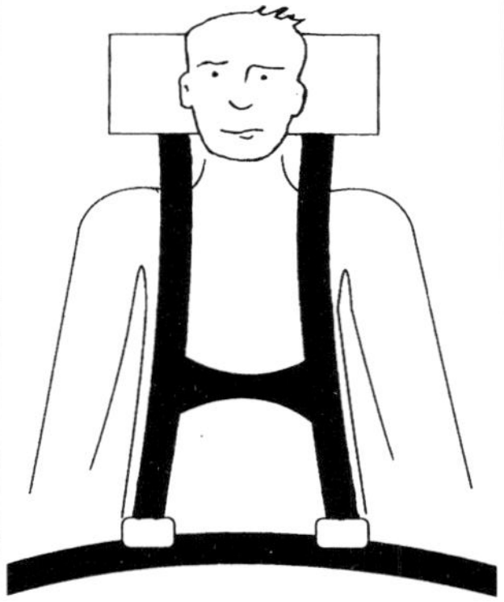	• runs horizontally across occupants chest • position varied • postural support depends on width of strap • should not limit upper limb function • less cumbersome than H harness • various fastening mechanisms and materials 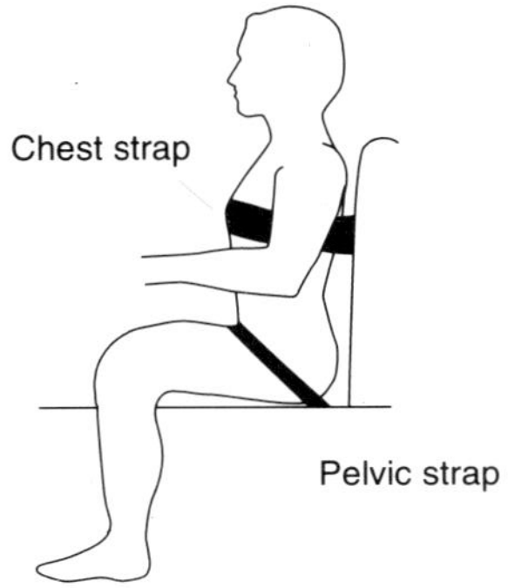	• prevents rearward or forward slip of feet • role depends on position in relation to tibia – anterior / posterior • various materials, fastening mechanisms, widths • heel loops can be used as alternative 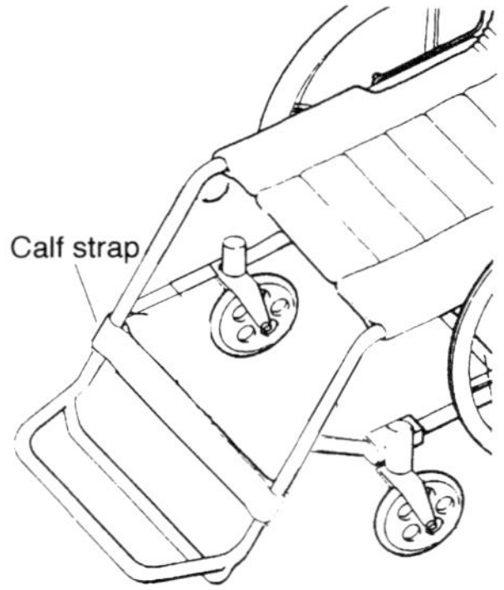

Chest strap

Pelvic strap

Calf strap

Figure 9   Continued

Footplate modifications	Extended footplates	Angle variation
	• increased in width, depth or both • assists in maintaining foot position • can have rear cut away to allow castor run • non-slip surfaces often used 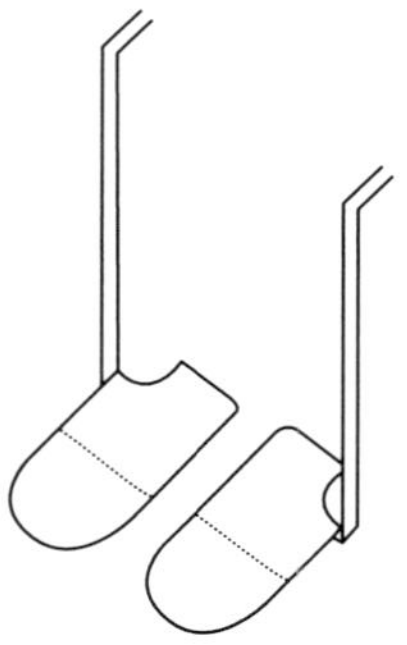	• generally 90–100° in position • reduced in 'tuck position' • access improved in 'tuck' position • angle of hanger caters for hamstring tone/length • castor tracking may be blocked when angle is reduced, outrigger castor may be required 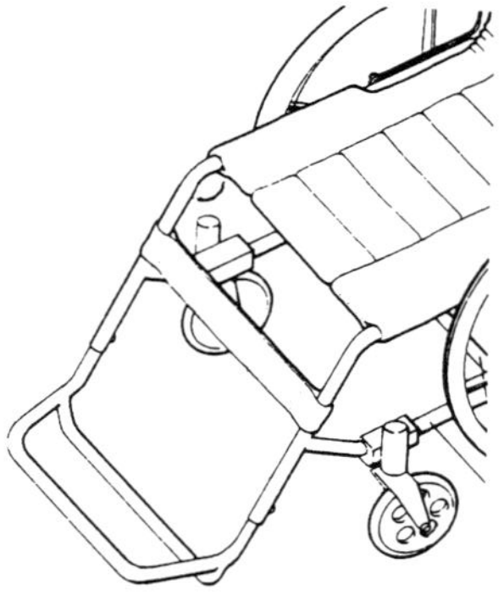

Steps to Wheelchair Prescription

To determine the exact mobility and positioning needs of the child with disability, a logical process of gathering and interpreting information should be followed (see Figure 10). Collaboration and consultation with the child, parents or carers, therapists involved, biomedical engineers, teachers and other school staff is necessary as the decision on the type of wheelchair or adaptive seating required will ultimately be a team decision. The decision may require liaison with other therapists who deal more regularly with the child or the assistance of professionals from specialized seating clinics for difficult cases. The child, as the focus of the team, should be involved in the decision-making process with their preferences for individual features, such as colour, identified. The appearance of the chair and the appearance of the child in the chair are extremely important. The trialling of different chairs or adaptations to the chair will assist in choosing the wheelchair that will best meet the

needs of the individual child. Once the wheelchair has been provided, education on use of equipment, review to ensure goals are being met and ongoing review to monitor suitability of equipment with changes due to growth and development of the child, are necessary.

ASSESSMENT

A thorough assessment considering numerous aspects which will guide the prescription must be undertaken; these are detailed in Figure 11.

DETERMINATION OF SEATING GOALS

It is necessary to determine which of the goals for seating are appropriate for each individual. No one seating system can meet all goals. Prioritization of goals may be required as certain goals will contraindicate others. The goals for seating should be clearly documented and used to guide the final prescription. They are as follows:

- improve functional status
- improve posture (body alignment and symmetry)
- correct or accommodate deformity
- normalize tone and reflex activity
- relieve pressure
- improve comfort
- increase sitting endurance
- improve communication and peer interaction
- improve appearance
- improve visual access to environment
- meet goals of parents / caregivers
- other

MEASUREMENTS

Once the child's body dimensions have been taken they will need to be transferred on to the appropriate prescription form for the selected chair. Manufacturers usually have a unique prescription form which indicates how wheelchair measurements are to be determined. If adaptive seating systems are to be used, this must be considered when translating body dimensions into wheelchair measurements for prescription.

Body dimensions should be taken with the child in an optimal position, seated on a firm surface with hips and knees at 90° (if deformity allows) and the feet

Figure 10   Steps to Prescription of Wheelchair and Adaptive Seating

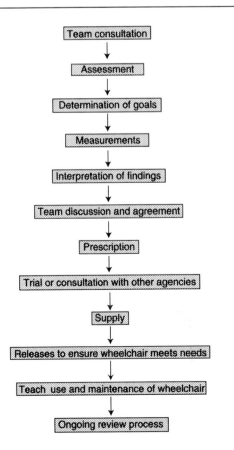

Team consultation
↓
Assessment
↓
Determination of goals
↓
Measurements
↓
Interpretation of findings
↓
Team discussion and agreement
↓
Prescription
↓
Trial or consultation with other agencies
↓
Supply
↓
Releases to ensure wheelchair meets needs
↓
Teach use and maintenance of wheelchair
↓
Ongoing review process

Figure 11   Assessment

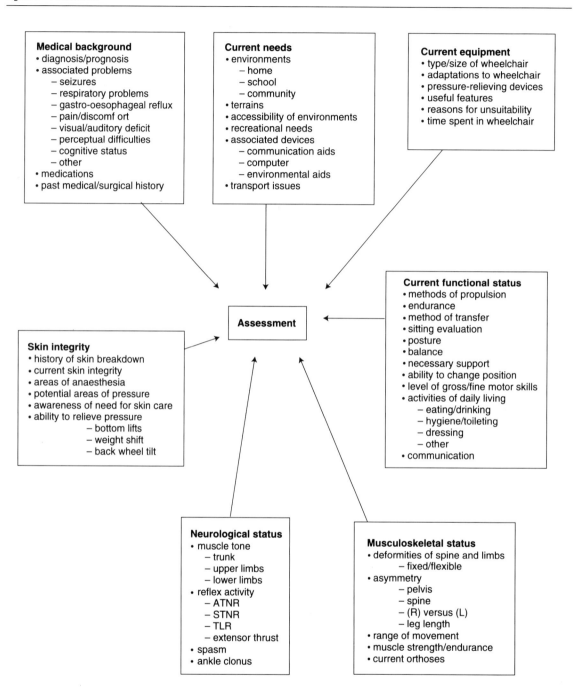

Medical background
• diagnosis/prognosis
• associated problems
  – seizures
  – respiratory problems
  – gastro-oesophageal reflux
  – pain/discomf ort
  – visual/auditory deficit
  – perceptual difficulties
  – cognitive status
  – other
• medications
• past medical/surgical history

Current needs
• environments
  – home
  – school
  – community
• terrains
• accessibility of environments
• recreational needs
• associated devices
  – communication aids
  – computer
  – environmental aids
• transport issues

Current equipment
• type/size of wheelchair
• adaptations to wheelchair
• pressure-relieving devices
• useful features
• reasons for unsuitability
• time spent in wheelchair

Assessment

Current functional status
• methods of propulsion
• endurance
• method of transfer
• sitting evaluation
• posture
• balance
• necessary support
• ability to change position
• level of gross/fine motor skills
• activities of daily living
  – eating/drinking
  – hygiene/toileting
  – dressing
  – other
• communication

Skin integrity
• history of skin breakdown
• current skin integrity
• areas of anaesthesia
• potential areas of pressure
• awareness of need for skin care
• ability to relieve pressure
  – bottom lifts
  – weight shift
  – back wheel tilt

Neurological status
• muscle tone
  – trunk
  – upper limbs
  – lower limbs
• reflex activity
  – ATNR
  – STNR
  – TLR
  – extensor thrust
• spasm
• ankle clonus

Musculoskeletal status
• deformities of spine and limbs
  – fixed/flexible
• asymmetry
  – pelvis
  – spine
  – (R) versus (L)
  – leg length
• range of movement
• muscle strength/endurance
• current orthoses

appropriately supported. Key measurements are shown in Figure 12.

Assistance to maintain pelvic position and trunk alignment should be provided for the measuring. Bergen and Colangelo (1985) suggests the correction of pelvic/trunk position may be difficult for those with tonal problems and may be supplemented with those in supine.

Seat Depth can be determined by measuring from behind the buttocks to the rear of the knee. This measurement is crucial in achieving correct pelvic position and adequate pressure distribution to the pelvis and thighs. If leg length discrepancy is significant the seat depth must accommodate the shortened leg; an asymmetrical seat is often required. The anterior seat edge should clear the popliteal

Figure 12   Key Measurements for Wheelchair Prescription

Body dimensions

a buttock to behind knee
b hip width
c height to inferior angle of scapula
d lower leg length
e elbow height

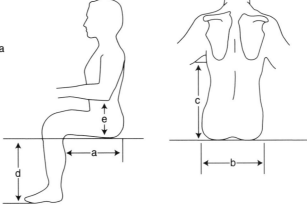

Wheelchair Measurements

A seat depth
B seat width
C backrest height
D seat to
E armrest height
F seat height from floor

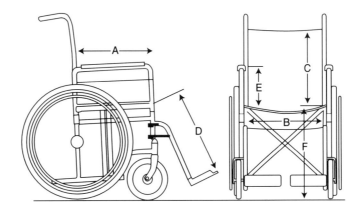

* note: further body dimensions are required for adaptive seating

fossa and calf. Wheelchair cushions should protrude past the front edge of the seat upholstery, but still be clear of the calf.

Seat Width   is based on the width across the hips at the widest point. To determine the appropriate width it is necessary to consider the following factors:

- points of reference of manufacturer's measurement specifications, e.g. width may be measured from outside frame tubes, edge of seat upholstery, or armrest uprights
- need to accommodate seating adaptations (e.g. contoured backrests) and orthotic devices worn (e.g. thoraco lumbar sacral orthosis (TLSO), reciprocating gait orthosis (RGO))
- ability or need for child to access propulsion wheels

- allowance for growth and weight increases of children

The overall width of the wheelchair needs to remain as narrow as possible for improved access and manoeuvrability.

Backrest Height   is determined largely by the amount of support the child requires, and personal preference. For children who self-propel, the backrest needs to be clear of the inferior angle of the scapula. A higher backrest offers more support and comfort; however, increased trunk mobility allowed by a lower back height offers advantages particularly for sport. If a cushion is to be used, this needs to be taken into account when determining the backrest height.

Important Considerations for Seated Mobility

It is important for the physiotherapist to consider not only the benefits of seated mobility, but also the potential for problems. These may include risk of skin and pressure problems, weight gain, reduced potential for reaching a particular level of ambulation, increased flexion contractures at hips and knees and spinal deformity. These can in part be balanced by encouraging the child to spend time both out of the chair and out of the seated position each day.

SKIN CARE

Characteristics of children particularly at risk include:

- limited ability to relieve weight
- anaesthetic skin
- asymmetrical weight distribution or poor sitting posture
- fixed deformity – spine, pelvis, foot/ankle
- slim body build
- past history of pressure areas
- prolonged periods in the chair

Children with spinal disabilities have a combination of many risk factors, especially anaesthetic skin, deformity, prolonged sitting and incontinence. This population has a high incidence of skin breakdown and ulceration (Harris and Banta 1990). At-risk areas in terms of skin breakdown for children with spinal disabilities include ischial tuberosities, coccyx, greater trochanter, the apex of a kyphosis and feet/ankles that are not plantigrade. The greater trochanter may be at risk if the child has significant pelvic obliquity. This will also mean that the ischium under the lower side of the pelvis will be under greater pressures. If correctable, seating should aim to improve the symmetry of the pelvis. If fixed, adaptive seating should accommodate the deformity and/or a specialized pressure cushion be prescribed. This management must be accompanied by a practical skin care regime.

Feet and ankles are at risk of skin breakdown if no shoes are worn and if the foot is in a position of fixed deformity. A square plantigrade foot, flat on the footplate will take some of the weight of the leg without significant pressures. Shoes protect the feet

from bumps and scrapes from walls and furniture and from friction as the feet move over rough footplates. Decisions can be made during the prescription process about the most suitable type of footplate.

A number of children with high-level spina bifida lesions have significant fixed kyphosis (see Figure 13). The apex of this curve is particularly at risk in terms of skin breakdown and must be accommodated in the seating. A loosely slung backrest with sheepskin may be appropriate or a contoured foam backrest with little or no pressure at the apex of the curve may be considered. Attempts to correct a fixed kyphosis will not only cause skin problems but will also make stable upright sitting difficult for the child to achieve.

Preventive management and safe and effective skin care involves the following:

- a regime of regular inspection
- good hygiene
- use of an appropriate sitting surface (cushion)
- appropriate positioning in the chair
- frequent and consistent weight relief (bottom lifts, lateral weight shift, periods of time tilting (wheelies) and not sitting)
- care to prevent injury during transfers

PRESSURE CUSHIONS

Children with anaesthetic skin or those unable to move readily in the chair should have cushioning to distribute pressure away from the 'at risk' bony areas of the ischial tuberosities and sacrum. Cushions may be of medium-density foam or, for the higher risk child, a more specialized pressure cushion with air or gel pieces to distribute the pressure should be used. These cushions should be trialled to assess the child's posture and stability on the cushion, as well as checking the pressure-relieving qualities of the cushion. Cushion-cover tension should not be high as this can totally negate the pressure-relieving qualities of the cushion. Dissipation of heat and moisture are also important factors and using two cushions or covers is usually helpful as incontinence may make control of these factors more difficult. Specialized seating clinics or therapists working in the area may be consulted for further information to help with decision-making.

An ischial or sacral pressure area usually means the

Figure 13 Adolescent with Spina Bifida. A, Fixed kyphosis; B, skin breakdown over apex of deformity; C, kyphosis accommodated with adaptive seating to remove pressure from apex of curve

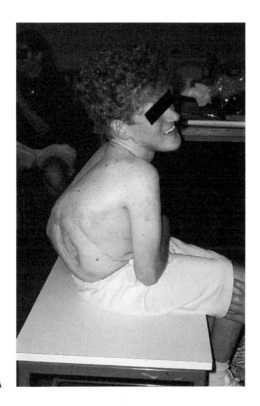

A

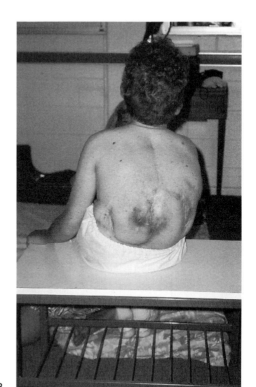

B

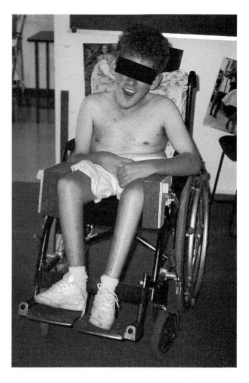

C

child should not sit, but rather lie prone or in side-lying until the skin is healed (see Figure 14). This can be a very slow process. Prevention is the key to effective skin care.

Problem-Solving for Seating

Monitoring of position, fit and function in the wheelchair should be undertaken regularly. Common problems that may be encountered during assessment or review are outlined and explored in Figure 15.

Case 1

Matthew is a 15-year-old boy with Duchenne muscular dystrophy who has been independently mobile in a powerdrive wheelchair (PDC) for 5 years. He attends the local state high school. His current PDC has a flat padded backrest and flat padded

Figure 14   Skin care. A, pressure area on anaesthetic skin; B, prone trolley — allowing independent mobility while pressure area heals

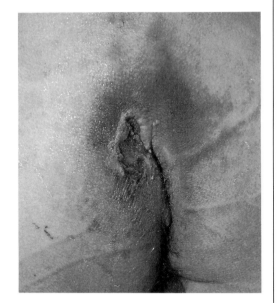

A

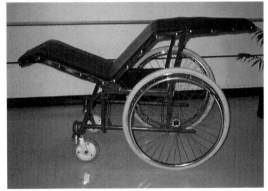

B

seat and a seat belt. The chair has a manually adjustable backrest recline. An appointment was arranged with his community-based physiotherapist and wheelchair company representative for review of his seating as recent deterioration in his muscle power, especially in his head and trunk, were problematic. Matthew underwent spinal instrumentation for his thoracolumbar scoliosis 18 months ago. The spinal fusion had corrected his marked scoliosis; however, the increased rigidity and muscle weakness make Matthew's sitting control unstable.

Matthew reports he feels unsafe in his chair as he has difficulty repositioning his trunk when displaced both forwards and later-

ally. His increasing muscle weakness also makes his neck tired during the day, especially after school. Another significant problem is that he has pressure marks on his feet from the metal footplate. Other relevant findings include marked equinus contracture of both feet, fixed flexion deformities at knees and hips, and increased lumbar lordosis persistent after surgery.

Both Matthew and his parents feel he needs further support in sitting. They have increased the recline of his backrest by a few degrees – this decreases his trunk instability, but appears to give him back pain after a period of time. Improved safety and comfort were the goals of the seating review.

PROBLEM-SOLVING EXERCISE

1. What factors could be contributing to Matthew's back pain?
2. What options are available to decrease pressure problems in his feet?
3. How can support, safety and comfort be increased?

Case 2

Chris is a 6-year-old boy with cerebral palsy in the form of a spastic quadriplegia and has recently started the first year at the local primary school. Chris's intellectual abilities are well within the normal range, though he has some limitation to his expressive language ability.

Chris is presently seated in a standard manual wheelchair with slung upholstery, armrests and a 1" leather pelvic strap which sits high on his stomach. He leans to the (R) and sits with marked lumbar flexion. Chris's mother has been concerned about his posture in the wheelchair. His school therapists agree that his seating is inadequate and arranged a team review with his mother to consider the options available.

Figure 15 Problem-Solving

Problem	Possible causes	Possible solutions
Posterior pelvic tilt *[diagram labelled "Posterior pelvic tilt"]* 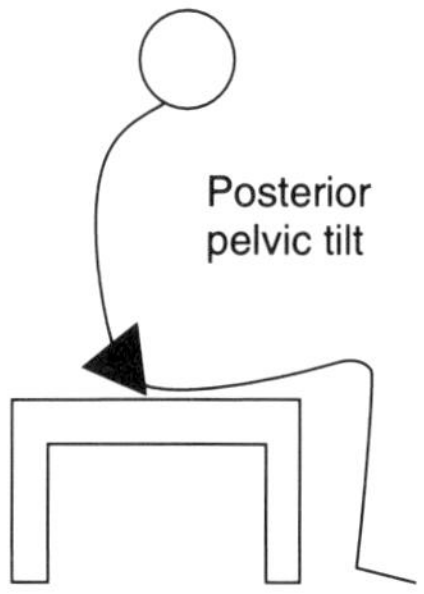	• decreased dynamic sitting control • fixed kyphosis • poor positioning in wheelchair • trunk hypotonia • influence of primitive reflexes • increase in extension tone • decrease ROM of hip flexion • decreased hamstring length • seat depth too long • slung seat • no pelvic strap/incorrect position • footplates too high • stretched backrest upholstery • backrest angle >90°	• teach caregivers correct positioning • position patient with appropriate orientation • pelvic strap correctly positioned • ischial block • knee blocks • firm seat • lumbar roll/space between seat and backrest • appropriate seat length • position feet to accommodate short hamstrings • wedge seat to decrease extensor tone • feet to weight-bear through heels • appropriate seat/back angle
Anterior pelvic tilt 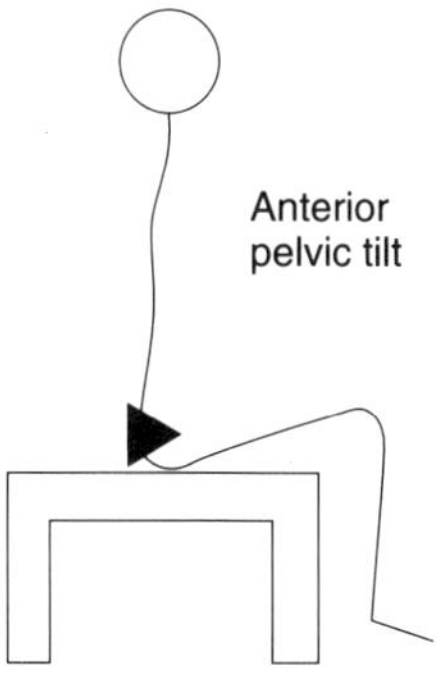 *[diagram labelled "Anterior pelvic tilt"]*	• hypotonia • muscle weakness • fixed flexion at hips • excessive anterior wedge in seat	• reposition pelvic strap • open out seat/backrest angle • rearward tilt in space • check footplate height • reduce anterior wedge in seat
Pelvic obliquity 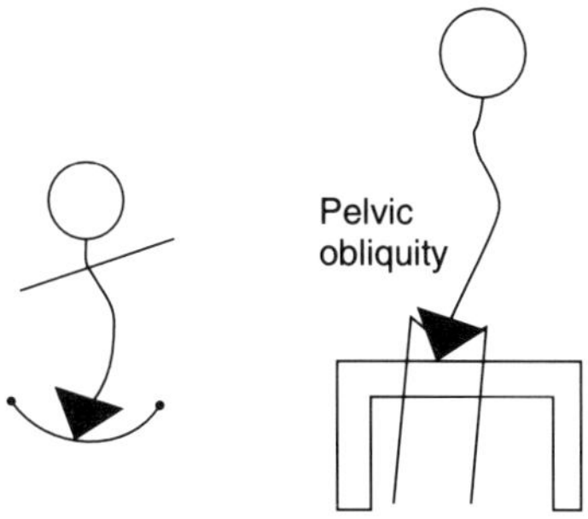 *[diagram labelled "Pelvic obliquity"]*	• Asymmetrical muscle tone strong ATNR • 1 hip does not flex to 90° • fixed scoliosis • seat too long • Dislocated/subluxated hip • slung seat • chair too wide/narrow	• ischial block • pelvic strap • midline positioning of head • firm seat • lateral pelvic blocks (hip guides) • asymmetrical seat may assist • build up in seat may improve obliquity

Figure 15 Continued

Pelvic rotation 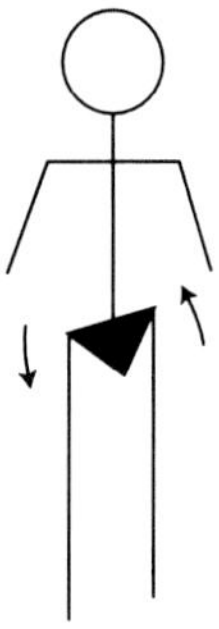	• asymmetrical muscle tone
	• primitive reflexes – ATNR
	• scoliosis with rotational component
	• leg length discrepancy
	• seat depth too long
	• subluxed/dislocated hips
		• midline positioning of head
		• midline positioning of pelvis
		  – pelvic strap
		  – hip guides
		  – knee blocks
		  – firm seat
		• accommodate leg length discrepancy
		• aim for forward orientation of trunk and head if deformity is fixed

Scoliosis 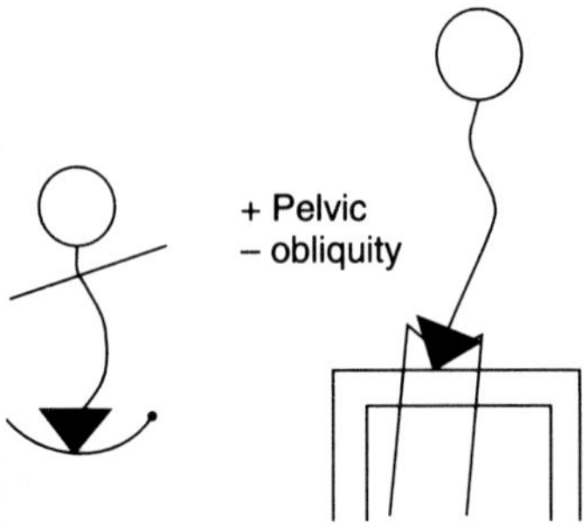 + Pelvic – obliquity	• hypotonic trunk/muscle weakness • asynum muscle tone • ATNR/path reflexes • fixed deformity • combined with pelvic deformity	• midline positioning of head in space • use of tilt-in-space system • customized backrest for correction or accommodation of deformity • midline pelvic position – pelvic blocks (hip guides) • firm seat appropriate length • firm backrest to accommodate deformity if fixed
Increased lordosis 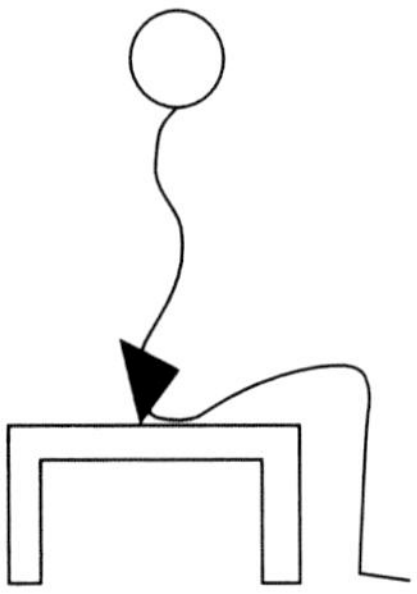	• muscle weakness • fixed/flex • tight hip flex • active hip flex • anterior pelvic tilt	• flat seat rather than anterior wedge • pelvic strap as per anterior pelvic tilt • tilt chair back in orientation • open out seat/backrest angle

Figure 15 Continued

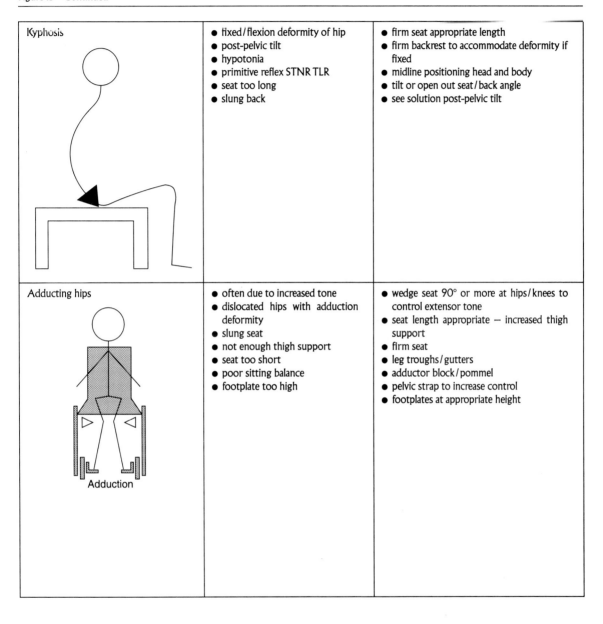

Kyphosis	• fixed/flexion deformity of hip • post-pelvic tilt • hypotonia • primitive reflex STNR TLR • seat too long • slung back	• firm seat appropriate length • firm backrest to accommodate deformity if fixed • midline positioning head and body • tilt or open out seat/back angle • see solution post-pelvic tilt
Adducting hips Adduction	• often due to increased tone • dislocated hips with adduction deformity • slung seat • not enough thigh support • seat too short • poor sitting balance • footplate too high	• wedge seat 90° or more at hips/knees to control extensor tone • seat length appropriate – increased thigh support • firm seat • leg troughs/gutters • adductor block/pommel • pelvic strap to increase control • footplates at appropriate height

Figure 15   Continued

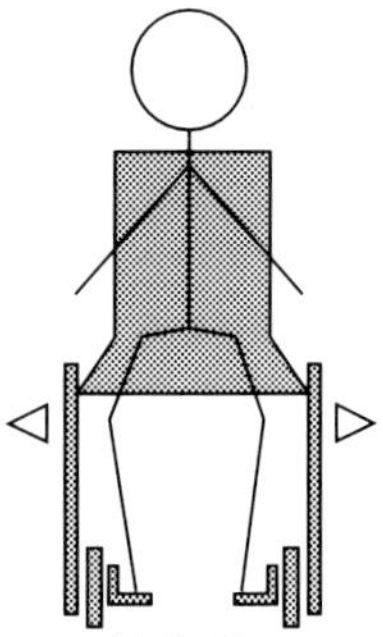 Abducting hips	• muscle weakness / low tone • fixed abduction contracture • insufficient thigh support • footplates too high • foot deformity	• lateral thigh blocks • leg troughs / gutters • appropriate seat length • footplates appropriate height
Abduction		
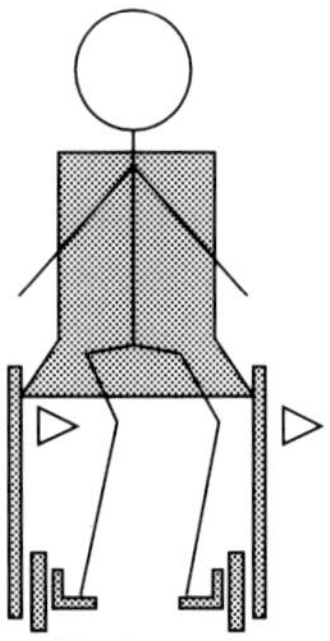 Windsweeping	• asymmetrical muscle tone • fixed adduction deformity one side • sublux / dislocated hip • pelvic / spinal deformity • footplates too high • decreased sitting balance • leg length discrepancy	• pommel / adduction block • lateral thigh block • appropriate seat length • leg troughs • seat appropriate for leg length discrepancy • pelvic strap
Windswept		

Assessment findings include a strong (L) symmetrical tonic neck reflex (ATNR) pattern with greater flexor tone on his (R) side. Chris has no significant spinal deformity, but a windswept posture to the (R). He underwent releases of adductor and hamstring muscles bilaterally 2 years ago. His (L) hand is more functional than the (R). Chris has eating difficulties due to extensor tone, tongue thrust and head position associated with his ATNR pattern and poor seated posture.

PROBLEM SOLVING EXERCISES

1. What changes can be made to achieve the goals of improved posture and function while seated in the chair?
2. Should you consider a powerdrive wheelchair for Chris?
3. What findings support your choice?

Case 3

Kate, aged 14 years, has a spastic quadriplegia as a result of a head injury at 3 years of age. She lives in a small country town where she attends the local high school. Kate's receptive language skills are reasonable, and she is able to indicate 'yes' or 'no' with different tongue positions. Furthermore she is able to use a communication board with her (R) hand if well positioned.

Kate is currently seated in a tilt-in-space wheelchair with an anterior wedged foam seat and deep curved backrest. She is, however, constantly sliding forward into a posterior pelvic tilt position. This places her in a very flexed posture and increases the difficulty Kate has in holding her head up for any period of time. Positioning Kate's pelvis back in the chair and maintaining a symmetrical position has become extremely difficult in the last months, and this affects Kate's ability to communicate. Kate's sitting tolerance has been limited by both discomfort and frustration with the increasing difficulties she has

been having with communication. Kate's therapists have referred her to a specialized seating clinic.

Significant orthopaedic assessment findings include:
- limitation of (L) hip flexion to 70°
- bilateral tight hamstrings limiting the range of knee extension in sitting
- severe fixed thoracic kyphosis

PROBLEM-SOLVING EXERCISES

1. Who are the team members who should be involved in Kate's seating?
2. Identify the seating goals for Kate.
3. Given the assessment findings, identify the major problems with Kate's current adaptive seating inserts.
4. Choose adaptive seating options that will improve Kate's position, comfort and function. State why each was chosen.
5. Discuss why trialling Kate in her new adaptive seating is so important.

Case 4

Liam is turning 16 and was in a motor vehicle accident 3 years ago which resulted in T10 paraplegia. Liam has had a lightweight manual wheelchair which is not only becoming too small, but no longer meets his needs. Liam and his parents have returned to the Children's Hospital where he was an inpatient following the accident, to receive assistance in deciding on a new chair.

Liam is keen to begin playing basketball with the local sporting wheelies team and he wants his new chair to be suitable for this as well as meeting his mobility needs for home and school.

PROBLEM-SOLVING EXERCISES

1. Who could be involved in the wheelchair prescription?

2. Discuss ways to increase Liam's knowledge of options in lightweight manual wheelchairs and his involvement in the prescription process.

3. Choose a chair type with options that will be suitable for Liam, stating why you have chosen each option.

Case 5

Ariel presented as a floppy 19-month-old child with poorly controlled seizure activity. Between seizures Ariel was attentive, smiling and interacting well with her parents. Following a seizure, however, the hypotonia would increase and she became lethargic, sleeping for extended periods of time. Ariel had a 7-month-old baby brother and the two children shared a twin pram for outside mobility. Ariel had two older siblings who attended school and Ariel's mother walked these children to school. This resulted in Ariel spending a significant period of time in her pram each day. Both Ariel's parents and her physiotherapist were concerned that positioning in the pram was difficult.

PROBLEM-SOLVING EXERCISES

1. What styles of mobility devices would be appropriate for a child this age?

2. What factors other than physical findings will be influential in the choice of mobility equipment style?

3. How could Ariel be supported in sitting to improve her posture and function?

4. Consider options available which would accommodate post-seizure lethargy.

Lower Limb Orthoses

The use of orthoses and other assistive devices (e.g. walking frames, standing frames) in the management of children with disability, should contribute towards meeting the goals identified for physiotherapy intervention and thus assist in meeting the needs of the child and family. In particular, lower limb orthoses are used extensively to assist in meeting mobility and functional requirements by allowing the child with disability to stand and ambulate. The benefits of standing and ambulation have been discussed at length in the literature and include both physiological and psychosocial benefits (DeSouza and Carroll 1976, Rosenstein *et al.* 1987, Mazur *et al.* 1989, Charney *et al.* 1991, Stuberg 1992).

The main functions of orthoses are as follows:

- to support the body weight
- to correct dynamic deformity, or slow the progression of deformity; or prevent deformity from occurring
- to control range of movement
- to stabilize joints and limbs
- to improve alignment and in turn biomechanical function
- to positively alter tonal influences
- to assist in the management of pain by providing support
- to assist in joint protection in post-operative rehabilitation
- to facilitate function

Principles of Orthotic Prescription

When considering orthotic prescription the clinician must remember that each component of the lower limb does not function in isolation. The foot is a significant example of this principle. The hindfoot, generally comprised of the talus and calcaneus, has a key role in the total alignment of the foot and in turn the lower limb. The talocrural joint is a pure hinge joint which only allows for plantarflexion and dorsiflexion. The oblique subtalar joint has the key role of coping with the multiaxial movements and forces of the foot. The subtalar joint connections to the midtarsal area transfer these forces to the rest of the foot and direct forces up to higher structures in the lower limb. Establishment of correct alignment at the hindfoot is an important function of any lower limb orthoses. Orthotic devices may provide stability to a joint in one plane while allowing movement in another. Fit and alignment with the anatomical joint is critical.

All orthoses are force systems that act on the body segments. The forces that are generated by an orthosis are limited by skin and subcutaneous tissue tolerance (Rose 1986). The interface between orthoses, skin and subcutaneous tissue is subjected to pressure and shear.

Orthoses should be designed to contour to the limb well and cover an adequate surface area to disperse pressure and forces. Pressure (force per unit area) can be reduced by either increasing the area of application or diminishing the force. Intermittent pressure is tolerated by the skin at much higher levels than constant pressure. Continuous pressure will damage superficial circulation, especially if this is compromised in any way. If the pressure is intermittent and applied slowly, it initially causes thickening and formation of callosities. This is a protective reaction and will completely disappear once the cause is removed. If applied quickly over a short period, skin breakdown may occur. Interface forces should be applied to areas that are more able to sustain pressure and sharp bony prominences with thin or traumatized subcutaneous tissue should be avoided. Shear stress to these areas often causes problems (Rose 1986). The fibro-fatty subcutaneous layer allows the skin to slide over bony points and this protects the tissue from shear forces in normal circumstances. If the skin is adhered to the bone, or if the subcutaneous layer is thinned this does not occur and the tissue is at risk of breaking down.

Heat retention, particularly with close-fitting thermoplastic orthoses, not only causes discomfort but can also cause an increase in the oxygen requirements in tissues of patients with poor peripheral circulation. This may lead to localized tissue necrosis. Sweating and maceration also increase the risk of skin breakdown and invasion of yeasts, fungi and bacteria (Rose 1986). Skin problems are far more likely to occur in those children with anaesthetic skin (see Figure 16) and it becomes very important to teach skin care with regular monitoring and problem-solving for these children and their families.

Orthotic intervention should not be considered for purely cosmetic reasons, for example to make a non-weight-bearing, non-functional foot appear less deformed. Fixed deformity cannot be corrected by orthotic devices, but can be accommodated within the device. Orthoses should not be prescribed as a substitute for appropriate surgery. There is an appropriate time for each intervention and a time for a combination of both.

Clinical Assessment

Thorough assessment is vital to choosing the equipment which is best suited to the child and their presenting problem. Primary aims must be identified to guide the process of appropriate prescription. Orthopaedic, biomechanical, developmental and neurological factors will largely determine the prescription process. Clinical assessment requires subjective information and objective assessment.

Subjective information includes:

- interventions
  - previous and present equipment
  - conservative management, e.g., inhibitory serial casting
  - surgical history

Figure 16 Foot Deformity and Anaesthetic Skin – ulceration from weight-bearing in rigid splint

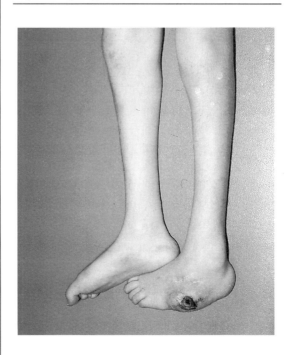

- current problems
- goals of intervention

Objective assessment (with the child appropriately dressed) includes:

- observation of the patient in standing, during gait and other functional activities, with and without equipment as appropriate
- musculoskeletal assessment to establish:
  - passive ranges of movement of joints
  - extensibility of muscles
  - evidence of fixed deformity
  - muscle strength
  - balance of agonist / antagonist
  - leg length
- skin sensation and integrity
- neurological / neurodevelopmental assessment
  - influence of tone and reflexes at rest / function.
  - posture and balance
  - sensorimotor status
- footwear and orthotic wear patterns

Physical findings cannot be considered in isolation. Family needs, life style, environment, compliance with the therapy programme and cultural aspects should also be incorporated into the prescription process. Factors influencing the prescription process are shown in Figure 17.

Characteristics of Orthoses

The various characteristics of orthoses need to be considered in relation to how they might impact on the child and family. Not all characteristics are compatible at any one time or in any one situation. However, if you consider goals, relevant assessment findings, and the features of the orthoses, assist in an appropriate choice.

Characteristics of orthotic devices to consider when prescribing are as follows:

functional outcome	static and dynamic comfort
weight	stability / stiffness / flexibility
energy demands during use	ease of donning and doffing
ease of toileting	potential for pressure problems
potential for heat retention	potential for skin reaction

noise during function	time for manufacture / replacement
reliability	adjustability
cost	cosmesis

Materials used for orthoses commonly include thermoplastics, foams, leather and metal. These materials provide the orthoses with various properties. The use of thermoplastics has significant advantages in orthotic design and function.

An understanding of the available orthotic options and other standing / ambulatory devices is necessary for appropriate selection of the aid required, and for the prescription process to be completed. Commonly used lower limb orthoses and aids are discussed.

Footwear

The components that make up a 'good' shoe such as a firm heel counter, adequate cushioning in the sole, arch support and appropriate 'last' shape (listed as important for sportspersons in literature), are applicable also to children. Cost, however, does not necessarily indicate the efficiency of a shoe.

Footwear no matter how well made is readily shaped and distorted by the forces of the body and reactions to the ground. Many thermoplastic orthoses can be fitted into most shoes. As the rigid orthosis holds the foot in the corrected position then the components of the shoe and cost become less crucial to the control of the foot. Despite this, a well-fitting shoe is still important. Most orthoses require shoes to be a half-size bigger than the regular size for the child. Firm leather shoes and boots are often too rigid when combined with moulded orthoses indicating the need to use softer sport-style shoes. These are also more cosmetically acceptable to children and families.

Leather-style footwear usually in a boot form can still provide valuable assistance to some biomechanical problems. The leather upper, heeled boot provides a number of advantages:

- the upper is more resistant to deforming processes, but not unchanging
- the heel provides a firm basis for mounting of calliper ferrules
- sole modifications if used can be fitted, e.g., wedges, flares
- the heel height in a boot may allow or improve weight-bearing through the heel, especially for

Figure 17 Factors Influencing Prescription Process

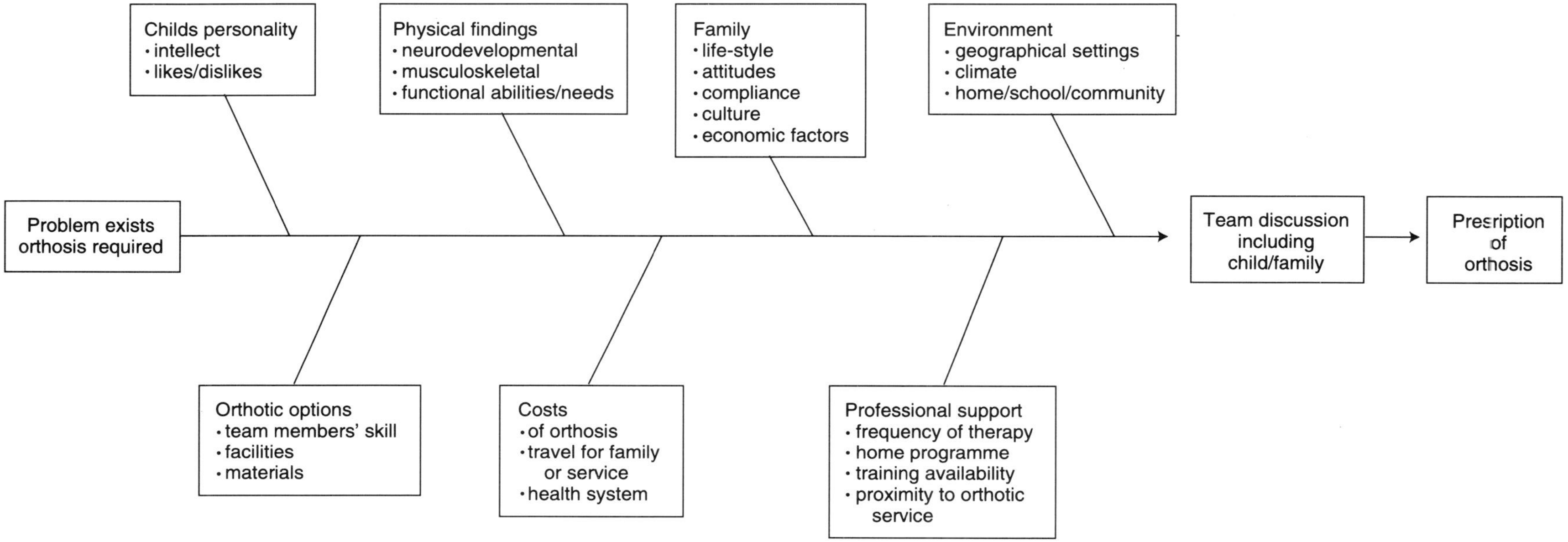

those children with reduced dorsiflexion during gait. This increased weight-bearing may assist in normalizing tone.

Disadvantages of this type of boot include:

- the boot can 'hide' abnormality in the foot
- the materials can be deformed by forces
- it can be expensive and cosmetically unappealing

Although boot footwear was previously used, more recent research now questions effectiveness. Wedging of the calcaneal area of a simple shoe innersole is still used to influence heel varus and valgus but this deformity must be mobile.

Build-ups for leg length differences should be assessed carefully. Modern synthetic materials used for the sole of shoes may cause difficulties in attaching the build-up. This issue should be discussed with the orthotist or technician undertaking the work. The actual length difference found on assessment may not need to be added to the shoe. The build-up required is often decided by using blocks under the shorter leg. Appropriate correction is judged by posterior superior iliac spine (PSIS) alignment.

Minor length differences may require no intervention at all. Build-ups should always be placed along the entire sole of the shoe, not just the heel, as this places the child's ankle in a plantarflexed (equinus) position. For large build-ups it is important to consider using lightweight materials such as cork to keep the shoe as light as possible and prevent the build-up itself contributing to abnormal gait. As with all equipment, the influence of the build-up in the growing child requires monitoring. In some cases the build-up may be reduced and in the long-term removed.

Foot Orthoses

These orthoses include numerous items varying in their manufacture material, the extent of foot contact and in turn control (Lockard 1988). As noted earlier, the foot is a complex structure in which each component is highly interrelated to the other components. An orthosis such as a calcaneal cup, directly contacts one or limited components to influence the alignment problems of the foot. More complex problems may require an orthosis that controls the majority of the foot such as a UCBL (Figure 18). It is stressed again that fixed deformity cannot be corrected by orthotic intervention.

The use of foot orthoses is controversial and considered to be one of the most overprescribed orthoses in paediatrics. This is often due to their use in the management of the non-neurological, physiological or flexible flatfoot. Clinicians must remain cognisant that it is normal for a child to present with a flat or minimal arch and pronated foot posture up to 4 years of age. Orthotic intervention is indicated in the flexible flatfoot only if persistent pain or malalignment limits normal function. Orthopaedic consultation is recommended to exclude conditions such as vertical talus, accessory navicular, tarsal coalition and tarsal/metatarsal bar. Foot orthoses should not be applied for cosmesis alone.

Hindfoot alignment can be influenced by simple innersole wedges, but often heel cups, calcaneal cups or UCBL inserts are useful. The plastic is moulded to hold the hindfoot and importantly the subtalar joint in a normal position for age and the inserts are worn in normal footwear. See Figure 18.

For midfoot or arch support there is a wide range of materials such as foam, rubber or sorbathan which may be commercially available. Some customized shoe inserts used to correct deformity are manufactured from various materials such as foam, thermoplastics, pelite, rubber and leather, and may include full foot support.

Figure 18   Foot Orthoses: Manufacture of UCBL from cast

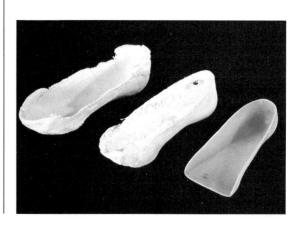

It should be noted that rigid orthoses used to hold or correct significant deformity can induce marked pressure problems in the area of skin contact. These moulded orthoses tend to increase the rigidity of the foot, require regular replacement due to growth and are expensive. As highlighted previously, these items due to the range of materials and design should be prescribed with care and thought.

Ankle–Foot Orthoses (AFO)

This term refers to a number of individual devices which are made with various materials and styles, but in general their effect influences the position and function of the foot and ankle. AFOs may also influence the rest of the lower limb and the overall function of the child. These orthoses address mobility problems resulting from a variety of conditions (Cusick 1988). A selection of AFOs is shown in Figure 19.

The following orthoses are described: below knee iron (BKI); and thermoplastic AFOs which include solid AFO, ground-reaction AFO, hinged AFO and tone-reducing orthosis (TRO).

BELOW KNEE IRON (BKI)

The BKI or short calliper has been used for many years to aid in the control of lower limb problems particularly in children with cerebral palsy and spina bifida. Its application with an anterior strap is based on the three-point brace system with the calf band and ferrule pins of the heel of the shoe posteriorly opposing the anterior force of the leather anterior strap located at the level of the talocrural joint.

The BKI provides some lateral stability to the ankle whilst allowing active plantarflexion and dorsiflexion. The anterior strap places the ankle in dorsiflexion and thus limits the range of plantarflexion available. This limits toewalking gait and encourages active dorsiflexion. The dorsiflexed ankle position may also assist in limiting hyperextension of the knee in some children. The addition of range stops can predetermine the range of either dorsiflexion or plantarflexion allowed. The BKI can be considered as a dynamic orthosis allowing some movement of the ankle dur-

Figure 19 Ankle Foot Orthosis. A, Selection of AFOs—solid AFO, boot and BKI, TRO, GRAFO; B, more recently developed hinged AFO

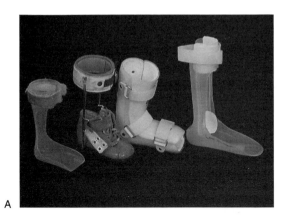

A

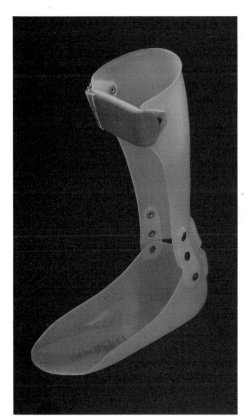

B

ing gait and other activities such as squatting and climbing.

A T-strap attachment to the boot may be fitted to the BKI to assist in the support of an overpronating or pes planus component of foot deformity. The correction offered by this is somewhat limited if it is attached to the outside of the boot upper material. Some attempts at internal attachment have been a little more successful.

The BKI may be of benefit in children with some hypertonia following inhibitory plaster casting, as it supports the weakened ankle, encourages dorsiflexion and allows functional activities. A BKI is contraindicated for a foot influenced by strong abnormal tone or for a foot which barely achieves a plantigrade position. The use of a BKI may cause pain or encourage midfoot hypermobility or 'broken foot' appearance.

In this case, the talocrural joint has limited dorsiflexion, and the orthosis induces a dorsiflexion force resulting in movement occurring at the subtalar and midtarsal area. Regular monitoring of true talocrural joint dorsiflexion range is therefore necessary. This example highlights the importance of correcting any hindfoot deformity (e.g. valgus position) and reestablishing subtalar alignment before assessing the range of dorsiflexion available in the foot when prescribing any orthotic device incorporating the foot. Figure 20 shows correct and incorrect assessments of the foot of a child with cerebral palsy.

The boot used with a BKI can also 'mask' foot deformity and where movement is occurring in the foot. This orthosis therefore is not a good option for a child with significant 'broken foot' posture. It can be very effective, however, with mild to moderate foot malalignment and tonal problems. Shoe condition and sole wear patterns must be monitored regularly.

THERMOPLASTIC AFO

The thermoplastic AFOs have a foot component and a tibial component. These may be one continuous piece or two pieces, as in the hinged AFO. The rigidity/flexibility of the AFO is determined by a number of factors including the type and thickness of the material used, amount of enclosure of the foot and tibial component, length of plantar surface contact and shoe style chosen.

Thermoplastic moulding provides a close fit and thus pressure distribution and movement control. Hypermobile feet and ankle deformities can be realigned and held effectively, incorporating the effects of foot orthotics such as subtalar control and arch support. Thermoplastic materials resist deforming forces bet-

Figure 20   Child with Cerebral Palsy. A, Medial view of pathologically aligned foot; B, incorrect assessment of ankle range of movement; C, appropriate assessment of ankle range with heel aligned

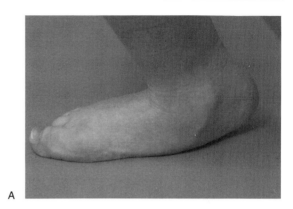

A

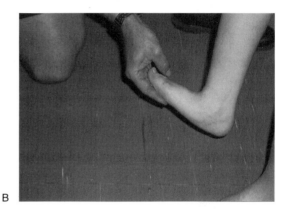

B

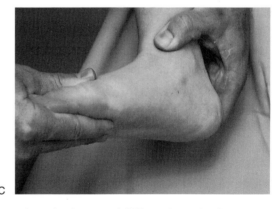

C

ter than the boot and BKI, and can be fitted into 'normal' footwear. Pressure on the common peroneal nerve should be avoided by finishing 10–15 mm distal to the head of fibula.

The manufacture of thermoplastic orthoses requires specific materials, facilities and skills. Due to the child's growth and close fit, regular replacement is necessary and this has financial implications.

SOLID AFO

This is one of the most commonly used orthotic devices and has application to numerous conditions and problems. Use of this orthosis has shown improvements in muscle function, gait patterns and efficiency for disabled children (Jones and Knapp 1987, Thomas et al. 1989).

A standard solid AFO prevents ankle movement and is generally set into 2–3° of dorsiflexion. It is designed to limit footdrop posture or excessive plantarflexion as commonly seen in children with cerebral palsy. Foot alignment is well controlled. Dorsiflexion range needs to be monitored carefully. If plantargrade is not achieved the heel can lift out of the orthosis and pressure problems can arise. A solid AFO used for standing and walking should not be set into plantarflexion as this would have implications for body alignment and gait. In the case of limited dorsiflexion, inhibitory casting or surgical intervention would be required before orthotic use.

The rigidity or support provided by the foot component can be adjusted by the height of the medial and lateral walls of the orthosis and the amount of plantar surface support. In children with excessive toe grasp and extensor thrust the plantar support should extend under the metatarsal heads and toes.

The angle of the tibial component can be set at 5–7° of dorsiflexion to limit the common problem of knee hyperextension or 'back kneeing' which can be common in hemiplegia patients, or in patients after surgical lengthening of the hamstrings. It is vital to establish whether the hyperextension posture of the knee is due to lack of control of the quadriceps or as a compensatory response to excessive plantarflexion or equinus posture of the ankle. In this case the child extends the knee to obtain heel contact during the gait cycle. See Figure 21.

Children in the solid AFO who rely on its use throughout their daily activities will normally develop some calf muscle wasting and families should be advised of this prior to application. Children with variable tone such as athetosis and ataxia can have difficulties with moulded orthoses due to rub and excessive movement in the device.

Figure 21 Control of Hyperextension. A, Hyperextending knees; B, control of hyperextension with solid AFO set in dorsiflexion. Nonslip soles negate the need for shoes. Note use of posterior walker.

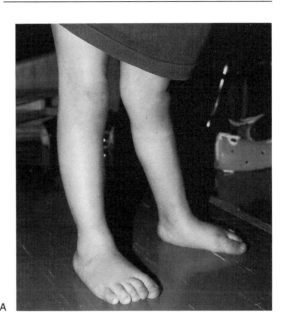

A

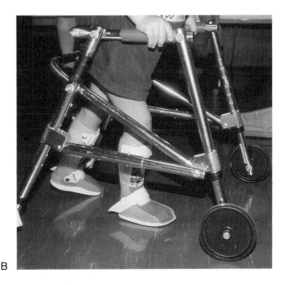

B

GROUND REACTION AFO (GRAFO)

This style of AFO has the same foot aspects of all thermoplastic AFOs but the tibial component is set on the anterior surface of the tibia. The mechanics of this device is that at heelstrike and stance phase the tibial component limits the amount of forward travel of the tibia and limits dorsiflexion range at the ankle, thereby assisting the knee extension capabilities of the patient. This style of AFO is used often for children with spina bifida or cerebral palsy who pre-

Figure 22 Child with Cerebral Palsy. A, In crouch gait; B, note improved posture of child with GRAFO

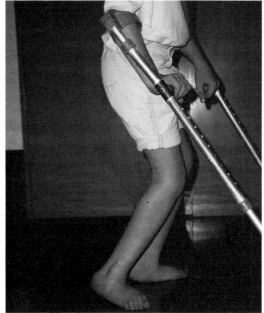

A

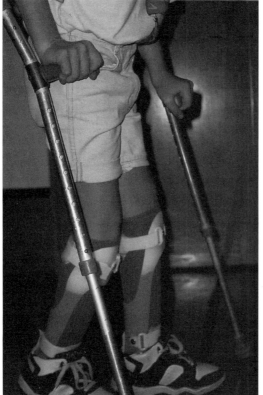

B

sent with an excessive crouched or flexion posture at hips, knees and ankle (Figure 22).

Children with spina bifida and L4 lesions, and children with cerebral palsy who stand with knee flexion due to overlengthened tendoachilles benefit particularly from this AFO (Knutson and Clark 1991). The child must, however, have adequate knee control as the AFO places them in a more extended position. The angle of the tibial component can be altered as with the solid AFO but dorsiflexion range is limited generally to 2–3°. The more plantarflexion in the orthosis, the greater the extension force applied to the knee, with knee stability enhanced. Resistance to forward progression, however, is increased (Yang et al. 1986).

HINGED AFO

This device applies the basic principles of the solid AFO but allows for more dynamic activity at the ankle and in turn the whole lower limb. This provides significant functional advantages for the child in various positions, e.g. squatting, slopes and rough ground (Cusick 1990). The BKI allows some of these dynamic functions. The hinge is set to allow plantarflexion/dorsiflexion at the ankle. The range of each movement can be set with the adjustment of the hinge or the application of a lip in the thermoplastic to limit range. There are various hinge styles available (Knutson and Clark 1991). The amount of range allowed is decided during the prescription process, but most commonly plantarflexion range is limited by the device. Some modification to the allowed motion may be possible with adjustments to the orthosis. The hinges are commonly applied to the standard AFO design; however, they may be used with ground-reaction AFOs if the range of both dorsiflexion and plantarflexion are set. Hip and knee mechanics will alter with the range variations.

This orthosis allows the child to move through half-kneeling, squat to stand and climb, but more importantly it allows for a more normal gait cycle by permitting ankle movement. Research has shown that a hinged AFO is more energy efficient and presents a more normal gait pattern than the solid AFO (Middleton et al. 1988). Care needs to be taken with its application to the athetoid child due to excessive movement and rub. The child with rigid spasticity may also have difficulty with foot position because of tonal influences; however, the use of the hinged AFO in this population is not totally contra-indicated. The child must have easily obtainable ranges of both dorsiflexion and plantarflexion as set in the orthosis manufacture. Limited range of movement can lead to the heel lifting in the orthosis causing rub and poor gait mechanics.

TONE-REDUCING ORTHOSES (TRO)

This thermoplastic orthosis is based upon the principles of the solid AFO but is used more as a therapy tool than an all-day mobility device. The development of this device, especially in Australia, can be attributed to the work of the Queensland Spastic Welfare League. It was designed for use after inhibitory plaster casting with the angle of dorsiflexion set between 5 and 12°. This enables the improved dorsiflexion range gained during casting to be maintained and use of the calf muscles in outer range whilst the child is active. This position also strongly reinforces a heel-strike gait thus improving both tone and gait pattern.

The orthosis is worn from 1 to 2 hours daily to maintain the range achieved. The TRO usually consists of a solid AFO with an anterior leaf which is held in place by at least three velcro attachments, thus totally enclosing the lower leg and foot. This leaf is integral to control of tone and to the strength of the device, especially with older or heavier children. A hole may be cut through the sole at the heel to increase proprioceptive input to the heel and allow the position of the heel in the orthosis to be checked. The entire orthosis usually has a thin foam lining for increased comfort. *Caution*: A dorsiflexion angle set at > 12° can induce an abnormally flexed posture in the lower limb and in turn increase hamstring activity and thus be detrimental to the child.

Knee–Ankle–Foot Orthoses (KAFO)

The knee–ankle–foot orthosis or long leg brace may be used to control motion and alignment of knee and ankle and to support the body weight when standing. The KAFO may be indicated for problems including weakness or paralysis of the lower limb, involuntary movement, hypertonicity, hyperextension of the

Figure 23 Long Leg Callipers in Long Leg Sitting, note knee pads to maintain extension

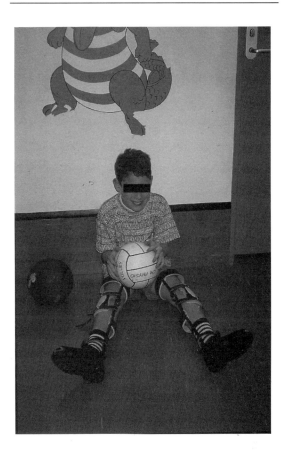

knee, genu valgum or varum and knee flexion contracture.

The more traditional bilateral KAFO or bilateral long leg calliper (LLC) consists of leather-covered metal thigh (and calf bands) with steel stirrups which affix into boots. The boot is attached and an integral part of the orthoses. This style of KAFO was commonly used as a therapy tool in the management of hyper-tonicity rather than an ambulating orthosis in the child with cerebral palsy or for the child with marked knee extension weakness.

With the knee held in a more extended position with a knee pad, emphasis on hip extension and abduction strengthening can be undertaken. Hamstring length-ening can easily be incorporated into the therapy programme with activities in long sitting (Figure 23). The more recent KAFOs are moulded plastic foot/calf back shells (solid AFO) attached by one or two metal uprights (usually incorporating a knee hinge) to an intimately fitting plastic thigh band. This orthosis

Figure 24 KAFOs: A Child with Spina Bifida Ambulating with Elbow Crutches

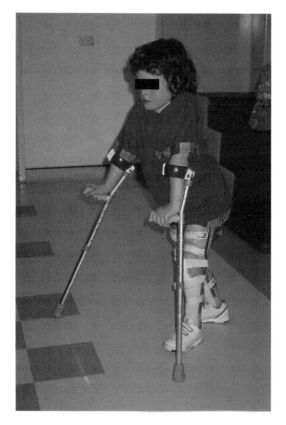

can be used with a variety of shoes. The features of thermoplastic AFOs and BKIs have already been discussed and these principles can be applied to assist with prescribing either callipers or plastic-moulded KAFOs. See Figure 24.

A cushion-heeled shoe is recommended with the plastic/metal solid ankle KAFO (Krebs *et al.* 1988) as this permits a few degrees of 'plantarflexion' of the shank relative to the floor. The knee can be supported to prevent it from giving way in the presence of weak or non-functioning quadriceps and also to assist in the control of genu varum or genu valgum and improve alignment of the leg.

Knee pads over patella or an anterior strap over the proximal tibia may be used to hold the knee in extension. Genu valgum/varum straps may be incorporated into knee pad and buckle around either the medial or lateral upright to assist in the control of valgus or varus and achieve more vertical alignment. A variety of knee joints and knee locks or a free-swinging knee joint may be used, depending on the needs of the child.

In the past, children with spina bifida with an apparent valgus thrust at the knee during gait (weight acceptance), were often braced above the knee with KAFOs. Recent investigations using three-dimensional gait analysis indicates that the valgus thrust in many of these children is mainly a visual effect — confounded by excessive internal rotation of the pelvis, progressive knee flexion and an externally rotated flail foot (Ounpuu *et al.* 1992).

Krebs *et al.* (1988), in a study to determine whether there were any significant differences between thermoplastic/metal and leather/metal KAFOs found most children preferred the plastic/metal orthoses. These authors suggest that the advantages of the newer plastic/metal KAFO over the traditional leather/metal KAFO include:

- lighter in weight
- faster and more easily donned and doffed
- improved hindfoot varus/valgus control
- more effective control of hip and knee motion in the sagittal plane
- different shoes can be used
- speed advantages in timed ADL tests (possibly related to weight advantage)
- more cosmetically acceptable.

The disadvantages of the thermoplastic/metal KAFOs which may be relevant for some children include:

- hotter during summer months
- skin irritations more common
- less tolerant of growth because of close fit
- limited ankle motion may cause difficulties on slopes and rough ground

Orthoses Which Offer Control of the Hip Joint

Attachments to the KAFO are necessary for some children to maintain proper body alignment, to control weightbearing and to prevent, control or facilitate motion at the hip.

TWISTERS

Twister cables or elastics may be used judiciously when there is abnormal internal rotation at the hip joint, tibial torsion or muscle imbalance which results in

Figure 25 Twister Cables Attached to AFOs to Correct Intoeing

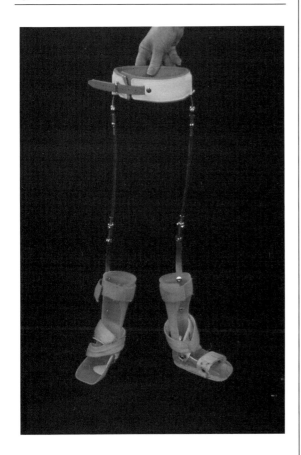

marked intoeing during stance and gait (Figure 25). The use of these orthoses is generally limited to children with lower level paraplegia more commonly of congenital origin. The aim is to achieve a more normal gait pattern by correcting or improving the rotational alignment and orientation of the lower limb. The twisters are designed to store energy in the cables or elastic. This is supplied when the orthosis is applied and produces a potentially corrective force.

Excessive internal tibial torsion in children with spina bifida has been classified as dynamic, when it is secondary to an imbalance between medial or lateral hamstrings, or fixed (Golski and Menelaus 1976). This torsion is associated with an in-toed gait with the patient tripping easily. External tibial torsion is always fixed and often accompanied by progressive valgus of the hindfoot and midfoot (Fraser and Menelaus 1993). The control of this deformity with an orthosis is rarely successful (Nicol and Menelaus

1983). Both torsional deformities result in awkward gait patterns with associated problems such as excessive shoe wear, difficulties with orthoses and secondary skin breakdown.

For those patients with internal tibial torsion, Fraser and Menelaus (1993) suggest that twister cables may improve the gait while they are being used, but have no influence on fixed deformity. Surgical intervention may be necessary.

Rotational or torsional deformities of the lower leg may also be controlled and compensated for with an orthosis that fixes long leg orthosis to the pelvis or trunk – the HKAFO. If the child has adequate hip and knee control, free hip and knee joints may be used to allow active movement in the sagittal plane during gait and also allow for crawling and sitting while wearing the orthosis. Hip rotation straps may be applied to the KAFO to control the amount of hip motion in the transverse plane, i.e. amount of internal rotation, and to encourage more active hip extension (see Figure 26).

HIP–KNEE–ANKLE–FOOT ORTHOSES (HKAFO)

The hip–knee–ankle–foot orthosis may be used to control movement and alignment at each of these joints allowing the child to maintain an upright position against gravity and to become mobile in this position. This orthosis has been used commonly with patients with congenital or acquired paraplegia. Hip joints and a pelvic or waist band are attached to the lateral uprights of KAFOs in the standard traditional HKAFO (Figure 27).

Most HKAFO hip joints have a single axis motion in the sagittal plane, i.e. flexion and extension, while controlling abduction/adduction and rotation. If the hip locks are undone a free range of flexion and extension at the hips may be possible. Aligning the orthotic hip joint with the greater trochanter of the femurs is necessary. More recently, a lock allowing hip abduction for toileting has been designed.

When using the traditional HKAFO with pelvic band and locked hip joints, the child learns to swivel, hop-to and finally achieve a swing-through gait pattern. If the hip joints are unlocked in children without active hip extension they will need to compensate for this lack,

Figure 26 Rotator Strap Attached to Long Leg Callipers. A, No knee hinges; B, child with spina bifida ambulating — intoeing corrected and hip extension facilitated

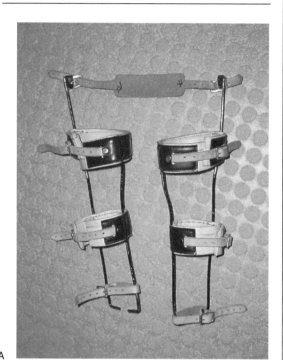

A

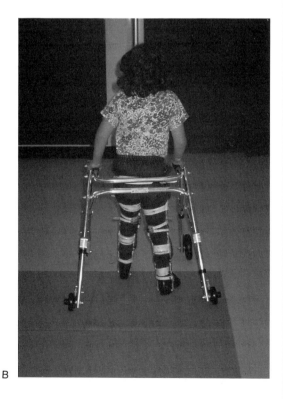

B

Figure 27 HKAFO — Gait Training with Anterior Walker for Child with Spina Bifida (with active hip flexion)

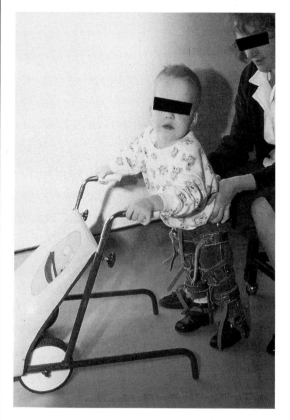

by either excessive use of the upper limbs for weight bearing, or by maintaining erect posture by hyperextending the lumbar spine and shifting the centre of gravity posteriorly. If active hip flexion is possible, one or both hip joints may be unlocked and a reciprocal gait pattern attempted.

A thoracic brace may be attached to the HKAFO for a child with limited trunk control. This usually results in a child with extremely limited mobility. A range of other orthoses including parapodium and reciprocating orthoses are often found to be more successful for these children.

Reciprocating Orthoses

In an effort to provide patients with high-level spinal paraplegia the opportunity to ambulate, a range of reciprocating orthoses have been developed. These types of HKAFOs allow both congenital and acquired paraplegic patients to stand and achieve a reciprocal gait pattern using crutches or a walking frame. The orthoses discussed include the reciprocating gait orthosis (RGO), the hip guidance orthosis (Parawalker) and the Walkabout device with KAFOs.

RECIPROCATING GAIT ORTHOSIS (RGO)

The reciprocating gait orthosis (RGO) provides stability for the joints of the lower limbs while supporting the trunk and pelvis. The RGO allows ambulation in a reciprocal pattern and dynamically couples flexion of one hip with extension of the contralateral hip. This effectively compensates for the lack of hip extensor power and the resultant forward pelvic tilt and lordotic posture (Douglas et al. 1983) seen commonly in children with high level spina bifida or spinal cord injury.

The Louisiana State University (LSU) RGO consists of bilateral HKAFOs connected by an extended pelvic band with two cables cross-connected to opposite sides of each hip joint (Douglas et al. 1983). A single cable and horizontal cable, rather than the dual cable system, were early modifications to the original orthosis.

More recently the cables have been replaced by a centrally pivoting bar and tie rod arrangement. This RGO called the isocentric RGO maintains the same function as the original RGO. Many clinics are beginning to use the isocentric RGO in preference to the cabled RGO as physiological cost index (PCI) has been shown to be reduced (Winchester et al. 1993) and breakages are thought to be less common.

Using a walking frame or elbow crutches, ambulation in the RGO is achieved by a diagonal weight shift to one leg and a leaning back with the upper part of the trunk (trunk and hip extension or 'tuck') to facilitate hip flexion, and hence stepping of the unweighted leg. This is repeated for the opposite side and thus a reciprocal stepping gait with both stance and swing phases begins. No active motor function in the lower limbs (thoracic level of lesion) is necessary; however, symmetrical activity in the hip flexors (lumbar level of lesion) is beneficial (Guidera et al. 1993). Alignment (static and dynamic) in the orthosis is necessary.

Gait training needs to begin in the parallel bars, with the physiotherapist moving the child passively through the movement of walking and then encouraging active participation, working towards smooth, even strides. The child progresses to a walking frame, then to elbow crutches as able. The resulting gait pattern is more acceptable to patients and parents. Increased speed, smoothness and reciprocating gait pattern have been identified as the major reasons for the popularity of this orthosis with patients (Yngve et al. 1984). The hip and knee locks are able to be released to allow the child to sit. See Figure 28.

Careful patient selection and close monitoring are necessary for those patients who are to use the RGO. Strong personal and family motivation appear essential. Patients with obesity, scoliosis, spasticity and upper extremity weakness have been found to be less likely to successfully ambulate using this orthosis (Guidera et al. 1993). These authors suggest other criteria for successful ambulation with the RGO to include good trunk control and standing balance, knee contractures less than 30°, hip contractures less than 45° and previous standing and walking.

Advantages of the RGO include:

- lightweight
- reciprocal gait pattern
- reduced energy consumption
- cosmetically acceptable

Disadvantages include:

- expensive
- many contraindications
- independent donning difficult
- difficulty sit ↔ stand

PARAWALKER OR HIP GUIDANCE ORTHOSIS (HGO)

Not unlike the RGO, the ParaWalker or hip guidance orthosis (HGO) provides low-energy reciprocal ambulation for both children and adults with high-level spinal cord lesions (Butler and Major 1987). This device was developed at ORLAU in the UK and is only available through accredited prescribing and manufacturing agencies. This makes it less accessible to some children.

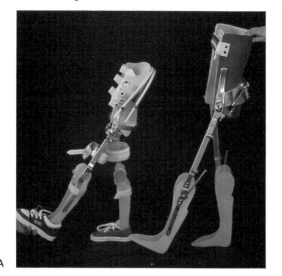

A

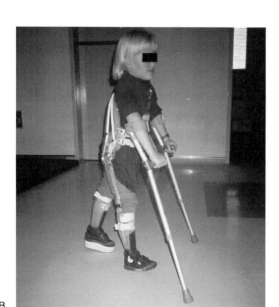

B

Figure 28 Reciprocating Gait Orthosis. A, Dual cables LSU RGO and isocentric RGO – facilitating stepping; B, child with flail lower limbs ambulating in RGO with elbow crutches – note upright stance and heel rise on (L) leg; C, isocentric RGO – note central pivot mechanism; D, note sitting function in RGO

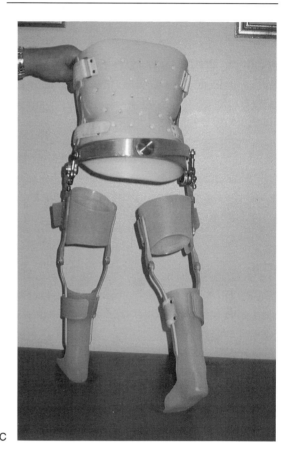

C

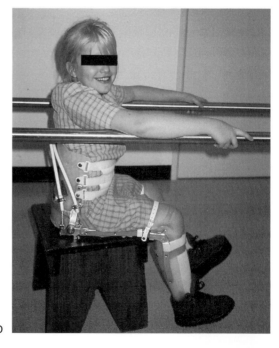

D

Callipers stabilize knees and ankles and attach to a close-fitting rigid body brace with special hip joints with limited range of flexion and extension available. The low friction hip joint allows motion only in the one plane. The hip joint locks release manually to allow sitting. The knees release automatically as contact is made with the back of the chair via the bale lock knee release mechanism or a manually operated knee release mechanism. The callipers are attached to a shoe plate which incorporates a rocker sole and is set in dorsiflexion. The rigid body brace helps maintain the relative abduction of the legs during the swing phase of the gait cycle. Figure 29 shows the Para-Walker.

Figure 29 ParaWalker: posterior view

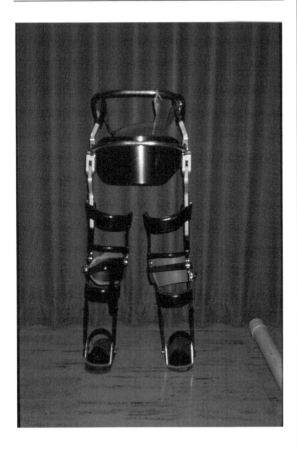

Figure 30 Walkabout: note low frictional joint creating spacing between KAFOs. Abdominal bracing belt not attached

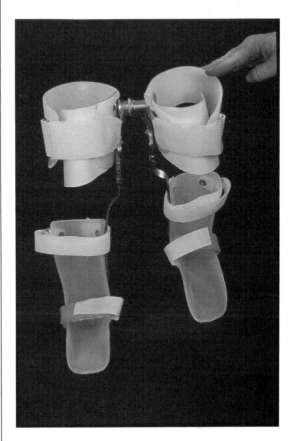

The body weight is always partially supported by the stance leg and the pathway of the centre of mass of the body approximates that of normal walking. Butler and Major (1987) suggest that many patients find the reciprocal style of walking more aesthetically pleasing than a swing-through gait. Good arm and latissimus dorsi function is necessary to use crutches with the ParaWalker. The design and the ability to modify the orthoses mean that a wide range of deformities can be accommodated and this characteristic in addition to the strength and the stability of the ParaWalker are features that allow this orthosis to be useful for patients who may not be accommodated with the RGO.

WALKABOUT

This Australian-made device attached to KAFOs was originally designed for use by adult paraplegics following spinal cord injury (Kirtley 1992). A non-detachable version has been produced for the paediatric population. While the use of this device for both children and adults warrants further investigation, this device has proven to be useful as a walking orthosis for some patients. See Figure 30.

This stainless steel low-friction joint is attached to the medial uprights of KAFOs and acts to space the legs apart controlling both abduction/adduction and rotation at the hip. Two inguinal straps connect the device and thus KAFOs to an abdominal bracing belt. Hip stability and stance are achieved because hyper-extension of the lumbar spine keeps the body's centre of gravity posterior to the hip joints (Kirtley 1992). Tension of the anterior straps assists in controlling the lumbar lordosis. Unlike the other reciprocating orthoses, the centre of rotation of the Walkabout does not align with the anatomical hip joint because of its position between the legs.

Kirtley (1992) suggests the following indications for use of the Walkabout:

- mobile thoracolumbar spine

- able to achieve an upright erect trunk
- to fit suitably into KAFOs
- no fixed flexion contracture at the hips
- appropriate upper limb function and strength

Caution: if localized hyperextension or 'shelving' of vertebrae in the lumbar spine is present or occurs above or below spinal rods or fusion, the device may not be suitable.

EQUIPMENT WHICH OFFERS FREE-STANDING

There are a range of standing devices which will be discussed under this heading. These include, standing frame, parapodium, swivel walker, and multiuser standing frames. The free-standing allowed by these devices, gives the child an opportunity to play in a well supported position. Fine motor activities and self-feeding are ideal to do during this standing time. Other social benefits should be considered. Standing should be an active time for the child.

These devices generally consist of a rigid body structure on a support base which provides stabilization of the trunk and lower limbs. The support is achieved via a three-point bracing system with a chest pad and knee support anteriorly and pelvic support posteriorly. The alignment should be viewed from front, side and rear. Generally the chest pad is at the level of xiphoid, pelvic support at the level of the ischial tuberosities, knee blocks at tibial plateaus with the knee straight, not hyperextended, footplates positioning the malleoli posterior to the knee. The pelvis should not be rotated. Standing is usually not contra-indicated for the child with a dislocated or subluxed hip. Pain must always be considered.

Standing periods and number of sessions per day may vary considerably depending upon the ability of families to manage, and the tolerance and endurance of the child.

STANDING FRAME

This may be used as an initial standing device for children who cannot maintain a good standing posture or cannot stand without external support.

It is commonly used in the management of arthrogryposis, high- and mid-level spina bifida and a variety of neurological conditions. The standing frame, as the

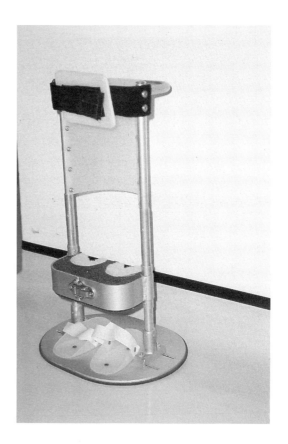

Figure 31 Standing Frame – three-point bracing system

initial standing device is also useful as an assessment and training tool. The child's ability in the standing frame assists the physiotherapist, orthotist and orthopaedic surgeon in deciding how and when to progress the child to other types of orthoses or assistive devices. Figure 31 shows a standing frame.

The timing for introduction of the first standing orthoses has caused some debate in the literature. Drennan (1976) recommended that the orthoses be prescribed at the neurodevelopmental age when children normally learn to stand and walk – from 9 months onwards. Carroll (1974), however, advocates beginning standing when the child starts to demonstrate interest in being upright, which allows for the individual developmental differences. Taylor and Sand (1975) recommend that orthoses for standing are introduced from 11 to 15 months old, or the developmental equivalent, as children of this age group were found to accept most readily the confinement of the frame. After the age of 22 months more children strongly resisted the orthosis.

The free-standing allowed by these devices, gives the child an opportunity to play in a well-supported position, with hands free from the need to prop. Dynamic use of the standing frame should also be encouraged whenever appropriate, as development of head and trunk righting and dynamic control can be facilitated.

In the child with spinal paraplegia, protective reactions can also be encouraged with controlled falling on the trampoline or on a soft mat. These activities help to make the child confident in the upright position and this provides a good basis for future ambulation. The bracing around the trunk may be reduced as the child becomes more confident and trunk control increases. The child can begin to weight-shift and swivel in the standing frame (if designed appropriately) using parallel bars or a walking frame.

Jumping and progressing to a swing-through gait pattern can be achieved by children with adequate upper limb strength and function. The size and shape of the base plate should be modified as the child begins to ambulate.

PARAPODIUM

This orthosis is usually prescribed for children with spina bifida with high-level lesions, particularly if they have reduced trunk control. Once children attend preschool, the option of sitting or standing in their orthosis is advantageous and this is the major functional difference between the parapodium and the basic standing frame. See Figure 32.

The use of the parapodium has declined with the introduction of reciprocating orthoses; however, it remains very useful and the most appropriate device for some children. A child is able to swivel or may achieve a swing-to or swing-through gait. Crutches or a walking frame are required for ambulation.

The advantages of the parapodium include:

- relatively easy to don / doff unless significant flexion contractures
- allows for free-standing
- possibility of hands-free swivelling
- provides trunk support for those with poor trunk control
- allows child to sit in orthoses

- relatively easy to adapt to deformity and leg length discrepancies and can be adjusted for growth

The disadvantages may include:

- appearance of the orthoses may cause concern
- high energy requirements
- restrictive
- lack of reciprocal pattern of gait

SWIVEL-WALKER

The swivel-walker is similar to the parapodium, but the baseplate is mounted on swivelling footplates. This device is most commonly used for children with high-level paraplegia resulting from spina bifida who have poor motor control. The mechanics are arranged so that, as the child rocks from side to side, one footplate is cleared from the ground causing the whole device to swivel forward automatically on the other footplate.

The line of gravity of the swivel-walker and the child is aligned so that it falls just ahead of the footplate-bearing centres (Butler et al. 1982). The inertial reaction is supplied by the child swinging trunk and upper arm from side to side. The child can swivel forwards, backwards and turn, all with hands free – crutches and walking aids are not required. The swivel-walker, therefore, offers the opportunity for the more severely impaired child who is unable to use a reciprocating orthoses or parapodium, to achieve upright stance and mobility (Butler et al. 1982). Those with poor upper limb function, in particular, will be able to achieve some independent ambulation using this device. The swivel-walker is usually reserved for this group of children. Mobility is slow, however, and only possible on level surfaces (Rose et al. 1983).

MULTIUSER STANDING FRAMES

These items differ from parapodiums and other individualized standing frames as they are available for a number of patients due to their multiadjustability. They are commonly used with the more severely disabled child to allow upright positioning and weight-bearing. See the prone table shown in Figure 33.

Generally these devices have an anterior forward-angled support surface. Various components and

Figure 32 Parapodium. A, Learning to swivel using posterior walker; B, early training for swing through gait; C, allows flexion at hips and knees for sitting

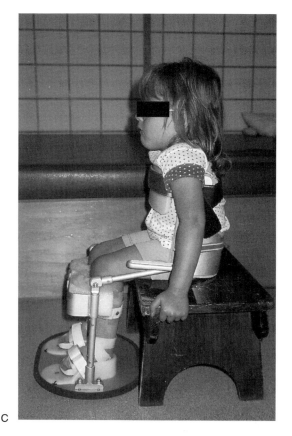

C

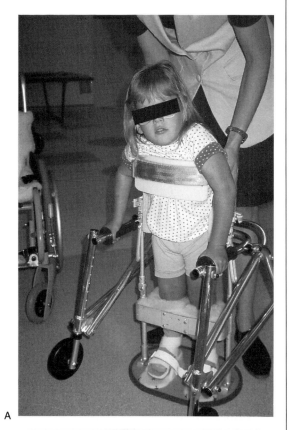

A

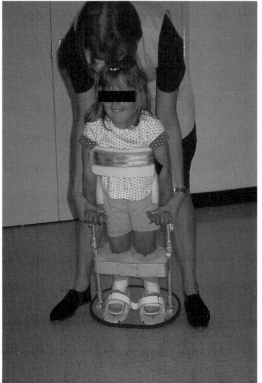

B

support straps can be added or deleted to provide varying levels of support. Care should be taken to ensure the anterior support does not impinge on the child's airway. The child is initially positioned with the frame in a marked forward position and then gradually adjusted into an almost vertical or vertical position. Progression to the upright position may need to be graduated in the early use of these devices.

Though the majority of these devices position the child in prone, the supine-supporting tilt-table may be used as an alternative in the older heavier child. A tray is often incorporated to assist in propping to improve posture and as a platform for activities. These devices may be mounted on wheels.

Initial Use of Orthoses

To ensure that an orthosis is successfully introduced to the child and family, there are a number of key points to remember:

- Reconfirm the aims of the orthoses.
- Check the fit and function of the orthosis — adjustments can be made as necessary at this time.

Figure 33 Prone Table – used for assisted partial weight-bearing for severely disabled child. Note currently in hip spica

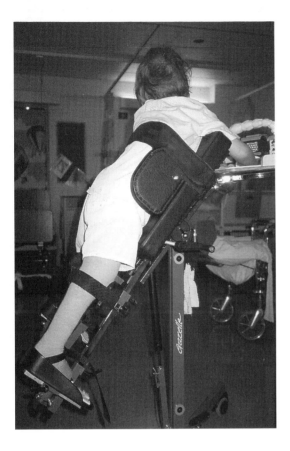

- Instruct and practise carers in applying orthosis. As a general rule socks are worn under the orthosis to limit skin problems, and should be clean, dry, wrinkle-free and not bulky.
- Discuss skin care and the need for regular monitoring of skin condition. This is especially important during the early use of the orthoses.
- Ensure carers are aware of safety issues/problems to watch for and know who to contact should these problems arise.
- Set a programme of initial wear and gradually increase towards required time in the orthoses.
- Discuss the expected daily use of the orthoses so the family have a clear idea of how long, how often, and where the orthoses is to be used.
- Establish a timetable of further gait/function training as appropriate.
- Set a review time.

Ideally, the physiotherapist and orthotist are both present for the final fitting of the orthosis. When an orthosis has been provided there is a responsibility to ensure that the therapy programme incorporates the advantages of the orthoses and that further skills needed to use the orthoses correctly are introduced.

Review of Orthoses

It is important for clinicians to review and evaluate the effectiveness of the prescription.

Subjective responses to the orthoses by both children and their parents will reflect their willingness to use and wear the equipment. These responses would include reactions to appearance, comfort, ease of donning, perception of stability and functional influences.

Orthotic efficacy is often judged by the extent to which this piece of equipment improves gait (Krebs et al. 1988). ADL tests, looking at effect of use of orthotics on function such as timed walking, dressing including ability and time to don and doff equipment, stair and ramp climbing can be utilized by the clinician.

Aids To Assist Mobilizing

ANTERIOR WALKER

Both the anterior and posterior walkers provide continuous support to the child while allowing a variety of gait patterns. The child tends to lean forward to push the anterior walker. The body is forward and in a flexed position, at the trunk, hips and other joints (Logan et al. 1990). This changes the alignment of the joints and changes the dynamics of balance for the child. At times the walker can 'get away from the child'. As a result the child may 'chase the walker' and fall. The use of rear stoppers or slides may prevent this problem.

POSTERIOR WALKER

Posterior walkers are becoming more popular and are positioned behind the child during ambulation. A study by Logan et al. (1990) showed that use of posterior walkers encouraged a more upright posture allowing the centre of mass to move over the base of support, rather than in front of the child, as with an anterior walker. Trunk and hip flexion were significantly decreased. This more erect posture mirrors normal stance far more closely. Gait analysis

Figure 34 Walking Aids: Elbow Crutches with Hoop

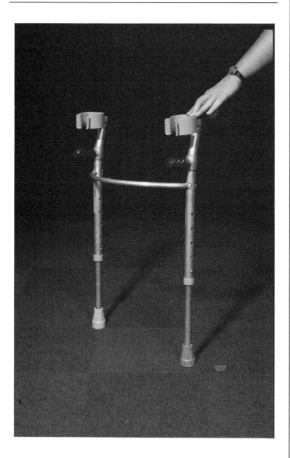

showed decreased time in double support, longer swing phase and increased stride length. From a practical point of view, the child is able to walk straight up to a table for table-top activities without having to negotiate to move the walker out of the way. As a safety mechanism, these walkers may have a ratchet device on the rear wheels allowing the child to lean against the walker when stationary.

WHEELS/STOPPERS

For those walking frames without wheels, the child must pick up the walker and move it forward as he progresses. During this pick-up stage, the child must momentarily stand and maintain an upright position. This may be an effective way to help progress the child towards independent stance and ambulating with crutches or sticks. The disadvantage with this is that the child must perform a 'step to' gait pattern. The hopper frame can be used either in front or behind the child.

ELBOW CRUTCHES/STICKS

Walking frames require an even surface, minimal slope, cannot be used on stairs and may be bulky to transport. With improved balance and motor planning the child progresses towards the use of crutches/sticks and, in turn, greater independence. Rough terrains and stairs become more accessible. As a means of progressing to elbow crutches, the interim use of joined elbow crutches may be useful. In general, the height of all walking aids should be at the level of wrist/greater trochanter; however, individual variations may be necessary. See Figure 34.

IMPROVIZED AIDS

Various household and clinic items can be used as aids and orthoses to overcome limitations to access to more advanced or technological items, or can be used purely to trial the influence of equipment. Often these everyday items are more accepted by both the child and the family than a specialized aid. Some examples of make-do items include:

- felt with adhesive backing cut to provide wedges to heels and arch supports to gauge the effect of intervention
- lower limb casts applied to the lower limb setting joints at desired angles to assess the influence of a solid AFO
- magazines held in place by rubber bands make good leg or arm wraps
- canvas leg or arm bands with ribbing and velcro fastening can also provide limb stability and support
- the use of semirigid/rigid fibreglass casts and low-heat thermoplastics for weight-bearing or resting splints to control tone or pain
- a double line of chairs or broomsticks set up on chairs can be used as a substitute for parallel bars
- rope rails around the garden can provide interim support
- children's wooden block trolleys, chair frames, prams, pusher cars can be used instead of specialized walking frames.

Your imagination and exploration of environment are the only limits to providing this style of equipment. The best inventors are often parents and other family members of the child. If you can provide the outline and theory of what you are trying to achieve then someone else may find a solution.

CASE 6

Nicholas is a 7-year-old boy with cerebral palsy in the form of spastic quadriplegia. His lower limbs are more affected than his upper limbs with his left side more affected than the right. Nick presented to physiotherapy because his gait had deteriorated recently and he was wearing out the toe of his boots. He was independently mobile using an anterior walker wearing bilateral BKIs and boots. Nick had a crouch posture in sustained stance. He remained flexed and walked up on his toes achieving heel contact only on the (R) foot during the midstance phase of the gait cycle. He had moderate tone in his adductors and hamstrings. Plantigrade position was only just obtainable at both ankles. The equinovalgus posture of both feet was able to be passively corrected to just short of plantigrade with the hindfoot held in neutral.

PROBLEM-SOLVING EXERCISES

1. Should the use of the BKI be continued? If not, what findings support your decision?
2. What role could the anterior walker play in Nicholas's difficulties?
3. What other orthoses might be considered suitable for Nicholas?

Case 7

Tobi is 3 years old and has a spinal cord lesion at T4 following a tumour invading his spinal canal. This was discovered at 13 months of age. His lower limbs are completely flail and his abdominals poorly innervated, resulting in poor trunk control. Tobi was initially prescribed a standing frame and he enjoyed using this on a daily basis. His upper limb and fine motor function showed improve-

ment due to his stable trunk position whilst standing. Tobi quickly became mobile in the frame and is now able to swivel and jump in the standing frame using an anterior walker.

PROBLEM-SOLVING EXERCISES

1. What orthosis might Tobi progress to next? Support your decision.
2. Describe gait training for Tobi in this orthosis and progression of walking aids.

Recommended Reading

Redford, JB (ed.) (1986) *Orthotics Etcetera*, 3rd edn. Baltimore, MD: Williams & Wilkins.

Rose, GK (1986) *Orthotics: Principles and Practice*. London, UK: William Heinemann Medical Books Ltd.

REFERENCES

Andersson, BJG, Ortengren, R (1974) Lumbar disc pressure and myoelectric back muscle activity during sitting. *Scandinavian Journal of Rehabilitative Medicine* 6: 122–127.

Andersson, BJG, Ortengren, R, Nachemson AL et al. (1975) The sitting posture: electromyographic and discometric study. *Orthopaedic Clinics of North America* 6(1): 105–119.

Basmajian, JV (1985) *Muscles Alive: Their Functions Revealed by Electromyography* 5th edn. Baltimore: Williams and Wilkins.

Bergen, A, Colangelo, C (1985) *Positioning the Child with Central Nervous System Deficits*, pp. 3–48. New York: Valhalla Publications.

Butler, PB, Major, R (1987) The ParaWalker: A rational approach to the provision of reciprocal ambulation for paraplegic patients. *Physiotherapy* 73: 393–397.

Butler, PB, Farmer, IR, Poiner, R et al. (1982) Use of the ORLAU swivel walker for the severely handicapped patient. *Physiotherapy* 68(11): 324–326.

Carroll, N (1974) The orthotic management of the spina bifida child. *Clinical Orthopaedics* 102: 103–114.

Charney, EB, Melchionni, JB, Smith, DR (1991) Community ambulation by children with myelomeningocele and high level paralysis. *Journal of Paediatric Orthopedics* 11: 579–582.

Cusick, BD (1988) Splints and casts: managing foot deformity in children with neuromotor disorders. *Physical Therapy* 68(12): 1903–1912.

Cusick, BD (1990) *Progressive Casting and Splinting for Lower Extremity Deformities in Children with Neuromotor Dysfunction*. Tuscon, AZ: Therapy Skill Builders, pp. 240–244.

DeSouza, LJ, Carroll, N (1976) Ambulation of the braced myelomeningocele patient. *Journal of Bone and Joint Surgery* 58A: 1112–1118.

Douglas, R, Larson, PL, D'Ambrosia, R et al. (1983) The LSU reciprocating gait orthosis. *Orthopaedics* 6(7): 834–839.

Drennan, JC (1976) Orthotic management of the myelomeningocele spine. *Developmental Medicine and Child Neurology* 18 (suppl. 37): 97–103.

Fraser, RK and Menelaus MB (1993) The management of tibial torsion in patients with spina bifida. *Journal of Bone and Joint Surgery* 75B: 495–497.

Golski, A, Menelaus, MB (1976) The treatment of intoed gait in spina bifida patients by lateral transfer of the medial hamstrings. *Australian New Zealand Journal of Surgery* 46: 157–159.

Guidera, KJ, Smith, S, Raney, E et al. (1993) Use of the reciprocating gait orthosis in myelodysplasia. *Journal of Pediatric Orthopedics* 13: 341–348.

Harris, MB, Banta, V (1990) Cost of skin care in the myelomeningocele population. *Journal of Pediatric Orthopedics* 10: 355–361.

Hughes, CJ, Weimar WH, Sheth, PN et al. (1992) Biomechanics of wheelchair propulsion as a function of seat position and user-to-chair interface. *Archives of Physical Medicine and Rehabilitation* 73: 263–269.

Jones, ET, Knapp, R (1987) Assessment and management of the lower extremity in cerebral palsy. *Orthopedic Clinics of North America* 18(4): 725–738.

Kirtley, C (1992) Principles and practice of paraplegic locomotion: experience with the Walkabout walking system. *Australian Orthotic Prosthetic Magazine* 7: 4–7.

Knutson, LM, Clark, DE (1991) Orthotic devices for ambulation in children with cerebral palsy and myelomeningocele. *Physical Therapy* 71: 947–960.

Krebs, DE, Edelstein, JE, Fishman, S (1988). Comparison of plastic/metal and leather/metal knee–ankle–foot orthoses. *American Journal of Physical Medicine* 67: 175–185.

Lockard, MA (1988) Foot orthoses. *Physical Therapy* 68: 1866–1873.

Logan, L, Byers-Hinkley, K, Ciccone, CD (1990) Anterior versus posterior walkers: a gait analysis study. *Developmental Medicine and Child Neurology* 32: 1044–1048.

Mazur, J, Shurtleff, D, Menelaus, M et al. (1989) Orthopaedic management of high level spina bifida: early walking compared with early use of a wheelchair. *Journal of Bone and Joint Surgery* 71A: 56–61.

Middleton, EA, Hurley, GR, McIlwain, JS (1988) The role of rigid and hinged polypropylene ankle–foot–orthosis in the management of cerebral palsy: a case study. *Prosthetics and Orthotics International* 12: 129–135.

Nicol, RO, Menelaus, MB (1983) Correction of combined tibial torsion and valgus deformity of the foot. *Journal of Bone and Joint Surgery* 65B: 641–645.

Ounpuu, S, Davis, R, Banta, J et al. (1992) The effects of orthotics on gait in children with low level myelomeningocele. *Proceedings of NACOB II The Second North American Congress on Biomechanics, Chicago.*

Taylor, N, Sand, PL (1975) Verlo orthosis: experience with different developmental levels in normal children. *Archives of Physical Medicine and Rehabilitation* 56: 120–124.

Rose, GK (1986) *Orthotics: Principles and Practice.* London: William Heinemann Medical Books Ltd.

Rose, GK, Stallard, J, Sankarankutty, M (1983) A clinical review of the orthotic treatment of myelomeningocele patients. *Journal of Bone and Joint Surgery* 65B: 242–246.

Rosenstein, BD, Green, WB, Herrington et al. (1987) Bone density in myelomeningocele: the effects of ambulatory status and other factors. *Developmental Medicine and Child Neurology* 29: 486–495.

Stuberg, WA (1992) Considerations related to weight-bearing programs in children with developmental disabilities. *Physical Therapy* 72: 35–40.

Thomas, SE, Mazur, JM, Child, ME et al. (1989) Quantitative evaluation of AFO use with myelomeningocele children. *Zeitschrift fur Kinderchirurgie* 44: 38–40.

Trefler, E, Hobson, DA, Taylor, SJ et al (1993) *Seating and Mobility for Persons with Physical Disabilities.* Tucson, AZ: Therapy Skill Builders.

Waksvik, K, Levy, R (1979) An approach to seating for the cerebral palsied. *Canadian Journal of Occupational Therapy* 46(4): 147–153.

Winchester, PK, Carollo, JJ, Parekh, RN et al. (1993) A comparison of paraplegic gait performance using two types of reciprocating gait orthosis. *Prosthetics and Orthotics International* 17: 101–106.

Yang, GW, Chu, DS, Ahn, JH et al (1986) Floor reaction orthosis: clinical experience. *Orthotics and Prosthetics* 40: 33–37.

Yngve, DA, Douglas, R, Roberts, JM (1984) The reciprocating gait orthosis in myelomeningocele. *Journal of Paediatric Orthopaedics* 4: 304–310.

Zacharchow, D (1988) *Posture: Sitting, Standing, Chair Design and Exercise.* Springfield, IL: Charles C Thomas Books.

12

Gait Analysis in the Assessment of Orthotic Devices

SUSAN SIENKO THOMAS

Joint Kinematics
•
Joint Kinetics
•
Electromyography
•
Gait Analysis for Children with Cerebral Palsy
•
Gait Analysis for Children with Myelomeningocele

Over the last 10–15 years, computerized gait analysis has become an accepted tool to assist the physician in the clinical decision-making process for children with neuromuscular disorders (Gage 1987, DeLuca et al. 1991, Rose et al. 1991). Each component of the gait analysis assessment is used to assess the child's movement disorder and to provide insight into the optimal treatment plan for that individual. This treatment plan may include physiotherapy, orthotic devices and/or surgical intervention. To date, a significant amount of gait analysis research is available which documents the alterations in the gait pattern of children with neuromuscular disorders following surgical intervention (Gage et al. 1984, Hadley et al. 1992, Ounpuu et al. 1993a, b).

Yet despite the vast use of gait analysis in the assessment of surgical interventions, it is not common in the assessment of orthotic or prosthetic devices. With the proliferation in the design of energy storage feet and advances in gait analysis technology, a significant amount of research in prosthetics is now being performed to assess the dynamic contribution provided by the available energy storage feet (Winter and Sienko 1988, Barth et al. 1992, Schneider et al. 1993). This knowledge has led to further advances in the prosthetic design, as well as improving the gait pattern of amputees by prescribing the optimal foot for the individual.

In contrast, despite increased use of gait analysis clinically in the determination of orthotic recommendations for children with neuromuscular disorders, minimal research is available regarding the contribution to the gait pattern of various orthotic devices. Only recently has gait analysis been used to provide insight into the function of the orthotic device. In order to understand the benefit of using gait analysis in the assessment of orthotic devices and how the information may contribute to changes in orthotic design and treatment recommendations for children with neuromuscular disorders, a thorough understanding of the components involved in gait analysis is required.

Joint Kinematics

Kinematics is the general term given to variables that are involved in the description of movement, independent of the forces that cause the movement. They include linear and angular displacements, velocities and accelerations (Winter 1990). Joint motion is usually assessed in three planes: sagittal, coronal and transverse. Assessment of the sagittal plane divides the body into left and right parts, while the coronal plane divides the body into anterior and posterior parts. The transverse plane is slightly more complex as it is the horizontal plane which cuts through the body at right angles to the sagittal and coronal planes (Winter 1991).

Joint kinematics are defined as the relative motion of

each joint to the other beginning at the pelvis in the sagittal plane (Kadaba *et al.* 1990). They are displayed as a percentage of the gait cycle, in which the gait cycle is defined as the period of time from foot contact to ipsilateral foot contact, or 100% of a cycle. Mann (1982) classified the percentage of the gait cycle as follows: 0% = heel strike; 15% = flat foot; 30% = heel rise; 60% = toe off; 60+ % = swing phase; 100% = heel strike.

The kinematic variables most commonly used in the assessment of pathological gait are in the sagittal plane. These variables are the magnitude of pelvic tilt, hip and knee flexion/extension and ankle plantar/dorsiflexion.

The coronal and transverse planes provide information about more complex movements. Assessment in the coronal plane allows for movements such as pelvic

Figure 1 Representation of Normal Kinematics in the Sagittal, Coronal and Transverse Planes of an Adult Subject. NB: These illustrations depict findings of an adult subject — representation of kinematics of the child and adolescent subject can be found in Sutherland (1984).

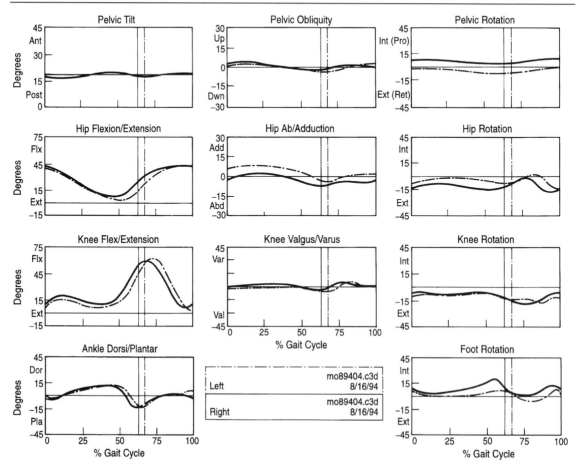

obliquity, hip ab/adduction and knee valgus/varus to be documented, while the transverse plane allows for assessment of pelvic, hip, knee and ankle rotation. The information gained from the assessment of kinematics provides the basis from which a preliminary decision regarding the gait abnormality is made. Normal kinetics of an adult are shown in Figure 1.

The Use of Joint Kinematics in the Assessment of Orthotics

Joint kinematics can be used in a variety of different ways to determine the effect of an orthotic device. Modifications in orthotic prescription may be made as a result of the findings from the gait analysis. For example, if one were trying to determine whether a child wearing a hinged ankle–foot orthosis (AFO) actually benefited from the device, an assessment of sagittal plane ankle motion would determine whether the AFO allowed the child to move into dorsiflexion during stance, thus utilizing the hinged effect. If, however, there was no change in ankle motion throughout the entire stance phase, then it may not be beneficial to have a hinged AFO, and a solid AFO may be a more appropriate treatment recommendation for the child.

In addition to AFO modifications, new orthotic recommendations may be made as a result of the findings from the gait analysis. Gait abnormalities, such as knee hyperextension which can be documented through sagittal plane knee motion, may be improved through the addition of an AFO positioned in dorsiflexion. The increase in dorsiflexion by the AFO limits the amount of knee extension possible through the plantarflexion/knee extension couple. Assessment of sagittal plane knee motion, both with and without the orthotic device, would determine the benefit of the orthotic as well as any further changes in the device which may further improve knee kinematics. Gait analysis, with and without the orthotic device, can aid in determination of primary and secondary problems. For example, the child with cerebral palsy may demonstrate plantarflexion in the barefoot condition. However, when the orthotic device is applied a relatively neutral position of the foot is assumed, while subsequent increases in knee and hip flexion are seen. This finding would indicate that the problem may be tight hamstrings which cause the child to assume a plantarflexed position, rather than a tight achilles causing increased hip and knee flexion. The use of kinematics in the assessment of orthotic devices provides the therapist and the orthotist with information regarding the gait abnormality and the changes or compensations which result from the application of an orthotic device.

Joint Kinetics

Kinetics is the general term given to the forces that cause the movement. These include both internal (muscle activity, ligaments or friction in the muscles and joint) and external (ground reaction) forces (Winter 1990). Joint moments and powers are the two types of kinetic assessments commonly used in the clinical assessment of pathological gait. Owing to the relative newness of joint kinetics in the assessment of abnormal gait, moments and powers are commonly represented in the sagittal plane only (see Figure 2).

A joint moment is defined as a force acting at a distance about an axis of rotation which causes an angular acceleration about that axis (Gage 1992, Ounpuu et al. 1991). Moments are equal to the force multiplied by the distance from the centre of rotation, and are represented in units of Newton metres (N m). Moments can be represented as either internal or external. External moments about a joint are the result of the ground reaction force and are not commonly used in the clinical interpretation of gait analysis data. Internal moments, however, are produced by muscle action and assist in the determination of the primary muscle group active at the joint. Joint power is the product of the net joint moment and the joint angular velocity, and is expressed in watts/kilogram (W/kg). Power curves provide useful information regarding which muscle groups are the primary source of power generation at a joint, thus influencing surgical intervention. If the sources of propulsive power can be identified, then surgical intervention on those muscle groups which are criti-

Figure 2 Representation of Normal Kinematics and Kinetics in the Sagittal Plane of an Adult Subject. NB: These illustrations depict findings of an adult subject — representation of kinetics of the child and adolescent subject can be found in Ounpuu *et al.* (1991).

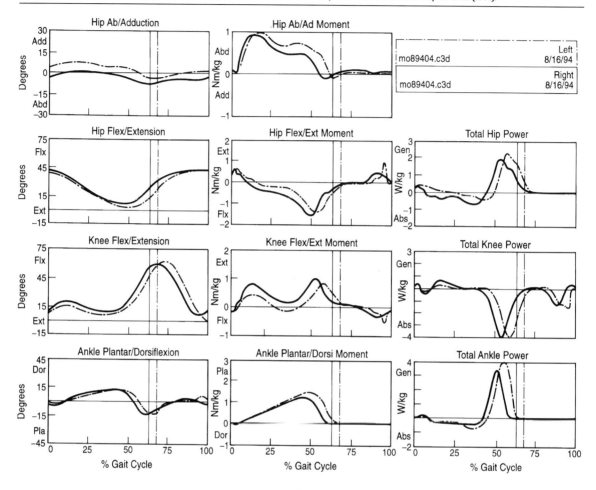

The Use of Joint Kinetics in the Assessment of Orthotics

Although relatively new in the clinical assessment of patients, joint kinetics can be used to determine the effect that an orthotic has on normalizing joint moments and maintaining joint power, specifically at the ankle (Gage 1994). One of the main concerns in the use of an orthotic device on a child with cerebral palsy is that it does not allow the child to generate enough power at the ankle. The reduction in power from the ankle, as a result of the orthotic device, may hamper forward progression and require other muscles such as the hip flexors to create more power to achieve the same forward propulsion. As joint kinetics cal to power generation can be kept to a minimum (Gage 1992).

become part of the normal clinical repertoire in the assessment of pathological gait and research begins to use these advanced tools, a greater understanding of the results will be determined and further clinical applications will be made in the areas of surgical and orthotic recommendations.

Electromyography

Electromyography (EMG) is the primary signal which describes the neural input to the muscular system. It gives information regarding which muscle or group of muscles is responsible for a muscle moment or whether antagonistic activity is taking place (Winter 1990). In the clinical setting, EMG is used to determine when a muscle or muscle group is active; however, it cannot accurately measure the magnitude of

Figure 3 Representation of Normal Electromyographic Activity of an Adult Subject during Gait Cycle. These illustrations depict the findings in an adult subject — representation of the EMG patterns in the child can be found in Sutherland (1984).

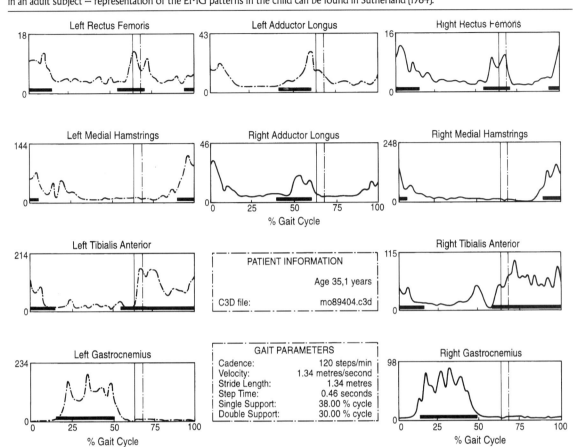

the activity (Gage 1992).The normal EMG activity of an adult during the gait cycle is shown in Figure 3.

Dynamic EMG is used to determine which muscle is responsible for the gait dysfunction in situations where there are several possibilities which may be causing the abnormality (Gage 1992). Electromyographic activity can be matched with joint moment and power information to corroborate the muscle group responsible for the movement. By comparing the timing of the child's EMG activity to the internal moments, the onset and cessation of muscle activity should correspond with those of the moments about the appropriate joint.

The Use of Electromyography in the Assessment of Orthotics

Prior to the use of joint kinetics in the assessment of abnormal gait, electromyography was used to deter-

mine which muscle group was predominant during various phases of gait. In the assessment of orthotic devices, electromyography can be used to determine the changes in electromyographic activity with the application of an orthotic device. Clinical assessment of the EMG patterns in both the orthotic and barefoot conditions are used to determine whether there is a normalization of electromyographic pattern when an orthotic device is worn. For specific orthotic devices, such as the tone-reducing AFOs, electromyographic patterns can be used to determine whether the orthotic device decreases the abnormal cocontraction between the agonists and antagonists. With the advances in technology and further understanding of joint kinetics, electromyography is now used as a supplement to confirm joint moment findings and provide insight into whether the muscle is generating, absorbing, or transferring power.

Gait Analysis for Children with Cerebral Palsy

As a result of the increased use of gait analysis in the assessment of children with cerebral palsy, there is an increase in the amount of research available regarding the effects of orthotic devices on the gait pattern of children with cerebral palsy. Early studies using gait analysis to determine the effects of the AFO on children with cerebral palsy revealed that in addition to improving ankle motion, which was the purpose of the orthotic device, there were significant improvements in velocity and stride length (Thomas et al. 1989b). Furthermore, improvements were found in hip and knee motion with a decrease in the amount of cocontraction between muscle groups which subsequently decreased energy consumption.

Ounpuu et al. (1993c) assessed the effects of the posterior leaf spring orthosis on ankle kinematics, moments and powers. The results revealed that there was a significant increase in ankle dorsiflexion during swing when using the posterior leaf spring orthosis, which resulted in better preposition of the ankle at initial contact and an increase in the incidence of ankle dorsiflexion moment during loading response. The peak power generation was significantly less when wearing the posterior leaf spring orthosis in comparison to the barefoot condition. The amount of energy absorbed at the ankle, however, was increased when this particular orthosis was worn. Thus, the posterior leaf spring orthosis was capable of storing energy; however, it did not return it to augment push-off. Radka et al. (1994), compared the effects of dynamic AFOs, solid AFOs and the barefoot condition in children with cerebral palsy by comparing changes in joint motion, electromyography and stride characteristics. Both AFOs increased stride length and the knee and ankle motions during gait when compared to the no AFO condition. However, no further effects on proximal motions and muscle activity were found when using the dynamic AFO. Based on these findings, either AFO was recommended for children with cerebral palsy. Research is continuing to advance the understanding of orthotic devices.

Gait Analysis for Children with Myelomeningocele

Assessment of children with myelomeningocele using various orthotic devices is relatively new, with few published articles. Only recently have articles been written documenting the benefit of using gait analysis in the assessment of the child with myelomeningocele, most specifically in the assessment of the optimal orthotic prescription for the child (Thomas et al. 1988, 1989a, Mazur 1989).

Initial assessment of sagittal plane gait and electromyography in children with myelomeningocele revealed an increase in gait parameters such as velocity, cadence and stride length, a decrease in excess hip, knee and ankle motion, with a subsequent decrease in excess muscle activity when using an AFO (Thomas et al. 1989a). Ounpuu et al. (1992) furthered the investigation by adding the assessment of kinetic variables and finding that AFOs improved the gait pattern in children with low-level myelomeningocele, although not significantly.

Using gait analysis to assess the change in gait in children with myelomeningocele following the application of knee–ankle–foot orthoses (KAFO), Ounpuu et al. (1993d), found that when the brace was worn there was a decrease in the knee extension moment, a decrease in power absorption and a decrease in excessive range of motion at the ankle. Ounpuu et al. (1993d) also found that despite a 'visual' valgus thrust noted during observation of gait, adductor moments at the knee did not verify this visual illusion.

Hunt et al. (1993) evaluated the changes in velocity and electromyographic patterns in children with myelomeningocele using two different types of orthotic devices. Findings revealed that velocity was significantly greater with the hinged AFOs than either the barefoot or solid AFO condition. Both orthotic devices decreased the activity found in the medial hamstrings and vastus lateralis, which may be indicative of the decreased need for this activity to maintain knee extension during stance. The primary difference in orthotic devices was found in gastrocnemius, where the hinged AFO condition showed greater activity from this muscle than when the solid AFOs were worn. Recommendations from this study stated that the improvements in velocity and gastrocnemius activity were desired results and that limited motion AFOs for selected children with myelomeningocele may be warranted.

Summary

The use of gait analysis in the assessment of orthotic devices is relatively new. However, advances in gait analysis have allowed for assessment of orthotic devices as part of the clinical assessment providing optimal individual patient care. Continued research in the area of orthotic devices for children with myelomeningocele, cerebral palsy and other conditions of gait disorder will allow therapists and orthotists to design orthotic devices which enhance kinematic and kinetic variables, thus facilitating improvements in gait patterns.

REFERENCES

Barth, DG, Schumaker, L, Sienko Thomas, S (1992) Gait analysis and energy cost of below-knee amputees wearing six different prosthetic feet. *Journal of Prosthetics and Orthotics* 4: 63–75.

DeLuca, PA (1991) Gait analysis in the treatment of the ambulatory child with cerebral palsy. *Clinical Orthopaedics* 264: 65–75.

Gage, JR (1987) Gait analysis for decision making in cerebral palsy. *Bulletin of the Hospital for Joint Disorders Orthopaedic Institute* 43: 147–163.

Gage, JR (1992) Computer based decision making. In: Sussman, MD (ed.) *Spastic Diplegia*, pp. 187–202. Rosemount, IL: American Academy of Orthopaedic Surgeons.

Gage, JR (1994) The clinical use of kinetics for evaluation of pathological gait in cerebral palsy. *Journal of Bone and Joint Surgery* 76A: 622–631.

Gage, JR, Fabian, D, Hicks, R, Tashman, S (1984) Pre- and postoperative gait analysis in patients with spastic diplegia: a preliminary report. *Journal of Pediatric Orthopaedics* 4: 715–725.

Hadley, N, Chambers, C, Scarborough, N et al. (1992) Knee motion following multiple soft-tissue releases in ambulatory patients with cerebral palsy. *Journal of Pediatric Orthopaedics* 12: 324–328.

Hunt, KG, Knutson, LM, Soderberg, GL (1993) The effects of fixed and hinged ankle–foot orthoses on gait myoelectric activity in children with myelomeningocele. *Developmental Medicine and Child Neurology* suppl. 69, abst. 25, p.16.

Kadaba, MP, Ramarkrishnan, HK, Wooten, ME (1990) Measurement of lower extremity kinematics during level walking. *Journal of Orthopaedic Research* 7: 849–860.

Mann, RA (1982) Biomechanics. In: Jahss, M (ed.) *Disorders of the Foot*, vol. I, pp. 37–67. Philadelphia: WB Saunders.

Mazur, JM, Thomas, SS, Wright, NE et al. (1989) The use of gait analysis in the evaluation of patients with myelomeningocele. *Developmental Medicine and Child Neurology* suppl. 59, abst. 12, p. 7.

Ounpuu, S, Gage, JR, Davis, RB (1991) Three-dimensional lower extremity joint kinetics in normal pediatric gait. *Journal of Pediatric Orthopaedics* 11: 341–349.

Ounpuu, S, Davis, RB, Banta, JV (1992) The effects of orthoses on gait in children with low-level myelomeningocele. *Proceedings of North America Congress on Biomechanics*, Chicago, IL, pp. 323–324.

Ounpuu, S, Muik, E, Davis, RB et al. (1993a) Rectus femoris surgery in children with cerebral palsy. Part I: The effect of rectus femoris location on knee motion. *Journal of Pediatric Orthopaedics* 13: 325–330.

Ounpuu, S, Muik, E, Davis, RB et al. (1993b) Rectus femoris surgery in children with cerebral palsy. Part II: A comparison between the effect of transfer and release of the distal rectus femoris on knee motion. *Journal of Pediatric Orthopaedics* 13: 331–335.

Ounpuu, S, Bell, KJ, Davis, RB et al. (1993c) An evaluation of the posterior leaf spring orthosis using gait analysis. *Developmental Medicine and Child Neurology* suppl. 69, abst. 10, p.8.

Ounpuu, S, Davis, RB, Bell, KJ et al. (1993d) An evaluation of orthoses on gait in children with low-level myelomeningocele. *Developmental Medicine and Child Neurology* suppl. 69, abst. 24, pp. 15–16.

Radka, S, Skinner, SR, Dixon, D (1994) A comparison of gait with solid and dynamic ankle–foot orthoses in children with spastic cerebral palsy. *Developmental Medicine and Child Neurology* suppl. 70, p. 26.

Rose, S, Ounpuu, S, DeLuca, PA (1991) Strategies for the assessment of gait in a clinical setting. *Physical Therapy* 71: 961–980.

Schneider, K, Hart, T, Zernicke, RF et al. (1993) Dynamics of below-knee child amputee gait: SACH foot versus Flex foot. *Journal of Biomechanics* 26: 1191–1204.

Sutherland, DH (1984) *Gait Disorders in Childhood and Adolescence*, 202 pp. Baltimore: Williams and Wilkins.

Thomas, SES, Wright, NE, Mazur, JM et al. (1988) Quantification of gait of children with myelomeningocele using motion analysis. *Developmental Medicine and Child Neurology* suppl. 57, abst. 86, p. 41.

Thomas, SES, Mazur, JM, Child, ME et al. (1989a) Quantitative evaluation of AFO use with myelomeningocele children. *Zeitschrift fur Kinderchirurgie* 44: 38–40.

Thomas, S, Mazur, JM, Wright, NE et al. (1989b) Quantitative assessment of AFOs for children with cerebral palsy. *Developmental Medicine and Child Neurology* suppl. 59, abst. 11, p. 7.

Winter, DA (1990) *Biomechanics and Motor Contol of Human Movement*, 277 pp. New York: John Wiley and Sons.

Winter, DA (1991) *The Biomechanics and Motor Control of Human Gait: Normal, Elderly and Pathological*, 2nd edn. Ontario: University of Waterloo Press.

Winter, DA, Sienko, SE (1988) Biomechanics of below knee amputee gait. *Journal of Biomechanics* 21: 361–367.

Section E:

Physiotherapy Practice in Cardiorespiratory Conditions Presenting from Infancy to Adolescence

PROLOGUE: JULIE MACDONALD

Prologue

JULIE MACDONALD

It becomes apparent throughout the following chapters that for the physiotherapist to manage children with cardio-respiratory problems successfully s/he must have an extremely sound theoretical knowledge of the distinctive cardiorespiratory system of the neonate, infant, child and adolescent. Furthermore, a knowledge of the psychosocial development of children and adolescents is essential as physiotherapists must always instigate treatment techniques which not only address the specified cardiorespiratory problem, but are also developmentally appropriate for the individual.

Each chapter highlights the fact that the physiotherapist must accurately assess and reassess each paediatric patient with cardiorespiratory problems and consider very carefully his/her selection of treatment techniques for specified problems. Indeed, Chapter 14 which explores the effect of various respiratory physiotherapy techniques on intracranial and cardiovascular dynamics in neonates particularly illustrates why the physiotherapist should exercise the utmost care when selecting the most appropriate respiratory techniques for an individual patient.

Although a wide number of paediatric cardiorespiratory conditions are introduced in these chapters, undoubtedly there are many other conditions which may cause cardiorespiratory problems. The problem-solving approach generated throughout these chapters, however, will assist the reader in understanding the basis of physiotherapy assessment and management of the child with cardiorespiratory difficulties.

Most importantly, preventative and long-term management of children with chronic respiratory illnesses is addressed in the following discussions. Such management ideas are relevant in the older child and adolescent with chronic respiratory difficulties, particularly as the individual's motivation and compliance with a physiotherapy respiratory treatment regimen may wane during this stage of development.

13

Cardiorespiratory Physiotherapy Management – Neonate and Infant

KYM MORRIS

Lung Development
•
Characteristics of Respiration
•
Respiratory Physiotherapy Assessment of the Neonate and Young Infant
•
Principles of Neonatal Respiratory Physiotherapy Management
•
Physiotherapy Management of Common Respiratory Conditions
•
Surgical Conditions

Physiotherapy plays an important role in the respiratory care of the neonate and infant. In order to gain the particular skills in implementing an effective and appropriate management programme it is necessary to have a clear understanding of lung development, its relationship to particular conditions of the preterm and term neonate and infant, and the basic principles of respiratory physiotherapy management.

Lung Development

The development of the respiratory system begins early in fetal life and continues long after birth. The nature of this development has been the topic of many studies over the years.

Prenatal Development

Merenstein and Gardner (1989) have set out and described the stages of development in the respiratory system based on a compilation of previously published works. They divided lung development into four stages:

- embryonic period – first 5 weeks after conception
- pseudoglandular phase – 5–16 weeks gestation
- cannicular phase – 13–25 weeks gestation
- terminal sac period – 24 weeks to birth

and closely examined each of these stages in the following manner.

The Embryonic Period is viewed as the period from conception to approximately 5 weeks gestation when the primitive lung bud evaginates from the cervical region of the endodermal tube, and the main and lobar bronchi are formed. Aberrations in development at this stage may lead to such conditions as tracheo-oesophageal fistula. The pulmonary arteries invade the lung tissue following the airways and divide as the airways divide. The pulmonary veins arise independently from the lung parenchyma and return to the left atrium, thus completing the pulmonary circuit.

203

The Pseudoglandular Phase follows on from the embryonic period and is completed by approximately 16 weeks gestation. During this phase there is dichotomous, asymmetric bronchial branching such that bronchial formation is completed and the number of branches of conducting airways is equal to the number in adults (i.e. the conducting portion of the tracheobronchial tree is established). Any further conducting airway growth is through an increase in size and length of the airways not by an increase in numbers.

Along the tracheobronchial tree there is evidence of muscle fibres, elastic tissue and early cartilage formation while at approximately 12 weeks, mucous glands are formed and these increase in number until 25–26 weeks when cilia begin to develop. During this phase, the diaphragm also develops (Merenstein and Gardner 1989).

The Cannicular Phase occurs from 13 to 25 weeks gestation and is the phase of further development and vascularization of the future respiratory portion of the lung. From 22 weeks, rapid proliferation of the pulmonary capillary bed, an increase in the surface of the respiratory epithelium, and formation of alveolar buds and sacculi occur.

Respiratory epithelium contains cells that become differentiated into type I and type II pneumocytes. Type I pneumocytes produce an extremely thin squamous epithelial layer that lines the alveoli and fuses to the underlying capillary epithelial cells, providing the air–blood interface for gaseous exchange. Type II pneumocytes (cuboid cells) are the site of surfactant synthesis and storage. Merenstein and Gardner (1989) report that after this phase is completed extrauterine life becomes viable as alveolar cells appear in increasing numbers making respiration possible. However, Farrell (1982) suggests that sustained inflation of the lung after the first breath requires surfactant which is not present in adequate amounts before 32 weeks gestation, yet from 22 weeks surface-active phospholipid (lecithin) has been detected.

The Terminal Sac Period is traditionally said to end at birth, with a respiratory unit consisting of three orders of respiratory bronchioles. A generation of transitional ducts and terminal clusters of alveo-lar sacs with less than 70×10^6 alveoli are present at birth. These terminal alveoli are shallow and wide-mouthed in the newborn and do not assume a cup-shaped configuration until several months after birth. The shallow wide-diameter alveoli tend to prevent atelectasis in the first few months of life, but they also offer less surface area for gas exchange. From 34 weeks phosphatidylglycerol appears and there is a dramatic increase in the principal surfactant compound phosphatidyl-choline (Merenstein and Gardner 1989).

In order to provide a clearer picture of the state of lung development at birth the terminal sac period may be expanded to comprise:

- saccular phase – 28–36 weeks gestation
- alveolar phase – 36 weeks to term to postnatal

The saccular phase is one of marked change in lung appearance (Langston *et al.* 1984). There is a considerable decrease in the prominence of interstitial tissue, with the saccular walls becoming narrower and more compact. Secondary crests also subdivide the distal air space structures (saccules) into smaller units (sub-saccules).

The alveolar phase is marked by the acquisition of alveoli. Alveoli may be present as early as 30 weeks gestation in some neonates, but according to Langston *et al.* (1984) are not found in *all* lungs until 36 weeks. This process of alveoli development continues into the post-natal period.

The actual alveoli dimensions and number and volume of alveoli have been the topic of many studies. Findings of studies by Emery and Mithal (1960), Thurlbeck (1982) and Langston *et al.* (1984), however, suggest large differences in the total alveolar number at term. Generally, these studies similarly describe alveoli present at birth with a rapid increase in number in the first couple of years of life, a slowing at approximately 4 years of age, then ceasing by about 8 years. The alveoli were shown to enlarge and become deeper to maximize the exposed surface area for gas exchange.

Post-natal Development

Although the infant is capable of sustaining respiratory effort and the lung is able to provide oxygenation and ventilation at term birth, lung development is still incomplete (Thurlbeck 1982, Langston *et al.* 1984). During this period there is development of the atrium, the alveolar sacs and alveoli. At birth, cartilage, mucous glands, goblet cells, ciliated cells and smooth muscle of conducting airways are all present. These all are apparent only in the trachea and bronchi, and are not normally present in the bronchioles. Smooth muscle increases with growth especially around peripheral airways, therefore bronchospasm can occur even in young infants. As a result of this continuing lung development, young infants who suffer severe lung disease may not necessarily have permanent severe lung damage (Merenstein and Gardner 1989).

Characteristics of Respiration

There are similarities between the respiratory system of the normal newborn and an adult (Dunn and Lewis 1973). In all age groups, air passes into the lungs through the nasal and oropharyngeal pathways and travels via the larynx, trachea, bronchi, respiratory bronchioles and alveolar ducts to the alveoli. Gas is exchanged between the alveoli and circulatory system by way of diffusion across the thin walls of the alveoli. The pleural spaces within the thorax surround each lung and, under normal conditions, maintain a negative pressure which helps to keep the lung expanded. The cleansing mechanisms of the lung keep the tract moistened and aid the passage of mucus toward the upper respiratory tract so it can be swallowed or coughed up.

There are some differences, however, which may place the neonate and very young infant in a very vulnerable position when faced with unusual respiratory disturbances. These characteristics are summarized below:

- There is minimal development of alveoli for gas exchange.
- The ratio of conducting airways to the respiratory portion of the lung is larger in the infant and child than in the adult.
- The airway resistance is higher in the newborn and in the young child than in the adult and as the conducting airways are small in the infant they

can be more easily obstructed at the larynx and beyond than in an adult by mucus secretion, inflammation or a foreign body.

- The abdominal muscles of infants are poorly developed resulting in ineffective coughing to clear the airways of mucus.
- In the neonate and young infant the chest wall is very compliant and is cylindrical in shape with ribs slanting horizontally. Consequently diaphragm excursion may cause subcostal retraction rather than rib elevation.
- The neonate and young infant depend on a diaphragmatic pattern of breathing as the ribs slant horizontally and the intercostal muscles are poorly developed.
- The respiratory rate is much higher in infants with the normal resting infant rate at approximately 40 breaths per minute compared with 12 breaths a minute in adults.
- The infant is an obligatory nasal breather producing a direct airway from the nasal cavity to the lungs, so anything obstructing the nares tends to compromise respiration.
- The trachea is short and squat compared with that of an adult thereby aiding entry of bacteria and irritants into the lung.
- The cough and gag reflexes needed to clear and protect the airways are not present until about 32–34 weeks gestation (Burns *et al.* 1987) and even then the infant may fatigue easily due to immature musculature.
- The infant is highly susceptible to diaphragm fatigue due to immature fibre differentiation and compensates for respiratory difficulty by increasing the rate rather than the depth of ventilation (Henderson-Smart 1992).
- Preterm infants less than 35 weeks gestation exhibit periodic respiration, that is, brief apnoeic spells lasting no more than 10–20 seconds with no alteration in other body functions. This is apparently due to respiratory centre immaturity (Stebbens *et al.* 1991, Henderson-Smart 1992). Frequent handling of the infant during care procedures may predispose them to more severe apnoea with associated bradycardia and acidosis (Long *et al.* 1980, Gorski *et al.* 1990).
- The neonate, particularly the preterm neonate, has

a predisposition to hypothermia because of the lack of insulation, its relatively large surface area and immature thermoregulation mechanism. This can affect the respiratory drive and subsequent oxygen uptake (Rutter 1992).

Although these characteristics are normal for the neonate and young infant they may predispose to respiratory distress. All aspects of intervention undertaken in the respiratory care of this age group therefore require the utmost appreciation of these characteristics.

Respiratory Physiotherapy Assessment of the Neonate and Young Infant

As always, the first step to appropriate respiratory physiotherapy intervention is careful assessment before starting each and every treatment session.

HISTORY

This should include:

- Communication with primary caregiver and medical staff – previous medical history; current ventilatory support and stability thereof; tolerance of handling; and previous treatment if any
- Medical chart review – medications, e.g. forms of pain relief, sedation, respiratory stimulants
- Recent investigations – chest X-rays, ultrasound (US) scans, arterial blood gases (ABGs), blood count

OBSERVATION

Nothing replaces the importance of clinical observation by an experienced clinician – it is vital and is often the major form of assessing the neonate and young infant. In neonates, especially preterm neonates, the powerful tool of observation reduces the amount of handling necessary. In infants this tool may reduce the extent of the 'stranger response'. It is important to include in this observation, colour, respiratory effort (nasal flaring, recession, use of accessory muscles), respiratory rate and vital behavioural state. Furthermore, note all monitoring of infant.

AUSCULTATION

Auscultation in the neonate, particularly the preterm neonate, may not be as precise as in the older child or adult due to the small chest cavity and reduced density of the chest wall. Consequently, breath sounds are easily transmitted and anatomical specificity may be diminished. It is important to establish what are normal breath sounds throughout the lung fields and detect any adventitious sounds, such as crackles, wheezes and rubs. Other breath sounds, such as stridor and expiratory grunting, may be heard without the aid of the stethoscope. Owing to the inconclusiveness of auscultation it is very important to evaluate findings in conjunction with chest X-ray results and other assessment findings in planning an appropriate treatment programme for this age group.

PALPATION

This includes examining for:

- presence of any bony aberrations
- chest expansion and symmetry, particularly if mechanically ventilated
- presence of any subcutaneous emphysema or oedema

OTHER ASPECTS TO ASSESS

Assess the general neurodevelopmental status of the patient – some chronic respiratory conditions may result in varying degrees of hypoxic episodes. Also, evaluate the family and home situation, especially with regard to the family's knowledge and ability to participate in treatment programmes once discharged home.

Aims of Respiratory Physiotherapy

- Clear excess or accumulated secretions from the respiratory tract by monitoring the secretions during routine suction.
- Prevent respiratory complications such as atelectasis, infections and retained secretions by using positioning, suctioning and active techniques.

- Assist re-expansion of any collapsed pulmonary segments and clear any areas of consolidation.
- Maintain adequate oxygenation at all times.
- Improve overall respiratory function with the use of positioning.

Principles of Neonatal Respiratory Physiotherapy Management

Early prophylactic neonatal respiratory physiotherapy intervention always emphasizes:

- positioning and regular change of posture to prevent pooling of secretions
- monitoring tolerance of handling and suctioning procedures
- monitoring airway secretions

Nursing Positions

These are the resting positions used to rotate the baby through in a 24-hour period. Particular positions and the regular change of position are of vital importance in relation to lung ventilation/perfusion, neuromuscular development, craniofacial and other forms of positional deformation.

Prone positioning in premature and very young infants has been documented to have beneficial effects on cardiorespiratory (Campbell 1984, Bozynski et al. 1988) and gastrointestinal functions (Hewitt 1976, Orenstein and Whitington 1983) and sleep patterns (Brackbill et al. 1973, Casaer 1979).

Supine positioning is certainly very useful in terms of easy observation and access for the health team. There is sufficient evidence, however, to support the premise that supine should not be used as a routine resting position. For example, a study by Masterton et al. (1987) which examined the effect of prone and supine positioning on energy expenditure and behaviour of 74 low-birth-weight neonates found that infants nursed in prone had lower metabolic rates and spent less time awake than in the supine position, thereby suggesting that prone is the position of choice for the low-birth-weight infant.

Similarly, Dellagrammaticas et al. (1991) found that the prone position was superior to supine in the areas of respiratory performance and gastric emptying in stable very-low-birth-weight neonates. Improved gastric emptying and consequently less pooling of milk in the fundus of the stomach reduces the risk of milk aspiration. Furthermore, a study by Bjornson et al. (1992) on the effects of body position on the oxygen saturation of ventilated preterm infants supported the findings of Dellagrammaticas et al. (1991) as all of the infants in the Bjornson et al. study exhibited higher oxygen saturations in prone than both supine and side lying.

Supine lying may also contribute to postural extension such as shoulder retraction, neck hyperextension and poor abdominal development. Postural asymmetries related to reflex activity also are more common with prolonged supine lying as the infant's head tends to remain on the side to which it is placed. Plagiocephaly (cranial moulding) may also develop as a consequence. In spite of these problems, there are instances where supine positions are indicated.

From a development viewpoint, lateral positioning facilitates flexor muscle development and midline orientation. Lying on the right side also reduces pooling of milk in the fundus of the stomach.

Infants may routinely be nursed elevated to alleviate problems of abdominal contents interfering with diaphragmatic movement, and spontaneous reflux due to immature sphincter control with continuous or frequent feeding regimens. The best increase in end expiratory lung volume and oxygenation is achieved at 45 degrees (Dellagrammaticas et al. 1991).

On the evidence of the available literature it appears that neonates, particularly ventilated very-low-birth-weight neonates, would be best nursed prone with the head and trunk tilted upwards. Indeed the positioning of prone with 20–30° head elevation has been proven to be perhaps the single most important technique in managing gastro-oesophageal reflux GOR (Myers and Herbst 1982).

In order to prevent accumulation of secretions in any dependent area, overstretch on developing muscles of the arms and legs and craniofacial moulding, the infant's position must be regularly altered, maintain-

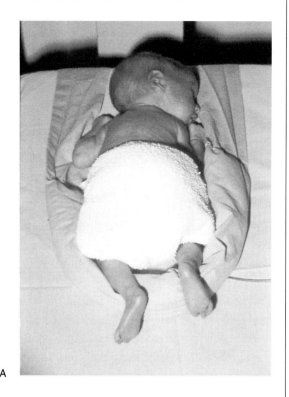

A

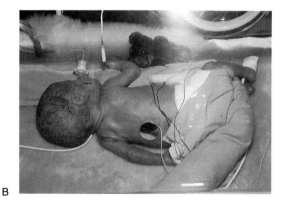

B

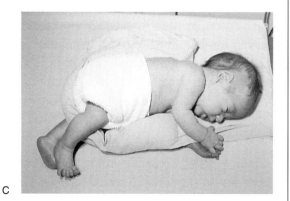

C

ing the same position for not more than 4–6 hours at a time, depending on the individual infant. Initially these positions may consist of prone, ¼ turn from prone, and then ½ turn (lateral) positions when tolerated (see Figure I).

There have been some reported concerns regarding the effect of head position on intracranial pressure (ICP) (Goldberg *et al.* 1983). It is suggested that head position influences ICP significantly probably due to venous congestion caused when the neck is turned, and hydrostatic pressure changes when the head of the bed is elevated. These ICP fluctuations due to head position changes may be deleterious to the infant at risk for intracranial haemorrhage or cerebral oedema. This topic is discussed in more detail in the next chapter. In these situations use of the ¼ turn from prone and particularly the ½ turn positions can assist in keeping the neck more central.

The positioning of infants for sleep is under some controversy in relation to its association with sudden infant death syndrome (SIDS), particularly the prone position. SIDS is a condition of multiple causes and risk factors. However, research over the past 6 years suggests that using the prone sleeping position for full-term healthy babies may increase the risk of SIDS to vulnerable babies by 2–4 times (AAP Task Force 1992).

The advice now given to parents with babies under 6 months of age is 'put your baby on its back or side to sleep'(National SIDS Council of Australia 1993). The advice generally infers a preference for supine over side in that the supine position is more stable, whereas the baby may roll from the side into prone. Some parents have become so concerned that they never put their baby on its tummy. The lack of this valuable experience may hamper the baby's developmental milestones. All advice given to parents on sleeping postures for their baby in the first 6 months should be followed by stressing the importance of alternating the side-to-side position and allowing the baby short intervals of time (5–10 minutes) on the stomach daily during wakeful periods.

All this must be taken in perspective, appreciating that there are several exceptions to the rule with the critically ill neonate and young infant. These exceptions are well supported by research as discussed earlier. Apart from the benefits of prone positioning for infants with acute respiratory distress or chronic neonatal lung disease or gastro-oesophageal reflux, infants with certain upper airway anomalies such as Pierre Robin syndrome do better in the prone position. Other infants, because of their anatomical makeup, such as in spina bifida or lower limb deficiency, need to be positioned prone to prevent soft tissue contractions.

Postural Drainage

Treatment positions are usually different from nursing positions as they are designed to drain specific areas of the lung by using gravity to assist movement of secretions from the smaller airways to the larger bronchi (Dunn and Lewis 1973). The anatomy of the neonate is similar to that of an adult, but the neonate's lungs have not differentiated into alveolar sacs. If a particular area is involved or suspected, the aim is to position the infant precisely for that area where possible, but often modifications are warranted.

It is rare to place a premature infant in a head down position at any time due to the fragility in their intracranial vasculature and risk of spontaneous gastro-oesophageal reflux. Care should be taken also when considering positioning with full rotation of the neck.

Tipping is contraindicated in the presence of:

- respiratory distress
- fluctuations in blood pressure
- post-operative abdominal or thoracic surgery
- recent intracranial haemorrhage
- hypoxia/episodes of apnoea and/or bradycardia
- abdominal distension
- suspected or confirmed gastro-oesophageal reflux
- marked facial/cranial bruising
- suspected raised intracranial pressure.

Postural drainage positions may also need to be modified in the presence of other apparatus such as monitoring equipment, intravenous or arterial lines and other drains and tubing attached to the infant.

Active Techniques

These are the manual physiotherapy techniques of percussion and vibration which are applied to the chest wall to loosen secretions and allow easier removal when the infant coughs, sneezes or has the airway cleared with a suction catheter. Manual hyperinflation (or bagging) is another technique that may occasionally be used with full-term neonates and infants but certainly not with preterm infants. Along with the risk of producing pneumothoraces, manual hyperinflation has the potential to decrease cardiac output which may increase the risk of cerebral haemorrhage (Paratz and Burns 1993).

Since vigorous therapy is very fatiguing, active techniques are only implemented after thorough assessment of an infant's tolerance of handling and positioning. Extreme care must be exercised in infants with osteoporotic ribs, cerebral bleeds, marginal levels of oxygenation and particular feeding regimens.

With percussion, a rhythmical cupping action is applied over the chest wall using the cupped hand or fingers (illustrated in Tecklin 1994), or a paediatric resuscitation face mask in order to cause pressure changes within the airways and loosen secretions. See Figure 2.

Vibration is performed by placing the fingers on the chest and producing a fine shaking action but ensuring very little pressure is exerted on the chest. This technique is good for infants with fragile paper-thin skin, where intercostal catheters (ICCs) are in situ,

Figure 2 The active technique of cupping with paediatric resuscitation face mask

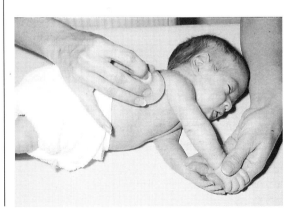

Figure 3 The active technique of finger vibration using pad of fingers not tips

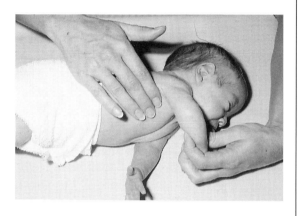

infants who are very small, or those who do not tolerate cupping. It is the most hazardous to administer because of the danger of fracturing ribs. It is useful in improving the tidal volume, especially in infants following abdominal surgery. See Figure 3.

The indications for commencement of active techniques (Crane 1981) include:

- crackles present on auscultation
- increase in amount and viscosity of secretions
- signs of atelectasis or infiltrate on chest X-ray

REPORTED EFFECTS AND EFFICACY OF TECHNIQUES WITH VERY PRETERM INFANTS

Some studies have indicated that physiotherapy resulted in hypoxaemia (Holloway *et al.* 1969, Fox *et al.* 1978). In the reporting of their results, however, it was not possible to distinguish the effects of active physiotherapy techniques from the effects of suctioning alone. In contrast, Finer and Boyd (1978) demonstrated a significant increase in arterial Po_2 following chest physiotherapy.

Etches and Scott (1978) and Dall Alba and Burns (1990) found that active chest physiotherapy techniques led to increased removal of secretions thus supporting the use of these measures to decrease the amount of secretions in the airways. Raval *et al.* (1987) reported that active chest physiotherapy techniques increased the incidence of intraventricular haemorrhage, whereas a more recent study by Paratz and Burns (1993) found that intracranial pressure was increased

with suction, but not with active physiotherapy techniques.

Different techniques of physiotherapy have been investigated in preterm infants. Finer and Boyd (1978) found a significant increase in arterial Po_2 with the technique of postural drainage and percussion compared with postural drainage alone. Hartrick *et al.* (1982) reported no increase in cardiorespiratory disturbances with postural drainage, percussion, vibration or suction. Vibration with an electric toothbrush was found by Curran and Kachoyeanos (1979) to produce a significantly higher Pao_2, clearer breath sounds and better tissue perfusion than percussion using a padded nipple.

Tudehope and Bagley (1980) compared the effects of cupping with a Bennett's face mask, vibration with an electric toothbrush and contact heel percussion. They found that all babies had an increase in Po_2 following percussion, particularly with a Bennett's face mask.

Though these studies present variable benefits of respiratory physiotherapy it is important to be aware that medical practice and care for very preterm infants is changing and improving all the time and indeed some of these studies may no longer be applicable to current forms of respiratory physiotherapy intervention. Furthermore, active techniques are used often in combination during a treatment session. The physiotherapist is guided by how the infant presents and their ongoing tolerance of the particular technique being administered. The skill of continued observation and monitoring of the infant's colour, respiratory effort, blood pressure and body temperature during each and every treatment session is vital.

Frequency of Treatment

This is dependent on the baby and its condition. Treatment is aimed at fitting in with major handling times. Physiotherapy treatment is usually done 15–20 minutes before a feed is due with treatment lasting for 1½–3 minutes per postural drainage position with a maximum of 2–3 positions for each treatment.

Ventilated infants, and infants on nasopharyngeal continuous positive airway pressure (CPAP) routinely have 4–8 hourly suction and position change, and active techniques when indicated. Hourly and second hourly physiotherapy is only indicated if there is severe collapse / consolidation or gross secretions. Hourly treatment is then only performed for a maximum of 6–8 hours before reverting to second hourly treatment. Hourly treatment does fatigue the baby and may lead to further complications.

Removal of Secretions

The use of the cough to clear secretions from the large airways may not be considered a reliable method in the neonate or very young infant. The presence and strength of the protective cough reflex depends on gestational age. It develops at approximately 32–34 weeks gestation, but is not consistent / mature until 38 weeks gestation (Burns *et al.* 1987). Even then endurance is low and the infant will tire easily.

Although suctioning is a standard procedure used in airway maintenance, it is potentially dangerous (Crane 1981, Perlman and Volpe 1983, Paratz and Burns 1993). The primary purpose of suction is to facilitate the removal of airway secretions where an effective cough is not possible, therefore preventing obstruction and optimizing oxygenation and ventilation.

The dangers of suction are well-documented (Shorten *et al.* 1991) and include:

- bacteraemia
- atelectasis
- pneumothorax
- tachycardia
- apnoea and bradycardia
- mucosal trauma
- systemic hypertension
- increase in intracranial pressure

To minimize the hazards of suctioning, different methods have been proposed. These include preoxygenation and hyperventilation to reduce hypoxaemia (Cheng and Williams 1989); assessing infant's blood pressure to reduce risk of precipitating a cerebral haemorrhage (Paratz and Burns 1993); limiting the depth, duration and suction pressure of the applied suction to reduce hypoxaemia and mucosal damage (Poole *et al.* 1974); using saline instillations to thin secretions and aid their removal (Shorten *et al.* 1991); and administering sedation as well as limiting handling

to decrease the effects of intervention on the cardiovascular system and thus cerebral blood flow (Fox *et al.* 1978). These factors appear to have contributed to a reduction in suction-related problems, but the technique of suction still remains a potentially dangerous procedure which must be performed with caution.

BRONCHIAL LAVAGE

Bronchial lavage is another method of removing secretions which may be used with neonates and young infants. As the name suggests it is used selectively to lavage and then suction from a main bronchus. It may be used to clear an obstructing plug of mucus or meconium, or to collect bronchial secretions to test for cytomegalovirus or other similar organisms. The volume of lavage used is much larger than that for routine suctioning – up to 2 ml/kg body weight. To ensure accurate placement of lavage and suction catheter it is necessary to have the infant positioned to give access to the main bronchus, i.e. by turning the head to the opposite side and depressing the ipsilateral shoulder. This positioning of the infant needs to be maintained whilst lavage is being instilled and suctioning is undertaken.

Suggested Guidelines to Suctioning a Ventilated Neonate or Very Young Infant

Oral

- suction oropharynx prior to tube or nasal suction
- distance from tip of nose to lowest aspect of ear
- size fg 8 catheter
- if cough reflex present infant may fatigue easily

Endotracheal tube (ETT)
may need to

- preoxygenate by 5–10% greater Fio_2
- increase respiratory rate by 5–10

Procedure
(This must be a sterile procedure and involve two staff members where possible)

- determine distance of ETT
- add extra length for suction port and connector
- instil lavage with blunt needle through suction port
- use sterile gloved hand to introduce suction catheter through suction port
- using marked measures on catheter advance catheter to predetermined distance
- repeat procedure with second lavage, sterile glove and catheter.

Important points

- one glove, one catheter per entry into ETT to retain sterility
- 10 seconds duration
- 20 kPa suction pressure
- nasal suction generally avoided unless obvious secretions, as trauma and oedema may embarrass ventilation of the preterm infant, who is an obligatory nasal breather

HUMIDIFICATION AND WARMING OF INSPIRED GASES

This is vital to decrease risks of hypothermia, dehydration and thickened secretions. All supplemental oxygen should be warmed to 34–37°C depending on the source of the oxygen and the gestational age of the infant, and humidified to about 90% saturation. If the temperature of inspired oxygen is kept at 36.5–37°C for mechanically ventilated infants there is a decreased risk of ETT blockage and small airway plugging, decreased air leaks and consequent pneumothorax. This in turn results in decreased risk of intraventricular haemorrhage.

Particular care is warranted when treating an infant on a radiant heat table to avoid an increase in insensible water loss. In ventilated infants and infants on NPCPAP, additional humidification is used before suctioning in the form of a NaCl lavage. For an ETT, use a lavage of 0.25 ml NaCl in the preterm infant and 0.5 ml in a term infant. Diluted $NaHCO_3$ may be used to loosen thick secretions alternated and finishing with NaCl to reduce the burning effect of this alkaline solution on the respiratory mucosa. Nebulized

NaCl is used in non-intubated infants to loosen thick secretions.

Causes of thickening of secretions are as follows:

- infection
- fever
- trauma to bronchial cilia from long-term ventilation
- post-operatively with atelectasis
- insensible water loss
- poor humidification of inspired gases

Insensible water loss may be eliminated by the use of:

- bubble sheet
- glad wrap
- bonnets and booties where permissible

Physiotherapy Management of Common Respiratory Conditions

The following is an outline of a number of respiratory conditions frequently seen in the neonate and young infant population and physiotherapy involvement.

Retained Fetal Lung Fluid (RFLF) or Transient Tachypnoea of the Newborn (TTN)

This condition occurs in 1–2% of all newborns with tachypnoea being its main feature. The chest X-ray exhibits a streaky, often asymmetrical appearance. The fluid usually absorbs within 24–72 hours with rapid improvement in respiratory status. Active chest physiotherapy is not indicated in this condition although a positioning regime should be instigated which emphasizes minimal handling. Often these are babies who are born close to term and certainly settle better in the prone position.

Respiratory Distress Syndrome (RDS)

Respiratory distress syndrome (RDS) occurs in 1% of all births and has a characteristic clinical course (Farrell and Avery 1975, Stark and Franz 1986, Levene et al. 1987, Merenstein and Gardner 1989, Greenough et al. 1992, Wood 1993). It is most often associated with prematurity at birth. Other predisposing factors include maternal diabetes, antepartum haemorrhage, second twin, hypoxia, acidosis, shock, male sex and possibly caesarean section (Levene *et al.* 1987, Greenough *et al.* 1992, Wood 1993). The primary contributing factor in RDS is immaturity of the surfactant system, and since functional maturity of this system does not occur until late gestation, the incidence of RDS relates to the degree of prematurity.

In 1959, Avery and Mead demonstrated that a deficiency of pulmonary surfactant is the cause of RDS. As surfactant modifies surface tension to keep the alveoli expanded and stabilize them at a uniform volume, a deficiency in surfactant leads to widespread atelectasis. In turn, alveolar collapse and obstruction of conducting airways leads to a mismatch of ventilation and perfusion and consequently profound hypoxaemia (Levene *et al.* 1987). Surfactant may have other functions as well, including the prevention of pulmonary oedema, infection, lung injury from toxic substances such as oxygen (Soll and Lucey 1991), and the prevention of airway mucus obstruction (Rubin *et al.* 1992).

In recent years much research has gone into investigating methods of accelerating lung maturation and hence reducing or preventing the presentation of RDS and its complications. Steroid therapy (betamethasone or dexamethasone) administered to the mother 24–48 hours before the delivery of the fetus of less than 34 weeks gestation is used to facilitate lung maturation prior to birth. The use of exogenous surfactant preparations administered to the neonate via the ETT has also been widely investigated (Long and Sanders 1988, Bose *et al.* 1990, Rubin *et al.* 1992). The two forms of surfactant preparations, synthetic or natural surfactant extracts, are now in wide use in neonatal intensive care units whilst research continues. There is still some debate about the most appropriate time to provide this form of therapy – either as a prophylactic strategy immediately following birth (Soll *et al.* 1990, Corbet *et al.* 1991), or as a rescue form of therapy (Long *et al.* 1991).

Symptoms of RDS usually occur within 2–3 hours after birth progressively deteriorating within the first 24–48 hours. Clinical signs include tachypnoea (respiratory rate greater than 60 per minute), expiratory grunting, intercostal and sternal recession and nasal flaring. Respiratory failure occurs as a result of fatigue. Tachypnoea is an attempt to increase alveolar gas exchange while recession is due to the result of attempts to ventilate stiff lungs (Polgar 1973). The expiratory grunt is caused by expiration against a partially closed glottis (Polgar 1973, Robertson 1984). This has the effect of maintaining a positive pressure within the lung throughout expiration and thus helping to maintain the patency of the alveoli (Robertson 1984). The actual diagnosis of RDS is made using standard criteria of progressive respiratory insufficiency and hypoxaemia in the first hours of life in a premature neonate with accompanying roentgenographic signs of bilateral interstitial pulmonary infiltrates and air bronchograms (Levene *et al.* 1987).

PHYSIOTHERAPY MANAGEMENT

Physiotherapy management for this condition in neonates is directed towards preventing complications that affect airway efficiency by focusing on assisting airway clearance, improving ventilation and decreasing the work of breathing (Crane 1981). This is done by regular suction and positioning of the neonate and adding active respiratory physiotherapy techniques when indicated.

In the exudative phase (acute stage) of the illness, physiotherapy management consists of positioning and regular change of position with regular suctioning to maximize diaphragmatic movement, enhance aeration and perfusion, reduce atelectasis, and maintain oxygenation. Change in ETT secretions must also be monitored. There are usually minimal secretions in the exudative phase due to laying down of the hyaline membranes along the bronchial and alveolar epithelium and loss of cilia action. A typical regime may consist of 6/24 suction and position change but each infant needs to be assessed individually.

In the recovery phase, the hyaline membranes become fragmented and the end result of the necrosis and exudate are phagocytosed by the pulmonary macrophages. Physiotherapy involvement consists of positioning as in the acute stage, and adding in more changes in position as the infant becomes tolerant, to reduce pooling of secretions and to reduce free and interstitial air (note importance of $\frac{1}{4}$ turn from prone position). It is also necessary to continue to monitor ETT secretions. The break up of hyaline membranes and the end result of necrosis increases bronchial secretions. These secretions tend to thicken due to stasis and pooling, and make spontaneous clearance less adequate. Active respiratory physiotherapy techniques within the infant's tolerance are added to enhance removal of debris and facilitate re-expansion of areas of collapse.

From this subacute stage there are those infants who resolve and continue to improve, and there are those who fail to resolve and progress to the proliferative phase with interstitial lung oedema and fibrosis. Alternating areas of atelectasis and overinflation begin to appear with air trapping. Further progression of this process results in the chronic phase, which Northway et al. (1967) initially described as bronchopulmonary dysplasia (BPD). Tudehope (1993) notes that the incidence of BPD relates to the severity of the initial RDS and the degree of prematurity (p. 86).

Chronic Neonatal Lung Disease (CNLD)/Bronchopulmonary Dysplasia (BPD)

Tooley (1979) assigned the term 'chronic lung disease' to those neonates who had radiological abnormality of lung parenchyma and who required an $Fio_2 > 0.21$ for more than 30 days (p. 851). BPD, which is characterized by hypoxia, hypercapnia and oxygen dependency, is a major presentation of chronic neonatal lung disease (CNLD). Indeed, Bancalari et al. (1979) defined BPD as a disease affecting infants who require intermittent positive pressure ventilation for >3 days and supplemental oxygen for >28 days and whose chest radiographs revealed parenchymal densities (p. 819). This disease causes thickening of the bronchial epithelium, hypertrophy of smooth muscle and interstitial oedema and fibrosis which produces uneven aeration, atelectasis, emphysema and compression of the respiratory ducts. Clinically, the infant exhibits persistent chest retractions, crackles and wheezes on auscultation, gross hyperinflation of the chest with an increased A–P diameter of the chest (in an attempt to gain maximum efficiency of the diaphragm), and may show signs of congestive heart failure from a prolonged L–R shunt.

PHYSIOTHERAPY MANAGEMENT

The physiotherapy management in this phase consists of respiratory management as for the recovery phase of RDS to facilitate opening up of compressed airways and collapsed segments and to gain more even oxygenation. This is essential for lung healing and growth which may take up to 2–3 years. Positioning is aimed at: (a) promoting feed tolerance and avoiding the high risk of reflux, i.e. use of elevation and avoiding left side lying which may result in pooling in the fundus of the stomach; and (b) promoting the development of muscle tone and strength in the flexor components of the body of the low-birth-weight infant, i.e. use of $\frac{1}{4}$ turn from prone and later side lying with swaddling.

Acute Collapse/Consolidation

Acute collapse usually occurs as a result of mucous plugging, infection or aspiration of milk or blood.

PHYSIOTHERAPY MANAGEMENT

Physiotherapy management of this condition consists of short frequent treatments to the specific area of opacification. Selective positioning between treatments is critical to complement the treatment positions. Use of the appropriate postural drainage positions may be the aim, but there may be other considerations that will influence these positions. The techniques of cupping, vibration and suction are administered according to the infant's tolerance, and additional humidification may be important to help mobilize the plugs of mucus.

Meconium Aspiration

Meconium aspiration is most likely to occur in the term infant as the passage of meconium is uncommon under 34 weeks gestation. The infant may show signs of growth retardation. Meconium is an extreme irritant to the airways and cause of pneumonitis. Clinically, signs of respiratory distress appear and the chest is typically hyperinflated and barrel shaped. On chest X-ray there are coarse mottled densities with areas of increased radiolucency in both lung fields or, alternatively, there may be one specific area of involvement. A pneumothorax or a pneumomediastinum are frequent complications.

PHYSIOTHERAPY MANAGEMENT

Active respiratory physiotherapy techniques are begun as soon as the infant is stable enough to treat the specific areas of concern. Pulmonary hypertension may influence the time of commencement and the type of respiratory physiotherapy techniques used as these infants generally have a very poor tolerance of handling. The frequency of treatment depends on the infant's tolerance of handling, response to treatment, severity of aspiration and specific areas of concern.

Treatments are usually short with the emphasis being on quality of treatment rather than quantity of positions treated each time. Therefore, the regime is planned to eliminate any unnecessary turning and handling. Humidification is of vital importance to enhance the mobilization of meconium, with the use of bagging and vibrations after instilling the lavage being beneficial in removing plugs of mucus.

Pulmonary Interstitial Emphysema (PIE)/Pneumothorax

Pulmonary interstitial emphysema is a condition mainly noted in preterm infants with RDS. It is a result of entrapment of gas in the interstitium of the lung from overinflated and ruptured alveoli. The causes may be due to excessive interstitial fluid relating to permeability problems, the ETT down the right main bronchus therefore causing hyperinflation of the right lower lobe, or as a result of trauma from ETT suctioning producing granulous tissue which acts as a 'ball valve' phenomena causing blowing out of the lower lobes. This condition is frequently observed with, or just before, a pneumothorax or pneumomediastinum.

PHYSIOTHERAPY MANAGEMENT

The physiotherapy management of PIE and also for undrained pneumothoraces involves: positioning to decrease airflow to the affected lung/segment, i.e. that side dependent, or positioning prone with the head turned to the ipsilateral side; avoiding use of cupping but using vibrations if active techniques are indicated; suction ensuring a premeasured catheter is used. Once an intercostal catheter is in situ, it is important to position with the drain and the lung involved uppermost; if the drain is placed anteriorly,

the baby is nursed supine with the ipsilateral side uppermost.

Surgical Conditions

Congenital Diaphragmatic Hernia

With diaphragmatic hernias, there is often extensive impairment of both the ipsilateral and contralateral lungs with fewer small bronchioles and bronchiolar divisions and fewer pulmonary arteries. The number of alveoli per unit area is normal, but there is a decrease in number of acinar units (i.e. lung distal to the terminal bronchiole). The ipsilateral lung is considerably smaller in volume, but the alteration in airway branching is similar in both lungs. The left lung is more commonly involved (Tudehope and Thearle 1984).

Clinically, there are ventilation and perfusion problems, post-operative atelectasis and pooling of secretions, and peripheral oedema impairing chest wall movement. These babies are usually drug-paralysed post-operatively and environmental noise is kept to a minimum to reduce stress on the repaired diaphragm. These babies tend to be fragile with handling.

PHYSIOTHERAPY MANAGEMENT

The aim of physiotherapy is to keep the contralateral lung clear and inflated and also to assist inflation of the affected side. This involves specific and regular position changes with the active respiratory physiotherapy techniques of cupping and vibrations being gradually incorporated. Passive movements and effleurage may also be used to decrease oedema and increase chest movement.

Tracheo-oesophageal Fistula

Clinically, these babies have excess saliva and mucus production and a high incidence of aspiration pneumonia. Post-operatively, they are nursed prone with head and trunk elevated 45°. A naso-oesophageal tube is in situ on continuous low suction to keep the anastomosis dry, and the infant is fed via a naso-jejunal tube.

PHYSIOTHERAPY MANAGEMENT

The aim of physiotherapy is to treat the areas of aspiration and post-operative atelectasis. Frequent oral suction is necessary using a premeasured catheter to avoid trauma to the anastomosis.

Cardiac Conditions

Apart from the considerations of the effect of surgery and the incision site, physiotherapists need to be aware of the cardiovascular status of the neonate, in particular the capillary return, skin temperature and peripheral pulses, the blood pressure, the presence of any arrythmias, cardiac support drugs, and internal lines.

PHYSIOTHERAPY MANAGEMENT

The problems associated with this surgery usually result from the prolonged intubation. The early use of positioning as tolerated and regular secretion clearance is vital with the addition of active techniques when necessary and when tolerated.

Pierre Robin Syndrome

Pierre Robin syndrome consists of micrognathia (small jaw) with associated pseudomacroglossia (large tongue) and high arched or cleft palate. Under the influence of gravity the tongue assumes a retruded position obstructing the pharynx. The obstruction of the airway, particularly on inspiration, usually requires treatment in order to avoid suffocation. The safe position is with the baby prone such that the tongue falls forward to relieve respiratory obstruction. Sufficient mandibular growth usually takes place within a few months to relieve the risk of obstruction.

A long nasal CPAP tube is used to maintain patent airway but mechanical ventilation is not required. It is initially inserted by the doctor as this tube is required to sit just above the epiglottis. Once the correct length is established, the tube can be changed by the appropriate staff member.

Post-extubation Atelectasis

Post-extubation collapse has occurred frequently in newborn infants who have received mechanical ventilation for respiratory failure in the newborn period.

Wyman and Kuhns (1977) used chest X-rays during and after intubation to show that no babies developed lobar collapse during intubation, but 11 out of 27 developed collapse post-extubation. This collapse is thought to have been due to retained secretions and mucosal oedema caused by the endotracheal tube (Finer et al. 1979), the build-up of secretions due to trauma from repeated suctioning and ciliary dysfunction and tissue damage leading to the infants' inability to move secretions (Wyman and Kuhns 1977), or from the secretions forming around the tube and massing together to occlude the lobar bronchus as the tube is extracted.

PHYSIOTHERAPY MANAGEMENT

To minimize the incidence of post-extubation collapse, a specific procedure incorporating regular suction and position change needs to be used to aerate particularly the right upper lobe.

Bronchiolitis

This condition is usually as a result of the respiratory syncytial virus and is the most common lower respiratory tract infection in infants under 1 year of age and in particular under 6 months. The main features are symptoms of a cold followed 1–2 days later by an irritating cough, distressed rapid wheezy breathing and difficulty feeding. The chest is commonly barrel-shaped due to pulmonary hyperinflation and costal recession occurs during inspiration. On auscultation, there are fine inspiratory crackles with intermittent expiratory wheezes.

PHYSIOTHERAPY MANAGEMENT

The physiotherapy management of bronchiolitis involves minimal handling and the treatment of any specific areas of collapse/consolidation once the infant is stable. The use of humidification often plays a key role in assisting with the mobilization of secretions.

Aspiration Pneumonia

Aspiration pneumonia may be due to:

- disorders of sucking and swallowing
- oesophageal malfunctioning leading to reflux into the pharynx

- abnormal communication from the airways to the oesophagus, e.g. tracheo-oesophageal reflux

The symptoms include a cough, rattling / wheezy breathing, tachypnoea, malaise, hyperinflated chest, crackles and wheezes, and may be fever and / or cyanosis.

PHYSIOTHERAPY MANAGEMENT

The physiotherapy management includes feeding facilitation, maintaining food / air entry by positioning with the head up, and the treatment of any localized problems.

Summary

This chapter provides a summary of lung development and the unique characteristics of the neonatal and infantile cardiorespiratory systems which can place this age group at risk of respiratory distress. Assessment and principles of respiratory physiotherapy intervention have been reviewed and discussed. The common respiratory conditions for this age group are highlighted and appropriate forms of respiratory physiotherapy management are described. Respiratory physiotherapy does have a part to play in the respiratory care of the neonate and very young infant providing that role continues to be evaluated and kept up to date with the changing medical management of this age group.

REFERENCES

American Academy of Pediatrics (AAP) Task Force on Infant Positioning and SIDS (1992) *Pediatrics* **89**: 1120–1126.

Avery, ME, Mead, J (1959) Surface properties in relation to atelectasis and hyaline membrane disease. *American Journal of Disease in Childhood* **97**: 517–523.

Bancalari, E, Abdenour, GE, Feller, R et al. (1979) Bronchopulmonary dysplasia: clinical presentation. *Journal of Pediatrics* **95**: 819–823.

Bjornson, KF, Deitz, JC, Blackburn, S et al. (1992) The effect of body position on the oxygen saturation of ventilated preterm infants. In: *Pediatric Physical Therapy*, pp. 109–115. Baltimore: Williams and Wilkins.

Brackbill, Y, Douthitt, TC, West, H (1973) Psychophysiologic effects in the neonate of prone versus supine placement. *Journal of Pediatrics* **82**: 82–84.

Bose, C, Corbet, A, Bose, G et al. (1990) Improved outcome at 28 days of age for very low birth weight infants treated with a single dose of a synthetic surfactant. *Journal of Pediatrics* **117**: 947–953.

Bozynski, MEA, Nagile, RA, Nicks, JJ et al. (1988) Lateral positioning of the stable ventilated very-low-birth-weight infant. *American Journal of Diseases in Childhood* **142(2)**: 200–202.

Burns, Y, Rogers, Y, Neil, M et al. (1987) Development of oral function in preterm infants. *Physiotherapy Practice* **3**: 168–178.

Campbell, SK (1984) *Pediatric Neurologic Physical Therapy. Clinics in Physical Therapy*, vol. 5, 430 pp. New York: Churchill Livingstone.

Casaer, P (1979) *Postural Behaviour in Newborn Infants. Clinics in Developmental Medicine* no. 72, 112 pp. London: Spastics International Medical Publications.

Cheng, M, Williams, PD (1989) Oxygenation during chest physiotherapy of very low birth weight infants: relations among fraction of inspired oxygen levels, number of hand ventilations and transcutaneous oxygen pressure. *Journal of Pediatric Nursing* **4**: 411–418.

Corbet, A, Bucciarelli, R, Goldman, S et al. (1991) Decreased mortality rate among small premature infants treated at birth with a single dose of synthetic surfactant: a multicenter controlled trial. *Journal of Pediatrics* **118**: 277–284.

Crane, L (1981) Physical therapy for neonates with respiratory dysfunction. *Physical Therapy* **61**: 1764–1773.

Curran, LC, Kachoyeanos, MK (1979) The effects on neonates of two methods of chest physical therapy. *Mothercraft Nursing* **4**: 309–313.

Dall Alba, PT, Burns, Y (1990) The relationship between arterial blood gases and removal of airway secretions in neonates. *Physiotherapy Theory and Practice* **6**: 107–117.

Dellagrammaticas, HD, Kapetanikas, J, Papadimitriou (1991) Effect of body tilting on physiological functions in stable very low birthweight neonates. *Archives of Disease in Childhood* **66**: 429–432.

Dunn, D, Lewis, AT (1973) Some important aspects of neonatal nursing related to pulmonary disease and family involvement. *Pediatric Clinics of North America* **20**: 481–497.

Emery, JL, Mithal, A (1960) The number of alveoli in the terminal respiratory unit of man during late intrauterine life and childhood. *Archives of Disease in Childhood* **35**: 544–547.

Etches, PC, Scott, B (1978) Chest physiotherapy in the newborn: effect of secretions removed. *Pediatrics* **62**: 713–715.

Farrell, PM (1982) Overview of hyaline membrane disease. In: *Lung Development: Biological and Clinical Perspectives*, vol. II. New York: Academic Press.

Farrell, PM, Avery, ME (1975) Hyaline membrane disease. *American Review of Respiratory Disease* **111**: 657–688.

Finer, NN, Boyd, J (1978) Chest physiotherapy in the neonate: a controlled study. *Pediatrics* **61(2)**: 282–285.

Finer, NN, Moriarty, RR, Boyd, J et al. (1979) Post-extubation atelectasis: a retrospective review and prospective controlled study. *Journal of Pediatrics* **94**: 110–113.

Fox, WH, Schwartz, JG, Shaffer, TH (1978) Pulmonary physiotherapy in neonates: physiologic changes and respiratory management. *Journal of Pediatrics* **92**: 977–981.

Goldberg, RN, Joshi, A, Moscoso, P et al. (1983) The effect of head position on intracranial pressure. *Critical Care Medicine* **11**: 428–430.

Gorski, PA, Huntington, L, Lewkowicz, DJ (1990) Handling preterm infants in hospitals. *Clinics in Perinatology* **17**: 103–112.

Greenough, A, Morley, CJ, Robertson, NRC (1992) Acute respiratory disease in the newborn. In: Robertson, NRC (ed.) *Textbook of Neonatology*, 2nd edn, pp. 385–504. London: Chuchill Livingstone.

Hartrick, J, Fluitt, L, Parrott, J et al. (1982) A controlled study of chest physiotherapy methods in the newborn infant. *Australian Paediatric Journal* **18**: 141.

Hewitt, VM (1976) Effect of posture on the presence of fat in tracheal aspirate in neonates. *Australian Paediatric Journal* **12**: 267–271.

Henderson-Smart, D (1992) Respiratory physiology. In: Robertson, NRC (ed.) *Textbook of Neonatology*, 2nd edn, pp. 349–367. London: Churchill Livingstone.

Holloway, R, Adams, EB, Desai, SD et al. (1969) Effect of chest physiotherapy on blood gases of neonates treated by intermittent positive pressure respiration. *Thorax* **24**: 421–426.

Langston, C, Kida, K, Reed, M et al. (1984) Human lung growth in late gestation and in the neonate. *American Review of Respiratory Disease* 129: 607–613.

Levene, MI, Tudehope, D, Thearle, J (1987) *Essentials of Neonatal Medicine*, 402 pp. Oxford: Blackwell Scientific.

Long, WA, Sanders, RL (1988) New treatment methods in neonatal respiratory distress syndrome: replacement of surface active material. In: Guthrie, RD (ed.) Neonatal Intensive Care. *Clinics in Critical Care Medicine* 13: 21–56.

Long, JG, Phillip, AGS, Lucey, JF (1980) Excessive handling as a cause of hypoxaemia. *Pediatrics* 65: 203–207.

Long, W, Thompson, T, Sundell, H et al. (1991) Effects of two rescue doses of a synthetic surfactant on mortality rate and survival without bronchopulmonary dysplasia in 700- to 1350-gram infants with respiratory distress syndrome. *Journal of Pediatrics* 118: 595–605.

Masterton, J, Zucher, C, Schulze, K (1987) Prone and supine positioning effects on energy expenditure and behaviour of low birth weight neonates. *Pediatrics* 80: 689–692.

Merenstein, Gardner (1989) *Handbook of Neonatal Intensive Care*, 404 pp. 2nd edn. St Louis: CV Mosby.

Myers, WF, Herbst, JJ (1982) Effectiveness of positioning therapy for gastro-esophageal reflux. *Pediatrics* 69: 768–772.

National SIDS Council of Australia (1993) *Help Reduce the Risks of Cot Death* (leaflet).

Northway, WH, Rosan, R, Porter, DY (1967) Pulmonary disease following respiratory therapy of hyaline membrane diseases and broncho-pulmonary dysplasia. *New England Journal of Medicine* 276: 357–368.

Orenstein, SR, Whitington, PF (1983) Positioning for prevention of infant gastroesophageal reflux. *Journal of Pediatrics* 103: 524–537.

Paratz, JD, Burns, YR (1993). Intracranial dynamics in pre-term infants and neonates: implications for physiotherapists. *Australian Journal of Physiotherapy* 39: 171–178.

Perlman, JM, Volpe, JJ (1983) Suctioning in the preterm infant: effects on cerebral blood flow velocity, intracranial pressure, and arterial blood pressure. *Pediatrics* 72(3): 329–334.

Polgar, G (1973) Practical pulmonary physiology. *Pediatric Clinics of North America* 20: 303–322.

Poole, JL, Abrahams, N, Fisk, GC (1974) Paediatric endotracheal suction. *Anaesthesia and Intensive Care* 11: 131–141.

Raval, D, Yeh, TF, Mora, A et al. (1987) Chest physiotherapy in preterm infants with RDS in the first 24 hours of life. *Journal of Perinatology* 7: 301–304.

Robertson, B (1984) Pathology and pathophysiology of neonatal surfactant deficiency. In: Robertson, B, Van Golde, LMG, Batenburg, JJ (eds) *Pulmonary Surfactant*, pp. 383–418. Amsterdam: Elsevier Science.

Rubin, BK, Ramirez, O, King, M (1992) Mucus rheology and transport in neonatal Respiratory Distress Syndrome and the effect of surfactant therapy. *Chest* 101: 1080–1085.

Rutter, N (1992) Temperature control and its disorders. In: Robertson, NRC (ed.) *Textbook of Neonatology*, 2nd edn. pp. 217–231, London: Churchill Livingstone.

Shorten, DR, Byrne, PJ, Jones, RR (1991) Infant responses to saline instillations and endotracheal suctioning. *Journal of Obstetric, Gynecologic, and Neonatal Nursing* 20: 464–469.

Soll, RF, Lucey, JF (1991) Surfactant replacement therapy. *Pediatrics in Review* 12: 261–267.

Soll, RF, Hoekstra, RE, Fangman, JJ et al. (1990) Multicenter trial of single-dose modified bovine surfactant extract (Survanta) for prevention of Respiratory Distress Syndrome. *Pediatrics* 85: 1092–1102.

Stark, AR, Franz, ID (1986) Respiratory Distress Syndrome. *Pediatric Clinics of North America* 33: 533–544.

Stebbens, VA, Poets, CF, Alexander, JR et al. (1991) Oxygen saturation and breathing patterns in infancy. *Archives of Disease in Childhood* 66: 569–573.

Tecklin, JS (1994) *Pediatric Physical Therapy*, 2nd edn, 468 pp. Philadelphia: JB Lippincott Co.

Thurlbeck, WM (1982) Postnatal human lung growth. *Thorax* 37: 564–571.

Tooley, WH (1979) Epidemiology of bronchopulmonary dysplasia. *Journal of Pediatrics* 95: 851–858.

Tudehope, DI (1993) Editorial comment: bronchopulmonary dysplasia. *Journal of Paediatrics and Child Health* 29: 86–89.

Tudehope, DI, Bagley, C (1980) Techniques of physiotherapy in intubated babies with the respiratory distress syndrome. *Australian Paediatric Journal* 16: 226–228.

Tudehope, DI, Thearle, MJ (1984) *Primer of Neonatal Medicine*, 272 pp. Brisbane: William Brooks.

Wood, BP (1993) The newborn chest. *Radiologic Clinics of North America* 31: 667–676.

Wyman, ML, Kuhns, LR (1977) Lobar opacification of the lung after tracheal extubation in neonates. *Journal of Pediatrics* 91(1): 109–112.

14

The Effect of Respiratory Physiotherapy Techniques on Intracranial and Cardiovascular Dynamics in the Neonate/Infant

JENNIFER PARATZ

Control of Brain Circulation in the Preterm Infant
•
Volume–Pressure Relationships
•
Cardiovascular Dynamics
•
The Effect of Certain Respiratory Physiotherapy Techniques on Intracranial and Cardiovascular Parameters

Although respiratory physiotherapy has been demonstrated to be beneficial in terms of the pulmonary system, there can be potentially detrimental effects on intracranial and cardiovascular parameters, particularly in the extremely premature infant.

Premature infants have a high rate of cerebral lesions such as peri-intraventricular haemorrhage or periventricular leukomalacia. The incidence of peri-intraventricular haemorrhage has been quoted as 29–42% (Volpe 1989) and is one of the major causes of neurological handicap. Associated factors for cerebral lesions appear to be respiratory distress syndrome and extreme prematurity. Rapid alterations in arterial blood pressure, arterial blood gases and cerebral blood flow velocity have also been cited as causes of these lesions.

Full-term infants are more vulnerable to neurological conditions such as post-asphyxial encephalopathy. Post-asphyxial encephalopathy can arise from impaired placental exchange (Williams et al. 1993), birth trauma, respiratory distress syndrome or apnoeic spells. A severe asphyxial insult is defined as

an Apgar score ≤3 at 5 minutes after birth, an umbilical artery metabolic or mixed acidosis (pH <7.0), neonatal neurological sequelae such as seizures, coma or hypoxaemia and multiple organ dysfunction (Carter et al. 1993). Following this lesion, intracerebral dynamics will be disrupted and any changes in arterial blood gases or arterial blood pressure may increase the damage.

Control of the cerebral circulation in the preterm and term infant is highlighted in the following discussion. The essential immaturity in these control mechanisms will explain the vulnerability of this population to cerebral lesions.

Control of Brain Circulation in the Preterm Infant

Autoregulation is a process inherent in vital organs such as the brain, heart and kidney whereby perfusion to that structure is maintained at a constant level despite changes in blood pressure. Cerebral auto-

Figure 1. The pressure–volume curves were generated by injecting and withdrawing CSF from (A) a normal infant (left) and (B) a teenager (right). The slope of the infant's pressure–volume curve is steeper than that of the teenager, resulting in less ability to buffer increments of volume. PVI, pressure volume index. Reprinted with permission from Shapiro and Marmarou (1982).

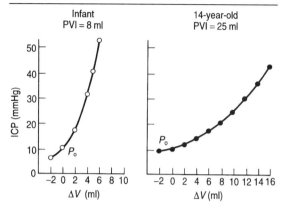

regulation is dependent on myogenic, metabolic and neurogenic mechanisms with a complicated interplay between brainstem neurones and transmitter substances. These are essentially immature in the extremely premature infant.

Autoregulation also has a functioning range quoted at various limits of 30–100 mmHg (Hollinger 1987, Raemakers et al. 1990). Arterial blood pressure in extremely premature infants often does not come into the autoregulatory range and so alterations in blood pressure can cause ischaemia or hyperperfusion. Autoregulation has been quoted as not present in the very premature infants (< 30 weeks or < 1500 g) (Jorch and Jorch 1987), but appears to be present in full-term infants. A difficult delivery with a mild degree of asphyxia or hypoxaemia can often temporarily disrupt autoregulation leaving the infant subject to irregular perfusion of the brain.

Volume–Pressure Relationships

Volume–pressure relationships are also important to appreciate when planning intervention in the neonate or infant. The skull contains cerebrospinal fluid (CSF), brain tissue and blood. If there is an increase in one of these contents, there is a compensatory decrease in another of the contents. This mechanism is controlled

partly by the sympathetic system (Busija and Heistad 1984), but is only effective to a certain point of volume loading (Figure 1B).

If there is a continued increase in blood, oedema or CSF, pressure in the brain will increase exponentially. In the infant there is less reserve (Figure 1A) with a high intracranial pressure (ICP) resulting from a small volume increase. Increased ICP can also result in a low cerebral perfusion pressure from the equation:

Cerebral perfusion pressure = Mean arterial pressure – Intracranial pressure (ICP)
where
Mean arterial pressure = Diastolic arterial pressure + (1/3 (Systolic arterial pressure – Diastolic arterial pressure)

A low cerebral perfusion pressure (considered to be less than 32 mmHg in the infant) (Colditz et al. 1988) will indicate that the level of tissue oxygenation to the brain is inadequate.

Arterial blood gases are important controllers of cerebral blood flow, with hypercarbia and hypoxaemia increasing cerebral blood flow and subsequently increasing ICP. Hyperoxia, especially an Fio_2 (fraction of inspired oxygen) of 1.0 is able to decrease cerebral blood flow by 30% in the infant. There is some dispute, however, as to how early from both a gestational and post-natal age chemical reactivity in the cerebral circulation, i.e. reactivity to arterial blood gases develop in the preterm and term infant (Jones et al. 1988, Van Bel et al. 1988, Pryds et al. 1990). Anatomical differences such as absence of the blood–brain barrier, immaturity of the blood vessels and the fragile tissue of the germinal matrix (Hegedus and Molnar 1985, Joo 1987) also predispose the preterm infant to haemorrhage and/or ischaemia of the brain.

If the infant has post-asphyxial encephalopathy, there is often disturbed autoregulation, cerebral oedema and decreased cerebral perfusion pressure. Obviously any further increase in blood pressure or arterial blood gases during respiratory physiotherapy, will further disturb intracerebral dynamics.

Cardiovascular Dynamics

Cardiovascular dynamics can also be immature in the infant. Preterm infants are especially prone to bradycardia. This has been described as a peripheral chemoreceptor reflex to falling oxygen saturation when apnoea is present (Upton & Milnar 1992). Bradycardia can also affect brain circulation, and Perlman and Volpe (1983) have described a decrease in systolic flow velocity in the anterior cerebral artery when heart rate decreases below 80 beats/min.

During fluctuations in heart rate, left ventricular output is maintained by stroke volume (Agato *et al.* 1991, Winberg and Ergander 1992). The neonatal heart has been shown to be immature in terms of structure, function and sympathetic innervation (Gilbert 1980) and will go into cardiac failure if preload is excessively increased. Obviously, very frequent bradycardias or decreased oxygenation can affect the response of the heart. Furthermore in respiratory distress syndrome, there can be hypoxia and acidaemia which depress the myocardium and, together with low blood volume and decreased responsiveness of the peripheral vessels, there is decreased perfusion and oxygenation of tissues such as the heart. The preterm infant will therefore have very decreased reserve and poor tolerance of handling.

The Effect of Certain Respiratory Physiotherapy Techniques on Intracranial and Cardiovascular Parameters

At certain times the infant is more vulnerable to cerebral lesions. Administration of artificial surfactant during severe respiratory distress syndrome has been shown to result in decreased or irregular cerebral blood flow velocity (Cowan *et al.* 1992) and so if the infant has immediately had surfactant, it would be wise not to administer physiotherapy. Mechanical ventilation (IPPV) has been cited (Cowan and Thoresen 1987) as increasing the chance of a cerebral lesion, but this is usually if the infant is breathing out of synchronization with the ventilator. Haemodynamic changes associated with pneumothorax also often lead to a cerebral lesion such as peri-intraventricular haemorrhage.

Various studies have quoted suction as causing decreased oxygenation, and alterations to blood pressure. These effects may be associated with cerebral vasodilatation, increased cerebral blood flow, increased ICP and perhaps decreased cerebral perfusion pressure.

Bradycardia frequently develops during suction and cardiac arrest has been reported (Cordero and Hon 1971).

Studies directly assessing the effect of suction on intracranial parameters have been completed by Perlman and Volpe (1982, 1983). Increases in ICP, mean arterial pressure and cerebral blood flow velocity were reported during endotracheal suction. Resistance index decreased after suction, indicating a dilatation of the vessel. There was a range of 26–35 weeks and infants under 32 weeks would have been especially vulnerable to increases in cerebral blood flow velocity and blood pressure due to their immature cerebral anatomy.

A further study which directly measured intracranial dynamics during suction was completed by Gavryushov *et al.* (1988). Twenty-seven ventilated infants (GA 38.3 +/ −3 weeks) had transcutaneous oxygen levels ($TcPo_2$), transcutaneous carbon dioxide levels ($TcPco_2$), blood pressure and cerebral blood flow velocity measured during endotracheal suction and manual hyperinflation. The authors stated that six of these infants who were in 'circulatory shock' became hypoxaemic with increased blood pressure during suction. Cerebral blood flow velocity also increased in these infants. In four of six of these infants, massive peri-intraventricular haemorrhage was diagnosed. The actual gestational age of the infants (nearly term) is older than the usual incidence of peri-intraventricular haemorrhage, but if as stated these infants were in circulatory shock, autoregulation was lacking, and these six infants would have been especially vulnerable to increases in arterial blood pressure. Although cerebral blood flow velocity increased significantly, it still cannot be proven that endotracheal suction actually led to a peri-intraventricular haemorrhage.

Manual hyperinflation or manual bagging is a technique used occasionally with full-term neonates and infants. It has little place in the care of preterm infants due to the high risk of pneumothoraces. The technique, using some form of anaesthetic bag connected to 100% oxygen, aims to give an increased minute volume, to provide oxygenation before suction and expand atelectatic alveoli. This technique has the potential to decrease cardiac output through the application of increased positive pressure. This is offset by a sympathetic compensatory response. Restoration of cardiac output, however, results only if the sympathetic nervous system is capable of this response.

Evidence exists that sympathetic innervation and control of cardiac contractility and rhythm are abnormal in the preterm infant and neonate (Rogers et al. 1980). A decrease in cardiac output, as mentioned previously can decrease cerebral blood flow causing either ischaemia or widespread cerebral vasodilatation exposing the brain to potential haemorrhage. The fact that manual hyperinflation is sometimes performed with 100% oxygen could also be dangerous, as this could reduce cerebral blood flow to ischaemic levels. Greisen et al. (1987) found significant neurodevelopmental deficits in infants who had been severely hypocarbic so it can be highly detrimental to hyperventilate these babies to a $PaCO_2$ of <15 mmHg.

Greisen et al. (1985) measured adrenaline, noradrenaline and mean arterial pressure in 13 preterm, ventilated infants just before and just after respiratory physiotherapy, consisting of vibration and endotracheal suctioning. It was reported that after the procedure, both adrenaline and noradrenaline were significantly higher than baseline levels. The adrenaline response was reduced by phenobarbitone. Mean arterial pressure was not affected by the procedure and did not correlate with the rise in catecholamines. Owing to the lack of a blood–brain barrier, in this population the catecholamines would be able to affect cerebral blood flow.

In a study designed to investigate the efficacy of respiratory physiotherapy Ravel et al. (1987) divided their subjects into two groups. The treatment group received postural drainage, percussion and suction, while the control group were given suction only. Five out of 10 of the treatment group suffered a grade III or grade IV peri-intraventricular haemorrhage whilst subjects in the control group demonstrated grade I or grade II peri-intraventricular haemorrhage. This study appears at first to support the supposition that respiratory physiotherapy causes peri-intraventricular haemorrhage. On closer examination, it is apparent that treatment was given to the infants at a mean post-natal age of 4.9 hours (range 1–12 hours). The infants were also in the early stage of respiratory distress syndrome. In most neonatal units today, preterm infants would not be treated with active physiotherapy at this early stage (except in the case of meconium aspiration), but would receive positioning and suctioning only (Bertone 1988). The actual treatment regime described by Ravel et al. (1987) consisting of percussion in both the head up and head down position, is very aggressive and not normally prescribed for infants of this post-natal age. As these infants were unlikely to have autoregulation, the cerebral blood flow would have undergone a dramatic decrease and increase over a few minutes, an event very likely to cause peri-intraventricular haemorrhage. It is not surprising therefore that there was no increase in secretion removal or improvement in oxygenation in the treatment group. The infants would be in the acute phase of respiratory distress syndrome, and would not be producing secretions. As these infants are so vulnerable to handling at this stage, PaO_2 would also decrease.

Use of certain positions for drainage may be associated with undesirable effects in preterm infants and modification of standard positions may be necessary (Crane 1985). Drainage in the head down position has been shown to increase systolic blood pressure to a greater extent than treatment in horizontal positions (Crane et al. 1978), and Cowan and Thoresen (1986) have found that tilting the head down only 6–10° results in increases in transfontanelle pressure. An increase in systolic blood pressure, especially in an infant lacking autoregulation, can be associated with intraventricular haemorrhage and for this reason, head down positions are not used in very premature infants who are at most risk of this condition.

Although benefits of prone lying appear to result in increased PaO_2, decreased blood pressure, and heart rate and be conducive to a positive behavioural state, which supposedly should benefit intracranial dynamics, there is some concern that head rotation in prone may cause trapping of cerebrospinal fluid and subsequently increase intracranial pressure (Goldberg et al. 1983). Cowan and Thoresen (1986) found that lying prone with the head turned to right or left, occluded the jugular venous drainage and reduced the blood velocities in the superior sagittal sinus. If the head is not in the midline, deformation of upper airways and nasal resistance to airflow may also affect oxygenation and deformation of the upper airway may increase airway resistance and consequently work of ventilation (Martin et al. 1988). In some nurseries, the infants are nursed one-quarter off prone to prevent this strong neck rotation. Elevation of the head has been shown to reduce ICP significantly on a group of newborn with post-haemorrhagic hydrocephalus (Urlesberger et al. 1991).

From the available literature and knowledge of the techniques it does appear that physiotherapy has the potential to cause alterations in cerebral venous pressure, cerebral blood flow velocity and cerebral perfusion pressure. The fact that the peak incidence of peri-intraventricular haemorrhage is usually in the first 24 hours (Dolfin et al. 1983), that is, prior to the commencement of active physiotherapy does undermine the proposal (Ravel 1987) that physiotherapy is responsible for this particular cerebral lesion.

REFERENCES

Agato, Y, Hiraishi, S, Oguchi, K et al. (1991) Changes in left ventricular output from fetal to early neonatal life. Journal of Pediatrics 119: 441–445.

Bertone, N (1988) The role of physiotherapy in a neonatal intensive care unit. The Australian Journal of Physiotherapy 34(1): 27–34.

Busija, DW, Heistad, DD (1984) Factors involved in the physiological regulation of the cerebral circulation. Reviews of Physiology, Biochemistry and Pharmacology 101: 162–196.

Carter, BS, Haverkamp, AD, Merenstein, GB (1993) The definition of acute perinatal asphyxia. Clinics in Perinatology 20(2): 287–304.

Colditz, PB, Williams, GL, Berry, AB et al. (1988) Fontanelle pressure and cerebral perfusion pressure continuous measurement in neonates. Critical Care Medicine 16: 876–879.

Cordero, L, Hon, EH (1971) Neonatal bradycardia following nasopharyngeal stimulation. Journal of Pediatrics 78: 441–443.

Cowan, F, Thoresen, M (1986) The effects of interruption to the cranial venous drainage on cerebral haemodynamics in the newborn infant. In: Rolfe P (ed). Neonatal Physiological Measurements: Proceedings of the Second International Conference on Fetal and Neonatal Physiological Measurements, pp. 86–96. London: Butterworths.

Cowan, F, Thoresen, M (1987) The effects of intermittent positive pressure ventilation on cerebral arterial and venous blood velocities in the newborn infant. Acta Paediatrica Scandinavica 76: 239–247.

Cowan, F, Whitelaw, A, Wertheim, D et al. (1992) Cerebral blood flow velocity after rapid administration of surfactant. Archives of Diseases in Childhood 67: 840–845.

Crane, LD (1985) Physical therapy for the neonate with respiratory disease. In: Irwin, S, Tecklin, J (eds) Cardiopulmonary Physical Therapy, pp. 305–333. St Louis: CV Mosby Co.

Crane, LD, Zombek, M, Krauss, AN, Auld, PAM (1978) Comparison of chest physiotherapy techniques in infants with HMD. Pediatric Research 12: 559.

Dolfin, T, Skidmore, MB, Fong, DK (1983) Incidence, severity and timing of subependymal and intraventricular haemorrhages in preterm infants in a perinatal unit as detected by real time ultrasound. Pediatrics 7: 541–544.

Gavryushov, VV, Alimov, AV, Milenin, OB et al. (1988) Blood gas composition, blood pressure and brain circulation during tracheobronchial aspiration in the newborn. Anesteziologiia i Reanimatologiia 4: 6–9.

Gilbert, RD (1980) Control of fetal cardiac output during changes in blood volume. American Journal of Physiology 238: H80.

Goldberg, R, Joshi, A, Moscosco, P et al. (1983) The effect of head position on intracranial pressure in the neonate. Critical Care Medicine 11(6): 428–430.

Greisen, G, Frederiksen, PS, Hertel, J, Christensen, NJ (1985) Catecholamine response to chest physiotherapy and endotracheal suctioning in preterm infants. Acta Paediatrica Scandinavica 74: 525–529.

Greisen, G, Munck, H, Lou, H (1987) Severe hypocarbia in preterm infants and neurodevelopmental deficit. Acta Paediatrica Scandinavica 76(0): 401–404.

Hegedus, K, Molnar, P (1985) Histopathological study of major intracranial arteries in premature infants related to intracranial haemorrhage. Journal of Neurosurgery 62: 419–424.

Hollinger, I (1987) Paediatric neuroanesthesia anesthesiology. Clinics of North America 5(3): 541–564.

Jones, MD, Koehler, RC, Traystman, RJ (1988) Regulation of cerebral blood flow in the fetus, newborn and adult. In: Guthrie, RD (ed). Neonatal Intensive Care, pp. 123–152. New York: Churchill Livingstone.

Joo, F (1987) Mini review: current aspects of the development of the blood–brain barrier international. Journal of Developmental Neuroscience 5(5): 369–372.

Jorch, G, Jorch, N (1987) Does the autoregulatory capacity of cerebral blood flow depend on gestational age? Monatsschrift fur Kinderheilkunde 135: 744–747.

Martin, RJ, Siner, B, Carlo, WA, Lough, M, Miller, MJ (1988) Effect of head position on distribution of nasal airflow in preterm infants. Journal of Paediatrics 112: 99–103.

Perlman, JM, Volpe, JJ (1982) The effects of oral suctioning (OS) and endotracheal suctioning (ES) on cerebral blood flow velocity (CBFV) and intracranial pressure (ICP) in the preterm infant. Pediatric Research 16: 303A.

Perlman, JM, Volpe, JJ (1983) Suctioning in the preterm infant: effects on cerebral blood flow velocity, intracranial pressure and arterial blood pressure. Pediatrics 72(3): 329–334.

Pryds, O, Anderson, GE, Friis-Hansen, B (1990) Cerebral blood flow reactivity in spontaneously breathing, preterm infants shortly after birth. Acta Paediatrica Scandinavica 79: 391–396.

Raemakers, VT, Casaer, P, Daniels, H et al. (1990) Upper limits of brain blood flow autoregulation in stable infants of various conceptional age. Early Human Development 24: 249–258.

Ravel, D, Yeh, TF, Mora, A et al. (1987) Chest physiotherapy in preterm infants with RDS in the first 24 hours of life. Journal of Perinatology 7(4): 301–304.

Jennifer Paratz

Rogers, MC, Nugent, SK, Traystman, RJ (1980) Control of cerebral circulation in the neonate and infant. *Critical Care Medicine* **8(10)**: 570–574.

Shapiro, K, Marmarou (1982) Mechanisms of intra-cranial hypertension in children. In: McLaurin RL (ed). *Paediatric Neurosurgery: Surgery of the Developing Nervous System*, pp. 255–264. New York: Grune and Stratton.

Upton, CJ, Milner, AD (1992) Apnoea and Bradycardia. In: Roberton, NRC (ed). *Textbook of Neonatology*, pp. 521–528. London: Churchill Livingstone.

Urlesberger, B, Muller, W, Ritschl, E *et al.* (1991) The influence of head position on the intracranial pressure in preterm infants with posthaemorrhagic hydrocephalus. *Child's Nervous System* **7**: 85–87.

Van Bel, F, van de Bor, M, Baan, J *et al.* (1988) The influence of abnormal blood gases on cerebral blood flow velocity in the preterm newborn. *Neuropediatrics* **19**: 27–32.

Volpe, JJ (1989) Intraventricular haemorrhage in the preterm infant – current concept Part II. *Annals of Neurology* **25(2)**: 109–116.

Williams, CE, Mallard, C, Tan, W *et al.* (1993) Pathophysiology of perinatal asphyxia. *Clinics in Perinatalogy* **20(2)**: 305–319.

Winberg, P, Ergander, U (1992) Relationship between heart rate, left ventricular output, and stroke volume in preterm infants during fluctuations in heart rate. *Pediatric Research* **31(2)**: 117–120.

15

Cardiorespiratory Physiotherapy Management – the Young and School-Aged Child

JULIE MACDONALD

The Efficacy of Physiotherapy Management of Cardiorespiratory Problems

•

The Young Child's Cardiorespiratory System

•

Vulnerability of the Child's Airways and Lungs

•

The Physiotherapist's Role in Preventing Cardiorespiratory Problems

•

The Physiotherapist's Clinical Assessment of Cardiorespiratory Problems

•

Physiotherapy Techniques for Cardiorespiratory Problems

•

Case Studies

The physiotherapist can play a significant role in the care of the young child with an acute and/or chronic cardiorespiratory condition, if she/he acts responsibly. The therapist, for example, must undertake a careful assessment of each patient, establish the particular problems of this individual and critically evaluate whether one or more physiotherapy techniques may assist in the resolution of varying cardiorespiratory problems, such as an inefficient breathing pattern, retained excessive mucopurulent secretions, atelectasis, paroxysmal coughing, poor thoracic mobility, decreased exercise tolerance. It is only when such a careful analysis of the problems of each patient and the establishment of a treatment regimen designed specifically to address identified problems is undertaken, that the physiotherapist's intervention is likely to be effective.

The Efficacy of Physiotherapy Management of Cardiorespiratory Problems

During the last decade, a very strong attempt to establish a scientific basis to the physiotherapy management of the patient with cardiorespiratory problems has been made. Numerous comparative studies of various physiotherapy techniques have been undertaken to establish the most effective mode of treatment for patients with cardiorespiratory difficulties. Unfortunately, the breadth of techniques which the physiotherapist has the opportunity to employ, when treating a patient with cardiorespiratory problems, makes this a formidable task and has led to a conflicting body of literature in many instances. For example, positioning, postural and autogenic drainage, percussion, vibrations, directed breathing exercises, the forced expiratory technique (FET), directed/assisted coughing, low-pressure and high-pressure positive expiratory pressure (PEP)-mask-therapy, intermittent positive pressure breathing, continuous positive airway pressure, exercise and respiratory muscle training and incentive spirometry are just some of the range of techniques which can be incorporated into the physiotherapy management of patients with cardiorespiratory problems.

Further difficulties associated with this examination of the efficacy of physiotherapy management of cardiorespiratory patients relates to the heterogeneous nature of the cardiorespiratory population. Sophisticated statistical tools, such as meta-analysis, have been employed in an attempt to assess quantitatively the findings of many trials involving physiotherapy cardiorespiratory techniques. Still, problems arise due to difficulties associated with the source studies, such as poor study design, poor patient compliance, poor outcome measures and definitions (Thomas and McIntosh 1994). Indeed, patient compliance and the methodological difficulty of testing the pulmonary function of the young child undoubtedly explain to a large extent the lack of clinical studies assessing the efficacy of physiotherapy management of the toddler and preschool child with cardiorespiratory problems.

The problematic nature of evaluating the efficacy of physiotherapy treatment regimens in the management of the patient with cardiorespiratory difficulties suggests that the clinical physiotherapist must be more discriminating in the selection of appropriate treatment techniques for particular patients. For example, in a review of numerous clinical physiotherapy treatment trials, Kirilloff *et al.* (1985) suggest that certain treatment regimens undertaken by the physiotherapist appear to be beneficial for those patients with an acute and chronic respiratory illness who have large volumes of secretions and in patients with lobar atelectasis. In contrast, similar physiotherapy treatment regimens appear to be of little benefit for patients with an exacerbation of chronic bronchitis or patients with pneumonia who are producing slight secretions.

The clinical physiotherapist treating the patient with cardiorespiratory problems should heed the advice that, although there are guidelines, each patient must have a programme designed specifically for him/her taking into consideration many issues. For example, relevant factors, such as the patient's age, the severity of the condition, any concomitant pathology, family background and social situation, must be considered by the therapist before designing a treatment regimen for a particular patient (Schoni 1989).

The success of the physiotherapist's role in the intervention of cardiorespiratory problems is therefore dependent upon numerous factors and the therapist must be clear in what they are attempting to achieve with a particular patient. At times, due to the general health of the child, the therapist's role may be limited. Sound problem-solving skills and the ability to adapt to varying circumstances, however, can certainly influence the success of any appropriate intervention.

The Young Child's Cardiorespiratory System

Developing effective problem-solving abilities requires sound theoretical knowledge. The young child with cardiorespiratory problems has distinctive anatomical and physiological features. These features should always be considered by the therapist when assessing, designing and implementing an appropriate physiotherapy intervention.

One of the most significant anatomical and physiological features of the young child is the profound postnatal lung growth and development. Perhaps the most overt expression of the growth and development of the child's cardiorespiratory system is the dramatic increase in the anteroposterior, transthoracic and vertical diameters of his/her chest wall. The shape of the child's chest starts to change towards the end of the first year of life as the ribs, which were initially horizontally orientated, take up a more oblique position. This downward descent of the ribs continues over the next 2 years and is completed a few years later (Engel 1947). See Figure 1.

The significant increase in number and size of respiratory structures, such as the respiratory bronchioles, alveolar ducts and alveoli, plays a major role in the increasing size of the chest wall diameters (Scarpelli 1990). The number of respiratory bronchioles and

Figure 1: The infant's squat chest changes considerably as the ribs take up a more oblique orientation in the young school-aged child

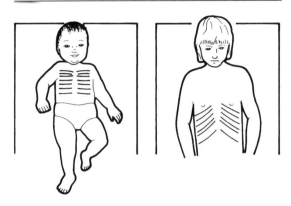

alveolar ducts increases from 1.5 million at birth to 14 million by age 8 years (Inselman and Mellins 1981). There is also a 10-fold increase in the number of alveoli from birth to 8 years of age (Angus and Thurlbeck 1972). Significant postnatal development of intra-acinar arteries and veins occurs after the formation of the new alveoli (Inselman and Mellins 1981).

The conducting airways are complete in number at birth but increase in size, though at different rates. This disproportionate growth pattern of the young child's airways is particularly demonstrated by the varying growth rate of the diameters of the trachea and the main bronchi. During infancy and childhood the diameters of the main bronchi are relatively small in relation to the tracheal lumen. However, towards puberty the bronchial diameters enlarge until by adulthood their joint calibre exceeds that of the trachea by 40% (Engel 1947).

This disproportionate lung growth is further highlighted by the fact that the lumen of the terminal bronchiole increases only slightly during early childhood (Engel 1947). Measurements by Hogg and colleagues (1970) indicate that the calibre of the peripheral conducting airways (airways beyond the fifteenth generation) changes very little during the first 5 years of life and that they have low conductance. These investigators emphasize that the peripheral conducting airways of the child under 5 years are extremely sensitive to narrowing.

The inflammatory process of a lower respiratory illness may readily narrow and obstruct the young child's peripheral airways causing significant pro-blems with ventilation distribution and gas exchange. The high density of mucous glands in children, particularly under 4 years of age, and the glands' large size in relation to the bronchial wall and the small diameter of airways further contribute to the often severe manifestations of obstructive pulmonary disease during infancy and childhood (Scarpelli 1990). Since the collateral ventilation pathways (the pores of Kohn and Lambert's channels) do not appear to be well developed until late childhood, it is not surprising that atelectasis is often a further difficulty associated with lower respiratory illnesses in the young child.

A longitudinal study of the respiratory status of children in the first 3 years of life suggests that variations in the structure and function of the child's lungs may be predisposing factors for recurrent wheezing illnesses during the early years of life (Martinez et al. 1991). In addition, there appear to be different dysynaptic growth patterns of airways and lung parenchyma in boys and girls (Pagtakhan et al. 1984). Taussig et al. (1981) similarly suggest a possible sex difference in the mechanical properties of the lung in young children. Their study of partial and maximal expiratory flow–volume curves in girls and boys aged between 3 and 13 years demonstrated significantly higher flows at functional residual capacity in girls. These investigators suggest that this difference in the mechanical properties of the lung may relate to the prevalence of severe lower respiratory illnesses, including asthma, in young boys. This difference in maximal flows between boys and girls may provide some further insight into the study by Rona and Chinn (1993). These investigators extensively studied the effects of passive smoking on children (aged 6.5–12 years) and found that maternal smoking was significantly associated with reduced forced expiratory flow rates of 25–75% and forced expiratory flow rates of 75–85% in boys but not in girls.

Vulnerability of the Child's Airways and Lungs

Numerous investigators suggest that, in view of the developing nature of the child's cardiorespiratory system, their airways and lungs are particularly vulnerable to injury by various agents (Samet *et al.* 1983). For example, Weiss *et al.* (1985) suggest that respiratory tract infections in children, such as croup, bronchiolitis and lower respiratory tract infections may not be self-limiting. These investigators' findings suggest that children who have had such illnesses are likely to have increased levels of airways responsiveness later in childhood. More epidemiological and longitudinal studies need to be undertaken before any relationship between respiratory tract infections in childhood and chronic airways obstruction in adulthood can be drawn. There are suggestions, however, that early childhood cardiorespiratory illnesses may affect normal lung development.

There are studies which support the hypothesis that family history has an influential role in the development of respiratory function during infancy. All infants with a family history of asthma have an increased risk of having asthma by the age of 2 years (Young *et al.* 1994). Furthermore, studies by Martinez *et al.* (1991) and Young *et al.* (1994) suggest that there are infants with abnormal lung function soon after birth (flow limitation during tidal expiration) which predisposes them to wheezing respiratory illnesses starting in the first year of life and a higher risk of being diagnosed with asthma.

Environmental agents, such as cigarette smoke, may significantly influence the incidence of obstructive respiratory disease during the early years of life. Pedreira *et al.* (1985) suggest that there is an increased incidence of tracheitis and bronchitis in infants exposed to smoking in the home. Indeed, the negative effects of passive smoking upon rate of lung development in children cannot be dismissed lightly. Tager *et al.* (1983) note that their longitudinal study into the effects of passive smoking upon the rate of development of lung function in children suggests that, after 5 years of exposure to maternal smoking, the lungs of children grow at only 93% of the rate of growth in non-smoking children with mothers who do not smoke.

Several studies further suggest that passive smoking may increase the risk of childhood asthma. For example, Martinez *et al.* (1988) note that their findings suggest that male children with smoking parents have significant increased bronchial responsiveness and atopy. Weitzman *et al.* (1990) reveal that maternal smoking is associated with higher rates of asthma in children and an earlier onset of the disease. Similarly, Martinez *et al.* (1992) note that children of mothers with 12 or fewer years of education and who smoked 10 or more cigarettes per day were 2.5 times more likely to develop asthma and had 15.7% lower maximal mid-expiratory flow than children of mothers with the same education level who did not smoke or smoked fewer than 10 cigarettes per day.

The Physiotherapist's Role in Preventing Cardiorespiratory Problems

The physiotherapist who has a sound understanding of the vulnerability of the young child's airways and lungs to environmental agents can play an essential role in educating the community about this. More specifically, the physiotherapist can introduce such education into his/her patient's treatment regimens. Physiotherapists dealing with the young child with cardiorespiratory problems should not only be addressing the immediate management of a particular problem, such as excess mucopurulent secretions. If and when appropriate, they should introduce an education programme to the child and parents to prevent or at least decrease the severity of any further obstructive airway difficulties.

The physiotherapist can also provide essential support to the health profession's attempt to educate the community about various cardiorespiratory conditions, such as asthma, a most prevalent chronic childhood cardiorespiratory disorder (Bauman *et al.* 1992). Life style education of children identified with asthma certainly needs to be implemented further. Health workers are still not successful in emphasizing the potential risks of cigarette smoke, particularly to the young. For example, a longitudinal study of asthmatic children found that 33% of their asthmatic cohort are now adult smokers (Roorda *et al.* 1993). Health workers, including physiotherapists, must highlight further the deleterious effects of smoking upon respiratory symptoms. Patient and parental education should be a major component of the physiotherapist's management of young children with cardiorespiratory problems, particularly if their problems are chronic.

The Physiotherapist's Clinical Assessment of Cardiorespiratory Problems

The most essential component of the physiotherapy management of the child with cardiorespiratory problems is a thorough assessment of the individual. If the assessment is inadequate, an inappropriate problem list and treatment regimen will be devised for the patient. An assessment should be carried out both before and on completion of every treatment session. If an assessment is not undertaken on completion of a treatment, the physiotherapist will not know if the treatment techniques selected for this individual effectively addressed his/her specific problems. In addition, during the treatment, the physiotherapist should continually observe the individual's cardiorespiratory status and be ready to adapt or remove a particular technique from the treatment regimen if the patient's problems are worsening.

The physiotherapist's cardiorespiratory assessment of the child should incorporate relevant aspects from the following.

BACKGROUND INFORMATION

Relevant details from medical chart. These include: (a) present admission details, e.g. date of admission, what is the diagnosis, severity of the condition, concomitant pathologies; (b) past medical and surgical history; (c) family history; and (d) investigations if applicable, e.g. pulmonary function testing which can be effectively performed with most children as young as 5–6 years of age. There are certain methodological difficulties in assessing the pulmonary function of infants and young children. However, several techniques can establish lung volume, respiratory patterns and flow rates. Other information on microbiology (sputum cultures), chest X-rays and acid-blood gases may be helpful.

Relevant details from monitoring chart (generally at foot of patient's bed). These are: (a) vital signs; (b) medications and times of administration; (c) dietary/feeding times; and (d) peak flow readings (if patient uses one).

Presence of monitors and other attachments. Examples are: electrocardiograph (ECG), intracranial pressure (ICP), arterial blood pressure, oximetry, central lines (infusaport), nasogastric tube, indwelling catheters. If the child is ventilated, note the mode of intubation and type of ventilator.

OBSERVATIONS

When observing a young child, the physiotherapist should attempt to make it a relaxed situation as the child may quickly become self-conscious and change their typical resting posture and breathing pattern. While making observations the therapist should attempt, if age appropriate and fully conscious, to ask the child relevant questions about their cardiorespiratory difficulties. When asking a child about their difficulties, phrase questions in an age-appropriate manner. The therapist may refer questions to the child's parents but must remember that it is the child who is experiencing the symptoms. It is particularly important to ask the individual who is experiencing pain/distress to describe this. Parents can provide important details of their child's symptoms, for example, confirming exercise tolerance. However, one should not dismiss the advantages of gaining significant insight and achieving good rapport with the child when you include them in your assessment and management. A further advantage is that in asking the child questions one can concomitantly assess their cardiorespiratory status from their ease of breathing. Generally, the child with significant breathing problems will not be interested in speaking to any extent, as it places further demands on their respiratory reserve. One must be aware, however, of the shy child who finds hospitalization overwhelming and will not speak freely.

The Child's Cough. As the child begins to relax and talk to the physiotherapist he/she is more likely to have a spontaneous cough which is often quite different from the type of cough you hear when you ask the child to cough, as then they generally merely clear the back of the throat. When the child does spontaneously cough, you should note the nature of the cough. Is it weak, moist, tight, paroxysmal or harsh? (The child who has had a tracheo-oesophageal fistula (TOF) correction in the past, often has an extremely harsh cough.) Do they become tachypnoeic, dyspnoeic or wheezy during or after a coughing bout? Do they produce any sputum through their cough? If so, describe its colour, texture and quantity. At times, the young child is unable to cough the sputum out of their mouth but rather swallows it. Observe and note if they swallow after coughing and if their next cough is clearer.

The Child's General Colour. Note particularly the area around the mouth and lips as a bluish hue may be indicative of arterial hypoxaemia. Also note body shape (amount of musculature), height and weight, and any evidence of splinting of chest due to pain. To clearly observe the child's chest, one must attain anterior, posterior and lateral views. Note any relevant scars (surgery/trauma). Look at the child's distal extremities and note any signs of clubbing which can suggest persistent arterial hypoxaemia.

The Child's Resting Posture. Observe whether the shoulders are elevated and rounded. Also look for evidence of kyphotic thoracic spine, scoliosis, barrel-shaped chest or any other indication of thoracic cage immobility. Other chest variations include: pectus excavatum or funnel chest; pectus carinatum or pigeon chest; Harrison's sulcus, a visibly evident ridge running along the lower ribs, often demonstrated in children who have experienced significant breathing difficulties early in life. Look for evidence of intercostal/subcostal recession.

Respiratory Rate and Heart Rate. The young child has a higher resting oxygen (O_2) consumption and carbon dioxide (CO_2) output per kilogram of body weight than the adult. The young child's spontaneous respiratory rate is higher (double) than that of the adult's since as body size increases there is a concomitant decreasing resting respiratory frequency. Heart rate is similarly higher in the young child and progressively decreases during childhood. Note any significant variations in rate.

Breathing Pattern. Take note of: nasal/mouth breathing; predominantly diaphragmatic or upper chest breathing; and overuse of accessory respiratory muscles, such as scalene, sternocleidomastoid, pectoralis major, trapezius, external intercostal muscles.

Efficacy of Abdominal Musculature and Internal intercostal Muscles. These have an essential role as accessory muscles of forced expiration. To examine these muscles, introduce blowing and huffing type games to children. Children as young as 3–4 years of age have been successfully taught to do forced expiratory technique (FET) manoeuvres.

PALPATION

Note the following: (a) temperature of skin, (b) evidence of any pain on palpation, (c) the amount of bibasal expansion, if there is symmetry, and (d) tactile fremitus.

LUNG SOUNDS

The therapist should assess the quality of lung sounds via the ear and using a stethoscope. Lung sounds can be effectively divided into breath sounds and added sounds, such as wheezing, crackles and stridor. Normal breath sounds should be barely audible at the mouth.

The young child with some breathing difficulties may demonstrate loud harsh breath sounds, perhaps an expiratory grunting noise. Added sounds, which are abnormal, are often very audible even at a distance from the patient. Stridor, particularly, is often a harsh audible noise. The inspiratory stridor associated with whooping cough is pronounced, and the young child who has tracheal scarring (TOF correction) often produces a significant noise during respiration. Wheezes, which are continuous musical sounds produced by airflow-induced oscillation of the airway walls (Earis 1992), can often be heard at the mouth of the child. In addition, crackles (intermittent explosive sounds) are sometimes heard at the patient's mouth. Although understanding of the origins of crackles is incomplete, Earis (1992) proposes the acoustic wave is produced either by equalization of the downstream and upstream pressures or by sudden alterations in the tension of airway walls.

The physiotherapist should be aware that the assessment of lung sounds via the stethoscope can be difficult, particularly when dealing with the young child. For example, the child may be irritable, restless, crying and uncooperative which may mask significant breath sounds and/or added sounds. In addition, there are problems associated with the sheer amount of information that the therapist can extract when assessing and comparing the lung sounds at varying auscultatory sites over the chest wall. For example, at a single auscultatory site during a single breath, many factors can be considered, such as the intensity and duration of the inspiratory and expiratory phase of respiration and also the presence, timing, profusion and quality of added sounds (Loudon and Murphy 1984). Indeed, recent trials suggest that there are problems of accuracy and reliability of physiotherapists using this assessment tool (Aweida and Kelsey 1990, Brooks et al. 1994).

Assessing the child's lung sounds may not be the most precise reflection of lung function and should be used in conjunction with other assessment observations. Increased or reduced breath sounds over various auscultatory sites of the chest wall can reflect varying pathologies. For example, consolidation of a lung field may heighten the transmission of breath sounds. Francis (1992) notes, however, that breath sounds are heightened only occasionally in either the older child with lobar pneumonia or the younger child with extensive consolidation. A pneumothorax will dramatically reduce the transmission of breath sounds.

Added sounds such as wheezes and crackles may be heard, particularly when the young child is experiencing some critical airway narrowing. Wheezing, however, need not always occur with children with airflow obstruction (Ignacio et al. 1993). The crackles associated with chronic obstructive airway disease and bronchiectasis are described as coarse and occur early in inspiration and in expiration, whereas the crackles associated with interstitial fibrosis are described as fine and occur in end inspiration (Earis 1992). The stethoscope is valuable in assessing any changes of lung sounds during a treatment regimen, and in evaluating the efficacy of the regimen.

EXERCISE TOLERANCE

The evaluation of the young child's level of activity/exercise tolerance is an essential component of the physiotherapist's clinical assessment of the cardiorespiratory patient. The physiotherapist may be involved in a formalized exercise testing programme where the patient is challenged and recordings are made of various cardiorespiratory changes, such as heart rate, respiratory rate, O_2 consumption and CO_2 production, respiratory exchange ratio. Design an age-appropriate challenge (if the child is not in any cardiorespiratory distress) to establish exercise performance, in an informal manner if sensitive objective equipment is unavailable. Be very aware of the potential for children to experience symptoms of exercise-induced asthma (EIA). The symptoms of EIA generally begin 6–10 minutes after exercise (Schulz and Olha 1986). The physiotherapist should ascertain via charting and subjective questioning of parent and child whether there is any shortness of breath and/or feelings of tightness in the chest when exercising. At times, however, this information is not available and precautions should always be taken.

A thorough clinical assessment of the patient's cardiorespiratory status enables the physiotherapist to identify and prioritize the problems experienced by the child. Furthermore, once an individual's specific problems are identified, the physiotherapist can then select the most effective techniques to address these problems. There are numerous techniques to address the various cardiorespiratory problems. The treatment techniques predominantly used for children are described next. It is essential that the physiotherapist views each patient's treatment regimen as a dynamic process which may be readily adapted to address patient's changing needs and/or problems.

Physiotherapy Techniques for Cardiorespiratory Problems

Postural Drainage

This technique is designed to assist in the mobilization of excess secretions. The child is moved into various gravity-assisted positions based on the anatomy of the bronchial tree. The patient remains in each position for approximately 10 minutes or until their cough is dry. Postural drainage is a passive technique, but once the child is able to cooperate it is used in conjunction with an active cycle of breathing, the forced expiratory technique (FET) and efficient coughing technique. See Figure 2.

Positioning (Modified Postural Drainage)

This is used to assist in the mobilization of excess secretions and resolution of atelectasis in children who are unable to sustain gravity-assisted positioning (head down positions). For example, the child with varying pathologies such as, gastro-oesophageal reflux, raised intracranial pressure and cardiac anomalies cannot be placed into head down positions because of the risk of exacerbating their pathology. The child who has recently had extensive lung/cardiac/abdominal surgery may also not be able to be placed into head down positions as it may compromise their status.

The child is positioned into alternate flat side lying for

Figure 2: A child demonstrating a postural drainage position (posterior lower lobes)

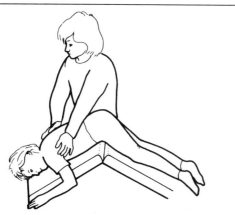

at least 20 minutes so as to avoid prolonged lying in one position. Once the child is able to cooperate this technique is used in conjunction with an active cycle of breathing, the forced expiratory technique (FET) and efficient coughing technique. If the child is ventilated this technique can be incorporated with vibrations, hyperinflation and suction.

Autogenic Drainage

This technique assists in the mobilization and removal of excess secretions, particularly the mucus in the more distal airways. It requires considerable concentration and understanding and is unsuitable for the toddler and young child. It may take a period of time to become confident with autogenic drainage, but once acquired it does provide the older child with greater independence in the treatment regimen. Throughout this technique an attempt is made by the patient to reach the highest possible airflow in the different generations of the lung. The child begins in a relaxed sitting position with the neck slightly extended and the hands placed over the thorax to heighten proprioceptive, tactile and auditory awareness of the mobilization of mucus. The patient is instructed to breathe in slowly through the nose to heat and moisten the air, thereby partly preventing coughing. Expiration is carried out in a relaxed manner described as 'sighing' with open mouth and glottis, thereby reducing expiratory pressure and preventing airway collapse and compression of bronchi.

There are three phases or breathing cycles in this technique. Phase one involves low lung volume breathing in an attempt to unstick mucus in the peripheral airways. Phase two, in which there is a deepening of inspiration and expiration (tidal volume level,) subsequently collects the mucus into the larger bronchi. During the last phase the patient breathes at higher lung volumes and through a short burst of coughing evacuates secretions from the central airways. This breathing cycle is repeated until the patient feels their airways are clear, which may take up to 45–60 minutes (Schoni 1989). In view of the emphasis upon the avoidance of excessive airway compression, this technique may be particularly effective for the patient with hyperreactive airways.

The Forced Expiratory Technique (FET)

This method facilitates the clearance of excess secretions, particularly those secretions in the more peripheral airways. Because FET incorporates a forced expiration at a low lung volume, the equal pressure point of dynamic compression of airways will move more peripherally, thereby mobilizing secretions in the more distal airways.

This technique requires cooperation from the child and it is generally felt effective for the child of 4 years and upwards. It is important to remember, however, that the attention span and planning ability of children vary widely. FET involves one or two forced expirations from mid-lung to low-lung volume followed by a period of relaxation and breathing control. This period of relaxation and breathing control is viewed as an integral component of the FET. During the breathing control phase the child's upper chest should be relaxed (any use of accessory respiratory muscles is discouraged). Breathing should be gentle, normal tidal volume with an unforced expiration. The forced expiration from mid-lung to low-lung volume phase is achieved by taking in a medium-sized breath and then breathing out forcefully by contracting abdominal and chest wall muscles with the mouth and glottis open – the sound created is like a forced sigh. Once the secretions reach the upper airways they can be cleared with a high-volume huff or cough. FET discourages any paroxysmal coughing episodes (Partridge *et al.* 1989).

Directed Breathing Exercises / Active Cycle of Breathing / Thoracic Expansion Exercises

These are designed to increase lung volume which may assist in the resolution of atelectasis and facilitate mobilization of excess secretions. The physiotherapist initiates these thoracic expansion exercises by placing her / his hands on the child's chest wall to provide the child with sensory awareness of expanding the lower chest. These exercises are often used in conjunction with percussion and expiratory vibration techniques. Generally the child undertakes approximately 3–4 thoracic expansion exercises while the physiotherapist percusses / vibrates the chest wall and then the child is instructed to relax (to prevent fatigue and hyperventilation) and commence a period of gentle breathing at normal tidal volume.

Percussion (Clapping) and Vibrations

The techniques achieve mechanical dislodgement of secretions. The physiotherapist generally performs them with cupped hands or with a small face mask. Commercially available products such as the Flutter device are based on a similar principle of causing vibration of the airway walls. Percussion and expiratory vibrations are performed over the affected area of the lung and are often used in conjunction with postural drainage or positioning. They are passive techniques and are therefore more likely to be selected in the management of the very young and the ventilated child with excess secretions who are unable to participate actively in their treatment regimen.

Directed / Efficient Coughing

This enables effective removal of secretions from central airways. The physiotherapist always discourages any vigorous or paroxysmal coughing episodes as such uncontrolled forced expiration causes distress which can exacerbate hyperreactive airways. The child must contract his / her abdominal muscles to produce an efficient cough as secretions in the central airways will only be mobilized when the expiratory flow rate is at a high velocity. A cough, which causes a dynamic compression of airways, should always be followed by a period of relaxation and gentle breathing.

Abdominal Push-assist Technique During Cough

The purpose of this technique is to improve the effectiveness of coughing in patients with spinal cord injuries. The therapist's hands are placed cupping the patient's abdominal contents, since the

Figure 3: The therapist's hands are placed over the abdominal contents when undertaking an 'abdominal push-assist technique during cough'

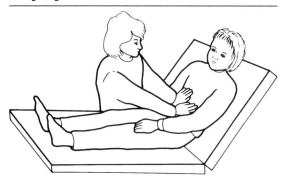

patient's expiratory effort is assisted by the therapist pushing the patient's abdominal contents up against his/her diaphragm. The therapist must be careful that the direction of this abdominal push-assist technique is posterior and cephalad. The technique must also not be undertaken too aggressively, otherwise the patient's ribs and abdominal contents may be compromised. It is helpful for the therapist to have his/her hands in position during the patient's inspiratory cycle in order to initiate the abdominal push simultaneously when the patient starts their maximal expiratory effort. Verbal coaching is also encouraged (Braun' *et al.* 1984). See Figure 3.

Positive Expiratory Pressure (PEP)-Mask-Therapy (Low Pressure and High Pressure)

This will help to increase lung volume and mobilize excess secretions. It involves the child using a face mask or mouthpiece and breathing out against a pressure of 10–15 cm H_2O. An attached manometer can be an effective feedback mechanism for the child. The outflow valve can be adjusted to maintain this level of resistance. The toddler and young child generally would not have the attention span or understanding to execute this technique effectively. The child (generally 8 years and upwards) undertakes this technique in a comfortable sitting posture with arms resting on a table, then proceeds to breathe through the mask/mouthpiece approximately 10 times. The child then removes the mask and undertakes a FET and a clearing cough if necessary. In high-

pressure PEP-mask-therapy the outflow valve is adjusted in order to generate greater expiratory pressures (e.g. 50–120 cm H_2O). PEP-mask-therapy for children demands effective training and close supervision.

Manual Hyperinflation (Bagging)

This will assist in the aeration of lung fields, pre-oxygenate before suctioning and simulate impaired cough mechanism by generating a high expiratory flow rate from large lung volume. The bagging technique should inflate the chest with a slow deep inspiration. After holding full inspiration for a short time, the bag is released quickly to allow the high expiratory flow rate. Hyperinflation generates an increased intrathoracic pressure which can reduce venous return by compression of the great veins. A fall in cardiac output and blood pressure can occur therefore during this procedure, so heart rate and blood pressure parameters should be monitored through the treatment.

Precautions: manual hyperinflation should be kept short if treating a child with head injuries as intracranial pressure increases with time. Furthermore, when treating infants and young children with this technique the physiotherapist should carefully monitor the peak inspiratory pressure via the attached pressure gauge. Manual hyperinflation would be contraindicated in patients with pneumothorax, surgical emphysema or with an intercostal catheter in situ to control an air leak, as this would exacerbate their pathology.

Suctioning

This is a necessary technique for those patients who have an inefficient cough and cannot clear excess secretions. The very young child will also require suctioning if a sputum culture is ordered. The ventilated child or the child with a tracheostomy will often require frequent suctioning, but suctioning should only be carried out when necessary.

The physiotherapist should be always aware that suctioning will not only remove secretions, but will also remove oxygen and, if appropriate measures are not taken, suctioning may cause respiratory distress.

Catheters with a Y-connection and intermittent suctioning will reduce this potential for hypoxia, as will the selection of smaller size of catheters (catheter size should never be a snug fit, but be significantly narrower than the diameter of the airway). Furthermore, the suctioning procedure should be kept short (no longer than 10 seconds). In the ventilated patient, hyperinflation before and after suctioning may also assist in the prevention of hypoxia. When suctioning the non-intubated child the physiotherapist must ensure that the child is secured in side-lying to prevent trauma and to reduce the risk of aspiration of vomitus if the catheter stimulates a gag reflex (Young 1984).

Intermittent Positive Pressure Breathing (IPPB)

This is used to aerate lung fields at optimal flow rates in children who have poor inspiratory capacity due to weakness of respiratory muscle, e.g. children with tetraplegia and Duchenne muscular dystrophy. Such an increase in inspiratory volume may assist in the removal of excess secretions since IPPB is generally used in conjunction with other techniques, such as vibrations, FET and efficient directed coughing. Humidification and medications can also be administered via IPPB.

The patient is generally placed in a comfortable sitting or high side-lying position. The child must initiate the inspiratory phase of IPPB through a mouthpiece or mask, but must then relax and not resist this procedure. This may be difficult for the young or anxious child. IPPB is contraindicated when patients have a pneumothorax or any potential for such pathology.

Incentive Spirometry

This can encourage greater inspiratory volume and expiratory flows through effective breathing pattern. It is essential that the child avoid any overuse of accessory respiratory muscles during this technique. In young children this may be adapted by sitting the youngster in a comfortable position and then encouraging him/her to participate in blowing games, for example blow bubbles to gain active increase in inspiration and controlled expiration. As the child matures and attention span and compliance improves he/she can be instructed in the independent use of commercially available tabulated equipment which can demonstrate improvement or regression in inspiratory and expiratory flows.

Respiratory Muscle Training

This is designed to: (1) increase the endurance and strength of the diaphragm, and (2) improve peak expiratory flow which is associated with a more efficient cough. It is generally employed when the child has some chronic weakness of the respiratory muscles, e.g. tetraplegia. The child must be developmentally advanced to have a sufficient attention span and understand commands. Respiratory muscle training is generally carried out through the use of a respiratory muscle training mouth–nose-mask (RMT-mask) with inspiratory and expiratory resistors which can be individually set. The individual is in sitting position while they apply the mask for a set period (e.g. 15 minutes) and the mask is used several times a day. The minimal amount of training required to be beneficial for individuals needs further studies (Biering-Sorensen et al. 1991). The use of a peak flow meter after each training session can demonstrate to the child improvements in their peak expiratory flow.

Aerobic Exercise/Demand Ventilation

This can be used to increase air entry which can assist in the mobilization of excess secretions and in the resolution of atelectasis. Furthermore, upper trunk exercise will facilitate thoracic cage mobility. An exercise conditioning programme in children can increase work tolerance and fitness.

The physiotherapist obtains from the clinical assessment of the child a baseline exercise ability and tolerance. The selection of particular exercises for children is naturally dependent on the child's developmental age and their interests. Ball games are useful as they encourage thoracic cage mobility as well as increasing ventilation. The physiotherapist must constantly be aware of the potential for exercise-induced asthma in some patients and should take necessary precautions.

Case Studies

The physiotherapist assesses children with many and varied cardiorespiratory conditions. This section concentrates initially on the child and his/her problems rather than the condition. A description of the condition is also provided. A number of problems experienced by a child with a particular condition, however, may be similarly experienced by a child with a different pathology. Respiratory problems such as retained mucopurulent secretions, inefficient breathing and coughing, and poor exercise tolerance can be similarly identified in the child with cystic fibrosis and in the child with suppurative lung disease following significant bacterial infection. Although these case studies provide a limited view of the type of cardiorespiratory conditions seen by the clinical paediatric physiotherapist, they illustrate the problem-solving approach which is required for every child.

Case Study 1

A 7-year-old girl, Alice, has recently been hospitalized due to an exacerbation of obstructive airways symptoms. As an infant, she was medically treated for failure to thrive (FTT), severe gastro-oesophageal reflux (GOR) and associated oesophagitis and lower respiratory tract infections. She was subsequently diagnosed with cystic fibrosis (CF) at 4 months of age by a confirmatory sweat test. She has continued to be hospitalized approximately three times a year for worsening respiratory symptoms. She underwent a fundoplication and gastrostomy 6 months ago in an attempt to improve her nutritional status through supplemental feeding. She is presently tracking along the third percentile for weight and height. Microbiology studies of Alice's sputum over the last few years consistently indicated Pseudomonas aeruginosa and Candida albicans colonization. Her last chest X-ray (taken 6 months ago while hospitalized for fundoplication and gastrostomy) showed signs of hyperinflation, and there were increased broncho-vascular markings throughout the lung fields. Alice's medication generally includes: inhaled β_2 agonist and steroid (via metered dose inhaler (MDI) + large volume spacer device), pancrease (6 with meals and 4 with snacks), salt tablets, multivitamin and vitamins K and E.

Alice has two older sisters who do not have cystic fibrosis, but the eldest girl, Veronica (14 years) has been diagnosed with a mild form of asthma. Both of Alice's parents work and both smoke. They find that they have to be quite organized, particularly trying to supervise Alice's physiotherapy programme before breakfast. Veronica supervises Alice's home programme of physiotherapy techniques which includes postural drainage, active cycle of breathing, percussion and FET and directed coughing in the afternoons while she organizes the family dinner. Parents and elder sister have expressed concerns about Alice's cooperation with her physiotherapy regimen. Alice is presently coping fairly well in grade 2 at school and it is generally felt by Alice and her parents that her hospitalizations have not significantly interrupted her learning. Her parents are quite happy with the school's support of Alice's medication regimen. Alice is not involved in any organized physical exercise/sport at present, but does participate in playground activities at school. She prefers, in her free time at home, to watch TV or play video games.

Alice attends the CF clinic at the hospital every 3 months where she is regularly examined by members of the CF team, such as the respiratory physician, dietitian, physiotherapist. Since last year she has been having regular pulmonary function testing at this clinic. This clinic most importantly also provides Alice and her parents with the opportunity to express any concerns. During her latest clinic visit, it was established by history and examination that Alice's *respiratory status had worsened. She was experiencing disturbed nights, waking several times, coughing up considerable amounts of much thicker and darker mucopurulent secretions, and she was finding that she got too tired and breathless to participate in schoolground activities. Her weight had dropped by 1 kg since her last visit. Furthermore, her latest pulmonary function testing, particularly her forced expiratory volume in one second (FEV$_1$) and her forced expiratory flow rates of 25–75% (FEF$_{25-75}$), had dropped significantly. It was generally felt that to relieve such worsening symptoms, hospitalization was necessary, so that she could commence intravenous (IV) antibiotics, have intensive physiotherapy, and would enable the dietitian to review her nutritional status.*

Physiotherapy for Cardiorespiratory Problems of Cystic Fibrosis

Before assessment and the instigation of any treatment regimen for Alice's cardiorespiratory problems the hospital physiotherapist should have:

- a background understanding of CF
- an appreciation of the various physiotherapy treatment techniques to relieve the cardiorespiratory problems associated with CF, and a knowledge of the findings of clinical studies examining the efficacy of physiotherapy techniques in the management of the CF patient.

BACKGROUND

CF is a genetic syndrome, predominantly affecting caucasians. This multisystem disorder, which has varying degrees of presentation can affect individuals differently. The clinical picture of CF includes respiratory, pancreatic and gastrointestinal complications, such as meconium ileus, distal intestinal obstructive syndrome, gastro-oesophageal reflux, severe oesophagitis. Lung disease in CF, however, accounts for more than 95% of the morbidity and mortality associated with this autosomal recessive disorder (Zach 1991).

Significant advances in the understanding of the genetics and cellular pathophysiology of CF have occurred. The CF gene has been located and the membrane protein coded by the CF gene, CF transmembrane conductance regulator (CFTR) which is involved in chloride conductance, is felt to be abnormal in the CF population (Cuthbert 1992). CF is autosomal recessive, i.e. it occurs when there are abnormalities of both CF genes. The most common mutation is the $\Delta F_{508\,allele}$ (Super 1992). Investigators have discovered many distinct mutations and describe CF as a genetically heterogeneous condition (Brock et al. 1991).

Such scientific advances have been particularly beneficial in the clinical field of genetic screening. As 90% of children with CF are born into families with no known family history, known relatives and spouses of those with CF can be screened for carrier status (Super 1992). Ranieri et al. (1994) suggest that a number of the problems associated with developing an acceptable neonatal screening strategy for CF have been reduced by direct gene analysis of CF mutations (ΔF_{508}, ΔI_{506}, $G_{551}D$, $G_{542}X$ and $R_{553}X$). For example, these investigators suggest that direct gene analysis of cystic fibrosis mutations in samples with immunoreactive trypsinogen concentrations in the highest 1% and in all neonates with meconium ileus or family history of CF has an improved sensitivity and specificity. Further research is needed to understand more clearly how such cellular pathophysiology gives rise to the clinical manifestations of CF (McPherson and Dormer 1994).

The underlying inherited defect in the respiratory mucosa of the individual with CF is thought to be due to a defective stimulation of chloride transport thereby facilitating increased bacterial adherence and colonization by bacterial pathogens such as *Pseudomonas aeruginosa*. Such colonization causes obstructive airway changes and proteolytic airway wall damage which will inevitably lead to alterations in lung structure and function (Zach 1991). Significantly, the bronchiectasis associated with CF is often masked by obstructive changes. Indeed, many children with CF, even those with mild symptoms, have moderate to severe non-specific airway hyperreactivity which can reduce forced expiratory flows (Ignacio et al. 1993).

TREATMENT

The immediate short-term aim of physiotherapy management of the child with CF is to remove excessive mucopurulent secretions so as to improve ventilation and reduce airway resistance and ventilation–perfusion mismatch (Prasad 1993). There is the suggestion also that, because the elastolytic activity in CF sputum is significantly high, the rapid removal of such secretions may decrease the rate of connective tissue degradation associated with this disease (Schoni 1989, Zach 1991). In addition, enhancing the rate of clearance of secretions in the CF child at specific times should have positive psychological and social benefits for the child as they will not need to cough so constantly, for example through school. Similarly, by increasing the removal of secretions before sleep the child should be less disturbed by coughing.

Considerable controversy has arisen regarding the efficacy of various physiotherapy regimens in the management of the patient with CF. For example, Falk et al. (1984) note significant increases in sputum yield in treatments involving PEP in contrast to treatments involving PD, percussion and FET manoeuvres. Hofmeyr et al. (1986), however, report significant increases in sputum production in treatments involving breathing exercises and FET manoeuvres in gravity-assisted positions in comparison to treatments involving PEP. Both of these trials involved adolescent and adult CF patients. Steen et al. (1991) who included younger patients (8–21 years) with CF report no significant differences in outcome between treatment programmes which included different techniques, such as PD, percussion and FET manoeuvres and PEP in various combinations. Tyrell et al. (1986) similarly note that there was no significant difference in symptom scores, sputum production or lung function in patients with CF (10–18 years) after one month of treatment involving either PD, percussion or PEP with FET manoeuvre.

Both Tyrell et al. (1986) and Steen et al. (1991) emphasize that a number of factors should influence the appropriate selection of techniques for the individual with CF. Indeed, although PD and percussion is time-consuming and compliance is often poor, PEP with FET manoeuvres requires motivation and self-discipline on the part of the child and parents (Tyrell et al. 1986). These investigators also suggest that children producing moderate or large amounts of sputum may require techniques in addition to PEP and FET manoeuvres or at least to increase their treatment time. Steen et al. (1991) further note that, although PEP with FET manoeuvres encourages patient independence and may improve patient compliance, there is still the problem of treating the toddler and young child who is not adept at using FET manoeuvre and has limited attention to tasks.

Exercising is undoubtedly advantageous for the child with CF. It is fun and demand ventilation should assist in the removal of secretions. Salh et al. (1989) suggest that physiotherapy and exercise should be considered complementary rather than exclusive in the treatment of CF. These investigators note that their study of adolescent and adult patients demonstrated that physiotherapy was more effective than exercise in inducing sputum expectoration.

Alice's Physiotherapy Management During Hospitalization

After completing a comprehensive assessment of Alice's cardiorespiratory status, the hospital physiotherapist has devised a prioritized short-term problem list so that she can most effectively instigate a specified treatment regimen. The short-term problem list is as follow:

1. *retention of excessive mucopurulent secretions*
2. *inefficient/paroxysmal coughing procedure*
3. *excessive use of accessory respiratory muscles*
4. *poor thoracic mobility*
5. *poor exercise tolerance*

The physiotherapist addressed Alice's short-term cardiorespiratory problems in the following manner. Emphasis was placed on instructing Alice in the active cycle of breathing so as to achieve more efficient air entry while posturally draining. She had to be encouraged to use the FET manoeuvre instead of going into paroxysmal coughing episodes. Percussion and vibrations were also introduced while draining in an attempt to remove the extremely sticky purulent secretions.

During treatments attempts were made using a mirror to stop the excessive use of accessory inspiratory musculature. A short exercise programme involving ball catching was instigated to improve thoracic mobility and evoke some demand ventilation (being careful not to exacerbate any wheezing). Treatments took approximately 40 minutes and were undertaken three times a day.

Alice responded well to her IV antibiotic therapy and physiotherapy regimen. Her respiratory symptoms and pulmonary function tests significantly improved over the next 10 days. There was also an increase in her weight. Prior to discharge, however, the physiotherapist must address the long-term problem of Alice's poor compliance with her home physiotherapy regimen. The therapist should also consider the fact that Alice does very little exercise at home, preferring to watch TV.

Undoubtedly the physiotherapist needs to address these home programme issues with Alice's parents and other people involved in her home treatment regimen. Although low-pressure PEP-mask-therapy with FET manoeuvres requires motivation and self-discipline on the part of the child and parents it was felt that this should be introduced to the parents and child as an option if Alice continues to demonstrate poor compliance with active cycle of breathing, PD with FET manoeuvre at home. A progressive daily aerobic exercise programme, particularly concentrating upon ball activities which will encourage thoracic mobility, is also demonstrated to the child and parents and written down in an exercise book. Exercise will improve air entry which will facilitate more effective

removal of secretions. The therapist should further emphasize the importance of having a smoke-free environment in the house. When Alice returns to the hospital on her next clinic day she will be asked to bring her home programme exercise book and demonstrate she has continued to work on these exercises.

Case Study 2

A 10-year-old girl, Jenny, who sustained a complete cervical spinal cord injury (C7–8) 5 years ago in a motor vehicle accident, has been hospitalized for the surgical correction of a thoracolumbar scoliosis. Her scoliosis has increased significantly over the last 12 months and there are major concerns that if it is not arrested soon it will compromise further her pulmonary function. In addition, several adaptations have had to be made recently to her wheelchair in an attempt to overcome the uneven pressures that the scoliosis is causing. The orthopaedic surgeon has explained to Jenny and her parents that due to the rigidity of the thoracic curve it will be best to perform the spinal arthrodesis (via segmental spinal instrumentation) in a two-part procedure. Initially, they will undertake an anterior release of contracted soft tissue (via thoracotomy) and, one week later, enter posteriorly to achieve spinal fusion. Jenny's physiotherapist had been advised 6 weeks earlier of this impending surgery, and both Jenny and her mother have been attending regular outpatient appointments with the physiotherapist in preparation for this surgery. Before the instigation of a preoperative physiotherapy regimen for Jenny, the physiotherapist looked into the respiratory difficulties associated with tetraplegia and various physiotherapy treatment approaches which have been undertaken with this population of cardiorespiratory patients.

Physiotherapy for Cardiorespiratory Problems of Spinal Injury

BACKGROUND

The individual with tetraplegia will have some changes in their pulmonary function due to the paralysis of some of their respiratory muscles (these changes are generally directly related to the level of the lesion). Since abdominal muscles are innervated by the six lower thoracic levels and the first lumbar level, the individual with a high spinal cord lesion generally will not be able to activate their abdominal muscles. They will not be able to generate the intrathoracic pressures needed to get airway narrowing and the accelerated expiratory flows (Braun et al. 1984). Their cough is very weak and very inefficient in removing secretions. A cough is made more effective if the individual commences the procedure with an increased inspiratory volume. The individual with tetraplegia, however, will often have paralysis of the internal intercostal muscles which thereby reduces inspiratory capacity. Clinical studies by Ohry et al. (1975) and Forner (1980) highlight the fact that the individual with tetraplegia will demonstrate reductions in inspiratory and expiratory flow rates, total lung capacity and vital capacity.

TREATMENT

Braun et al. (1984) attempted to address the problem of inefficient coughing in the spinal injured population by evaluating the efficacy of an abdominal push-assist technique during cough. They found a significant improvement in peak flow using this technique. These investigators do note, however, that there may be some potential problems associated with this manoeuvre such as damage to the ribs and abdominal contents if the abdominal pressure is too aggressive. In addition, they suggest that it could be ineffective if the technique is not synchronous with the patient's effort. A further study attempting to address the respiratory changes in the individual with spinal cord injuries looked at the possibility of respiratory muscle training by the use of mouth–nose-mask with inspiratory and expiratory resistors which can be individually set. Biering-Sorensen et al. (1991) note,

however, that all pulmonary function parameters except peak expiratory flow (PEF) remained the same after 6 weeks of training. They suggest that the significant increase in PEF might indicate that a more efficient cough will be possible which may assist in removal of secretions and prevent further respiratory complications.

Jenny's Physiotherapy Management Prior to Surgery

After completing a comprehensive assessment of Jenny's cardiorespiratory status (particularly noting Jenny's latest pulmonary function testing), the hospital physiotherapist devised a prioritized short-term problem list so that he can most effectively instigate a specified treatment regimen for this particular patient. The short-term problem list is as follows:

1. inefficient cough manoeuvre (very little evidence of any abdominal contraction – resulting in reduced expiratory flow rates)
2. decreased power of accessory respiratory muscles (particularly little evidence of contraction of intercostal muscles – causing reduced inspiratory capacity)
3. significant risk that patient will not be able to remove secretions easily if they become evident post-operatively

The physiotherapist addressed Jenny's preoperative cardiorespiratory problems in the following manner. Before any preoperative intervention the physiotherapist emphasized to Jenny and her mother that if they have any concerns regarding the operative procedure they should indicate these to him so that he can assist in clarifying various issues or refer them to relevant personnel who can. The physiotherapist trains Jenny and her mother in the abdominal push-assist technique during cough manoeuvre in an attempt to improve the efficiency of her cough, explaining that if her cough is moist postoperatively this procedure may assist in the removal of secretions. Adapted respiratory muscle training is carried out through the use of low-pressure PEP-mask-therapy and incentive spirometry. Peak flow meter measurements are taken before and after daily training sessions. Instruction is given on the use of intermittent positive pressure breathing (which may be used in the postoperative physiotherapy treatment regimen). In addition Jenny's exercise tolerance is encouraged as much as possible through demand ventilation, e.g. activities such as wheelchair basketball.

Jenny's Post-surgical Physiotherapy Regimen

After the surgical anterior release of contracted soft tissue Jenny returned to the ward. As soon as she was stabilized medically, and her pain adequately controlled, the physiotherapist assessed her cardiorespiratory status, re-established Jenny's particular problems and subsequently addressed these problems with short frequent treatments. Jenny's problems postoperatively were similar to those established preoperatively, though, postoperative pain was now an issue and her cough was slightly moist. The physiotherapist introduced the techniques (intermittent positive pressure breathing, PEP-mask-therapy, incentive spirometry, abdominal push-assist technique) which had been introduced preoperatively in an attempt to increase Jenny's inspiratory capacity and improve the efficiency of her cough manoeuvre. Adapted positioning and upper limb movements (within pain limits) were also undertaken in an attempt to increase air entry. Passive movements and functional positioning of paralysed lower limbs were also carried out at every session. Such physiotherapy treatments were undertaken frequently throughout the week following initial surgery. Her cough became dry after the third day postoperatively.

One week later, the second stage of Jenny's spinal fusion was undertaken. Her postoperative physiotherapy management continued very similarly to the previous week (instigating techniques such as intermittent positive pressure breathing, PEP-mask-therapy, incentive spirometry, abdominal push-assist technique) since the physiotherapist had assessed her problems as being essentially the same as her problems after her first-stage spinal surgery. After this second-stage surgery active rotatory movement of patient's trunk was contraindicated, but frequent positioning of patient was achieved via movement of the bed. Bilateral assisted upper limb movements were encouraged initially to avoid any excessive rotatory forces. Within several days her cough was no longer moist and by the seventh day postoperatively she was sitting in her wheelchair. The surgeon felt as a precautionary measure that she should wear a brace when out of bed. She rapidly progressed and was discharged by the end of the week. A review of her surgery in 2 weeks was organized.

Case Study 3

Kate is a 4-year-old girl who has had significant cardiorespiratory difficulties since birth. She was born prematurely (27 weeks gestation), required prolonged ventilatory support and was subsequently diagnosed with bronchopulmonary dysplasia (BPD)/ (chronic neonatal lung disease, CNLD). During her first 3 years of life Kate experienced numerous respiratory infections and recurrent wheezing episodes. Testing of Kate's pulmonary mechanics suggests some abnormalities in expiratory flow rates. During the last year, however, there has been some reduction in the severity of Kate's wheezy exacerbations. Ten days ago, Kate developed a fever, wheezing and

241

> *paroxysmal coughing episodes. She was hospitalized as she developed some moderate respiratory distress and initially required supplemental oxygen to maintain saturations above 90%. Her chest X-ray showed extensive consolidation within her (R) lower lobe and middle lobe. She was diagnosed with pneumonia and serology tests indicated Mycoplasma pneumoniae as the causative agent which is being treated with appropriate antibiotics. Her fever reduced within 48 hours and her wheezing decreased during the first week of hospitalization. She is continuing to receive inhaled β₂ agonist and steroids via nebulizer to reduce airway hyperreactivity. Kate continues to experience paroxysmal coughing episodes which make her quite dyspnoeic. At times her cough sounds moist. A follow-up chest X-ray still shows marked consolidation. Since Kate is now out of the acute phase of her pneumonia, but shows some delay in resolution of consolidation due to retained secretions, her physician has requested the physiotherapist to review this patient.*

Physiotherapy for Cardiorespiratory Problems of Bronchopulmonary Dysplasia

BACKGROUND

BPD is a 'chronic neonatal lung disease' which occurs in infants who are ventilated for >3 days, who require supplemental oxygen for >28 days and whose chest radiograph revealed parenchymal densities (Bancalari *et al.* 1979, p. 819). Northway *et al.* (1967) originally suggested that BPD was a 'prolongation of the healing phase of respiratory distress syndrome combined with a generalized pulmonary oxygen toxicity involving mucosal, alveolar and vascular tissues' (p. 367). Tudehope (1993) notes that the pathogenesis of BPD is complex and multifactorial, but lists the principal factors in the pathogenesis of BPD as: (1) premature birth with immature lung structure, surfactant deficiency and inadequate respiratory drive; (2) respira-

tory failure; (3) oxygen toxicity with immaturity of antioxidant system; (4) barotrauma from positive pressure ventilation, especially when associated with pulmonary air leaks such as pulmonary interstitial emphysema and pneumothorax; (5) pulmonary oedema associated with patent ductus arteriosus, congestive heart failure and crystalloid and colloid overload; (6) pulmonary infection with organisms such as cytomegalovirus, respiratory syncytial virus and *Ureaplasma urealyticum* (pp. 86–87). The long-term prognosis of children with BPD is variable and, although a normal lifestyle and pulmonary function are achievable, some children have chronic airflow limitation and hyperreactive airways (O'Brodovich and Mellins 1985).

Epidemiological studies suggest that youngsters with chronic conditions have more of the usual array of behavioural disorders. Undoubtedly, chronic physical conditions can produce changes in the way the child is perceived by others, which can subsequently affect how the child perceives him/herself. A child's irritability, passivity and anxiety, however, may be due to symptoms such as pain or respiratory difficulties rather than primary manifestations of a behaviour disorder (Creer *et al.* 1992).

Kate's Physiotherapy Management

After completing a comprehensive assessment of Kate's cardiorespiratory status, the hospital physiotherapist devised a prioritized short-term problem list so that she can most effectively instigate a specified treatment regimen for this particular patient. The short-term problem list is as follows:

1. *marked passivity – general reluctance to move, particularly decreased thoracic mobility and decreased exercise tolerance*
2. *decreased air entry – particularly (R) lower and middle lobes*
3. *retained secretions – evidence of moist cough*
4. *inefficient cough manoeuvre – leading to paroxysmal coughing episodes and wheezing symptoms*

The physiotherapist addressed Kate's short-term cardiorespiratory problems in the following manner. Initially, attempts were made to address Kate's passivity by encouraging her to move more frequently from her bed. It was organized to undertake physiotherapy intervention within the physiotherapy outpatient department which therefore demanded that Kate would walk a short distance and provided her with positive, fun surroundings. In the department appropriate game type activities, such as ball and quoits throwing, were instigated so as to encourage thoracic mobility and to improve air entry and exercise tolerance. Care was taken not to exacerbate any exercise-induced wheezing. Activities such as blowing bubbles were also introduced in preparation for training Kate in the FET manoeuvre. After instruction, Kate achieved a fairly effective mid-volume FET manoeuvre. Emphasis was also placed on instructing Kate in the active cycle of breathing so as to achieve more efficient air entry while posturally draining (R) lower and middle lobes. She had to be encouraged to use the FET manoeuvre instead of going into paroxysmal coughing episodes. Percussion and vibrations were not introduced as there were concerns that such techniques may exacerbate some wheezing while draining.

Kate responded well to the physiotherapist's intervention. Over the next 5 days, her paroxysms of coughing had reduced markedly and air entry had improved significantly. Upon discharge, the physiotherapist encouraged Kate's mother to continue with the ball activities at home, emphasizing the beneficial physiological and psychological effects of exercise. As Kate's discharge medication included inhaled β₂ agonist and steroid (via metered dose inhaler (MDI) + large volume spacer device), the physiotherapist reviewed Kate's technique of inhalation in the presence of her mother. The physiotherapist also emphasized in this discharge discussion the deleterious effects of passive smoking upon children's airways.

These case histories have only provided a glimpse into the various young children with cardiorespiratory problems who may benefit from physiotherapy intervention. For example, the young child who has sustained head injuries or spinal injuries and the child who has undergone extensive surgical procedures (e.g. heart and liver surgery) and requires assisted ventilation have not been addressed. Indeed, the physiotherapist will play an integral role in the management of the ventilated child. Pneumonia is common among patients with artificial airways in place, particularly the ventilated patient with a closed head injury (Hsieh et al. 1992).

The physiotherapist may also be involved in assessment and intervention for the child with congenital anomalies such as micrognathia or tracheal stenosis who requires the use of a long-term tracheostomy tube for relief of respiratory embarrassment. Physiotherapy treatments for the ventilated child and the child with a tracheostomy tube often involve maintaining adequate ventilation of the lung, assisting in the mobilization and removal of secretions and assisting in the resolution of atelectasis. Various techniques may be instigated, such as positioning, vibrations, hyperinflation and suction, though these techniques are subject to any contraindications associated with the individual patient's pathology.

There are many children with cardiorespiratory problems, however, who can benefit from a patient-specific physiotherapy treatment regimen. After considering the previous case histories you may like to address the following scenarios relating to the physiotherapy management of children with varying cardiorespiratory problems.

1. Discuss the physiotherapist's assessment procedure and possible treatment ideas for an 8-year-old child recently diagnosed with Guillain–Barré syndrome who now has a moist weak cough. Her vital capacity has decreased by 20% in the last 2 days. She requires considerable assistance to sit up from lying or to stand.

2. List the necessary precautions the physiotherapist would have to undertake when managing a chest infection in a 2-year-old child who has a severe form of osteogenesis imperfecta (OI).

3. The parent of a 10-year-old child who experiences exercise-induced asthma is asking the physiotherapist what sort of sport is best for her child. How would you answer this parent?

4. Discuss the physiotherapist's cardiorespiratory management of an 18-month-child with spastic quadriplegia who has a (R) LL consolidation. This little boy has very poor oro-motor control and severe gastro-oesophageal reflux.

Summary

This chapter has attempted to encourage readers to explore further the role of physiotherapy in the management of young children with cardiorespiratory problems. Greater clinical exploration of the efficacy of physiotherapy intervention with respect to toddlers and the preschool child with cardiorespiratory difficulties is necessary. As noted at the outset of this chapter, physiotherapy management of cardiorespiratory difficulties is much more likely to be most effective when the physiotherapist undertakes a careful analysis of the problems of each patient and establishes a treatment regimen designed to address the individual's specific problems.

REFERENCES

Angus, GE, Thurlbeck, WM (1972) Numbers of alveoli in the human lung. *Journal of Applied Physiology* 32: 483–485.

Aweida, D, Kelsy, CJ (1990) Accuracy and reliability of physical therapists in auscultating tape-recorded lung sounds. *Physiotherapy Canada* 42: 279–282.

Bancalari, E, Abdenour, GE, Feller, R et al. (1979) Bronchopulmonary dysplasia: clinical presentation. *Journal of Pediatrics* 85: 819–823.

Bauman, A, Mitchell, CA, Henry, RL et al. (1992) Asthma morbidity in Australia: an epidemiological study. *Medical Journal of Australia* 156: 827–831.

Biering-Sorensen, F, Knudsen, JL, Schmidt, A et al. (1991) Effect of respiratory training with a mouth-nose-mask in tetraplegics. *Paraplegia* 29: 113–119.

Braun, SR, Giovannoni, R, O'Connor, M (1984) Improving the cough in patients with spinal cord injury. *American Journal of Physical Medicine* 63: 1–10.

Brock, DJH, Shrimpton, AE, Jones, C (1991) Cystic fibrosis: the new genetics. *Journal Royal Society of Medicine* 84 (suppl. 18): 2–9.

Brooks, D, Wilson, L, Kelsy, C (1994) Accuracy and reliability of 'specialized' physical therapists in auscultating tape-recorded lung sounds. *Physiotherapy Canada* 45: 21–24.

Creer, TL, Stein, REK, Rappaport, L et al. (1992) Behavioural consequences of illness: childhood asthma as a model. *Pediatrics* (suppl. 90) 808–815.

Cuthbert, AW (1992) The biochemical defect in cystic fibrosis. *Journal of the Royal Society of Medicine* 85 (suppl. 19): 2–5.

Earis, J (1992) Lung Sounds. *Thorax* 47: 671–672.

Engel, S (1947) *The Child's Lung: Developmental Anatomy, Physiology and Pathology,* 332 pp. London: Edward Arnold.

Falk, M, Kelstrup, M, Andersoen, JB et al. (1984) Improving the ketchup bottle method with positive expiratory pressure, PEP, in cystic fibrosis. *European Journal of Respiratory Disease* 65: 423–432.

Forner, JV (1980) Lung volumes and mechanics of breathing in tetraplegics. *Paraplegia* 18: 258–266.

Francis, P (1992) Treatment of pneumonia in childhood. *Current Therapeutics* 33: 44–46.

Garwely, D, Covey, M, Levison, H (1980) Pulmonary function and bronchial reactivity in children after croup. *American Review of Respiratory Disease* 122: 95–99.

Hofmeyer, JL, Webber, BA, Hodson, ME (1986) Evaluation of positive expiratory pressure as an adjunct to chest physiotherapy in the treatment of cystic fibrosis. *Thorax* 41: 951–954.

Hogg, JC, Williams, J, Richardson, JB et al. (1970) Age as a factor in the distribution of lower airway conductance and in the pathologic anatomy of obstructive lung disease. *New England Journal of Medicine* 282: 1283–1287.

Hsieh, AH, Bishop, MJ, Kubilis, PS et al. (1992) Pneumonia following closed head injury. *American Review of Respiratory Disease* 146: 290–294.

Ignacio, S, Powell, RE, Pasterkamp, H (1993) Wheezing and airflow obstruction during metacholine challenge in children with cystic fibrosis and in normal children. *American Review of Respiratory Disease* 147: 705–709.

Inselman, LA, Mellins, RB (1981) Growth and development of the lung. *The Journal of Pediatrics* 98: 1–15.

Kirilloff, LH, Owens, GR, Rogers, RM et al. (1985) Does chest physical therapy work? *Chest* 88: 436–444.

Loudon, R, Murphy, RLH (1984) State of the art: lung sounds. *American Review of Respiratory Disease* 130: 663–673.

Martinez, F, Antognoni, G, Macri, F et al. (1988) Parental smoking enhances bronchial responsiveness in nine-year-old children. *American Review of Respiratory Disease* 138: 518–523.

Martinez, F, Morgan, WJ, Wright, AL et al. (1991) Initial airway function is a risk factor for recurrent wheezing respiratory illnesses during the first three years of life. *American Review of Respiratory Disease* 143: 312–316.

Martinez, FD, Cline, M, Burrows, B (1992) Increased incidence of asthma in children of smoking mothers. *Pediatrics* 89: 21–26.

McPherson, MA, Dormer, RL (1994) Cystic fibrosis gene and mucin secretion. *Lancet* 343: 7.

Northway, WH, Rosan, R, Porter, DY (1967) Pulmonary disease following respiratory therapy of hyaline membrane disease and broncho-pulmonary dysplasia. *New England Journal of Medicine* 276: 357–368.

O'Brodovich, HM, Mellins, RB (1985) State of the art bronchopulmonary dysplasia: unresolved neonatal acute lung injury. *American Review of Respiratory Disease* 132: 694–709.

Ohry, A, Molho, M, Rozin, R (1975) Alterations of pulmonary function in spinal cord injured patients. *Paraplegia* 13: 101–108.

Pagtakhan, RD, Bjelland, JC, Landau, LI et al. (1984) Sex differences in growth patterns of the airways and lung parenchyma in children. *Journal of Applied Physiology* 56: 1207–1216.

Partridge, C, Pryor, J, Webber, B (1989) Characteristics of the forced expiration technique. *Physiotherapy* 75: 193–194.

Patterson, JM, Budd, J, Goetz, D et al. (1993) Family correlates of a 10-year pulmonary health trend in cystic fibrosis. *Pediatrics* 91: 383–389.

Pedreira, FA, Guandolo, VL, Feroli, EJ et al. (1985) Involuntary smoking and incidence of respiratory illness during the first year of life. *Pediatrics* 75: 594–597.

Prasad, SA (1993) Current concepts in physiotherapy. *Journal of the Royal Society of Medicine* **86** (suppl. 20): 23–29.

Ranieri, E, Lewis, BD, Gerace, RL *et al.* (1994) Neonatal screening for cystic fibrosis using immunoreactive trypsinogen and direct gene analysis: four years' experience. *British Medical Journal* **308**: 1469–1472.

Rona, RJ, Chinn, S (1993) Lung function, respiratory illness and passive smoking in British primary school children. *Thorax* **48**: 21–25.

Roorda, RJ, Gerritsen, J, Van Aaleren, WMC *et al.* (1993) Risk factors for the persistence of respiratory symptoms in childhood asthma. *American Review of Respiratory Disease* **148**: 1490–1495.

Salh, W, Bilton, D, Dodd, M *et al.* (1989) Effect of exercise and physiotherapy in aiding sputum expectoration in adults with cystic fibrosis. *Thorax* **44**: 1006–1008.

Samet, JM, Tager, IB, Speizer, FE (1983) The relationship between respiratory illness in childhood and chronic air-flow obstruction in adulthood. *American Review of Respiratory Disease* **127**: 508–523.

Scarpelli Emile, M (1990) *Pulmonary Physiology: Fetus, Newborn, Child and Adolescent*, 500 pp. Philadelphia: Lea and Febinger.

Schoni, MH (1989) Autogenic drainage: a modern approach to physiotherapy. *Journal of the Royal Society of Medicine* **82** (suppl. 16): 32–37.

Schulz, JI, Olha, AE (1986) Exercise-induced asthma. *Physiotherapy Canada* **38**: 208–213.

Steen, HJ, Redmond, OB, O'Neil, D *et al.* (1991) Evaluation of the PEP mask in cystic fibrosis. *Acta Paediatrica Scandinavica* **80**: 51–56.

Super, M (1992) The gene defect in cystic fibrosis and clinical applications of the knowledge. *Journal of the Royal Society of Medicine* **85** (suppl. 19): 6–8.

Tager, IB, Weiss, ST, Munoz, A (1983) Longitudinal study of the effects of maternal smoking on pulmonary function in children. *New England Journal of Medicine* **309**: 699–703.

Taussig, LM, Cota, K, Kaltenborn, W (1981) Different mechanical properties of the lung in boys and girls. *American Review of Respiratory Disease* **123**: 640–643.

Thomas, JA, McIntosh, JM (1994) Are incentive spirometry, intermittent positive pressure breathing, and deep breathing exercises effective in the prevention of postoperative pulmonary complications after upper abdominal surgery? A systematic overview and meta-analysis. *Physical Therapy* **74**: 3–10.

Thurlbeck, WM (1975) Postnatal growth and development of the lung. *American Review of Respiratory Disease* **111**: 803–844.

Torres, A, Aznar, R, Gatell, JM *et al.* (1990) Incidence, risk and prognosis factors of nosocomial pneumonia in mechanically ventilated patients. *American Review of Respiratory Disease* **142**: 523–528.

Tudehope, DI (1993) Editorial comment: bronchopulmonary dysplasia. *Journal of Paediatric Child Health* **29**: 86–89.

Tyrell, JC, Hillier, EJ, Martin, J (1986) Face mask physiotherapy in cystic fibrosis. *Archives of Disease in Childhood* **61**: 598–611.

Weiss, ST, Tager, IB, Munoz, A (1985) The relationship of respiratory infections in early childhood to the occurrence of increased levels of bronchial responsiveness and atopy. *American Review of Respiratory Disease* **131**: 573–578.

Weitzman, M, Gortmaker, S, Walker, D *et al.* (1990) Maternal smoking and Childhood Asthma. *Pediatrics* **85**: 505–511.

Young, CS (1984) A review of the adverse effects of airway suction. *Physiotherapy* **70**: 104–106.

Young, CS (1984) Reccommended guide lines for suction. *Physiotherapy* **70**: 106–108.

Zach, MS (1991) Pathogenesis and management of lung disease in cystic fibrosis. *Journal of the Royal Society of Medicine* **84** (suppl. 18): 10–17.

FURTHER READING

Becroft, DMO (1971) Bronchiolitis obliterans, bronchiectasis and other sequelae of adenovirus type 21 infection in young children. *Journal of Clinical Pathology* **24**: 72–82.

Burrows, B, Taussig, LM (1980) As the twig is bent, the tree inclines (perhaps). *American Review of Respiratory Disease* **122**: 813–816.

Burrows, B, Knudson, RJ, Lebowitz, MD (1977) The relationship of childhood respiratory illness to adult obstructive airway diseases. *American Review of Respiratory Disease* **115**: 751–760.

Campbell, DA, Ruffin, RE (1991) Diagnosis of atypical asthma. *Patient Management* **15**: 29–33.

Canning, GJ, Levison, H (1988) Aerosols – therapeutic use and delivery in childhood asthma. *Annals of Allergy* **60**: 11–20.

Citta-Pietrolungo, TJ, Alexander, MA, Cook, SP *et al.* (1993) Complications of tracheostomy and decannulation in pediatric and young patients with traumatic brain injury. *Archives of Physical Medicine and Rehabilitation* **74**: 905–909.

Clark, CJ (1992) Asthma and exercise: a suitable case for rehabilitation. *Thorax* **47**: 765–767.

Craven, DE, Kunches, LM, Kilinsky, V *et al.* (1986) Risk factors for pneumonia and fatality in patients receiving continuous mechanical ventilation. *American Review of Respiratory Disease* **133**: 792–796.

Drummond, DS (1991) A perspective on recent trends for scoliosis correction. *Clinical Orthopaedics and Related Research* **264**: 90–102.

Enright, PL, Lebowitz, MD, Cockroft, DW (1994) Physiological measures: pulmonary function tests asthma outcome. *American Journal of Respiratory Critical Care Medicine* **149**: S9–S18.

Fahy, JV, Schuster, A, Heki, I *et al.* (1992) Mucus hypersecretion in bronchiectasis: the role of neutrophil proteases. *American Review of Respiratory Disease* **146**: 1430–1433.

Forastiere, F, Agabiti, N, Corbo, N *et al.* (1994) Passive smoking as a determinant of bronchial responsiveness in children. *American Journal Respiratory Critical Care Medicine* **149**: 365–370.

Graham, WGB, Bradley, DA (1978) Efficacy of chest physiotherapy and intermittent positive-pressure breathing in the resolution of pneumonia. *New England Journal of Medicine* **299**: 624–627.

Henry, RL (1994) Cystic fibrosis: new developments. *Current Therapeutics* **35**: 9–12.

Hogg, JC, Macklem, PT, Thurlbeck, WM (1968) Site and nature of airway obstruction in chronic obstructive lung disease. *New England Journal of Medicine* **278**: 1355–1360.

Kamm, RD, Drazer, JM (1992) Airway hyperresponsiveness and airway wall thickening in asthma. *American Review of Respiratory Disease* **145**: 1249–1250.

Konstan, MW, Stern, RC, Doershuk, CF (1994) Efficacy of the flutter device for airway mucus clearance in patients with cystic fibrosis. *Journal of Pediatrics* **124**: 689–693.

Kuzemko, JA (1987) *The Respiratory Disorders of Infants and Children: A Guide to Practical Management*, 101 pp. Kent: Castle House Publications.

Landau, LI (1991) Factors inhibiting satisfactory parent education in asthma in children. *Patient Management* **15**: 53–55.

Littlewood, JM (1992) Gastrointestinal complications in cystic fibrosis. *Journal of the Royal Society of Medicine* **85** (Suppl. 18): 13–19.

Martin, AJ, McLennan, LA, Landau, LI *et al.* (1980) The natural history of childhood asthma to adult life. *British Medical Journal* **280**: 1397–1400.

Miller, MR, Dickinson, SA, Hitchings, DJ (1992) The accuracy of portable peak flow meters. *Thorax* **47**: 904–909.

Muszynski-Kwan, AT, Perlman, R, Rivington-Law, BA (1988) Compliance with and effectiveness of chest physiotherapy in cystic fibrosis: a review. *Physiotherapy Canada* **40**: 28–32.

Ninan, TK, Russell, G (1992) Respiratory symptoms and atopy in Aberdeen schoolchildren: evidence from 2 surveys 25 years apart. *British Medical Journal* **34**: 873–875.

Oberwalder, B, Theisl, B, Rucker, A *et al.* (1991) Chest physiotherapy in hospitalized patients with cystic fibrosis: a study of lung function effects and sputum production. *European Respiratory Journal* **4**: 152–158.

Orenstein, DM, Reed, ME, Grogan, FT *et al.* (1985) Exercise conditioning in children with asthma. *Journal of Pediatrics* **106**: 556–559.

Pryor, JA, Webber, BA, Hodson, ME (1990) Effect of chest physiotherapy on oxygen saturation in patients with cystic fibrosis. *Thorax* **45**: 77.

Redline, S, Tager, IB, Castile, RG *et al.* (1987) Assessment of the usefulness of helium–oxygen maximal expiratory flow curves in epidemiological studies of lung disease in children. *American Review of Respiratory Disease* **136**: 834–840.

Robertson, CF, Bishop, J, Dalton, M *et al.* (1992) Prevalence of asthma in regional Victorian schoolchildren. *Medical Journal of Australia* **156**: 831–838.

Stiller, KR, McEvoy, RD (1990) Chest physiotherapy for the medical patient – are current practices effective? *Australian New Zealand Journal of Medicine* **20**: 183–188.

Stiller, K, Geake, T, Taylor, J *et al.* (1990) Acute lobar atelectasis: a comparison of two chest physiotherapy regimens. *Chest* **98**: 1336–1340.

Sutton, PP, Pavia, D, Bateman, JRM (1982) Chest physiotherapy: a review. *European Journal of Respiratory Disease* **63**: 188–201.

Tager, IB (1988) Passive smoking – bronchial responsiveness and atopy. *American Review of Respiratory Disease* **138**: 507–509.

Van Der Schans, CP, Piers, DA, Postma, DS (1986) Effect of manual percussion on tracheobronchial clearance in patients with chronic airflow obstruction and excessive tracheobronchial secretion. *Thorax* **41**: 448–452.

Van der Schans, CP, Van der Mark, ThW, de Vries, G (1991) Effect of positive expiratory pressure breathing in patients with cystic fibrosis. *Thorax* **46**: 252–256.

Wanner, A (1984) Does chest physical therapy move airway secretions. *American Review of Respiratory Disease* **130**: 701–702.

Wiens, L, Sabath, R, Ewing, L (1992) Chest pain in otherwise healthy children and adolescents is frequently caused by exercise induced asthma. *Pediatrics* **90**: 350–353.

Wollmer, P, Ursing, K, Midgren, B (1985) Inefficiency of chest percussion in the physical therapy of chronic bronchitis. *European Journal of Respiratory Disease* **66**: 233–239.

Woodhead, M, Tattersfield (1987) The unacceptable face of tipping. *British Medical Journal* **294**: 921–922.

Young, S, Arnott, J, Le Souef, PN *et al.* (1994) Flow limitation during tidal expiration in symptom-free infants and the subsequent development of asthma. *Journal of Pediatrics* **124**: 681–688.

16

Cardiorespiratory Physiotherapy Management – Adolescence

BRENDA BUTTON AND SUSAN SAWYER

Adolescence
•
Meeting the Challenge of Treating Chronic Degenerative Lung Disease
•
Physiotherapy for Adolescents with Cystic Fibrosis
•
A Multifunctional Clinical and Research Data Collection System

Optimal physiotherapy management of the individual with cardiorespiratory problems involves appropriate treatment techniques and patient compliance. Compliance is a function of the age group treated. This chapter explores ways of achieving positive physiotherapy outcomes by looking at adolescent development and special needs, appropriate therapy, motivation and compliance. The approach and ideas have developed over a 5 year period of involvement with adolescents with pulmonary conditions, within a multidisciplinary team at a major specialist paediatric respiratory centre.

In *acute* respiratory illness, physiotherapy is a short-term intervention that generally ends once normal function is restored. In *chronic* respiratory illnesses, such as cystic fibrosis and idiopathic bronchiectasis, there is an ongoing relationship between the patient and the therapist. Review and modification of management together with interaction, rapport, interest and support are required to sustain motivation and compliance as the patient's condition progresses. Indeed, physiotherapy for chronic respiratory illnesses demands sound physical, managerial and communicative skills. The approach should achieve the following: assessment of the patient's needs and response to intervention; promotion of the development, restoration and maintenance of the patient's optimal respiratory function; prevention of further respiratory disorder; and enhancement of the patient's quality of life (Le Roux 1991).

Adolescence

Adolescence is defined as 'a period of personal development during which a young person must establish a personal sense of individual identity and feelings of self-worth which include an alteration of his or her body image, adaptation to more mature intellectual abilities, adjustments to society's demands for behavioural maturity, internalizing a personal value system, and preparing for adult roles' (Ingersoll 1989 p. 2). As young people experience the biological changes from childhood to adulthood, they also experience profound changes in their social, cognitive (particularly in relation to their perspectives of the future) and psychological worlds.

The period of adolescence is frequently viewed by professionals and parents with ambivalence. The exuberance, enthusiasm and idealism of youth are admired, while there is fear that the impulsive behaviours and egocentric demeanor will result in long-term health and social consequences.

Health professionals who care for adolescents can play important roles in fostering a positive transition to adulthood. To be effective in caring for adolescents, however, both physical and psychosocial development need to be understood. Therapeutic interventions that do not incorporate these needs are likely to be ineffective (Ingersoll 1992).

STAGES OF ADOLESCENCE

Early Adolescence   is marked by rapid acceleration of physical growth and maturation, with much of the early intellectual and emotional energies targeted at a reassessment and restructuring of body image. At the same time acceptance by peers is paramount; getting along and not being viewed as different are motives that dominate much of the early adolescent's social behaviour.

Early adolescents have a limited concept of time in the abstract sense. Telling young people that today's behaviour may affect their health 5, 10 or 20 years from now has little meaning for them.

Middle Adolescence   is marked by nearly completed pubertal growth, the emergence of new thinking skills, an increased recognition of impending adulthood, and a desire to establish emotional and psychological distance from parents. The ability to conceptualize and engage in abstract thinking is developing throughout this stage.

Late adolescence   is marked by preparation for adult roles, including the clarification of vocational goals and internalizing a personal value system. The role of the health professional caring for adolescents should vary according to the developmental status of the patient (Ingersoll 1992).

Meeting the Challenge of Treating Chronic Degenerative Lung Disease

There are many challenges for physiotherapists managing patients with chronic degenerative physical illnesses. The physiotherapist will have to consider ways of achieving rapport and cooperation, a selection of treatment techniques, issues of motivation, compliance and developing independence, as well as clinical tools of measurement to monitor objectively the physical condition of patients.

A number of medical conditions could be used to illustrate the unique requirements of adolescents with chronic respiratory lung disease, such as cystic fibrosis, idiopathic bronchiectasis, chronic granulomatous disease and immotile cilia syndrome. In view of the significant cardiorespiratory problems which can develop in adolescents with cystic fibrosis, this condition has been chosen to describe approaches that will result in effective management of adolescent patients requiring regular chest physiotherapy to achieve the optimal quality of life and long-term survival.

Important Elements of Effective Physiotherapy Management of Adolescents

A POSITIVE ATTITUDE

The therapist's approach should be calm, confident, mature, knowledgeable and relaxed. Therapists should enjoy working with young people, and not feel intimidated by them. Respect for the world of adolescents (music, clothing, unconventional hairstyles) is necessary. Negative or patronizing comments are alienating. Poor motivation and compliance may be symptoms of therapists who are not respected or accepted by patients.

Lack of respect for the therapist may be because of:

- a lack of respect shown to the adolescent by the therapist
- insensitivity to some aspect of the patient's manner, physical appearance or condition
- a perceived lack of knowledge or expertise
- a breach of confidentiality

In order to develop good rapport with patients the therapist should approach adolescents confidently and not be fearful of initial 'testing' behaviour. A sense of humour and a lighthearted approach assist in initiating and maintaining rapport.

Some therapists resort to the authoritarian approach when anxious about maintaining control or the ability to achieve cooperation. This often results in a backlash of rebellious non-cooperation. This need for compliance can shift the focus from the patient's well-being and best interests to meeting the demands of the therapist. The patient therefore transfers the 'problem' to the therapist, losing sight of the reason why physiotherapy is required and who actually stands to benefit from it. Feelings of lack of control may surround both the therapist and the patient and lead to frustration on both sides.

INDIVIDUALIZATION OF TREATMENT REGIMENS

Optimal physiotherapy programmes require an individualized approach which considers medical problems, interests, personalities, life styles and social background. Adolescents require evidence that the regimen prescribed 'works' for them. They question the value of compliance with a regimen which 'makes them feel worse' (quotes from patients with significant gastro-oesophageal reflux during postural drainage) or which according to their judgement is ineffective.

A cooperative approach in the selection of an optimal individualized regimen is necessary. The patient is at the receiving end of the physiotherapy intervention and should be encouraged to relay feedback to the therapist. The therapist has professional knowledge, clinical judgement and measurement tools to interpret objectively the findings, and thus prescribe an optimal programme for each patient.

The patient is not a passive recipient of therapy, but an active participant in the health care process, who can be helped to understand the rationale for adherence to the regimen and develop a sense of control of the situation. Some adolescents will say 'this technique does not work for me'. The therapist may believe that the techniqe is effective, but it is the patient's word against the therapist's. The therapist needs to consider carefully and take seriously the patient's feedback. Objective data obtained from measurements taken before and after therapy assist in establishing the best regimen for the patient. The way the techniques are used may need modification to be more effective. Ongoing review and fine-tuning of regimens are necessary to ensure optimal care.

POSITIVE FEEDBACK

Positive feedback and short-term rewards lead to motivation and compliance. Health professionals and parents use different tactics to try to encourage their charges to adhere to their prescribed treatment regimens. How often do we hear parents of children with asthma reduced to the desperate plea of 'if you don't take your medicines you are going to die from asthma'. In view of the lack of future perspective held by the majority of children and young adolescents with asthma, who are unable to perceive the long-term consequences of poor adherence, such a statement is unlikely to be successful as a motivational strategy.

Alternative strategies, such as, 'if you don't take your medication you'll be too breathless to play in the basketball competition next week' are more likely to be successful. If the patient is personally convinced that the regimen prescribed is effective, adherence to the prescribed regimen is more likely. This will in turn lead to improvement in quality of life (for example, fewer school days are missed resulting in academic, social and sporting benefits).

ATTENTIVE INTEREST IN PATIENT'S WELL-BEING.

This 'attentiveness' requirement is a recognized form of egocentricity. The presumption that everyone is ordinately concerned with the adolescent's well-being gives rise to the 'invisible audience' that is constantly attentive to the adolescent's actions and well-being (Elkind 1967). There is a requirement for physiotherapists to listen sensitively to patients, assimilate and, if necessary, act on the information, which is not always clearly articulated. Physiotherapists spend relatively long periods of treatment time with patients, particularly during hospital admissions and regular outpatient visits. They are able to gain the trust of patients and are sometimes expected to assume the role of patient advocate.

Because of the 'hands on' nature of physiotherapy, which takes time, there are opportunities for conversation other than the formal gathering of information and instruction. During these informal conversations between therapist and patient (and sometimes parents) during treatment, issues, problems, concerns and anxieties sometimes emerge. The therapist will need to consider the best way to deal with these issues.

Patients expect the therapist to be interested in them. They value objective and subjective assessment and require time to discuss these findings and to relate them to their treatment regimen.

APPROPRIATE LANGUAGE AND CLEAR COMMUNICATION

Patients' ability to relate their concerns and to understand the messages offered by health professionals are impeded by their lack of vocabulary. Professionals must be willing to adapt health messages — efforts should be made to probe the level of understanding since there is a likelihood of initial miscommunication. Visual illustrations, such as graphs, diagrams, charts, pictures, slides, overheads, photographs and audiovisual aids, assist in achieving understanding of important information.

PEER INFLUENCES

During early and middle adolescence, in particular, the need to be accepted by one's peer group dominates social interactions. Peer influence can produce a positive socializing effect. In their attempts to establish autonomy from parents, adolescents turn to peers for support. Peer groups offer a context within which the young person can experiment with the alternative concepts of their selves, learn social skills and clarify value systems. Just as peers can exert pressure to engage in health-jeopardizing behaviours, similarly they can exert pressures that promote positive health behaviours. At the same time the adolescent is likely to view himself or herself as unique. As a result a 'personal fable' evolves in which adolescents see themselves as invulnerable. This sense of invulnerability contributes to adolescents' willing-

ness to engage in high-risk activities, including failure to use contraceptives, experimenting with drugs, reckless automobile driving, and non-compliance with therapy (Ingersoll 1992).

CONFIDENTIALITY

Confidentiality and respect for all information entrusted to physiotherapists by patients, parents and other members of the health team is required. Breach of confidentiality may result in alienation, lack of trust, loss of rapport and damaged credibility which in turn may result in decreased motivation and compliance. A reputation of untrustworthiness can be permanent.

When confidential information is entrusted to a therapist, he or she will need to decide whether the information may alter the management prescribed by another member of the health team. If that is believed to be the case, then a confidential exchange of information will need to take place. Members of the multidisciplinary team must be able to be trusted with confidential information.

Medicolegal issues of confidentiality need also to be considered. Patients have a legal right to confidentiality with all aspects of their health care and documentation.

WIN / WIN NEGOTIATION AND COMPROMISE

Motivation and compliance can be achieved through an approach which is cooperative, negotiative and pragmatic rather than authoritarian. A dictatorial approach tends to be counterproductive. It is sometimes necessary to negotiate a deal in which the therapist 'gives' on some issue of treatment, while the patient agrees to 'take on' some aspect of treatment resulting in both being winners (even though there has been a measure of compromise on the therapist's behalf). These compromises are often temporary. As the patient feels 'in control' and gains respect for the therapist, more can be expected of the patient.

Wherever possible, choices should be offered in an effort to produce a positive outcome, for example 'are you going to exercise in the morning or the afternoon?' or 'which do you want to do first, exercise or chest physiotherapy?' A choice between two productive outcomes leads to a sense of ownership over the decision and a feeling of control. Conversely asking the patient 'are you going to exercise today?' suggests a choice between something and nothing, and the reply may well be 'no, not today'.

In a condition like cystic fibrosis, the day-to-day management, year in year out is the important focus. Therefore a chest care programme that carefully considers the activities of the week and the particular interests of the young person must be developed. Activities such as walking or riding to school, physical education programmes, team sports, musical instruments that require blowing, domestic duties such as mowing the lawn and walking the dog can be incorporated into daily chest care. Assisting the adolescent work out a weekly programme considering all academic, domestic and health care issues in a cooperative way, and encouraging the adolescent to be open and pragmatic about what he or she can realistically achieve, will in the long-term produce the best outcome.

The therapist needs to establish the minimum intervention to achieve optimal outcome and incorporate all the individual's activities that will enhance mucociliary clearance to establish the most effective regimen. Compromise is sometimes necessary. Therapists tend to have high personal standards and may find compromise uncomfortable.

When treating adolescent patients with chronic respiratory illnesses, short-term goals need to be set in the light of long-term considerations. As adolescents mature and interests, activities and health status change, the physiotherapy programme will need to be altered and fine tuned.

ISSUES OF INDEPENDENCE AND CONTROL

Physiotherapists play a role in assisting patients and their families in the transition from dependence in childhood with physiotherapy management to independence in adulthood. From early childhood onwards there is a constant change in the involvement of the child and physiotherapist. Adolescence is another change in that relationship.

If a routine of daily health care is established in childhood before the many complex changes of puberty begin, compliance with health care regimens will have become a normal part of daily life, and will be less of an issue than if the handover of health care commences simultaneously with all the other changes of puberty.

Children in the prepubertal stage are generally keen to assume 'grown-up' tasks and responsibilities. They are able to understand physiological processes that are explained clearly with appropriate vocabulary and choice of language. It should be impressed upon these adolescents that independent physiotherapy techniques are 'grown up things to do'.

Non-compliance During the Transition From Dependence to Independence. Young people have lapses of motivation and compliance for various reasons. Their time-management skills may lack maturity. If daily routines (for example, eating well, physiotherapy, medication, aerobic exercise, school work and domestic chores) are regarded by the young person as having been imposed by authority figures, this may lead to rebellion.

Parents need to relinquish control gradually as the adolescent takes on more responsibility. The physiotherapist's role is to assist the adolescent in this process, imparting the necessary knowledge and practical skills, and simultaneously supporting and assisting the parents to 'let go' while still maintaining encouragement, interest and support.

Many parents find handing over responsibility and control difficult, because they want the very best outcome for their child. For example, parents who have, regularly and effectively, carried out daily postural drainage physiotherapy on their child over many years, feel justifiably uncertain about the quality of the independent physiotherapy technique and the ability of the adolescent to be self-motivated and compliant.

The therapist's role is to assist the adolescent to become skilled in techniques which will make them more independent, and to demonstrate to the parents that he or she is able to be responsible for regular health care. The parents should be encouraged to 'give the patient a chance' to develop the skill and may need to 'allow' the adolescent to experience the consequences of non-compliance or an ineffective technique.

Establishing a daily 'physiotherapy journal' with the adolescent assists in developing a chest care programme which is time-efficient and provides feedback in relation to all other school, sporting, social and domestic activities. The daily journal should be drawn up by the therapist and patient jointly, with spaces for the various components of the programme, as well as relevant comments, and self-assessment measures to be recorded.

Where non-compliance is believed to impact negatively on health status, the role of the health team is to assist the adolescent make the connection between non-adherence and the deterioration in physical condition, and to reinforce the importance of adherence with all aspects of treatments prescribed. The therapist should adopt a gentle, sensitive approach in order to retain respect and credibility on both fronts.

In order to prepare the parents and adolescent for the achievement of gradual independence, it is helpful to discuss these issues during the prepubertal stage around 9 to 11 years. The timing of the transition to independence will vary according to the maturity and personal circumstances of each patient.

Regular physiotherapy sessions have, in many families, become important social times to talk about the day's events, issues at school and anticipated social or recreational plans. When introducing the concept of independence with physiotherapy this issue should be sensitively considered.

The following examples illustrate how parents can be involved with independent techniques during transition.

Postural Drainage, Percussion and Breathing Exercises. Instead of parents carrying out percussion with each cycle during postural drainage and breathing exercises, they offer hands-on assistance with each alternate cycle, and observe the adolescent during the alternating independent cycles of the active cycle of breathing and forced expiration technique. This allows companionship, interest and the opportunity of observing the quality of the independent technique.

Positive Expiration Pressure (PEP) Therapy. The adolescent sits up at the kitchen counter or table and carries out PEP therapy while the parent prepares the morning or evening meal. This way there is companionship, and the parent continues to be involved.

Objective measurements which demonstrate the effectiveness of the independent techniques are of great assistance when educating the adolescents and reassuring the parents that the 'new independent way' of doing physiotherapy is as good as the 'old dependent way'.

MAINTAINING A FOCUS TOWARDS AS NORMAL A LIFE AS POSSIBLE

Chronic illnesses disrupt the lifestyles of families and particularly of the individual. Life is for living and enjoying, for people with or without cystic fibrosis. Therapy must take its place in the life of the person with cystic fibrosis, but must not become the whole focus of life. Therapists should encourage patients from an early age to incorporate routine preventative chest care in the same way that they look after their teeth and personal hygiene.

Physical therapy in cystic fibrosis, whether formal airways clearance techniques, inhalations or aerobic exercise, should be incorporated in the weekly programme at regular times that best suit each individual and lead to the least disruption of a normal lifestyle. Physiotherapy may be carried out first thing in the morning, after school, before dinner or last thing at night, considering meal times, amount of sputum produced daily, whether coughing at school is a problem, and how often therapy is required. Each adolescent's requirements should be individually considered.

Clinical experience suggests that the more one asks a patient to do, the less they are likely to achieve on a regular basis. Therefore working out the minimum amount of physiotherapy intervention that will achieve the optimal results for each individual will in the long-term produce the best outcome. This will require a trial and error approach, and thus regular assessment at outpatient clinic visits with ongoing fine tuning are important. Objective measurements will assist in developing the most time-efficient and effective physiotherapy programme that will allow as normal a lifestyle as possible.

CONTINUITY OF PHYSIOTHERAPY CARE

The primary therapist who knows the patient, the past history and the personality develops credibility, trust and rapport over a period of time. It is optimal if at least one member of the physiotherapy team has a long-term involvement with the patients with chronic illnesses. A non-integrated approach with advice from different therapists, with different approaches, may lead to confusion and frustration which may in turn affect motivation and compliance and reduce hard-won respect. This is often difficult to achieve in hospitals where staff rotate through the different areas or where there is a high staff turn-over, and may partly explain why patients managed in specialist cystic fibrosis centres, with continuity of care and the development of specialist skills, and the opportunity to carry out research, will tend to have a better outcome.

Achieving an Optimal Outcome

Specialist skills are required by cardiorespiratory physiotherapists to assess function, to select, use and teach manual therapy and handling techniques effectively; and to devise, teach and develop effective exercise programmes (le Roux 1991). The therapist should have a broad knowledge base of the many forms of respiratory techniques in order that s/he can select those best suited to meet the needs of individual patients and subsequently be able to teach the adolescent patient to become skilled in the application of the techniques.

Physiotherapy for Adolescents with Cystic Fibrosis

Assessment of Patient's Needs and Response to Intervention

A complete and accurate assessment of the adolescent's problems is the first step in the physical

management. Continuing reassessment in relation to intervention is an ongoing requirement.

Cystic fibrosis affects the regulation and transport of ions across cell membranes, resulting in thicker mucus secreted in the lungs and other exocrine glands of the body. This causes various problems, the most serious of which is a predisposition to pulmonary infections, leading to bronchiectasis, fibrosis of airways and ultimately respiratory failure and premature death. With an aggressive multidisciplinary approach incorporating drug therapy, physiotherapy, dietetics and counselling, over the last quarter of a century, the quality of life and mean survival age have improved considerably (Phelan and Bowes 1991). There is a large variation in the manifestation of the disease in different individuals and the response to interventions; therefore, physiotherapists need to develop an individualized treatment approach.

Further improvements in survival will rely on ongoing improvements in the different therapies. Physiotherapists need to play their part in the achievement of ever-improving physiotherapy management. An open-minded, enquiring approach together with sound clinical research are the keys to finding ways to better therapy, which may mean fine-tuning existing techniques or developing new modes of treatment.

The mean life expectancy in patients managed by multidisciplinary teams in major specialist centres is around 30 years in Australia. Cystic fibrosis is a complex and changeable condition. Within an individual there is also significant variation with 'ups and downs' calling for regular review and fine-tuning of the patient's overall management. Assessment of patients has been described fully in the previous chapter and will not be repeated. Particular issues that affect adolescents will be discussed.

AUSCULTATION

Adolescents believe this to be a very important assessment technique, and doctors and physiotherapists are judged according to how thoroughly and frequently lung sounds are assessed with a stethoscope. Lung sounds should be considered together with all the other assessment findings in order to interpret correctly the patient's problems. The interpretation of breath sounds is subjective; there may, therefore, be variation between health professionals.

The following comment from a patient illustrates the point. 'How does the doctor know I am ready for discharge from hospital, he hasn't listened to my chest?' Regular auscultation is also a part of meeting the 'attentiveness' requirement of patients as well as providing the health professional with important information.

Interpreting the findings to patients when they ask 'how do I sound' should be made cautiously and sensitively, avoiding inducing undue alarm and anxiety. In cystic fibrosis, a patient producing thick green sputum may have a clear-sounding chest on auscultation (probably because the tenacious sputum is adherent to the airways). This assessment technique should therefore not be used in isolation, but should be used as one of the tools in order to make as accurate an assessment as possible.

RESPONSE TO EXERCISE

Aerobic exercise fitness testing is one of the most useful cardiorespiratory assessment tools available to physiotherapists. There are a number of recognized exercise fitness tests. The cardiorespiratory condition of the patient will determine the most appropriate test (Godfrey 1974, Nixon and Orenstein 1988, Singh and Michael 1992). A range of information (from the general to the specific) is gained during the test, making this one of the most important and enlightening of all assessment procedures.

Problems will become evident during the test; for example, bronchoconstriction, increased sputum production, oxygen desaturation, muscle weakness and joint pain. The increase in respiratory effort and rate during exercise will often elicit spontaneous coughing, providing further important information relating to respiratory sounds and secretions.

The therapist is quickly able to develop an overall view of the patient's condition, and can monitor progress with regular testing. The tests themselves can become part of the cardiorespiratory fitness training programme.

PULMONARY FUNCTION

Flow loop volume curves provide overall and specific information relating to pulmonary function. These are carried out at intervals in most specialist centres during outpatient visits and hospital admissions and should be carefully analysed (Hibbert and Lannigan 1989). Pulmonary function before and after each physiotherapy treatment session provides the therapist with objective information relating to the effects of the selected techniques on the patient. In the author's experience in day-to-day clinical practice, FEV_1 and peak flow measurements provide useful information about the patient's response to the intervention and fill in the gaps between the weekly flow loop volume curves. FEV_1 is believed to provide information about the effects of treatment on the smaller airways while peak flow rates relate more to changes in the larger airways.

Analysis of results gained from these measurements provides the therapist with valuable insight into the effects of selected physiotherapy techniques on the individual patient's lungs. Unless the measurements are carried out correctly, the information is of little value. Commonly, patients need to be encouraged to inspire maximally before carrying out the expiratory manoeuvre through the pulmonary function device. Selection of reliable measurement devices is an important consideration. Adolescents take a keen interest in measurements of lung function, which become an important feedback mechanism.

SPUTUM

The weight of sputum is highly controversial as an outcome measure for research. In clinical practice, however, one of the most important roles of the cardiorespiratory therapist is to assist with the removal of pulmonary secretions. Thus, an assessment of the amount of sputum expectorated during treatment should be included in order to evaluate the effectiveness of the prescribed regimen.

Objective measurement. Dry sputum weights are ideal in the research environment. However, in clinical practice cost and time restraints make wet sputum weights the more realistic option. Contamination of sputum with saliva and gastric contents must be taken into account. Adolescents take a keen interest in these weights and receive important feedback in relation to the effectiveness of the prescribed treatment techniques.

Subjective measurement. This requires the patient to assess the amount of sputum on a scale of 1 to 10 produced during each physiotherapy treatment session. The amount is greater than usual, the usual amount or less than usual. For example, a score of 10 equals the largest amount of sputum ever produced during a physiotherapy session; 1 = the smallest amount, 0 = nil secretions. This allows the therapist to gain a perspective of the significance of the sputum weight in relation to the patient's baseline production. Where 50 g per session is a baseline norm in one patient, 5 g is a significant increase in a patient who is usually 'dry'. These are important measures when considering whether a patient needs intensive treatment, is ready for discharge during a hospital admission, or is at baseline function. The subjective and objective assessment of the amount of sputum in relation to pulmonary function measurements will increase the therapist's understanding of the patient's problems and assist in the selection of the most appropriate treatment regimen.

ASSESSMENT OF FEELING OF WELL-BEING

During assessment of patients in the outpatient or the inpatient setting the subjective assessment of general well-being in relation to objective measurements of function, gives the therapist additional information about the adolescent's perception of his or her state of health.

A scale of 1 to 10 is used: 1 = feeling (generally) 'the worst you have ever felt' and 10 = feeling (generally) 'the best you have ever felt'. In many centres the physiotherapist's opinion is sought by medical staff in relation to the timing of discharge. Therapists spend relatively long periods of time each day with patients during hospital admissions; they have a 'hands on' role and opportunities for general observation and informal discussion with patients.

Sometimes the therapist believes the patient is ready for discharge, but when assessing well-being realizes

that the patient scores himself or herself lower on the scale and there is a discrepancy between the two opinions. These may be health-related or social issues. Sometimes patients do not want to leave hospital for social reasons, and discussion regarding objective measures in relation to scores of well-being enhance communication and negotiation about the 'best' timing for discharge. This approach has been found to reduce opportunities for conflict to arise between the staff and the patients.

Promotion of the Development, Restoration and Maintenance of Optimal Respiratory Function

During the last decade a number of different airways clearance techniques have been developed, evaluated and introduced in different parts of the world raising many questions:

- how do the techniques work?
- are they as effective as the traditionally accepted methods?
- which patient's will benefit?
- do the techniques promote independence?
- are there negative aspects to the techniques?

Interpreting the results of research trials carried out in different centres which compare the different techniques is complex and confusing. Questions arise as to the way the techniques were carried out in the different centres. How studies were controlled and the issue of bias further complicate the interpretation of results. Indeed, sound, conclusive physiotherapy research is difficult to achieve in degenerative conditions, treated with a multidisciplinary medical approach incorporating drug therapy, physiotherapy, dietetics, psychology and sometimes surgery. In cystic fibrosis the complex array of physical problems that patients may present with poses many challenges for physiotherapists.

Problems in cystic fibrosis to be considered when prescribing an optimal physiotherapy programme: sputum that is thick, tenacious, copious or difficult to expectorate; airways that are collapsible, inflamed, hyperreactive or narrow, reducing airflow; lung segments that are hyperexpanded or collapsed; respiratory muscle fatigue from the increased work of breathing, or strain from excessive or paroxysmal coughing, causing pain or an ineffective cough; altered posture; gastro-oesophageal reflux, haemoptysis, pneumothorax, ventilation–perfusion mismatch, shunting or unstable vital signs.

AIRWAYS CLEARANCE TECHNIQUES

Many of the cardiorespiratory techniques used by therapists around the world have been discussed in the previous chapter. The focus in this chapter will be those most suited to adolescent patients, particularly in relation to issues of independence.

AEROBIC EXERCISE

The inclusion in the daily programme of enjoyable 'normal' activities that promote mucociliary clearance, increase cardiorespiratory fitness, alter lung volumes and induce the feeling of well-being and positive self-esteem is accepted by most physiotherapists as being an essential component of the regular programme of adolescents with chronic suppurative lung disease (Phelan *et al.* 1992). The following are popular examples: swimming, running, cycling, walking, team sports, jumping on the trampoline, dancing, martial arts, skating, skiing, horse riding, exercise to music classes, circuit training, windsurfing, rowing and other water sports (Figure 1).

Prevention of injury is particularly important in adolescents with underlying lung disease. The impact of immobility due to injury can be detrimental to respiratory function. A varied exercise programme reduces the risk of overuse injury. Shock-absorbent supportive footwear together with attention to stretching, warming up and cooling down with exercise will further reduce the risk of injury. A suitable programme which meets the particular needs of each individual should be developed and modified as necessary.

THE ACTIVE CYCLE OF BREATHING AND THE FORCED EXPIRATION TECHNIQUE – WITH OR WITHOUT POSTURAL DRAINAGE

This technique was originally developed in New Zealand (Thompson and Thompson 1968). It has been widely researched and advocated at the Royal Bromp-

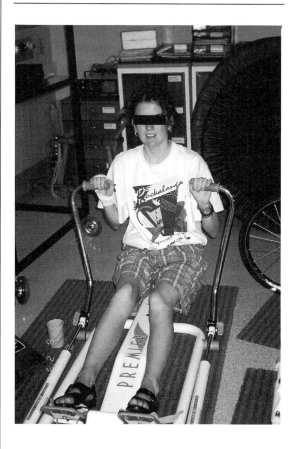

Figure 1 An adolescent patient with cystic fibrosis undertaking part of an exercise circuit programme

ton Hospital in London (Webber and Hofmeyr 1986) and is used in many international centres. It allows the patients independence with physiotherapy and is therefore suitable for adolescents.

The technique employs airway airflow during deep breathing exercises, forced expirations and coughing. It is thought to work by recruiting collateral channels during inspiratory holds, which allows air to enter alveoli and terminal bronchioles distal to secretions. Finally, it enhances mucociliary clearance when combined with postural drainage through the effects of gravity.

Some adolescent patients enjoy the social contact of parents or other family members assisting with percussion and vibrations, or believe that these added manual techniques improve the effectiveness of airways clearance and are able effectively to self-administer them or obtain assistance from family members.

A recent research study carried out in Sweden (Lannefors and Wollmer 1992), has suggested that the effects of position on mucociliary clearance in some patients during postural drainage may incorporate principles other than gravitational forces. In a number of patients with cystic fibrosis, mucociliary clearance was greater in the dependent lung than in the 'draining' lung. Further research is required and there is a need to include younger patients in such studies.

POSITIVE EXPIRATORY PRESSURE (PEP) THERAPY.

The idea of applying positive pressure during the expiratory phase of the respiratory cycle using a face mask, valves and resistors was developed, researched and introduced in Denmark early in the 1980s (Falk and Kelstrup 1984). This technique relies on the build up of a pressure gradient (back pressure) during expiration recruiting collateral channels and allowing air to enter alveoli and terminal bronchioles distal to secretions. The increased pressure generated during the expiratory phase of the cycle is the driving force behind secretions. Most adolescents at the Melbourne centre find ± 20 cmH$_2$O pressure, sustained for 3–5 seconds repeated in cycles and combined with the forced expiration technique, the most effective way to apply PEP. The pressure generated during a cough is believed to be around 200 cmH$_2$O. Therefore this technique uses about one-tenth of the driving force of a cough during part of each expiration while PEP is applied.

PEP therapy was shown to be as effective in the upright position as in postural drainage positions (Falk and Kelstrup 1984) making it one choice with adolescents reporting signs of gastro-oesophageal reflux (Button et al. 1994). The technique promotes independence and a sense of being in control. See Figure 2.

A complex technique of high-pressure PEP therapy has been developed and researched in Austria (Oberwaldner and Evans 1986). Adolescent patients using this technique report it to be effective and particularly time-efficient. The selection of the optimal pressures and resistors require objective measurements during the respiratory cycles using spirometry. This technique is reported to be especially beneficial to patients with 'floppy' or collapsible airways.

Figure 2 An adolescent patient with cystic fibrosis using PEP-mask-therapy

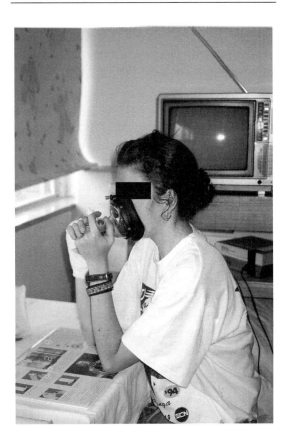

AUTOGENIC DRAINAGE

A technique of 'self drainage' incorporating breathing exercises has been developed over many years in Belgium (Dab and Alexander 1979). The technique aims to generate maximal airflow in each generation of bronchi without inducing airway collapse. It requires concentration and body awareness, discourages vigorous, paroxysmal or explosive coughing, and is often used in combination with other techniques. Autogenic drainage can be used independently and is therefore suitable for adolescents.

THE FLUTTER VRPI TECHNIQUE

This hand-held device was recently developed in Switzerland (Chatham and Marshall 1993). The patient blows out against an oscillating stainless steel ball which impedes airflow while simultaneously creating small high-frequency oscillations. Favourable reports from adolescent patients regarding effectiveness, together with recent published research, suggest that this technique should be considered (Konstan et al. 1994). Some patients report favourable results when used in combination with other techniques. The technique also promotes independence.

HYPERTONIC SALINE INHALATION – AN ADJUNCT TO AIRWAYS CLEARANCE TECHNIQUES

Inhaled hypertonic saline (HS) can cause airway narrowing in asthmatics. More recently non-isotonic aerosols have been used increasingly to perform bronchial provocation tests in asthmatic patients (Smith and Anderson 1990). HS can stimulate cough and create an osmotic gradient that draws water into the airways and has been shown to enhance mucociliary clearance. This effect of stimulating cough has been clinically used to induce sputum as an aid to better diagnose respiratory infections in patients who are immunosuppressed (Foot and Caul 1992). In adults with cystic fibrosis, mucociliary clearance has been enhanced following the inhalation of HS (Robinson and King 1994).

To determine whether inhalation of HS increases sputum production in patients with cystic fibrosis, 10 adolescents were studied in a controlled crossover design. Isotonic saline (IS) was the control. Results showed that HS 6% used before physiotherapy significantly increased sputum yield in adolescents with CF. A clinical score of the patients' own judgements of a cleared chest also yielded a significantly better result after HS than IS. This study suggests HS may be an effective and cheap part of the daily treatment of CF (Riedler *et al.* 1995).

Many adolescent patients with cystic fibrosis have requested to continue using HS as a part of their regular chest care programme. Some elect to use it only when secretions become thicker and difficult to expectorate, while others find regular daily use of greater benefit. The authors' centre has recently evaluated the use of HS among outpatients in a randomized controlled trial. HS resulted in a 15% increase in FEV_1 over a two-week period (Riedler *et al.* 1995).

Caution: Hypertonic saline (HS) is an effective bronchial challenge test and is capable of inducing an asthma attack in patients with hyperresponsive airways. It is usually used after inhalation of ventolin. Objective measurements are taken before and after inhalation of HS and the therapist auscultates for the onset of wheezing.

MASSAGE

Many adolescent patients develop tight and painful muscles in the upper body, especially around the neck and shoulders during acute exacerbations, with increased coughing and with changes in posture. Aerobic exercise programmes can cause pain and stiffness if overdone or if stretching, warming up and cooling down have been compromised. Massage and stretches to relieve muscle spasm, stiffness and tightness not only result in increased comfort, but also meet the 'attentiveness' requirement and enhance rapport with adolescent patients.

EXERCISES TO INCREASE THORACIC MOBILITY AND POSTURAL MUSCLE STRENGTH

During acute exacerbations when lung volumes decrease there is a corresponding change in the shape and size of the thoracic cage. During periods of intensive physiotherapy after a prolonged period of decreased pulmonary function some patients complain of chest wall pain. There is often a corresponding decrease in chest cage mobility and muscle weakness.

A programme incorporating thoracic mobilization and postural muscle strengthening results in decreased pain and increased strength in most patients with an improvement in postural awareness and alignment. The use of a mirror to demonstrate the improvement in overall appearance and increased height that results from corrected posture provides positive feedback and increased self-esteem.

RELAXATION TECHNIQUES

Disturbances of sleep from repeated coughing, pain and anxiety make the ability to achieve comfortable resting positions and relaxation an important part of a comprehensive cardiorespiratory rehabilitation programme. Laura Mitchell's 'Physiological Relaxation' technique is an effective and appropriate method for adolescents (Mitchell 1988).

HEAT OR ICE THERAPY – TENS – STRAPPING

Because aerobic exercise is an important part of an optimal cardiorespiratory rehabilitation programme, sprains and strains sometimes occur. Strapping, TENS, heat (hot packs, soaking in hot tubs, hot water bottles) and ice therapy are methods of achieving relief from sprains, strains and muscular pain while maintaining a 'normal life' focus.

EXERCISES AND MANAGEMENT OF STRESS INCONTINENCE

Some adolescent girls report stress incontinence with coughing. A programme of pelvic floor exercises and advice regarding pelvic floor bracing with coughing should commence. Teaching the patient to 'huff' effectively and avoid paroxysmal coughing is also important.

Prevention of Further Respiratory Disorder

Once optimal respiratory function has been restored, adherence to daily chest care is necessary if further disorder is to be prevented. Education and understanding of the disease process and the rationale for ongoing therapy, together with the establishment of an individualized regular physiotherapy programme in which the patient is encouraged to take control in order to achieve this objective, are essential to adherence with therapy.

EDUCATION

Education of adolescents in relation to health maintenance needs to be mostly informal and individually tailored, taking into account age, maturity and health status. Sometimes education needs to be provided more formally in a group setting. The use of audio-visual information, interaction with adult role models, multidisciplinary seminars and peer support groups are all ways of increasing knowledge and motivation. Opportunities to educate when individual patients or groups seek information and are receptive should be seized and fully used.

Enhancement of the Patient's Quality of Life

Regular clearance of pulmonary secretions, control of infections, appropriate diet, enzyme replacement and physical exercise are believed to be necessary to achieve optimal physical growth, development and well-being. Patients who are musically inclined may be encouraged to play wind instruments which incorporate deep breathing, respiratory control and sometimes positive expiratory pressure. This may involve interaction with a peer group in an orchestra or band, in a 'normal life' activity. Social development through interaction and participation, rather than withdrawal and isolation, together with academic and physical development (with minimal time away from school or work), will assist in the achievement of a 'normal life'.

Discussion about the future in terms of careers, sport, recreation, hobbies, relationships and future challenges should be encouraged during physiotherapy treatments. These conversations 'sow the seeds' of involvement in adult life. Patients should be encouraged to seek advice and counselling from career guidance experts regarding subjects, courses, suitability of the occupational environment and financial considerations.

A Multifunctional Clinical and Research Data Collection System

In order to achieve the four objectives of chest physiotherapy, the need for a system to collect, store and graphically portray data accumulated during treatment sessions was defined. The principles employed in this system can be adapted and applied to a wide range of physiotherapy situations with the outcome measures selected according to the needs of the patient population. This system can be used during hospital admissions or in the outpatient setting. At a glance, all aspects of the patient's management can be analysed. The system is efficient and comprehensive.

THE SELECTION OF OUTCOME MEASURES

Appropriate outcome measures are difficult to select in patient groups with complex chronic diseases. There is often controversy over which outcome measures are most appropriate. Each physiotherapist will need to select outcome measures and develop a data collection sheet relative to the medical conditions and needs of the patient population. The following outcome measures have been selected for a group of adolescents with cystic fibrosis:

Measurements of sputum produced during physiotherapy treatments

- subjective
- objective (see description earlier in the chapter)

Measurements of pulmonary function pre- and post-physiotherapy

- peak flow
- FEV$_1$

The best of three measurements is recorded before and after each physiotherapy treatment

Measurement of cardiorespiratory fitness

- 3-minute step test

These measurements are carried out regularly during the admission and are incorporated in the overall aerobic exercise fitness programme.

GRAPHIC PORTRAYAL

Each patient has a graph on which all information is displayed (see Figure 3A–D). This allows the therapist and patient to review and discuss different elements of the treatment regimen in an objective and interactive way. This visual information is useful on ward rounds for discussion with medical staff and parents, particularly when changing certain aspects of the treatment regimen and when training undergraduate and postgraduate students.

This data collection system can be helpful when considering:

- the normal development of adolescents
- the impact of chronic illness on normal development
- the specific aims and objectives of cardiorespiratory physiotherapy
- the overall physiotherapy management of patients with cystic fibrosis
- the need for positive feedback and objectivity

The system enables and provides:

- objective selection of an optimal physiotherapy programme for each patient

Figure 3 Measurements of an adolescent patient during an 11-day hospital admission. A, Sputum; B, peak flow; C, FEV$_1$; D, step test.

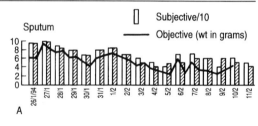

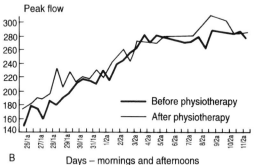

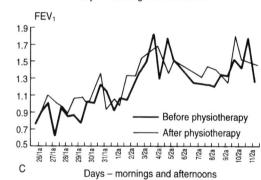

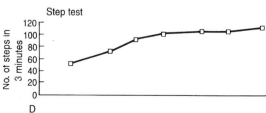

- monitoring of progress — prompt flagging of lack of progress or deterioration of the patient's condition
- general confidence that the selected treatment regimen is optimal (patient, parents, physician and therapist)
- an increase in motivation and compliance
- a teaching 'tool' for use with patients, families, the physiotherapy team and students
- the opportunity for evaluation of the physiotherapy service

- an increase in the quality of care of patients through objectivity
- a comprehensive recording system
- the opportunity for research in case studies and longitudinal studies

The system is simple, portable, readily available and easily stored in patient files or on computer discs. It can be used in the hospital system, in the outpatient setting or in the home to promote motivation and monitor the health status of patients. Different outcome measures can be selected and the system is adaptable to the individual needs of physiotherapists and patients.

Summary

The greatest teachers that postgraduate cardiorespiratory physiotherapists have are the adolescents referred for cardiorespiratory rehabilitation. Their willingness to try different techniques, analyse the effects, report their findings, and record thousands of measurements (always with a touch of humour) results in a greater collective understanding of the effects of the different techniques on different lungs.

Acknowledgements

The author would like to thank all the adolescent patients for the many lessons taught during physiotherapy sessions, and her own four adolescents Caroline, Lisa, Matthew and James.

The author gratefully acknowledges the expertise of the members of the multidisciplinary team of the Department of Thoracic Medicine, Royal Children's Hospital, who with many years of experience with adolescents with chronic lung disease, have taught by example.

REFERENCES

Button, BM, Heine, RG, Catto-Smith, AG et al. (1994) Postural drainage exacerbates gastroesophageal reflux in patients with lung disease: is positive expiratory pressure an alternative? *Pediatric Research* **36(1)**, part 2 pp 47A, 267.

Chatham, K, Marshall, C (1993) The flutter VRPI device for post-thoracotomy patients. *Physiotherapy* **79**: 95–98.

Dab, IF, Alexander, F (1979) The mechanism of autogenic drainage studied with flow volume curves. *Mongm Paedo.* **10**: 50–53.

Elkind D (1967) Egocentrism in adolescence. *Child Development* **38**: 1025.

Eng, P, Morton, J, Douglas, J et al. (1995) Efficacy of short-term ultrasonically nebulised hypertonic saline in patients with cystic fibrosis. *European Respiratory Journal* **8**, (suppl. 19): 510s.

Falk, M, Kelstrup (1984) Improving the ketchup bottle method with positive expiratory pressure, PEP and physical exercise. *European Journal of Respiratory Disease* **65**: 423–432.

Foot, AB, Caul, EO (1992) An assessment of sputum induction as an aid to diagnosis of respiratory infections in the immunocompromised child. *Journal of Pediatrics* **124(5)**: 689–693.

Godfrey, S (1974) *Exercise Testing in Children*, 168 pp. Philadelphia: WB Saunders.

Hibbert, E, Lannigan, A et al. (1989) Lung function values from a longitudinal study of healthy children and adolescents. *Pediatric Pulmonology* **7**: 101–109.

Ingersoll, GM (1989) *Adolescence*, 2nd edn. Englewood Cliffs: Prentice-Hall.

Ingersoll, GM (1992) Psychological and social development. In: McAnarney, ER, Kreipe, RE, Orr, DP et al. (eds) *Textbook of Adolescent Medicine*, pp. 91–98. Philadelphia: WB Saunders.

Konstan, MW et al. (1994) Efficacy of the flutter device for airways mucus clearance in patients with cystic fibrosis. *Journal of Pediatrics* **124(5)**: 689–693.

Lannefors, L, Wollmer, P (1992) Mucus clearance with three chest physiotherapy regimes in cystic fibrosis: a comparison between postural drainage, PEP and physical exercise. *European Respiratory Journal* **5**: 748–753.

Le Roux (1991) *Seminar Material*, Sheffield City Polytechnic.

Mitchell (1988) *Simple Relaxation: The Mitchell Method of Physiological Relaxation for Easy Tension*, 144 pp. London: John Murray.

Nixon, PA, Orenstein, DM (1988) Exercise testing in children. *Pediatric Pulmonology* **5**: 107–122.

Oberwaldner, B, Evans, JC (1986) Forced expirations against a variable resistance: a new chest physiotherapy method in cystic fibrosis. *Pediatric Pulmonology* **2**: 358–367.

Phelan, PD, Bowes, G (1991) Cystic fibrosis in Melbourne. *Thorax* **46**: 383–384.

Phelan, PD, Olinsky, A, Robertson, CF (1994) *Respiratory Illness in Children*, 414 pp, 4th edn. Oxford: Blackwell Scientific.

Riedler, J, Reade, T, Button, BM et al. (1995) Inhaled hypertonic saline increases sputum expectoration in cystic fibrosis. *Journal of Paediatric and Child Health* (in press).

Robinson, M, King, M (1994) Effect of hypertonic saline, amiloride and cough on mucociliary clearance in patients with cystic fibrosis. *American Journal of Respiratory Critical Care Medicine* **149(4)**: A669.

Singh, SJ, Michael, DL (1992) Development of a shuttle walking test of disability in patients with chronic airways. *Thorax* **47(12)**: 1019–1024.

Smith, CH, Anderson, SD (1990) Inhalational challenge using hypertonic saline in asthmatic subjects: a comparison with response to hyperpnoea, methacholine and water. *European Respiratory Journal* **3**: 144–151.

Thompson, B, Thompson, HT (1968) Forced expiration exercises in asthma and their effect on FEV_1. *New Zealand Journal of Physiotherapy* **3**: 19–21.

Webber, BA, Hofmeyr, JL (1986) Effects of postural drainage, incorporating the forced expiration technique, on pulmonary function in cystic fibrosis. *British Journal of Diseases of the Chest* **80**: 353–359.

Section F:

Physiotherapy Practice in Musculoskeletal Conditions Presenting from Infancy to Adolescence

PROLOGUE: JULIE MACDONALD

Prologue

JULIE MACDONALD

The physiotherapist has the training to provide optimal non-invasive clinical and functional assessments for infants, children and adolescents with a wide variety of musculoskeletal anomalies. In view of the many and varied musculoskeletal problems which may be experienced by the growing child, the paediatric physiotherapist must have sound clinical reasoning skills and an ability to develop age and developmentally appropriate treatment programmes which will most effectively address the identified problems.

Although a number of paediatric musculoskeletal conditions are introduced into the following chapters, it is apparent that the approach of physiotherapy management is based upon the child and his/her particular problems rather than being condition orientated. Space does not allow every paediatric musculoskeletal problem to be discussed in the following chapters. It is hoped, however, that insight into the assessment and problem-solving skills of the physiotherapist managing a child with a musculoskeletal anomaly, will provide a sound basis on which to design a treatment programme.

More adolescents are participating in sport competitively, very often at high levels, and are consequently sustaining musculoskeletal injuries for the physiotherapist to address. Preventative strategies are highlighted throughout Chapter 19 as well as treatment ideas for specific problems. Case studies are used to emphasize the problem-solving approach to treatment design.

17

Physiotherapy Management of Musculoskeletal Anomalies – Neonates and Infants

JULIE MACDONALD

Prenatal and Early Postnatal Growth and Modelling of the Musculoskeletal System
•
Common Muscular and Skeletal Deformities

Effective physiotherapy management of muscle and joint anomalies in neonates and infants is dependent upon thorough assessment procedures, accurate problem-solving abilities and the appropriate selection of techniques which specifically address the individual's identified problems. The infant's skeletal infrastructure, alignment, range of movement of joints and muscle activity are quite distinctive. The physiotherapist involved in the management of the infant with musculoskeletal problems must have a sound understanding of prenatal and postnatal development and growth of the musculoskeletal system.

It is essential that the physiotherapist appreciates the variable nature of musculoskeletal development as parents may express concern about what is merely a variation in normal development. Since management of the infant with muscle and joint problems is most effectively incorporated into a home programme, the physiotherapist must be skilled in communicating to parents and carers the infant's treatment programme. For example, the physiotherapist will often need to instruct parents and carers to carry out various

positioning, passive stretching and handling techniques and to facilitate specified movement and activities.

Prenatal and Early Postnatal Growth and Modelling of the Musculoskeletal System

Major development of all systems occurs during the embryonic period (2–8 weeks of gestation). Within a month of conception, the matrix of the future skeleton is laid down (Walker 1991). Early muscle fibres begin to appear at about the 11th week of gestation, but clear distinction between the two main histochemical fibre types (type 1 – slow twitch, oxidative – and type 2 – fast twitch, glycolytic) is not evident until the 18–20th prenatal week (Walker 1991). The formation of joints begins in the third prenatal month assisted by developing muscle activity (Bernhardt 1988).

Fetal positioning plays a significant role in the initial

alignment and joint mobility of the neonate. In utero, for example, the hips are predominantly flexed and laterally rotated and the feet are medially rotated. Such positioning produces greater lateral than medial rotation of the hips and femora, and medial rotation of the tibiae (Staheli *et al.* 1985). Progressive trunk flexion during the later months of prenatal life causes a kyphosis extending from the neck to the sacrum in the neonate (Cusick 1990). Other significant alignment features of the full-term neonate include an average 38–40° medial torsional twist of the femur (Cusick 1990), a 27° posterior tibial plateau slant (retroversion) and a 22° varus position of the calcaneus in relation to the tibia (Bernhardt 1988). In addition, the neonate presents with bow-legs. Heath and Staheli (1993) note that at age 6 months infants are maximally bow-legged and subsequently approach neutral knee angles (0°) by about 18 months.

Furthermore, the full-term neonate may show varying limitation of hip and knee extension and ankle plantarflexion (Walker 1991). The full-term neonate may also lack as much as 30° of elbow extension (Hesinger and Jones 1982a), and have slightly greater forefoot adduction than abduction (Bernhardt 1988).

Figure 1 shows the joint positioning in a full-term 2-month neonate. Such physiological limitation of joint mobility in full-term infants progressively resolves during the first year of life through the release from constraint and freedom of movement, and does not require any intervention. For example, Broughton *et al.* (1993) note that by 6 months of age the infant's knee flexion contracture is almost resolved. In contrast, the child's hip joint is still held in some degree of flexion throughout the first 2–3 years of life. Approximation of hip internal and external rotation occurs in the majority of children by 2 years of age (Phelps *et al.* 1985). There are, however, variations of joint mobility among different races (Cheng *et al.* 1991a,b). In addition, there appears to be a small percentage of any given population who demonstrate a generalized joint laxity affecting the axial and limb joints (Carr *et al.* 1993).

In contrast, the premature infant does not have the same amount of intrauterine moulding as the full-term neonate and demonstrates hypermobility at most joints (Walker 1991). Katz *et al.* (1990) suggest

Figure 1 Joint Positioning of 2-Month-old Infant Born Full-term

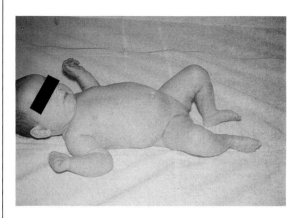

that the fact that metatarsus adductus is rare in the premature population and that medial tibial torsion does not occur in preterm infants (with gestational ages ≤30 weeks) further highlights the contrasting mobility and alignment of the premature and full-term neonate. These investigators support the view that postural deformities occur during the later weeks of pregnancy when the growing fetus can become constrained within the uterus. Figure 2 shows joint positioning in a preterm infant.

Abnormal Forces Causing Musculoskeletal Deformity

Development and growth of the musculoskeletal system is affected by many factors, such as genetics, nutrition, drugs, hormones and mechanical forces (LeVeau and Bernhardt 1984). Major morphological abnormalities occur only during the embryonic period (2–8 weeks gestation). Minor morphological abnormalities of the limbs can occur in the early fetal period, whereas deformation of normal tissue occurs more frequently in the third trimester when the fetus is subjected to greater constraint (Walker 1991). The physical forces acting on the skeleton are a major extrinsic influence in musculoskeletal development, as changes in such forces, prenatally and postnatally, will result in variations in the form of bones and joints (Carter *et al.* 1987). Indeed, because the primarily cartilaginous skeleton of the fetus and infant is highly compliant, it is not surprising that abnormal physical

Figure 2 Joint Positioning of 2-Month-old Infant (Adjusted) Born 27 Weeks Gestation

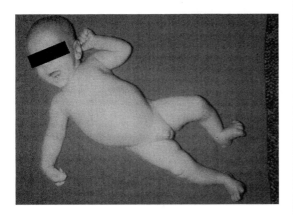

Figure 3 Swaddling Draws an Infant's Hips into Prolonged Extension and Adduction

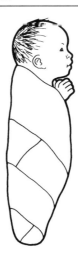

forces at this time can cause various chondral modelling errors (Cusick 1990).

Various ideas of how abnormal mechanical forces prenatally can lead to deformation of the musculoskeletal system are proposed. Abnormal extrauterine, intrauterine or uterine compression forces due to increased maternal abdominal tone, abnormal maternal skeletal structures, oligohydramnios, bicornuate uterus and multiple fetuses are some of the suggested causative agents of fetal constraint and subsequent deformity. The deformities include plagiocephaly, mandibular asymmetry, talipes equinovarus and calcaneovalgus, metatarsus adductus, tibial torsion and sternocleidomastoid contracture (infantile torticollis) (Bernhardt 1988).

Abnormal forces at or briefly following the birth process may also cause deformity of the neonate's musculoskeletal system. The neonate's shallow and incongruous hip joint is particularly vulnerable to abnormal extension forces. Breech delivery is often associated with hip dislocation (LeVeau and Bernhardt 1984). Kutlu et al. (1992) further note a significant relationship between dislocation and the practice of swaddling (the infant's lower extremities being constrained in extension and adduction) (Figure 3). Children with generalized joint laxity may be particularly susceptible to abnormal forces. Carr et al. (1993) emphasize that joint laxity is aetiologically important in neonatal hip dislocation.

Persistent sleeping or sitting postures are also proposed as providing deforming forces on the infant's musculoskeletal system. The relationship between habitual side-lying positioning and hip dysplasia (the upper adducted hip being dysplastic) indicates that an habitual sleeping posture postnatally can cause significant deformation of the infant's musculoskeletal system (Heikkila et al. 1985). These authors emphasize that acetabular dysplasia is only one aetiological factor of dislocation of the infant's hip and that dislocation is not liable to occur in the absence of some other factor or factors.

Walker (1991) suggests that such instances of deformation through habitual positioning demonstrate that movement plays an important role in modelling the joint surfaces during infancy. Active movement is an essential agent in the bone modelling process, and is influential in the development of bone mineral content (Margulies et al. 1986).

Bernhardt (1988) similarly suggests that habitual positioning can create and/or exacerbate pre-existing torsional deformities in the lower extremities. For example, sleeping in the prone knee–chest position with extremity medial rotation could be related to medial rotation deformities of the hip or tibia, tibia bowing, ankle equinus and metatarsus varus. In contrast, sleeping in the prone knee–chest position with the limbs in lateral rotation may encourage the potential for genu valgus and metatarsus valgus. The prone or supine frog-leg position may be correlated with lateral rotatory deformity of the hips and tibiae. Habitual W sitting (reverse tailor sitting) may contribute to abnormal medial torsion of hips and tibiae.

Common Muscular and Skeletal Deformities

The role that mechanical forces may play in muscles and joint problems in the neonate and infant is of interest since it is possible to manage deformity within the musculoskeletal system of the neonate and infant through the avoidance of abnormal loading and the application of therapeutic (corrective) forces. For example, all parents should take extreme care when moving the neonate's hips into marked extension and adduction. Similarly, the physiotherapist should emphasize to parents that they should encourage their infants and children to adopt variable sleeping and sitting postures.

Techniques, such as gentle progressive mobilization, casting and splinting, may be necessary in the treatment of varying neonatal musculoskeletal anomalies. These techniques are primarily based on the stretch creep rule, which relates to the creep (elongation over time) that occurs within the tissue as a tension load is applied (LeVeau and Bernhardt 1984). Most contractures can be elongated without breakage of skeletal structures by application of sufficient force for a prolonged period (Ikeda 1992). In conjunction with such techniques, the physiotherapist will generally employ active facilitation of movement which can enhance corrective bone modelling. For example, activation of the infant's hip lateral rotators and extensors provides essential torque forces needed across the proximal femur to reduce femoral antetorsion (Cusick 1990). Indeed, the dynamic forces created by muscle activation are foremost agents in the development of postnatal skeletal alignment.

A number of the more common neonatal musculoskeletal deformities which require mobilization and / or splinting and active facilitation of movement are discussed next.

Infantile Torticollis

The physiotherapist plays a significant role in the management of sternocleidomastoid contracture. The exact aetiology of infantile torticollis is unknown, but one of the latest hypotheses is that it may represent the sequela of an intrauterine or perinatal compartment syndrome (Davids et al. 1993). This deformity is often associated with other musculoskeletal problems, such as metatarsus adductus, developmental dysplasia of the hip, talipes equinovarus (postural) and talipes calcaneovalgus. Interestingly, Cheng and Au (1994) note that their findings suggest that the incidence of hip dysplasia increases in direct relation to the severity of torticollis.

It is always advisable to have the neonate assessed medically, before physiotherapy assessment and intervention, in case the asymmetrical head posture is due to other less common congenital conditions. For example, the infant may have a fixed or bony torticollis associated with Klippel–Feil syndrome and / or anomalies of the atlanto-axial articulation. Neurological, inflammatory and traumatic conditions may also cause an infant to adopt an asymmetrical head position (Hesinger and Jones 1982b). Furthermore, ocular problems can cause torticollis.

The neonate with torticollis generally presents for clinical assessment between 2 and 6 weeks of age holding their head in a characteristically asymmetrical position of forward flexion, ipsilateral flexion towards the affected muscle and lateral rotation away from the side involved. A large proportion of these infants will also present with concomitant craniofacial asymmetry of varying degrees (Cheng and Au 1994). Furthermore, a palpable benign mass can often be felt in the midsubstance of the sternocleidomastoid muscle (Davids et al. 1993). Cheng and Au (1994) note that 35.42% of their cohort demonstrated a palpable tumour. Figure 4 shows a sternocleidomastoid tumour.

During the assessment of the infant with torticollis, the physiotherapist may identify infants who have full passive range of motion of the neck, but continuously hold their head in a laterally flexed and rotated position. Some infants who have a side flexion contracture

Figure 4 Sternocleidomastoid Tumour

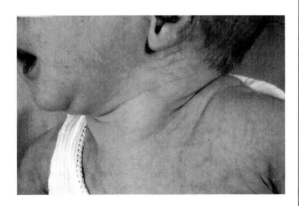

with no limitation of rotation demonstrate tightness in the upper trapezius, levator scapulae and even platysma. Other infants have significant sternocleidomastoid contracture, demonstrating varying passive range deficits. Cheng and Au (1994) suggest that the incidence of sternocleidomastoid tumour increases with the severity of neck motion deficit. If not treated, infantile muscular torticollis will cause progressive deformity of the skull and face. Shoulder girdle obliquity and scoliosis would also occur subsequently.

After the completion of a thorough musculoskeletal and neurodevelopmental assessment of the infant, the physiotherapist addresses the immediate problems of the abnormal posturing and contracture of sternocleidomastoid and/or other muscles. Stretching of tightened musculature may exacerbate an acute pain reaction and associated anxiety within the infant. Pain assessment in infants and children is extremely difficult as there are problems in accurately interpreting the intensity and nature of the infant's distress. Furthermore, the physiotherapist must consider the family's response to a child's distress and be aware that there are different cultural responses to an infant's pain (Savedra and Tesler 1989). The parents' impact on the infant's anxiety is central; it is desirable to involve parents as they can provide support, reassurance and appropriate distraction for the infant (Dolgin and Phipps 1989).

Parental education is the physiotherapist's highest priority, since the parents must instigate the programme of actively facilitating rotation of the neonate's neck towards and lateral flexion away from the contracture whenever the infant is awake. Such active movement is encouraged by placing the child such that he/she must turn to the affected side to see toys and faces or hear sounds. The parent should also encourage the child to turn to the affected side to feed. Active movement away from the contracture is a most effective means of stretching the contractured muscle, for it invokes the principle of reciprocal inhibition, thereby reducing pain-related muscle spasm. Encouraging the infant to look up, particularly in prone, will also encourage inhibition of sternocleidomastoid thereby facilitating a greater stretch of the contracture. Such active facilitation will encourage the infant to explore all of their visual field and thereby prevent secondary problems of spatial neglect. Furthermore, such active facilitation will ensure that normal postural reactions and patterns of movement are encouraged and, when delayed, facilitated.

The carrying position of the infant which will encourage stretch of contracted sternocleidomastoid should also be shown to and practised by parents. The therapist places one of her forearms through the infant's legs and then supports the infant's body on her forearm and places her hand on the infant's shoulder on the affected side. The therapist's other forearm/hand is free to instigate a gentle corrective stretch of the infant's laterally flexed neck to the upright. This gentle stretching of the infant's sternocleidomastoid muscle while being carried provides reassurance and support to the child and generally reduces the anxiety associated with the stretching of the sternocleidomastoid muscle. See Figure 5.

Figure 5 An Effective Carrying Position for an Infant with Torticollis

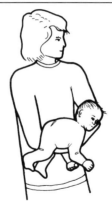

A further effective carrying position is in the crook of the arm so as to encourage some head righting to the upright. This carrying position provides the infant with a sense of reassurance and a stimulating visual field is a distracting element. Parents are also asked to encourage a sleeping position which will stretch the contracted muscle. For example, side lying on the unaffected side with no pillow generally encourages such a stretch, but the infant quickly outgrows the usefulness of such passive positioning when they start to move around and change position while sleeping.

In conjunction with this regimen of active and passive correction of the torticollis, the physiotherapist may also teach the parents passive stretching of the contracted sternocleidomastoid muscle while the infant is supine. There are difficulties associated with this procedure. Some clinicians believe that it is inefficiently undertaken by parents because they do not like to see the child upset. Often it is impractical where the child is cared for by a single parent without an extended family, since this procedure requires two people. For example, one pair of hands are placed on the child's shoulders and the other person's hands are placed around the child's chin and base of skull. A very gentle mobilizing force is applied in the side flexion direction away from the contracture and held for a short time (e.g. 5–10 seconds), and repeated a number of times (2–3). After completing those stretches, the operator then commences a passive rotation of the child's head towards the side of the contracture which is similarly held for a short time (e.g. 5–10 seconds), and repeated a number of times (2–3). This gentle passive stretching procedure is generally recommended to be undertaken twice a day. If the child becomes distressed muscle spasm will result and little stretch will occur. The physiotherapist should encourage parents and carers to talk reassuringly to the infant during this procedure and perhaps a further carer could distract the child's attention with a bright musical toy.

The physiotherapist should initially review the infant once a week, so as to assess progress. If the parents are very unsure, and there is little progress, more frequent treatment sessions should be arranged. Generally, the limitation of side flexion is the most difficult range to recover. As the infant reaches 3–4 months,

greater vestibular input, such as 'aeroplanes' (with the child supported horizontally over arms) can be included into the home programme to encourage head righting.

If these conservative measures of active facilitation and passive stretching of infantile torticollis are undertaken early and consistently, the outcome is extremely successful. Cheng and Au (1994) note that in their cohort 97% of all infantile torticollis resolved with conservative treatment in less than 6 months. These investigators, though, report some intermittent head tilt and mild craniofacial asymmetry after resolution. If contracture is still present at one year of age a surgical release of sternocleidomastoid is recommended (Davids et al. 1993). Active and passive stretching of contracted muscle should occur postsurgery to maintain the lengthened range.

Developmental Dysplasia of the Hip (DDH)

As noted previously, the infant with congenital muscular torticollis has an increased incidence of developmental dysplasia of the hip (DDH). The physiotherapist generally does not have such an active role in the management of DDH, but a comprehensive understanding of this condition is essential. Indeed, while undertaking a musculoskeletal assessment on a child, the physiotherapist may suspect this deformity. Indications are asymmetrical movement pattern, limited range of hip movement, asymmetrical gluteal and popliteal folds, and, in the toddler, a limping or waddling gait. The child should be referred for orthopaedic examination.

DDH covers a range of hip pathology, from acetabular dysplasia to subluxation and dislocation of the hip (O'Sullivan and O'Brien 1994). Despite screening every child at birth, using a combination of the Ortolani and Barlow tests, not all dislocated hips are diagnosed (Lennox et al. 1993). In addition, many hips dislocate at a variable time after birth and some do not dislocate until the child begins to walk (Coleman 1994). O'Sullivan and O'Brien (1994) emphasize that since developmental hip dysplasia can range from frank dislocation at birth to mild acetabular dysplasia presenting in adulthood, it may never be possible to predict an outcome based on stability and anatomy of the hip joint at birth.

Atar et al. (1993) suggest that the ideal management of developmental dysplasia of the hip involves early diagnosis, concentric reduction and maintenance of the reduction until hip stability is obtained and normal growth and development is observed. Commonly used splinting devices to maintain hip reduction are the Pavlik harness, the Von Rosen splint and the Frejka splint. The length of time that these splints are worn generally ranges between 3 and 8 months. There appears to be little difference in performance amongst the various splints. For example, Atar et al. (1993) note that there was a 10% failure of reduction with the Frejka splint and 12% with the Pavlik harness.

Lennox et al. (1993) similarly suggest that there is probably a group of patients, diagnosed at birth, in whom treatment by splinting fails to succeed. Operative procedures are necessary for such children and also for those who are diagnosed with DDH later in childhood. These operative procedures may involve closed reduction under anaesthesia with or without adductor tenotomy. If this fails to keep the hip reduced, an open reduction often in conjunction with a pelvic or femoral osteotomy is undertaken (Lennox et al. 1993).

A number of complications associated with the management of DDH include avascular necrosis of the femoral head, femoral nerve palsy, and traction or compression of brachial plexus or cervical roots (Mooney and Kasser 1994). Inappropriate fitting and positioning of splinting (e.g. Pavlik harness) undoubtedly may contribute to such complications, but Mooney and Kasser (1994) note that upper-extremity complications can occur even with a properly fitted and positioned Pavlik harness, particularly in the heavier or older infant. The physiotherapist may be treating a child being managed with a Pavlik harness, because, for example, the infant has a concomitant congenital muscular torticollis. If any anomalies are noted in the management of DDH the physiotherapist should contact the infant's orthopaedist immediately.

Metatarsus Adductus (Metatarsus Varus, Hooked Forefoot, Metatarsus Internus)

A further postural deformity often seen in association with congenital muscular torticollis and DDH is metatarsus adductus. Bleck (1983) describes metatarsus adductus as an adduction or medial deviation of the forefoot. The inner border of the forefoot of the infant with metatarsus adductus is concave and the lateral border is convex, but the heel appears normal. This deformity is generally noticed at birth or within the first 3 months of life (Rushforth 1978) and should be distinguished from other foot anomalies, such as metatarsus primus varus, an internally rotated foot, and the 'serpentine' foot (where valgus of the heel accompanies adducted metatarsals) (Bleck 1983). Many children with metatarsus adductus have an accompanying internal tibial torsion (Hesinger and Jones 1982a).

Bleck (1983) suggests classifying the severity of the metatarsus adductus deformity through the use of the 'heel bisector' line, which is a reference line for the centre of the hindfoot plantar surface. The 'heel bisector' line should cross between the second and third toes in the normally aligned foot. If this line crosses through the third toe, the deformity is viewed as mild; if it falls between the third and fourth toes or through the fourth, the deformity is classified as moderate; and between the fourth and fifth toes, it is seen as a severe deformity.

The flexibility of this deformity is a further means of classification. The extent of passive abduction of the forefoot against the stabilized hindfoot with reference to the 'heel bisector' line enables a statement to be made with respect to the flexibility of the deformity. For example, abduction beyond the heel bisector line is viewed as flexible; abduction only to the midline as partly flexible; and no abduction possible as inflexible, rigid or fixed (Bleck 1983).

A prospective study of the natural history of untreated idiopathic metatarsus adductus (hooked forefoot) suggests significant spontaneous correction of this deformity during early childhood. For example, Rushforth (1978) notes that at review only

14% of the metatarsus adductus cohort still demonstrated moderate and severe deformity. There is no agreement as to why spontaneous resolution occurs in the great majority of affected children, but Stark *et al.* (1987) suggests that the lengthening of the metatarsals and a changing mechanical axis may play a role. Unfortunately, there does not appear to be any definitive way to diagnose which feet will resolve spontaneously and which will persist (Hesinger and Jones 1982a). The initial severity of metatarsus adductus and flexibility of the foot are not good indicators of the likelihood of spontaneous correction (Bleck 1982). Hence, controversy has arisen over whether and/or when mobilization and splinting should be instigated in the treatment of metatarsus adductus.

In view of the poor public attitude toward deformity and the fact that surgical procedures are undertaken on children in whom the deformity persists and is severe, Bleck (1983) urges early use of mobilization, casting and splinting of moderate and severe metatarsus adductus. If treatment of moderate and/or severe metatarsus is to be successful it should be started before the child reaches 8 months of age, as a growth spurt occurs during this period (Bleck 1983). In addition, the foot is much more compliant during the early postnatal period.

The physiotherapist may be involved in assessing the neonate with metatarsus adductus and instituting a home programme of mobilization. Also important is instructing parents against the child adopting any habitual posturing since, as noted previously, sleeping in the prone knee–chest position with extremity medial rotation could exacerbate metatarsus adductus (Bernhardt 1988). Casting and/or splinting in conjunction with mobilization may be a further option for the neonate with a severe, rigid metatarsus adductus.

Talipes Calcaneovalgus (TCV)

The neonatal calcaneovalgus foot is the most commonly noted foot deformity and could result from too much force on the foot as it presses on the uterine wall during the latter months in utero (Bernhardt 1988). The foot is drawn into marked dorsiflexion, and the heel is in a valgus position (Hesinger and

Jones 1982a). Initially, the physiotherapist will assess the neonate and establish that this deformity is truly a postural deformity and is not associated with any neurological anomaly. Once it has been established that it is a postural talipes calcaneovalgus, the physiotherapist will demonstrate to parents gentle mobilizations of foot and ankle, encourage kicking movements and may at times provide a dorsolateral splint. This postural deformity readily resolves. See Figure 6.

Talipes Equinovarus (TEV)

The talipes equinovarus (TEV) deformity can be classified into:

- rigid/structural congenital TEV (clubfoot)
- postural TEV
- TEV associated with muscle imbalances secondary to an upper or lower motor neurone disorder (e.g. spina bifida, cerebral palsy) and muscle disease (e.g. muscular dystrophy)
- congenital TEV in association with other significant

Figure 6 An Infant with Talipes Calcaneovalgus (TCV)

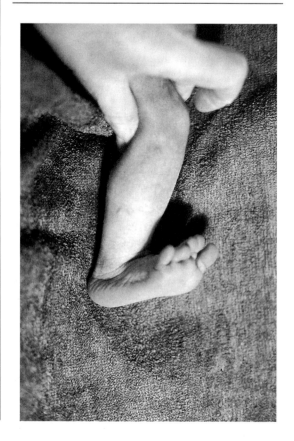

Figure 7 An Infant with Clubfoot

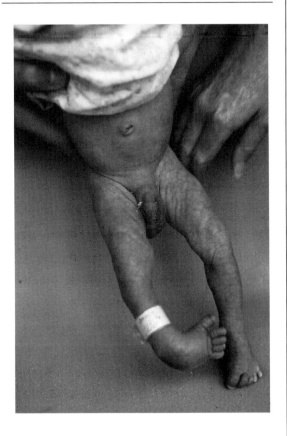

Figure 8 Various Foot Anomalies in Children with Spina Bifida

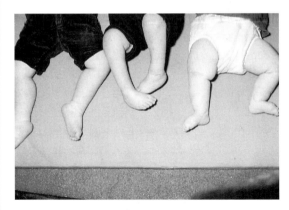

These investigators suggest that the clinical assessment of this deformity should be developed and studied more fully. Undoubtedly, the physiotherapist has the training to provide optimum non-invasive clinical and functional assessments for infants and children with such a musculoskeletal anomaly.

The initial assessment of the TEV deformity by the physiotherapist must be comprehensive. Birth history, family history and any other anomalies should be carefully noted. Observations are made of the neonate's general appearance, concentrating particularly on the feet, ankles, legs and hips – noting shape and evidence of any abnormal creases. The neonate with congenital TEV often has an extremely small tucked up heel, and very deep medial midtarsal creases. Photography is an extremely useful means of recording such observations.

The physiotherapist should spend a considerable amount of the assessment time, observing and facilitating any available active movement of the leg and foot (placing and supporting reactions of the feet can be particularly helpful in distinguishing any active dorsiflexion movement). Passive movements of the neonate's foot should be undertaken with great care. For example, the mobilizing force should always be gentle, and appropriately directed, so as to ensure that the abduction, eversion and dorsiflexion movements occur at the midtarsal, subtalar and talocrural joints respectively. The physiotherapist should be particularly careful to protect the neonate's distal tibial and fibular epiphyseal growth plates from any shearing strain during these manoeuvres. The neo-

teratological malformation (e.g. an infant who has multiple congenial contractures and major abnormalities of organs or of the central nervous system).

It is very important for the physiotherapist to distinguish the different types of TEV as the management regimens will differ considerably. For example, postural TEV can be treated very successfully with conservative means. The child with TEV associated with spina bifida will require significant skin care, may need specifically designed splints (sheepskin lined) and may require a surgical procedure during early childhood. The child with TEV in conjunction with other significant teratological malformation will most likely require surgical procedures in conjunction with conservative management and the management of other malformations may initially take greater priority.

ASSESSMENT OF TEV

Unfortunately, as Samson and Harris (1994) note, the physiotherapist's role in the assessment and management of clubfoot is not well defined in the literature.

nate's hip and knee should also be held in flexion while these passive forces are applied, so as to prevent any potential for subluxation / dislocation of the neonate's hip, and avoid any significant strain on the medial collateral ligament of the neonate's knee.

POSTURAL TALIPES EQUINOVARUS

A postural varus foot, which is commonly noted at birth, is not a clubfoot (Ponsetti 1992). The equino-varus deformity is easily corrected both actively and passively and appears a normal-looking foot. This deformity is successfully managed with gentle mobi-lization, encouragement of active dorsiflexion and eversion and often adhesive strapping (for example, buckle and strap) may be employed for a limited time. Once correction is maintained, there is no potential for relapse, unless there are other mitigating factors.

RIGID CONGENITAL CLUBFOOT

The rigid congenital clubfoot is a complex deformity and its equinus, varus, adductus and cavus (due to the first metatarsal being in more plantarflexion than the fifth metatarsal) components are difficult to correct (Ponsetti 1992). The incidence of true congenital club-foot is cited as one per 1000 live births and a sex ratio of one female to two males (Hesinger and Jones 1982a). Various hypotheses suggest possible pathogenetic mechanisms involved in the rigid congenital idio-pathic clubfoot (Sirca et al. 1990).

Pathology. Kawashima and Uhthoff (1990) note that the pathogenesis of clubfoot is multifactorial, but they suggest that a developmental arrest mainly of the talus at the 'physiological clubfoot stage', char-acterized by a medial deviation and plantigrade orientation of the talar neck and head during the 9th week of gestation is one of the main determi-nants of congenital clubfoot. Other studies suggest histochemical changes in various muscles of the clubfoot population, but there are no signs of denervation (Sirca et al. 1990).

Aronson and Puskarich (1990) suggest that the noticeably smaller calf circumference of the clubfoot leg combined with the normal leg length may indir-ectly suggest an in utero compartment syndrome as a more likely aetiology for clubfoot than an early germ-plasm defect, since germplasm deficiencies commonly result in shortening of the affected limb. Spero et al. (1994) further highlight the degree of variability in idiopathic clubfeet by describing a number of infants with congenital clubfeet who had tarsal coalition.

The bony malformation of clubfoot involves pro-nounced medial and plantar deviation of the talar neck and head (Hjelmstedt and Sahlstedt 1990). The calcaneus inverts under the talus, there is subluxation or dislocation of the talonavicular joint and changes in the position of the calcaneus and the navicular with respect to the talus and the forefoot is adducted (Yamamoto and Furuya 1990). Soft tissues resistant to realignment in the infant with clubfoot generally include musculature such as tibialis posterior, gastrocnemius, soleus, flexor hallucis longus, flexor digitorum longus and ligaments, such as deltoid, spring, bifurcated / Y-shaped, long and short plantar, dorsal talonavicular. Often the talocalcaneonavicular capsule is also quite fixed.

MANAGEMENT OF CLUBFOOT

It is important to assess the severity of the clubfoot deformity at birth, but at present it is extremely difficult to predict whether the deformity will be correctable through conservative management. Ikeda (1992) notes that studies demonstrate that clubfeet initially assessed as being severe can be cor-rected solely through conservative management. Pon-setti (1992) notes that in some clubfeet, tight soft tissues become easily stretchable with gentle manip-ulation and the alignment of the bones of the foot improves rapidly after the application of a few casts, whereas in other clubfeet the primary osseous defor-mities and tight soft tissues resist correction.

Table 1 demonstrates that conservative management of congenital clubfoot may include a variety of tech-niques such as passive stretching, manipulations, adhesive strapping, plaster series / casting and splint-ing and that numerous trials have met with varying degrees of success. Tibrewal et al. (1992) suggest that the assessment and treatment of clubfeet is presented in such varying ways that it is almost impossible to compare different regimens. However, the success of conservative management is often more dependent upon such factors as the age of the infant when conservative management is begun (the earlier the better, as the foot is more compliant), and the resistant nature of the clubfoot, than the specific type of conservative management. For example, the clubfoot with tarsal coalition will not be successful with conservative management alone and will require surgical intervention.

Regardless of treatment, there is definite trend for a clubfoot deformity to relapse until the child is about 7 years old (Ponsetti 1992). To prevent relapse, many clinicians suggest the use of night splints for a number of years. The toddler's walking posture should encourage dorsiflexion and pronation forces and parents can play with the child in squatting positions to facilitate a further stretch on the plantarflexors. Surgical procedures, such as heelcord lengthenings, posteromedial releases and tendon transfers, may be undertaken in those patients who relapse and have not responded to mobilization and casting.

The goal of conservative treatment for clubfoot is that the child will have a functional, pain-free, plantigrade foot, with good mobility and without calluses and does not need to wear modified shoes (Ponsetti 1992). Ikeda (1992) notes that all conservatively treated clubfeet are supple by adolescence, whereas early operative treatment often results in reduced motion of ankle and foot. Hence, most centres consider operative procedures only after conservative management has failed to obtain correction in a specified period of time, preferably not more than 3 months (Ponsetti 1992).

Interestingly, Aronson and Puskarlsh (1990) note that the group of patients with clubfeet that they followed for an average of 10 years exhibited relatively consistent deformity and disability, despite drastically varied treatment regimens, such as prolonged casting to posteromedial release. These authors emphasize that their clubfoot subjects had noticeably smaller calves and had a significant decrease in normal ankle motion, particularly lacking dorsiflexion range. They found that repeated heelcord lengthenings permanently weakened the plantarflexors and further reduced the calf girth. Furthermore, Yamamoto et al. (1994) and Yngve (1990) describe congenital clubfoot patients often demonstrating toe-in gait due to the incomplete correction of adduction deformity of the forefoot, equinus deformity of the hindfoot and internal tibial torsion. An operative procedure, such as tibial osteotomy, however, is rarely used in the treatment for clubfoot.

In view of the complex nature of congenital clubfoot it is important that the physiotherapist involved with such infants should be in close communication with the infant's orthopaedist. If conservative management of the congenital clubfoot is unsuccessful, a surgical procedure may be necessary, and conservative management should be continued after operative procedures. It is important for the physiotherapist to

Table 1

An Overview of Various Studies Examining the Outcome of Conservative Management of Clubfoot

Authors	Time span	No. of feet	Type	Follow-up
Yamamoto and Furuya (1990)	1974–1985	91	Plaster casting, splinting	66% good response 34% residual deformity
Bensahel et al. (1990a,b)	1974–1978	338	Manipulate, splinting, strapping	48% good response 29% fair 23% poor
Ikeda (1992)	1970–1985	36	Manipulate, strapping, orthosis, casting	95% good response
Karski and Wosko (1989)	1970–1987	323	Manipulate, casting	50% good results 50% require surgery
Nather and Bose (1987)	1972–1984	174	Manipulate, casting	58% good response 42% require surgery

continue to review the patient with congenital club-foot as initial correction may slowly erode, whether the correction was achieved by a conservative regimen, or by both conservative and surgical means.

Vertical Talus

This rigid, congenital 'rocker-bottom' foot anomaly is an uncommon condition. It may be associated with arthrogryposis, Turner's syndrome and other congenital anomalies, particularly those that involve the central nervous system. The vertical talus anomaly involves an equinus position of the hindfoot, talonavicular subluxation with forefoot abduction and dorsiflexion (Hesinger and Jones 1982a). Surgical intervention is necessary.

Case Study

Ben is an 8-year-old boy who participates in a youth gymnastics club twice a week, and plays soccer at school and a local club. He has won numerous awards for these sports. His mother, Jan, is particularly proud of Ben's athletic pursuits as he was born with a (R) rigid clubfoot and she often contacts the physiotherapist who was involved in the management of Ben's (R) clubfoot to inform her of his latest athletic award.

The physiotherapist recently carried out an extensive musculoskeletal assessment of Ben, as part of a clinical review of the efficacy of their centre's particular management of rigid TEV. It had been documented that Ben had commenced passive mobilization and application of a modified Denis Browne splint on day 2 postpartum. These splints were changed every second to third day initially and then weekly. Such splintage was continued until Ben was 5 months of age, when he was maintaining his (R) foot in abduction, eversion and dorsiflexion. A flexible strapping (buckle and strap) was then instigated, in conjunction with passive mobilization and facilitation of active dorsiflexion, eversion and abduction until the child began to walk. A night splint was then applied. Squatting and duck walking was encouraged. When Ben was 4 years of age, however, his (R) tendoachilles became tight very quickly. Casting could not halt this contracture. A tendon release was undertaken and the plantigrade position then held by casting for 6 weeks. Ben has had no further significant loss of range of motion since this operative procedure.

On review, Ben's ankle range of motion, muscle strength and stability, foot progression angle and calf circumference were examined. The physiotherapist also questioned Ben and Jan about any experiences of pain/discomfort associated with the clubfoot and if they had any difficulties finding comfortable footwear. They were also asked if they were presently happy about the outcome of intervention.

Ben certainly demonstrated a significant difference in his (R) calf circumference to his (L). Active and passive ankle dorsiflexion range was 15° less on the (R). On tests, such as single leg standing and sets of repeated rising on toes, however, there was no appreciable difference between legs, suggesting that muscle strength and foot stability was similar in both feet and legs. Foot progression angle suggests some (R) foot in-toeing. Ben and Jan report no pain or fatigue-like symptoms associated with his (R) foot and leg. Jan did note, though, that it was difficult at times to find a broad-fitting shoe for Ben, and that his shoes wore out more frequently than his sisters' shoes.

Both Ben and his mother are extremely happy with the correction of his (R) clubfoot. Ben certainly does not feel that this deformity places him at any disadvantage in his sporting pursuits. He presently demonstrates very little concern about his thinner calf or his in-toeing (R) foot. Jan reports that the difficulty finding Ben a broader style shoe is only a minor issue.

There are many other infants and young children with musculoskeletal problems whom the physiotherapist may have to assess and then select an appropriate treatment regimen for identified problems. In the following discussion a number of musculoskeletal conditions, for example arthrogryposis, osteogenesis imperfecta and other heritable diseases of collagen, nerve lesions and limb deficiencies are introduced and consideration is given to some of the musculoskeletal problems experienced by infants and children with such conditions. It must be remembered, however, that the physiotherapist does not manage a condition, but rather a child and his/her family, a unique group of people who have distinctive needs and wants. Indeed, although an infant may have a particular condition, the physiotherapist must identify the particular musculoskeletal problems experienced by this infant and establish a patient-specific treatment regimen.

Arthrogryposis

Arthrogryposis is a non-specific term referring to a large, heterogeneous group of patients who have multiple congenital soft tissue contractures (Sarwark et al. 1990). Over 150 specific arthrogrypotic entities have been identified. However, Hall (1985) suggests there are clearly many single gene, chromosome and multifactorial conditions yet to be described. A useful method of differentiating types of arthrogryposis is based on determining whether there is primarily involvement of just the limbs, limb involvement with other abnormalities, or limb involvement with major central nervous system dysfunction (Hall 1985).

A multidisciplinary approach is best for the initial care of a child with arthrogryposis. In conjunction with the geneticist, the neurologist, the orthopaedic surgeon and the occupational therapist, the physiotherapist plays a significant role in the management of the infant with an arthrogrypotic syndrome. Initially, the physiotherapist must undertake a thorough assessment of the infant, noting the extent of his/her contractures, the resting positioning, and the active and passive range of motion of all joints and the amount and quality of activity. An early and intensive regimen of passive and active movement and splinting

has been shown to be particularly effective in improving the overall function of the child with various arthrogrypotic conditions (Palmer et al 1985).

Certain types of arthrogrypotic disorders, however, will undoubtedly respond more effectively than others. For example, those conditions in which there is fibrotic replacement of muscle, such as amyoplasia, may not respond in the same way as conditions with hypoplastic or short tendons, such as distal arthrogryposis. Furthermore, conditions with coalitions, synostoses will generally have a poor response to passive and active movement (Hall 1985).

In view of the heterogeneous nature of arthrogryposis it is difficult to discuss widely the varying presentations and management of such infants. In an attempt to demonstrate more specifically the physiotherapist's management of the muscle and joint problems associated with arthrogrypotic disorders, the management of the infant with amyoplasia is presented, as it is one of the more common forms of arthrogryposis. Undoubtedly, physiotherapy management goals for the infant with amyoplasia, such as attaining the most functional range of motion of joints, achieving where possible the most effective muscle control of these joints, and introducing effective weight-bearing through the lower limbs, may often be very similar to the management of infants with other forms of arthrogryposis. It must be re-emphasized that each individual infant with an arthrogrypotic disorder will have specific needs which have to be addressed by the physiotherapist.

AMYOPLASIA

Amyoplasia has no known hereditary pattern and is characterized by multiple congenital contractures with a specific symmetrical positioning of the limbs. The deformities of amyoplasia are associated with fetal akinesia (Sarwark et al. 1990). Generally, infants with amyoplasia have wasted-looking shoulders with limited abduction and lateral rotation, elbows that are most commonly held rigidly in extension (though can also be held in flexion), wrists that are fixed in flexion, stiff, long-tapered fingers and thumbs which often adduct into the palm (Williams 1985). The lower extremity deformities associated with amyoplasia include rigid talipes equinovarus and predominantly

Figure 9 The Talipes Equinovarus (TEV) Anomaly in a Child with Amyoplasia

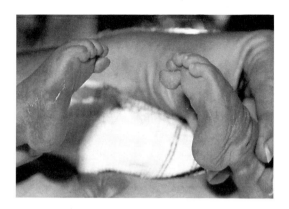

Figure 10 A Wrist Anomaly in a Child with Amyoplasia

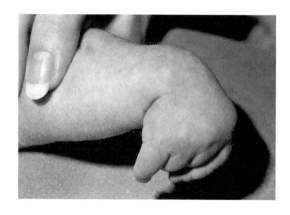

Figure 11 Multiple Joint Involvement in an Infant with Amyoplasia

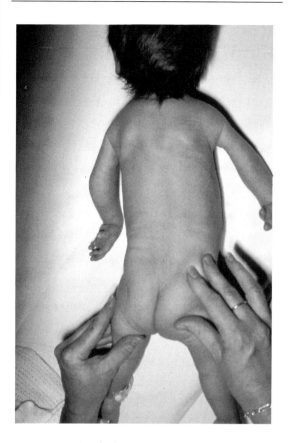

flexion contractures of the knee, though extension contractures can also occur. These infants generally have flexion, abduction and external contractures of the hip and approximately one-third of infants have unilateral or bilateral dislocation of the hip (Sarwark *et al.* 1990). See Figures 9 – 11.

Since prognosis is usually good for individuals with amyoplasia the physiotherapist will optimistically discuss short- and long-term treatment plan and goals with parents after completion of the infant's initial clinical assessment. Frequent passive range-of-motion exercises starting early in life and continued at home by parents (which are regularly reviewed by the physiotherapist) can be expected to improve range of motion in all joints, with best results in the wrist and hip (Sarwark *et al.* 1990). Gentle passive range-of-motion exercises are viewed as being prefer-

able to casting, for casting is thought to be associated with atrophy of musculature (Hall 1985).

Management of Lower Limb Contractures and Weakness. The physiotherapist's primary aim of treatment for the infant with amyoplasia is to achieve pain-free, stable and functional lower extremity joints with as much active control as possible. Attention is initially directed to the feet, followed by the knees and then the hips. A significant attempt is made by the physiotherapist and other members of the team to have achieved adequate correction of all lower limb contractures and asymmetries by the time the child is one year of age. The child will then be able to have the opportunity to commence standing and weight shifting at an age-appropriate time (Huurman and Jacobsen 1985). Throughout this period the physiotherapist is also persistent in encouraging the child's active movements, since the child's ability to walk is heavily dependent on the strength of the lower limb musculature.

The rigid TEV deformity associated with amyoplasia is initially treated conservatively (passive mobilization, splinting and casting). However, this deformity most often requires various surgical procedures, such as achilles tendon and posteriomedial releases. The physiotherapist will need to implement passive mobilization of the ankle postoperatively to maintain the newly gained range of motion. Recurrence of the TEV deformity is common and more radical operative methods may be required (Sodergard and Ryoppy 1994). Indeed, a functional, pain-free, plantigrade foot is an essential goal of treatment for the child with amyoplasia, as residual foot deformities are a major cause of the walking difficulties experienced by individuals with amyoplasia (Guidera and Drennan 1985).

Knee flexion contractures are similarly treated by conservative means initially. It is important that the parents continue regularly to carry out the home programme of passive stretches to the hamstring musculature and joint capsule. Surgical procedures such as hamstring and posterior capsule release may also be required (Thomas 1985). A postoperative physiotherapy programme of passive mobilization and facilitation of quadriceps musculature is subsequently implemented so as to maintain the newly gained range and to strengthen, where possible, weight-bearing musculature.

The hip flexion contracture is most effectively stretched out by placing the child in prone. Only carefully guided, gentle, passive range-of-motion exercises should ever be undertaken by the physiotherapist and parents and particular care should be taken when mobilizing the hip joint, as forceful extension may induce dislocation or fractures. The hip flexion contracture generally responds well to gentle conservative treatment. Once the newly gained range position is achieved, it is maintained with splinting (Huurman and Jacobsen 1985).

If the hips are bilaterally dislocated they are left untreated, since the child with bilateral dislocation is not functionally limited by this deformity (Palmer et al. 1985). A unilateral dislocation of the hip, however, may require surgical intervention as it will later give rise to pelvic obliquity and scoliosis (Huurman and Jacobsen 1985). Furthermore, a reduction of a unilateral dislocated hip in the child with amyoplasia can increase the child's functional ability to walk (Palmer et al. 1985). The physiotherapist initiates gentle soft tissue stretching until motion is gained in the hip. An open reduction with extensive soft tissue release is subsequently undertaken before the child's first birthday, but not before foot and knee deformities have been resolved. A physiotherapy programme of gentle stretches and active movement is commenced postoperatively in order to recover some of the lost preoperative hip range of motion (Huurman and Jacobsen 1985).

MANAGEMENT OF UPPER LIMB CONTRACTURES AND WEAKNESS

The physiotherapist expends a considerable effort in addressing the lower limb contractures and weakness of the child with amyoplasia, because of the importance to get the child into standing by the end of the first year of life. The concomitant upper limb contractures and weakness of the patient, however, are certainly not dismissed. In conjunction with the occupational therapist, the physiotherapist will attempt to address the infant's upper limb problems with the view to providing each individual with a functional ability to perform activities of daily living.

Hence, as soon as possible, the physiotherapist instigates a conservative treatment of gentle stretches of upper limb joints and facilitation of active movement. Range-of-motion passive stretches and facilitation of movement are demonstrated to parents who continue such a regimen regularly throughout the day. Reaching activities are encouraged through toys and verbal encouragement. The infant or child will often work out his/her own trick movements to reach a toy which should not be discouraged.

In contrast to the lower limb management, surgical procedures involving the upper limb are generally postponed until the child can tell the multidisciplinary team how he/she thinks he/she could perform more functionally. Children with amyoplasia are generally very alert and extremely competent in their ability to make the most of their movements and available range of motion. The physiotherapist and other members of the team should encourage such independent and creative undertakings in the child from a very early age.

Heritable Diseases of Collagen

The physiotherapist managing musculoskeletal conditions of the neonate and infant may be confronted by a number of genetic collagen diseases, such as the many variants of osteogenesis imperfecta, Marfan syndrome and Ehlers–Danlos syndrome (Prockop and Kivirikko 1984). Since collagen, the most abundant protein in the body, is a major constituent of skin, tendons, ligaments, bone and blood vessels, it is not surprising that an infant with a genetic 'collagen disease' may have significant musculoskeletal anomalies.

Osteogenesis Imperfecta (OI)

The infant with OI may exhibit obvious musculoskeletal anomalies, as this disease involves abnormalities of type I collagen which is a major bone protein (Edwards and Graham 1990). Indeed, the foremost feature of OI is brittle bone, but it also involves other tissues rich in type I collagen, such as ligaments, tendons, fascia, sclerae and teeth (Prockop and Kivirikko 1984). A biochemical confirmation of OI can be undertaken by skin biopsy. This collagen disease is classified into four main types on the basis of clinical criteria (Edwards and Graham 1990).

Type I OI is the most common (approximately 80% of all cases) and a milder form of the disease. Fewer fractures and bony deformities are seen in Type I than in other types of OI. This type of OI is associated with distinctly blue sclerae throughout life, presenile conductive hearing loss and significantly short stature. In contrast, Type II OI is the most severe form of the disease and is characterized by extreme bone fragility often leading to intrauterine or early infant death (Gahagan and Rimsza 1991).

Type III OI is a rare and variable form of the disease (Prockop and Kivirikko 1984). It presents with early and progressive clinical involvement. The sclerae may or may not be blue, deafness is common, and these patients may have dentinogenesis imperfecta (Gahagan and Rimsza 1991). Type IV is also a rare, variable

form of OI and is characterized by osteopenia leading to bone fragility of variable severity (Gahagan and Rimsza 1991).

The range of disability associated with OI extends from extremely severe to relatively mild. Major cause of death of the neonate with severe OI is respiratory insufficiency due to inadequate stability of the rib cage. Furthermore, there is the constant risk of respiratory insufficiency due to respiratory infections throughout life in the severe OI population (Albright 1981). The physiotherapist is limited in the techniques to remove excess secretions from the infant and child with OI because of the high risk for rib fracture. Undoubtedly, encouraging activity which will increase ventilation and improve respiratory muscle power is the most beneficial and prophylactic treatment regimen for the respiratory problems associated with OI.

The incidence of fractures in the severe OI population is extremely high during infancy. The physiotherapist is primarily involved in instigating a programme to prevent future fractures in the infant with OI, but should be very aware that the infant with OI will undoubtedly experience acute pain and associated anxiety when a fracture occurs. As noted previously, the parents' impact on the infant's anxiety is central (Dolgin and Phipps 1989). It is essential to emphasize to the parents the very important role that their support and reassurance can play in reducing their infant's anxiety. It is unfortunate that, although most children with OI are of average or above-average intelligence, they are often infantilized and isolated because of the fear of causing fractures (Binder et al. 1984).

The musculoskeletal problems of infants with severe forms of OI, such as brittle bones, recurrent fractures, lax joints and small weak muscles, will at some stage be assessed by the physiotherapist. Ideally, the physiotherapist should become involved in the management of the infant with severe manifestations of OI very early in the postnatal period and can advise parents on handling and positioning and maximizing the child's active movements. Parents may initally be apprehensive, but they can be taught that the infant with OI can be handled with little danger of fracturing, as long as the head and trunk are supported. The physiotherapist should emphasize that the infant and child with OI should be dressed in loose, light and absorbent clothes (because of tendency to have increased diaphoresis) with closures in the front and sides. Such clothing will assist in easy dressing and prevent excess stress on head or extremities and therefore prevent fractures (Binder *et al.* 1984).

Furthermore, parents should be informed that the infant with OI should rest on a padded surface or sheepskin and should be rotated regularly to avoid habitual posturing. Positioning the infant from supine to prone and either side with proper support will encourage more active movement and assist in the prevention of skeletal anomalies, particularly rib cage deformities. The physiotherapist should constantly emphasize to parents that active movement should never be restricted, but that considerable care should be taken so that the infant and child with OI do not hit hard surfaces. For example, the infant with OI will often become very active during his/her bath, so bathing should be done initially in a plastic basin and then small tubs lined with heavy towels (Werner *et al.* 1981).

Hydrotherapy is an excellent medium to encourage active movement and to begin weight-bearing for the infant and child with OI (Binder *et al.* 1984). Osteoporosis is often superimposed on the basic collagen defect in OI, which undoubtedly contributes to further fractures in the infant and child with OI. To reduce this associated osteoporosis, activity and very graduated weight-bearing are most important elements in the treatment regimen of infants and children with OI. Hydrotherapy is also beneficial for the cardiorespiratory system of infants and children as it can facilitate deeper breaths and controlled breathing patterns which will be particularly advantageous for the child with OI who is often subject to respiratory chest infections (Albright 1981).

As soon as the infant is interested in reaching (approximately 4 months of age), the physiotherapist should show parents how this ability can be used to strengthen the infant's upper extremities. The infant should be encouraged to reach in side lying, supine and supported sitting, which will also encourage visual field exploration and greater spatial awareness. Once sitting balance and upper limb strength is appropriate, mobility can be provided via

castor cart (sheepskin lined). Such mobility is essential in developing the child's motor planning abilities, spatial awareness and interaction with the environment.

Between 12 and 18 months of age the child with severe OI generally starts a standing programme. Stuberg (1992) suggests that children who have decreased bone mass or bone density should be considered candidates for standing programmes, but further studies are required to ascertain the duration and frequency of standing which would be most therapeutic for the child with OI. As noted previously, the infant with OI can be introduced to some partial weight-bearing during hydrotherapy. The benefits of the upright position are multiple. Weight-bearing has positive effects on bone development and there are significant psychosocial benefits associated with standing. For example, peer interaction is much more effective in standing and the child is less likely to be seen as an infant by parents and family. Furthermore, since the child with OI is frequently hypotonic, the upright position has added advantage of improving bowel function (Letts *et al.* 1988).

Unfortunately, when the child with severe OI assumes upright weight-bearing there is a significant risk that fracturing of lower extremity bones will occur. A vicious cycle can then commence, since when the child is immobilized further osteoporosis and weakness will eventuate and on resumption of weight-bearing fractures may recur. The use of specialized orthoses or vacuum pants (removable lightweight trousers lined with styrofoam beads that perform as a rigid system when air is evacuated from the trousers) is reported to provide support and decrease the risk of fractures during weight-bearing. Once the child has become accustomed to the vacuum pants the transition to a standing frame and ultimately to a knee–ankle–foot orthosis is facilitated (Letts *et al.* 1988).

Household and short-distance ambulation can be a possibility for children with less severe OI. These children will generally require some orthosis and a type of walker initially, but as their strength increases they may graduate finally to canes (Binder *et al.* 1984). Furthermore, it is important for the physiotherapist to remember that there are even milder forms of osteogenesis imperfecta. Any infant and child who may have sustained fractures through relatively minor injuries may be an individual with a milder form of osteogenesis imperfecta. Such an individual with a mild form of osteogenesis imperfecta may be difficult to differentiate from non-accidental trauma, particularly as a child with OI may have a normal physical examination, no radiographic abnormalities and a negative family history (Gahagan and Rimsza 1991).

Other Heritable Diseases of Collagen

The physiotherapist may be confronted by the infant with other heritable diseases of collagen, such as the Marfan syndrome and Ehlers–Danlos syndrome. These syndromes show considerable variability and it is most likely that it will be the infants with severe manifestations of these conditions that would be assessed by the physiotherapist. The child with a less obvious form of collagen disease may be referred to the physiotherapist for postural problems or clumsiness. The physiotherapist, therefore, should always consider such conditions if an infant or young child demonstrates profound joint laxity and hypermobility.

The Marfan syndrome is characterized by long, thin extremities, hypermobility, ectopia lentis and dilation and rupture of the aorta (Prockop and Kivirikko 1984). The hyperlaxity of these children is often particularly pronounced when weight-bearing. For example, they will demonstrate intractable pes planus/valgus (Bleck 1982).

Ehlers-Danlos syndrome is a heterogeneous group of disorders of collagen metabolism characterized by joint hypermobility and skin changes such as thinness, hyperextensibility and fragility. Specific types of this syndrome are defined according to clinical manifestations and mode of inheritance and biochemical deficiencies (Hamada et al. 1992). For example, Type VI and VII of the Ehlers–Danlos syndrome feature severe skeletal deformities (kyphoscoliosis and loose, often dislocated joints) (Eyre 1981). Furthermore, Hamada et al. (1992) report a form of Ehlers–Danlos syndrome associated with soft tissue contractures from birth. These contractures were resistant to mobilization and casting and required multiple surgical procedures to achieve a plantigrade foot.

The physiotherapist may be involved in educating parents with infants with various types of Ehlers–Danlos and Marfan syndrome about correct positioning to care for hypermobile joints and to prevent dislocation, as abnormal mechanical forces can be particularly damaging for them. Often when these children start weight-bearing the physiotherapist will be requested to review them in view of their severe rigid pes planus/valgus. Such children will generally require a stabilizing foot splint to maintain functional alignment and control deformity.

Nerve Lesions

The most common nerve lesion associated with the neonate and infant is the brachial plexus birth palsy. Although the reported incidences of this pathology vary, Hardy (1981) suggests 0.87 per 1000 live births. Despite vast improvements in obstetrical techniques and prenatal monitoring, birth palsy continues to occur in a substantial number of patients (Jackson et al. 1988). Jackson et al. (1988) describe several risk factors associated with this condition, such as high birth weight, prolonged maternal labour, dystocia of the shoulder, breech presentation and forceps delivery.

Although many of the infants initially seem to have a complete flail arm, within the first few weeks, it becomes apparent that brachial plexus birth palsy can be divided into three groups according to their major pattern of weakness (Jackson et al. 1988). For example: (1) the Erb's palsy (C5–6 lesion); (2) Dejerine–Klumpke paralysis (C8–T1); and (3) Erb–Duchenne–Klumpke, or a combined lesion (C5–T1) (Hesinger and Jones 1982b). In view of the risk factors associated with brachial plexus birth palsy, it is not surprising that neonates with such a palsy may also demonstrate other problems, such as mild facial palsies, subluxation of the shoulder, fractures of humerus and clavicles, torticollis, injury to the cervical spine and cord, radial nerve injury and Horner's syndrome (Eng 1971). Figures 12 and 13 show the resting position and lack of stabilizing shoulder musculature, respectively, in an infant with Erb's palsy.

Figure 12 The Resting Position of the Infant with Erb's Palsy

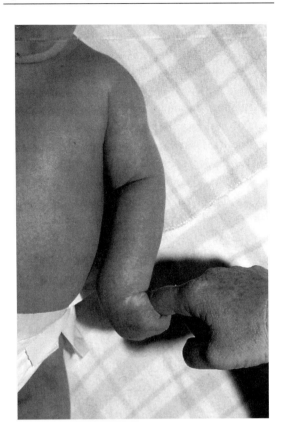

Figure 13 Lack of Stabilizing Shoulder Musculature in the Child with an Erb's Palsy

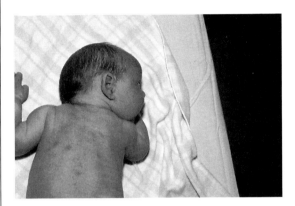

The prognosis for neonatal brachial plexus palsy is much better than previously thought. Most patients progress to complete recovery within 1 or 2 years (Covey et al. 1992). Jackson et al. (1988) suggest that patients who have a lesion of the upper part of brachial plexus have a relatively better prognosis. Serial muscle examinations, however, show that children with brachial plexus birth palsy who are treated with passive and active exercise develop additional muscle function with increasing age (Hoffer et al. 1978, Covey et al. 1992).

The physiotherapist will play a significant role in the conservative treatment of the child with neonatal brachial plexus palsy. Within the first 24–48 hours the physiotherapist will emphasize the importance of careful support to the upper limb involved during handling (e.g. feeding and bathing). The physiotherapist's initial clinical assessment of the neonate with brachial nerve palsy should particularly include the documentation of the active and passive and range-of-motion of upper extremity joints, muscle tone,

reflexes and the presence or absence of sensory deficits. In order to prevent contracture and maintain any viable muscle function the physiotherapist will commence passive and active range-of-motion exercises to the affected upper limb.

The parents are taught by the physiotherapist how to carefully keep a normal range of movement in the affected upper limb. Parents are informed that they should constantly compare range of movement of the affected upper limb with the unaffected side. Hence, the parents are instructed to undertake passive range-of-motion exercises of the affected upper limb 4–5 times a day and to encourage active movement of the upper limb particularly through the use of sensory input. Instructions on the care of the upper limb are also emphasized. The physiotherapist should review the parents' techniques at regular intervals and also ensure that the affected arm is encouraged in the same activities as the non-affected arm (e.g. hand to mouth, looking at fingers and, by about 4–5 months, holding two hands together). Furthermore, the parents are encouraged to facilitate bilateral shoulder girdle muscle activity while the infant is resting on his / her elbows, since normal scapular muscle activity is necessary to gain full return of functional movement in the upper limb. An assessment of returning muscle function, strength, motion and sensation should be also undertaken at regular intervals.

RECONSTRUCTIVE SURGERY

When the improvement in function has ceased, and if there is good sensory and motor function in the hand, the child with neonatal brachial nerve palsy may be considered for reconstructive surgery. The main aim of such surgery is to increase shoulder motion so as to improve function abilities. Most procedures seek to increase abduction and external rotation of the shoulder. Operative procedures to convert latissimus dorsi and teres major muscle into external rotators provide significant improvements in abduction and external rotation of the shoulder (Covey et al. 1992). Furthermore, a transfer of the teres major and latissimus dorsi to the rotator cuff has the advantage of being easily performed and enhances the stabilizing effect of the rotator cuff (Hoffer et al. 1978). Such surgery can also prevent deformities such as torsion of the humerus and flattening of the humeral head and glenoid fossa (Covey et al. 1992).

Several factors need to be considered before operating. For example, impaired sensation and muscle function in the hand, a deltoid muscle of grade 2 or less and a latissumus dorsi and teres minor graded less than 4 are considered as contraindication to such surgery (Hoffer et al. 1978). In addition, surgery should take place when the child is old enough to cooperate with the physiotherapist (3–4 years of age), since, after immobilization postoperatively the child commences an intensive physiotherapy regimen including gentle passive range-of-motion exercises and active humeral external rotation and shoulder abduction exercises (Covey et al. 1992).

OTHER CAUSES OF PERIPHERAL NERVE LESIONS AND THE ASSOCIATED MUSCULOSKELETAL PROBLEMS

As noted previously, Mooney and Kasser (1994) report an upper limb nerve palsy associated with the wearing of a Pavlik harness. It is apparent that the downward force of the shoulder straps, particularly in an infant who is active and on a high weight percentile could lead to abnormal traction or compression of the brachial plexus or cervical roots thereby causing weakness consistent with plexus neuropathy. Tollner et al. (1980) similarly report upper limb nerve palsy due to equipment, as a premature infant developed a radial nerve palsy following long-term measurement of blood pressure.

Lower limb peripheral nerve palsies in the neonate and

infant are certainly not common; however, the physiotherapist should be aware that they do occur. Hope et al. (1985) suggest that the weakness and lack of movement in an infant's leg was due to a traction injury to the lumbosacral plexus during a vigorous breech extraction. These investigators note that although neonatal lumbar plexus injury is much less likely than brachial plexus injury, it does occur. Furthermore, Hesinger and Jones (1982b) report sciatic nerve injuries due to direct, indirect and traction insults. Fischer and Strasburger (1982) alert us to the possibility of footdrop in the neonate due to compression of the common peroneal nerve at the lateral aspect of the knee from the placement of the footboard along the lateral aspect of the fibula to stabilize an intravenous needle at the medial aspect of the foot. They suggest that the use of more pliable restraints might prevent such nerve injuries. Furthermore, Mooney and Kasser (1994) report femoral nerve palsy associated with Pavlik harness secondary to prolonged hyperflexion.

The physiotherapist's assessment of lower extremity nerve palsies is similar to the procedures undertaken for the neonate with brachial nerve palsy. For example, the therapist should document closely the active and passive and range of motion of joints, muscle tone, reflexes and the presence or absence of sensory deficits. The primary goal of treatment is to avoid contractures of the joints involved by preserving a full range of passive motion and encouraging active movement. This regimen is taught to parents.

Prevention of peripheral nerve injuries is the responsibility of all health workers.

Limb Deficiencies

An examination of an extensive paediatric amputation population suggests that the majority of paediatric limb deficiencies are from congenital causes, and that the majority of multiple limb and unilateral upper limb deficiencies are congenital absences (Krebs and Fishman 1984). Congenital limb deficiencies are classified as being either a transverse/amputation type in which all skeletal elements distal to the level of loss are absent, or longitudinal in which some distal skeletal elements remain. For example, proximal femoral focal deficiency (PFFD), fibular dysplasia and tibial dysplasia are longitudinal deficiencies. Longitudinal deficiencies in the upper limb often involve the absence of the ulna (Krebs *et al.* 1991). Teratogens may play a role in transverse and longitudinal limb reduction deformities (Kricker *et al.* 1986). However, genetic factors are involved in a significant number of congenital limb deficiencies (Scott 1989).

The physiotherapist is a member of a multidisciplinary team managing the infant with limb deficiency. Team members can generally have an optimistic approach to the infant with limb deficiency as their prognosis for life is usually good, unless there are associated life-threatening defects (Dixon 1989). The families of the child with limb deficiency often experience much grief initially and the physiotherapist and other team members must be extremely supportive of the infant and the family (Marquardt 1983).

An extensive musculoskeletal assessment of the infant is undertaken by the physiotherapist. Documentation should include the extent and nature of the limb deficiency, the active and passive range of motion of all joints, muscle power and control, and the amount and quality of the infant's activity. It is essential that the physiotherapist observes closely the infant's level of sensorimotor and motor development. The preprosthetic and prosthetic physiotherapy programme for each individual should not merely address the site and level of limb deficiency, but most importantly suit the infant's stage of development.

A preprosthetic programme designed by the physiotherapist will emphasize active movement and range-of-motion activities which will increase the flexibility of limbs and trunk and strengthen the musculature of the remaining limbs and trunk (Krebs *et al.* 1991). Increasing the muscle control in the child with limb deficiency should be a high priority even during the preprosthetic programme, as clinical evidence suggests that the strength of shoulder flexion and abduction muscles is much lower than that of normal children on both the limb deficient and sound sides (Shaperman *et al.* 1992). Shaperman *et al.* note that the amount and types of play activity may account for differences in strength between children with and without limb deficiency.

The child's preprosthetic physiotherapy programme will also include activities which sponsor postural stability against gravity. Effective trunk control and equilibrium reactions are extremely necessary for the child to be maximally independent with or without a prosthesis (Krebs *et al.* 1991). Furthermore, training of potential and residual abilities of the individual with limb deficiencies is essential. The physiotherapist in conjunction with other team members and the family will initiate such training as soon as possible (Marquardt 1983).

Infants and children learn most effectively through play. Hence, the child's treatment regimen is generally most effective when the physiotherapist and occupational therapist have regular consultations. Undoubtedly, therapists dealing with the child with limb deficiency are concerned by biomechanical losses such as inequality of limb length, malrotation, inadequacy of proximal musculature and instability of proximal joints (Epps 1983). Therapists are concomitantly concerned to facilitate the infant's sensorimotor development. The residual tactile, proprioceptive and kinaesthetic awareness of the infant with limb deficiency needs to be facilitated so that the infant will experience and comprehend the spatial concept of the objects of his/her world. It is only through such a comprehensive programme that the child will achieve maximal functional independence (Marquardt 1983).

The timing of fitting the first upper and lower extremity prosthesis is dependent upon the young child's developmental readiness and abilities, as well as their functional need for a prosthesis (Krebs *et al.* 1991). The physiotherapist will work closely with the prosthetist. It is beneficial to have an early fitting of an upper limb prosthesis, since the infant is then able to use both arms for prone propping, creeping and pulling to standing which will subsequently encourage greater symmetry of movement (Krebs *et al.* 1991).

Once the infant shows interest in pulling to a standing position, he/she should be fitted for the first lower limb prosthesis. The prosthesis will assist the infant to acquire functional upright weight-bearing skills and eventually independent ambulation (Krebs *et al.* 1991). There is usually very little difficulty in the prosthetic fitting of children with congenital lower extremity stumps. Special prostheses even enable children with the complete loss of both lower extremities to stand and walk (Marquardt 1983).

In longitudinal lower limb deficiencies, surgery is often instigated before mobilization because of instability of proximal joints and inadequacy of proximal musculature (Epps 1983). For example, children with tibial dysplasia may undergo varying operative procedures (depending on the type of tibial dysplasia) when they are first able to stand (between 1 and 2 years of age). Once the disarticulation stump has healed, a prosthesis can be fitted and mobilization started (Pattinson and Fixsen 1992).

The physiotherapist will continue to incorporate the mobility training of the child with limb deficiency into a comprehensive developmental programme. The child will gain significant perceptual understanding as he/she physically translates his/her body in an upright orientation through space. Furthermore, profound psychosocial development can be sponsored through standing and walking programmes.

Summary

This chapter introduces a number of musculoskeletal problems experienced by the infant and young child and suggests some general ideas for treatment. There are various other issues which could be discussed, but the most effective physiotherapy management of muscle and joint anomalies in infants is dependent upon a comprehensive assessment and accurate problem-solving abilities. It is only when the infant's problems are identified and prioritized that the physiotherapist can subsequently construct a treatment regimen which will specifically address the individual's problems. Furthermore, in every physiotherapy musculoskeletal treatment regimen much consideration is given to the developmental stage of the infant and young child so as to ensure comprehensive management of the individual.

REFERENCES

Albright, JA (1981) Management overview of osteogenesis imperfecta. *Clinical Orthopaedics and Related Research* 159: 80–87.

Atar, D, Lehman, WB, Tenenbaum, Y *et al.* (1993) Pavlik harness versus Frejka splint in treatment of developmental dysplasia of the hip: bicentre study. *Journal of Pediatric Orthopedics* 13: 311–313.

Aronson, J, Puskarich, CL (1990) Deformity and disability from treated clubfoot. *Journal of Pediatric Orthopedics* 10: 109–119.

Bensahel, H, Catterall, A, Dimeglo, A (1990a) Practical applications in idiopathic clubfoot: a retrospective multicentric study in EPOS. *Journal of Pediatric Orthopedics* 10: 186–188.

Bensahel, H, Guillaume, A, Czukonyi, Z (1990b) Results of physical therapy for idiopathic clubfoot: a long-term follow-up study. *Journal of Pediatric Orthopedics* 10: 189–192.

Bernhardt, DB (1988) Prenatal and postnatal growth and development of the foot and ankle. *Physical Therapy* 68: 1831–1839.

Binder, H, Hawks, L, Braybill, G *et al.* (1984) Osteogenesis imperfecta: rehabilitation approach with infants and young children. *Archives of Physical Medicine and Rehabilitation* 65: 537–541.

Bleck, EE (1982) Developmental orthopaedics. III: Toddlers. *Developmental Medicine and Child Neurology* 24: 533–555.

Bleck, EE (1983) Metatarsus adductus: classification and relationship to outcomes of treatment. *Journal of Pediatric Orthopedics* 3: 2–9.

Broughton, NS, Wright, J, Menelaus, MB 1993 Range of knee-motion in normal neonates. *Journal of Paediatric Orthopaedics* 13: 263–264.

Carr, A, Jefferson, RJ, Benson, MKD'A (1993) Joint laxity and hip rotation in normal children and in those with congenital dislocation of the hip. *Journal of Bone And Joint Surgery* 75B: 76–78.

Carter, DR, Orr, TE, Fyhrie, DP *et al.* (1987) Influences of mechanical stress on prenatal and postnatal skeletal development. *Clinical Orthopaedics and Related Research* 219: 237–250.

Cheng, JCY, Chan, PS, Chiang, SC *et al.* (1991a) Angular and rotational profile of the lower limb in 2,630 Chinese children. *Journal of Pediatric Orthopedics* 11: 154–161.

Cheng, JCY, Chan, PS, Hui, PW (1991b) Joint laxity in children. *Journal of Pediatric Orthopedics* 11: 752–756.

Cheng, JCY, Au, AWY (1994) Infantile torticollis: a review of 624 cases. *Journal of Pediatric Orthopedics* 14: 802–808.

Coleman, SS (1994) Developmental dislocation of the hip: evolutionary changes in diagnosis and treatment. *Journal of Pediatric Orthopedics* 14: 1–2.

Covey, DC, Riordan, DC, Milstead, ME *et al.* (1992) Modification of the L'Episcopo procedure for brachial plexus birth palsies. *Journal of Bone and Joint Surgery* 74B: 897–901.

Cusick, BD (1990) *Progressive Casting and Splinting for Lower Extremity Deformities in Children with Neuromotor Dysfunction,* 410 pp. Bellevue: Therapy Skill Builders.

Davids, JR, Wenger, DR, Murbarak, SJ (1993) Congenital muscular torticollis: sequela of intrauterine or perinatal compartment syndrome. *Journal of Pediatric Orthopedics* 13: 141–147.

Dixon Jr., MS (1989) Pediatric screening and evaluation. In: Kalamachi A (ed.) *Congenital Lower Limb Deficiencies,* pp. 58–64. New York: Springer-Verlag.

Dolgin, MJ, Phipps, S (1989) Pediatric pain: the parents' role. *Pediatrician* 16: 103–109.

Edwards, MJ, Graham, JM (1990) Studies of type 1 collagen in osteogenesis imperfecta. *Journal of Pediatrics* 117: 67–72.

Eng, GD (1971) Brachial plexus palsy in newborn infants. *Pediatrics* 48: 18–28.

Epps, CH (1983) Current concepts review: proximal femoral focal deficiency. *Journal of Bone and Joint Surgery* 65A: 867–870.

Eyre, DR (1981) Concepts in collagen biochemistry: evidence that collagenopathies underlie osteogenesis imperfecta. *Clinical Orthopaedics and Related Research* 159: 97–107.

Fischer, AQ, Strasburger, J (1982) Footdrop in the neonate secondary to use of footboards. *Journal of Pediatrics* 101: 1003–1004.

Gahagan, S, Rimsza, ME (1991) Child abuse or osteogenesis imperfecta: how can we tell. *Pediatrics* 88: 987–992.

Guidera, KJ, Drennan JC (1985) Foot and ankle deformities in arthrogryposis multiplex congenita. *Clinical Orthopaedics and Related Research* 194 93–98.

Hall, J (1985) Genetic aspects of arthrogryposis. *Clinical Orthopaedics and Related Research* **194**: 44–53.

Hamada, S, Hiroshima, K, Oshita, S et al. (1992) Ehlers–Danlos syndrome with soft-tissue contractures. *Journal of Bone and Joint Surgery* **74B**: 902–905.

Hardy, AE (1981) Birth injuries of the brachial plexus: incidence and prognosis. *Journal of Bone and Joint Surgery* **63B**: 98–101.

Heath, CH, Staheli, LT (1993) Normal limits of knee angle in white children – genu varum and genu valgum. *Journal of Pediatric Orthopedics* **13**: 259–262.

Heikkila, E, Ryoppy, S, Louhimo I (1985) The management of primary acetabular dysplasia: its association with habitual side-lying. *Journal of Bone and Joint Surgery* **67B**: 25–28.

Hesinger, RN, Jones, ET (1982a) Developmental orthopaedics. I: The lower limb. *Developmental Medicine and Child Neurology* **24**: 95–116.

Hesinger, RN, Jones, ET (1982b) Developmental orthopaedics. II: The spine, trauma and infection. *Developmental Medicine and Child Neurology* **24**: 202–218.

Hjelmstedt, A, Sahlstedt, B (1990) Role of talocalcaneal osteotomy in clubfoot surgery: results in 21 surgically treated feet. *Journal of Pediatric Orthopedics* **10**: 193–197.

Hoffer, MM, Wickenden, R, Roper, B (1978) Brachial plexus birth palsies: results of tendon transfers to the rotator cuff. *Journal of Bone and Joint Surgery* **60A**: 691–695.

Hope, ED, Bodensteiner, JB, Thong, N (1985) Neonatal lumbar plexus injury. *Archives of Neurology* **42**: 94–95.

Huurman, WM, Jacobsen, SJ (1985) The hip in arthrogryposis multiplex congenita. *Clinical Orthopaedics and Related Research* **194**: 81–86.

Ikeda, K (1992) Conservative management of idiopathic clubfoot. *Journal of Pediatric Orthopedics* **12**: 217–223.

Jackson, ST, Hoffer, MM, Parrish, N (1988) Brachial-plexus palsy in the newborn. *Journal of Bone and Joint Surgery* **70A**: 1217–1220.

Karski, T, Wosko, I (1989) Experience in the conservative treatment of congenital clubfoot in newborns and infants. *Journal of Pediatric Orthopedics* **9**: 134–136.

Katz K, Naor, N, Merlob, P et al. (1990) Rotational deformities of the tibia and foot in preterm infants. *Journal of Pediatric Orthopaedics* **10**: 483–485.

Kawashima, T, Uhthoff, HK (1990) Development of the foot in prenatal life in relation to idiopathic club foot. *Journal of Pediatric Orthopedics* **10**: 232–237.

Kutlu, A, Memik, R, Mutlu, M et al. (1992) Congenital dislocation of the hip and its relation to swaddling used in Turkey. *Journal of Pediatric Orthopedics* **12**: 598–602.

Krebs, DE, Fishman, S (1984) Characteristics of the child amputee population. *Journal of Pediatric Orthopedics* **4**: 89–95.

Krebs, DE, Edelstein JE, Thornby, MA (1991) Prosthetic management of children with limb deficiencies. *Physical Therapy* **71**: 920–934.

Kricker, A, Elliot, JW, Forrest, JM et al. (1986) Congenital limb reduction deformities and use of oral contraceptives. *American Journal of Obstetrics and Gynecology* **155**: 1072–1078.

Lennox, IAC, McLauchlan, J, Murali R (1993) Failures of screening and management of congenital dislocation of the hip. *Journal of Bone and Joint Surgery* **75B**: 72–75.

Letts, M, Monson, R, Weber, K (1988) The prevention of recurrent fractures of the lower extremities in severe osteogenesis imperfecta using vacuum pants: a preliminary report in four patients. *Journal of Pediatric Orthopedics* **8**: 454–457.

Le Veau, BF, Bernhardt, DB (1984) Developmental biomechanics: effect of forces on the growth, development and maintenance of the human body. *Physical Therapy* **64**: 1874–1882.

Margulies, JY, Simkin, A, Leichter, I et al. (1986) Effect of intense physical activity on the bone-mineral content in the lower limbs of young adults. *Journal of Bone and Joint Surgery* **68A**: 1090–1093.

Marquardt, EG (1983) A holistic approach to rehabilitation for the limb-deficient child. *Archives of Physical Medicine and Rehabilitation* **64**: 237–242.

Mooney, JF, Kasser, JR (1994) Brachial plexus palsy as a complication of Pavlik harness sse. *Journal of Pediatric Orthopedics* **14**: 677–679.

Nather, A, Bose, K (1987) Conservative and surgical treatment of clubfoot. *Journal of Pediatric Orthopedics* **7**: 42–48.

O'Sullivan, ME, O'Brien, T (1994) Acetabular dysplasia presenting as developmental dislocation of the hip. *Journal of Pediatric Orthopedics* **14**: 13–15.

Palmer, PM, MacEwan, D, Bowen, JR et al. (1985) Passive motion therapy for infants with arthrogryposis. *Clinical Orthopaedics and Related Research* **194**: 54–59.

Pattinson, RC, Fixsen, JA (1992) Management and outcome in tibial dysplasia. *Journal of Bone and Joint Surgery* **74B**: 893–896.

Phelps, E, Smith, LJ, Hallum, A (1985) Normal ranges of hip motion of infants between nine and 24 months of age. *Developmental Medicine and Child Neurology* **27**: 785–792.

Ponsetti, IV (1992) Current concepts review treatment of congenital club foot. *Journal of Bone and Joint Surgery* **74A**: 448–452.

Prockop, DJ, Kivirikko, KI (1984) Heritable diseases of collagen. *New England Journal of Medicine* **311**: 376–386.

Rushforth, GF (1978) The natural history of hooked forefoot. *Journal of Bone and Joint Surgery* **60B**: 530–532.

Samson, PG, Harris, SR (1994) Congenital clubfoot: review of the literature on clinical assessment and physiotherapy intervention. *Physiotherapy Canada* **46**: 249–254.

Sarwark, JF, MacEwan, GD, Scott, CI (1990) Current concepts review amyoplasia (a common form of arthrogryposis). *Journal of Bone and Joint Surgery* **72A**: 465–469.

Savedra, MC, Tesler, MD (1989) Assessing children's and adolescents' pain. *Pediatrician* **16**: 24–29.

Scott Jr, CI (1989) Genetic and familial aspects of limb defects with emphasis on the lower extremities. In: Kalamachi A (ed.) *Congenital Lower Limb Deficiencies*, pp. 46–57. New York: Springer-Verlag.

Shaperman, J, Setoyuchi, Y, Leblanc, M (1992) Upper limb strength of young limb deficient children as a factor in using body powered terminal devices – a pilot study. *Journal of the Association of Children's Prosthetic Orthotic Clinics* **27**: 89–96.

Sirca, A, Erzen, I, Pecak, F (1990) Histochemistry of abductor hallucis muscle in children with idiopathic clubfoot and in controls. *Journal of Pediatric Orthopedics* **10**: 477–482.

Sodergard, J, Ryoppy, S (1994) Foot deformities in arthrogryposis multiplex congenita. *Journal of Pediatric Orthopedics* **14**: 768–772.

Spero, CR, Simon, GS, Tornetta, P (1994) Clubfeet and tarsal coalition. *Journal of Pediatric Orthopedics* **14**: 372–376.

Staheli, LT, Corbett, M, Wyss, C et al. (1985) Lower-extremity rotational problems in children: normal values to guide management. *Journal of Bone and Joint Surgery* **67A**: 39–47.

Stark, JG, Johanson, JE, Winter, RB (1987) The Heyman–Herndon tarsometatarsal capsulotomy for metatarsus adductus: results in 48 feet. *Journal of Pediatric Orthopedics* **7**: 305–310.

Stuberg, WA (1992) Considerations related to weight-bearing programs in children with developmental disabilities. *Physical Therapy* **72**: 35–40.

Tibrewal, SB, Benson MKD, Howard C et al. (1992) The Oxford club-foot programme. *Journal of Bone and Joint Surgery* **74B**: 528–533.

Thomas, B, Schopler, S, Wood, W et al. (1985) The knee in arthrogryposis. *Clinical Orthopaedics and Related Research* **194**: 87–92.

Tollner, U, Bechinger, D, Pohlandt, F (1980) Radial nerve palsy in a premature infant following long-term measurement of blood pressure. *Journal of Pediatrics* **96**: 921–922.

Julie MacDonald

Walker, JM (1991) Musculoskeletal development: a review. *Physical Therapy* **71**: 878–889.

Werner, P, Metz, L, Dubowski, F (1981) Nursing care of an osteogenesis imperfecta infant and child. *Clinical Orthopaedics and Related Research* **159**: 108–110.

Williams, PF (1985) Management of upper limb problems in arthrogryposis. *Clinical Orthopaedics and Related Research* **194**: 60–67.

Yamamoto, H, Furuya, K (1990) Treatment of congenital clubfoot with a modified Denis Browne splint. *Journal of Bone and Joint Surgery* **72B**: 460–463.

Yamamoto, H, Muneta, T and Furuya (1994) Cause of toe-in gait after posteromedial release for congenital clubfoot. *Journal of Pediatric Orthopedics* **14**: 369–371.

Yngve, DA (1990) Foot-progression angle in clubfeet. *Journal of Pediatric Orthopedics* **10**: 467–472.

FURTHER READING

Bleck, EE (1981) Nonoperative treatment of osteogenesis imperfecta: orthotic and mobility management. *Clinical Orthopaedics and Related Research* **159**: 111–122.

Catteral, A (1991) A method of assessment of the clubfoot deformity. *Clinical Orthopaedics and Related Research* **264**: 48–53.

Marinelli, PV, Oritz, A, Alden, ER (1981) Acquired eventration of the diaphragm: a complication of chest tube placement in neonatal pneumothorax. *Pediatrics* **67**: 552–554.

McHale, KA, Lenhart, MK (1991) Treatment of residual clubfoot deformity – the 'bean-shaped' foot – by opening wedge medial cuneiform osteotomy and closing wedge cuboid osteotomy. Clinical review and cadaver correlations. *Journal of Pediatric Orthopedics* **11**: 374–381.

Napiontek, M, Nazar, J (1994) Tibial osteotomy as a salvage procedure in the treatment of congenital talipes equinovarus. *Journal of Pediatric Orthopedics* **14**: 763–767.

Ouvrier, RA, McLeod, JG, Pollard, JD (1990) *Peripheral Neuropathy in Childhood*, 242 pp. New York: Raven Press

Staheli, LT (1990) Lower positional deformities in infants and children: a review. *Journal of Pediatric Orthopedics* **10**: 559–563.

Wientroub, S, Khermosh, O (1991) A new orthosis for the management of clubfoot and other foot and leg deformities in infancy and early childhood. *Journal of Pediatric Orthopedics* **11**: 485–487.

18

Physiotherapy Management of Musculoskeletal Problems – the Young and School-aged Child

JULIE MACDONALD

Musculoskeletal Assessment of the Young Child
•
Musculoskeletal Changes in the Young Child
•
Childhood Musculoskeletal Conditions Associated with Pain
•
Juvenile Chronic Arthritis (JCA)/Juvenile Rheumatoid Arthritis
•
Haemophilia
•
Other Childhood Musculoskeletal Conditions
•
The Young Child with Limb Deficiencies

The young child, like the infant, has quite distinctive postural features which gradually change over time. Every child, however, will demonstrate a variable presentation of these postural features. Factors, such as heredity, nutrition, hormones and force, all play a significant role in ensuring growth and development of the musculoskeletal system (Bernhardt 1988).

The influential role that prenatal and postnatal forces play in chondral and bone modelling in the infant is highlighted in the preceding chapter. Mechanical forces continue to dramatically affect musculoskeletal development throughout early childhood. Indeed, the dynamic forces created through physical activity have a significant effect upon bone modelling (Margulies et al. 1986). The physiotherapist involved in the management of childhood musculoskeletal problems is particularly aware of the influential role of physical activity in musculoskeletal development, as it provides the basis of many treatment regimens.

The physiotherapist should not only be fully cogni-

zant of the young child's distinctive postural features, but must also be constantly alert to individual differences. A child's 'so-called' muscle and/or joint problems may merely be an individual variation from the 'normal' presentation. It is imperative that the physiotherapist is able to distinguish between physiological variations and pathological anomalies. Furthermore, in view of the inherent variations of each individual's musculoskeletal system, it is essential that the physiotherapist designs a treatment programme which is specific to each individual patient.

Young children can be subject to a wide range of musculoskeletal problems. An attempt is made in this chapter to address some of the more common clinical presentations which confront the physiotherapist. Furthermore, insight into how chronic musculoskeletal problems can affect the paediatric patient will be provided. Major topics, such as childhood fractures and scoliosis, are discussed in the following chapter.

Thorough assessment procedures, accurate problem-solving skills, and the appropriate instigation of specific treatment techniques for the identified problems are essential for the effective physiotherapy management of the child with muscle and joint problems. The process of assessing the toddler and young child with musculoskeletal problems is complex. The physiotherapist should at all times attempt to create a comfortable, non-threatening environment for the young child, as social and physical contexts will significantly influence the child's performance (Haley *et al.* 1994).

Musculoskeletal Assessment of the Young Child

Initially, the physiotherapist will carefully observe the young child's activity and movements as he / she interacts with parents or siblings. A knowledge of the nature, quality and proficiency of the activities undertaken by children at various ages is essential for the physiotherapist. In view of the interdependence of the musculoskeletal and nervous systems, the physiotherapist is in a much better position to identify the actual nature of the child's problem if the status of both of these systems is assessed.

History-taking / Subjective Assessment

A comprehensive history will be obtained from the parents, particularly noting past medical and surgical history. If the child has a chronic condition, for example, juvenile chronic arthritis, a report of the present medical management would be invaluable. Pertinent questions should be referred to the child when he / she can understand simple questions. The child may be able to provide essential details regarding the physical symptomatology, the nature of the pain experienced, whether a joint or limb feels hot / burning, and whether there is numbness / pins and needles. Body outline figures can be effective tools in assisting children (5 years and above) to communicate the location of their pain, whereas younger children can be asked to point to the parts of the body where they hurt. The happy—sad face scales and numerical pain

ladders can be useful in assessing the intensity of pain in the child, though the older child may be able to provide a valuable description of symptoms (Savedra and Tesler 1989). A comprehensive history-taking should establish the functional abilities of the child. The physiotherapist should also explore the child's participation in sport, physical education and recreation activities.

Inspection / Palpation / Measurement

The physiotherapist's examination of the child's musculoskeletal system will involve inspection, palpation and various measurement procedures. In order to obtain the attention, cooperation and motivation of the toddler and preschool child, attempts should be made to turn the examination into a game. Furthermore, for the physiotherapist to undertake an effective inspection of the child's postural alignment, measure range of motion of joints, assess muscle strength and endurance, and identify muscle atrophy and joint effusion, it is essential that the child wears a minimal amount of clothing. Children generally feel comfortable in their swimming togs (bathing suits).

The examination should be a positive experience for the child. Throughout the examination the physiotherapist is attempting to discern anomalies in movement, but should also highlight the child's abilities wherever possible. Although the physiotherapist is greatly assisted by technological gait analysis systems, observational gait analysis is invaluable for the assessment of the young child's functional ambulation. The physiotherapist can document qualitative comments regarding the child's symmetry, stability and balance and weight shift on a variety of terrains and in different settings (Rose *et al.* 1985). The physiotherapist must have a sound appreciation of changing gait pattern of the growing child, as some parental concerns may merely be a gait feature of the particular age of the child. For elaboration on the normal development of gait, refer to Sutherland (1984) and Corradi-Scalise and Ling (1990). If the child has been prescribed specialized equipment (aids and / or orthotics) the physiotherapist's assessment should incorporate a comprehensive inspection and evaluation of postural alignment and gait both with and without the equipment.

Musculoskeletal Changes in the Young Child

Postural Alignment

The infant's medial femoral torsion (antetorsion) continues to decrease throughout childhood to about 8–16° by skeletal maturity. Similarly, the infant's slight medial to neutral tibial torsion develops into a lateral torsion during childhood, reaching 23–25° by maturity. The significant retroversion of the infant's tibial plateau (27° angulation in the newborn) gradually decreases through childhood (7° angulation at 10 years of age) (Bernhardt 1988). The bow-legged phase of the infant and toddler is replaced by a knock-kneed phase during early childhood. Heath and Staheli (1993) suggest that children at 4 years of age present the greatest mean knock-knee of 8° which gradually decreases to a mean of <6° at 11 years of age.

Joint Laxity and Extensibility

The degree of joint laxity generally diminishes with age, but there are ethnic differences in joint laxity. For example, Cheng et al. (1991b) note that throughout childhood Chinese children are far more lax than European children. These investigators suggest that differences in the basic ultrastructure and biomechanics of the joint and related structure may be the contributing factors in the variations of joint laxity among different races. The physiotherapist must consider age group and population variations before deciding that an individual has excessive joint laxity.

The normal ranges of popliteal angle in children (measured with the hip at 90° flexion) provide some indication of hamstring length, and demonstrate that muscle extensibility decreases with age. For example, findings by Katz et al. (1992) describe a mean popliteal angle of 6° between the ages of 1 and 3 years, whereas at age 4 this angle rose to 17° in girls and 27° in boys. At ≤5 years of age, the mean popliteal angle in this group of healthy children was 26° with little change up to 10 years. These investigators note that a popliteal

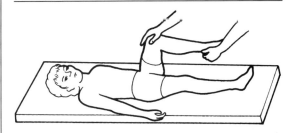

Figure 1 The Child's Hip and Knee are Flexed 90° and Then the Knee is Extended to Measure Popliteal Angle

angle ≤50° reflects considerable hamstring shortening and undoubtedly requires investigation. See Figure 1.

The toddler's externally rotated hips gradually become less marked during early childhood, as medial rotation of hip increases from a mean of 43° at age 2 to a maximum of 56° at age 9, but decreases again by 11 years. In contrast, lateral rotation of the child's hip decreases from a mean of 40° from age 2 to 30° at age 9 and slowly increases at age 10 (Cheng et al. 1991a).

Common Childhood Musculoskeletal Presentations

Genu varum (bow-legs), genu valgus (knock-knees), flexible pes planus (flat feet), in-toeing and out-toeing gait in children cause many parents considerable concern. Most will correct in time without treatment, but many children with such rotational variations are brought to the attention of physiotherapists. These children's parents generally only require information to allay their fears. Sometimes, the physiotherapist will advise the parents to seek a consultation from an orthopaedist and/or neurologist because the child's lower limb rotational profile does not fall within the normal range of variability and/or there is pain.

Torsional Variations

The changing rotational profile of the child's lower extremity has been noted, but since genu varum, genu valgus, flexible pes planus, in-toeing and out-toeing gait in children do cause concern, further discussion is warranted. The physiotherapist may inform parents that out-toeing in the toddler is due to the fact that the entire foot must laterally rotate to be in keeping with preponderance of lateral rotation of the hip at this time. By approximately 2 years of age the child's medial rotation of the hip is equivalent to the hip's lateral rotation range of motion and out-toeing is minimal. Similarly, the physiotherapist can inform parents that most children with in-toeing, who do not have neuromuscular disorder, will improve spontaneously by age 8 or 9 years. It is generally felt that this correction of in-toeing is due to the increased lateral rotation at the tibia and ankle level (Cheng et al. 1991a). Furthermore, internal femoral torsion continues to decrease throughout child-hood, primarily through the application of lateral torque forces to the femoral shaft.

Significantly, the use of twister cables, antirotation braces, exercises, orthoses, splints or shoes to decrease the existing degree of femoral or tibial torsion has not been substantiated by radiological or anatomical studies. Indeed, there are concerns that twister cables for femoral antetorsion may merely promote excessive lateral tibiofibular torsion or rotation (Cusick and Stuberg 1992). In view of the flexibility of the child's musculoskeletal system, the physiotherapist should ask parents to discourage any habitual positioning of medial rotation of the lower extremities (sitting and sleeping) which may exacerbate in-toeing. The physiotherapist can also explain to parents how hip extensor and lateral rotator muscles generate a lateral torque force across the femoral shaft and suggest physical activities to activate such musculature.

Genu Varum/Genu Valgum

Genu varum and genu valgus are stages in normal development of the lower limb. As noted previously, an initial varus position is followed by an extreme valgus stage which gradually resolves to a normal valgus position by middle to late childhood (Bern-hardt 1988). Genu valgum in the young preschooler with joint laxity appears particularly pronounced because of hyperextension of the knee. Certain chil-dren may demonstrate excessive bow-leg and knock-knee deformity. The physiotherapist should progres-sively record intercondylar and intermalleolar dis-tances of their patients to observe if these distances are decreasing. Bowen et al. (1992) suggest that if an intermalleolar distance of 10 cm at age 10 years exists and if genu varum persists in older children or adolescence operative correction, such as partial epiphysiodesis, should be considered.

In rare instances genu varum and genu valgus pre-sentations may be due to metabolic disease or skeletal dysplasias (Bleck 1982). A bow-leg deformity may also progress into infantile tibia vara or Blount disease which may require an early realignment osteotomy (Beck et al. 1987). The physiotherapist who establishes that a child has an excessive femoral–tibial angulation which is increasing should emphasize to the parents the importance of an orthopaedic consultation.

In general the aetiology of excessive femoral–tibial angulation presentations is uncertain. Intrauterine and habitual postnatal positioning are proposed to generate abnormal forces which cause growth to occur at an angle to the long axis of the tibia (Robertson 1987). For example, Le Veau and Bern-hardt (1984) suggest that genu varum can be pro-moted by a persistent prone sleeping position with the hips and knees flexed and the tibiae internally rotated. Similarly, such an habitual prone sleeping posture with tibiae externally rotated, and W sitting is felt to facilitate valgus positioning of the knees. Children should be encouraged to avoid any habitual postures. Ligamentous laxity can also exacerbate varum or valgus positioning.

In view of the location and malleability of the foot, excessive femoral–tibial angulation presentations can cause alterations in weight-bearing alignment. For example, genu varum may exacerbate talar adduction and in-toeing, whereas pes planus and out-toeing may occur due to genu valgus (Le Veau and Bernhardt 1984). Even when the physiotherapist is directed by the child and/or parents to a particular joint in their assessment, this joint should never be con-sidered in isolation, but rather as a part of a kinetic chain. For example, the physiotherapy assessment of flatfoot should entail comprehensive observa-tions and measurements of the whole lower extremity and pelvis.

Hypermobile Flatfoot

Other terms used for this condition are flexible pes valgus, flexible pes planus with plantarflexed talus and flexible pronation. The general term flatfoot describes a mixture of anatomical variations as well as a small core of pathological conditions (Rose *et al.* 1985). The physiotherapist must clearly distinguish flexible pes valgus from rigid flatfoot deformities due to structural (for example, congenital vertical talus) and neuromuscular abnormalities. Indeed, the malleability of the child's foot and its distal location make it extremely vulnerable to any disturbances in motor function in the trunk and lower extremity (Le Veau and Bernhardt 1984). For example, a tight heelcord due to hypertonicity of triceps surae musculature can displace calcaneus laterally into eversion with resulting pronation of the subtalar and midtarsal joints. Furthermore, the child with marked hyperlaxity and hypotonia (Marfan and Ehlers–Danlos syndrome) will often demonstrate intractable and severe pes valgus with a plantarflexed talus.

In contrast, flexible pes planus is a condition in which ankle mobility is full and the foot has a normal arch when non-weight-bearing, but collapses when weight-bearing (Bordelon 1983). On weight-bearing, the child with hypermobile flatfoot has an everted heel and a pronated forefoot, so that the second metatarsal deviates laterally from the heel bisector line (Bleck 1982) and when walking the hypermobile flatfoot produces out-toeing. No one test for flatfeet is completely reliable. Passive extension of the great toe at the metatarsophalangeal joint (which in the normal weight-bearing joint will elevate the medial longitudinal arch and cause lateral rotation of the tibia) in conjunction with a valgus index (which records any medial or lateral shift of the malleoli in relation to the centre of the heel imprint) are particularly helpful in diagnosis (Rose *et al.* 1985).

A large number of feet labelled flat are within normal variability. Furthermore, pronation or eversion of the foot is to some degree a stage in normal development of the human foot (Barry and Scranton 1983). In view of the considerable laxity in the supporting ligaments of the toddler's foot, and their wide-based, laterally rotated stance, it is not surprising that their feet pronate as a compensatory measure. In addition, the toddler looks particularly flatfooted because of the plantar fat pad which gradually resolves over the next few years. Toe-standing reveals an active longitudinal arch formation by approximately 12 months (Cusick 1990).

As the child's active supinatory balance reactions in the foot improve and relevant medial connective tissue strengthens, compensatory pronation of the foot decreases. Not surprisingly there is a tendency for the arch to improve spontaneously with age (Rao and Joseph 1992). Furthermore, the gradual reduction in the laxity of the joints during childhood contributes to the development of this longitudinal arch of the foot (Staheli *et al.* 1987). A small percentage of persons will carry this tendency toward foot pronation into adulthood (Barry and Scranton 1983). Significantly, although a low arch is often viewed negatively by many concerned parents, there is no evidence that flexible flat foot produces disability or later problems (Staheli *et al.* 1987).

In the otherwise normal young child with asymptomatic flexible flatfeet, the treatment involves providing parents with information about this condition, as there are no data to support aggressive intervention (Barry and Scranton 1983). Wenger *et al.* (1989) suggest that the wearing of corrective shoes or inserts for 3 years does not alter the natural history of flexible flatfoot in children. In addition, these investigators confirm the view that flexible flatfoot in young children slowly improves with growth.

The only absolute indication for treatment of flexible hypermobile flatfoot deformity in a child is when there is pain or severe deformity. The physiotherapist may be involved in instigating heelcord stretches and suggesting the use of orthoses which can cup the calcaneus and oppose the tendency to heel valgus. For example, Theologis *et al.* (1994) suggest that simple heel seats may provide an economical treatment for the child with excessive heel valgus and unacceptable shoe breakdown. In the persistently symptomatic child the surgical procedure which might be considered before skeletal maturity is achilles tendon lengthening (Barry and Scranton 1983).

Since active supinatory balancing responses assist in overcoming the pronatory loads of early walking, it is not surprising that there is a view that the wearing of shoes may interfere in the development of the medial longitudinal arch in children with flexible pes valgus. For example, Rao and Joseph (1992) suggest that wearing shoes in early childhood is detrimental to the development of the normal longitudinal arch. Furthermore, they note that this susceptibility for flat feet among children who wear shoes is most evident if there is an associated ligamentous laxity. The preponderance of flatfoot in their study also varied with the type of footwear, as closed-toe shoes inhibited the development of the arch more than slippers or sandals. These investigators suggest that this difference between the type of footwear may be that intrinsic muscle activity is necessary to keep slippers falling off, and that children who wear slippers or sandals generally remove them when playing. They suggest that children should be encouraged to play unshod. The physiotherapist supports the view that unrestrained physical activity is essential for normal musculoskeletal development.

Childhood Musculoskeletal Conditions Associated with Pain

Parents may also consult the physiotherapist because their children are complaining of varying musculoskeletal pains. As noted previously, the physiotherapist should always attempt to question the child about symptoms of pain. Children, like adults, can experience a wide variety of pains which are often categorized as acute, chronic, recurrent or cancer pain (McGrath and Hillier 1989). Acute musculoskeletal pain has a relatively short duration and can be incurred throug trauma, such as fractures, whereas chronic musculoskeletal pain is persistent and can be associated with diseases such as juvenile chronic arthritis and haemophilia. Although cancer is relatively rare in children, malignant bone tumours and soft tissue sarcomas constitute some of the causes of childhood cancer. Hence, the possibility of a tumour needs to be considered as a potential cause of paediatric musculoskeletal pain (Gebhardt et al. 1990).

The physiotherapist is particularly involved in the management of children with chronic musculoskeletal problems, such as juvenile chronic arthritis and haemophilia. However, it is imperative that he/she is aware of the varying musculoskeletal childhood pathologies which may evoke considerable painful symptoms and refers the child for appropriate medical intervention. Although the physiotherapist may play a limited role in the management of children with conditions such as irritable hip, Legg–Calve–Perthes (LCP) disease, slipped capital femoral epiphysis, osteomyelitis, septic arthritis and skeletal injury (e.g. fractures), he/she should have an appreciation of the pathology, presentation and the relevant medical management of these childhood musculoskeletal conditions.

Irritable Hip (Transient Synovitis of the Hip)

Irritable hip is described as a common self-limiting disorder of childhood (Bickerstaff et al. 1990). It is characterized by the sudden onset of a painful limp. The child may complain of pain in the hip, knee or anterior thigh and there can be a varying degree of restriction of movement of the hip (Landin et al. 1987). The diagnosis of irritable hip is only reached after the exclusion of a more serious pathology, such as septic arthritis, osteomyelitis, slipped capital femoral epiphysis, LCP disease and juvenile chronic arthritis (Royle 1992).

Landin et al. (1987) note that their findings suggest that the risk of a child being affected by at least one episode of acute transient synovitis of the hip is 3% and that more males are affected by this condition. Furthermore, these investigators suggest that the risk of recurrence is 20 times greater than the risk of having a single episode, and that only 10% of all LCP disease is preceded by an attack of transient synovitis of the hip.

The aetiology of transient synovitis of the hip remains unknown. An effusion is often identified by ultrasound in many children. The pressure from such an effusion may be the causative agent of the pain associated with this condition. However, there are children with irritable hip who do not demonstrate hip joint effusions on ultrasound examination (Bickerstaff et al. 1990). In view of the self-limiting nature of this condition, the relief of pain through bed rest is generally the only intervention necessary.

Legg–Calve–Perthes (LCP) Disease

The child with LCP disease generally presents with a painful limp and limitation of hip movements, especially internal rotation and abduction. Although the aetiology of LCP is unclear, the disease process involves an avascular necrosis of the capital femoral epiphysis (Crutcher and Staheli 1992). It is, however, a self-limiting disorder. In milder forms of this disease, the femoral head heals without residual deformity and is completely contained within the acetabulum.

Significant secondary hip joint pathology can ensue when there has been extensive femoral head involvement and the head is subsequently flattened during the healing stage of this disease (Crutcher and Staheli 1992). Kamegaya et al. (1992) suggest that the position of the femoral head, rather than sphericity is extremely important for acetabular growth and remodelling after primary healing of LCP disease. These investigators note that subluxation of the hip during LCP disease will affect final acetabular coverage at skeletal maturity.

LCP disease can affect children of varying ages, but the prognosis of this condition is often unsatisfactory with onset in children >8 years (Willett et al. 1992). For example, Willett et al. (1992) note that their findings suggest that 59% of children with LCP disease recover well without intervention, but poor results are common when the disease has onset in older children. The treatment of choice for the older child and the child with severe LCP remains uncertain (Crutcher and Staheli 1992).

The varied treatment regimens of LCP disease are based on the principle of femoral head containment and maintenance of hip motion. Non-operative containment methods include bed rest, traction, abduction orthosis or casts, whereas operative containment interventions include a varus or varus-derotational osteotomy of the proximal femur and/or an innominate osteotomy and an augmentation lateral shelf acetabuloplasty (Crutcher and Staheli 1992, Willett

et al. 1992). Generally, non-operative containment methods are selected for the younger child and for those children with less severe disease. Operative containment is viewed as the most appropriate course of action for the older child and for those patients with severe disease (Crutcher and Staheli 1992).

Coates et al. (1990) report that results of operative intervention (femoral osteotomy) for severe LCP disease in children aged 5 years and over at the time of diagnosis showed excellent clinical function at skeletal maturity. These investigators note that such results are considerably better than those obtained by non-operative methods. In children under 5 years femoral osteotomy procedures had poor long-term results when compared with hips treated conservatively.

The older child and the child with severe LCP disease will often present to the physiotherapist for a functional assessment and rehabilitation programme. Operative procedures can cause a number of musculoskeletal problems. For example, the proximal femoral osteotomy can result in weakness of hip abductor muscles and limb shortening thereby causing a limp. Furthermore, postoperative joint stiffness is a disadvantage of an innominate osteotomy (Crutcher and Staheli 1992). Although Coates et al. (1990) suggest that shortening of the limb can be seen as a consequence of the LCP disease itself, the child's asymmetrical gait should be addressed within the physiotherapist's comprehensive functional assessment of the child. Often the child may demonstrate only 1.5 cm of real limb shortening and 2.5 cm of apparent shortening due to hip hitching. A heel raise for the shortened limb may not be necessary if the physiotherapist instigates muscle retraining and postural realignment procedures and corrects the apparent shortening.

Furthermore, because active movement plays an essential role in the shaping of joints, the physiotherapist should address the associated musculoskeletal problems of LCP disease, such as hip stiffness and weakness of hip abductor muscles, with active movement within pain-free limits. Hydrotherapy is an excellent medium for the child with significant weakness and limitation of range-of-motion of the hip, as the warmth and buoyancy of the water can significantly facilitate active movement by reducing pain and fear-related muscle spasm. Muscle strengthening and gait retraining is often most effectively undertaken in the pool as the water can provide dynamic resistance. Hydrotherapy is very beneficial for the psychosocial development of the child with severe LCP disease as he / she will be able to undertake functional activities of walking and skipping and running much more freely and effectively in the pool and thereby regain confidence in functional abilities. A daily home programme consisting of a number of exercises which will increase hip strength and control should also be provided.

Slipped Capital Femoral Epiphysis (SCFE)

SCFE describes a displacement of the femoral neck from the capital femoral epiphysis which remains in the acetabulum. It is relatively rare, but it is one of the most common hip disorders in adolescence. Large adolescent males are more prone to this disorder (Cooperman et al. 1992).

Individuals with SCFE are classified as having either acute or chronic slips according to their symptomatology. For example, the slip is considered acute, if the child presents with a sudden onset of severe pain in the hip, with characteristic radiographic findings (Boyer et al. 1981). The slip is classified as chronic if the symptoms had a gradual or acute onset which persisted for several days with accompanying radiographic signs of periosteal new-bone formation (Aronson and Carlson 1992).

Acute and chronic SCFE are generally treated with in situ pinning. Single-pin fixation of SCFE is shown to provide adequate epiphyseal stability and promote premature physeal fusion with very little complications (Blanco et al. 1992, Ward et al. 1992). Postoperatively, the physiotherapist will instruct the patient on toe touch weight-bearing with crutches. The patient will then gradually progress to full weight-bearing ambulation over the next 6 weeks (Blanco et al. 1992).

Osteomyelitis / Septic Arthritis

Clinical symptoms of a limp or a refusal to bear weight in children may indicate infection. Ward et al. (1992)

note that only one-third of their study children with osteomyelitis of the calcaneum had systemic symptoms with pyrexia and very rarely was there evidence of a puncture wound. These investigators emphasize the importance of early diagnosis for osteomyelitis, as treatment with antibiotics alone is usually effective, but, if there is delay, complications and chronic disease are more likely to ensue.

Smoot et al. (1993) note that septic arthritis often follows establishment of a focus of metaphyseal osteomyelitis. Furthermore, these investigators suggest the hip joint in children is the most common site of septic involvement. Bacterial infections can also invade vertebrae, disc spaces and sacroiliac joints (Schaller 1984). The physiotherapist should immediately refer the child with a limp or a reluctance to weight-bear for medical assessment to exclude the possibility of infection.

Skeletal Injury – Fractures

Musculoskeletal trauma undoubtedly can result in the child complaining of pain and tenderness and demonstrating an acute loss of function. Indeed, a comprehensive history and radiographic findings will often quickly establish the cause of such symptomatology. The child who does not always appreciate the potential risks associated with his / her activities is extremely susceptible to traumatic injury. For example, falls causing femoral shaft fractures are particularly common in the young child (0–4 years), whereas forearm fractures are most common in the older child (10–14 years). Interestingly, Nafei et al. (1992) suggest that such trends in the type of childhood fractures may be due to the varying motor skills of children. For example, the young child may have unprotected falls as a result of incompletely developed protective reactions, whereas falls by the older child will more likely result in forearm injury due to falling on an outstretched arm. Fractures will have to be reduced if there is displacement, angulation or rotation of fracture fragments, and then immobilized. Femoral shaft fractures in children are treated via traction, spica casting or external fixation (Aronson and Tursky 1992). Generally there are minimal complications with such fractures. In contrast, fractures of the neck of femur, although uncommon in children, can be associated with considerable complications, such as avascular necrosis, non-union, premature physeal closure, chondrolysis and coxa vara (Forlin et al. 1992). Similarly, fractures of the radial neck in children are often associated with complications such as avascular necrosis and radial head enlargement. Complications often arise because the injury frequently involves the epiphyseal growth plate which can cause subsequent growth disturbances (D'souza et al. 1993). Alpar and Owen (1988) report that 15% of skeletal injuries involve damage to the growth plate which can cause subsequent growth disturbances. Since premature closure of the epiphysis and non-union are particularly common if there is delay in anatomic reduction and rigid internal fixation, the physiotherapist should always advise immediate medical assessment in cases of childhood trauma.

The physiotherapist involved with children who have sustained skeletal injury such as fractures should be aware of the potential risk of compartmental syndromes in children. The increased tissue pressure within a limited space compromises the circulation, function and the viability of the contents of the affected space. Any type of circumferential dressing, such as a cast may limit the space available to swelling tissues and thus exacerbate an increase in tissue pressure (Matsen and Veith 1981).

Clinical signs of compartmental syndrome may include pain out of proportion to the clinical situation, weakness, muscle pain on passive stretch and hypesthesia in the distribution of the nerves running through the compartment. The younger patient, however, is often unable to cooperate in the evaluation of muscle strength and sensation. If concerned, the physiotherapist should act quickly and notify medical staff as the child may require cast division and surgical decompression (Matsen and Veith 1981).

Malignancy – Bone Tumours

Although bone tumours account for a very small percentage of children presenting with musculoskeletal pain, the physiotherapist should be aware of this sinister condition. Pain is a predominant presenting complaint in paediatric cancer, particularly Ewing's sarcoma and osteosarcoma (Zeltzer and Zeltzer

1989). Although osteogenic sarcoma can occur in any age group, approximately 50% of the cases occur in the second decade and males are more frequently affected than females. The metaphyses of long bones are the usual sites of this common malignant tumour of bone, such as distal femur, proximal tibia, proximal humerus and proximal femur (Lane and Boland 1986).

The symptomatology associated with malignant bone tumours is variable. Some patients do not complain of any symptoms until a traumatic episode causes pain that does not subside, whereas other patients complain of a dull, aching constant pain that gradually worsens (Gebhardt et al. 1990). Clues to possible malignancy include severe joint or bone pain, pain at rest and swelling of either joints or bones (Schaller 1984). When the tumour is situated in the lower limb, a reluctance to weight-bear, atrophy of musculature and knee flexion contracture may also be evident (Gebhardt et al. 1990).

Current treatment of osteogenic sarcoma involves removal of the primary tumour and administration of adjuvant multiagent chemotherapy (Gebhardt et al. 1990). Advances in chemotherapy and orthopaedic surgical techniques such as limb salvage en-bloc resection (where removed portion of bone is replaced by an endoprosthesis) have significantly improved the functional abilities of many patients (Lane and Boland 1986). Furthermore, en-bloc procedures offer superior appearance, which is especially relevant for the older child's self-image (Krebs et al. 1991). Amputation is still the operative procedure of choice when there is neurovascular and skin involvement, pathological fracture and an inability to achieve a reasonable cuff around the tumour (Lane and Boland 1986).

The physiotherapist will be closely involved in the rehabilitation programme for such patients and management for a child with an acquired/congenital limb deficiency is discussed later in this chapter. The child and adolescent who has undergone surgical amputation of a limb because of malignancy generally requires considerable psychosocial support during the physiotherapy programme. Most often the child experiences not only pain related to the malignant disease, but also treatment-related pain. Children with malignant tumours require age-appropriate information about their disease, treatment and sources of pain and discomfort to enable both child and parents to cope and successfully participate in the rehabilitation programme (Varni *et al.* 1989). Furthermore, significant physical and psychological adjustments will have to be made by the patient who has undergone amputation or reconstruction following en-bloc resection. Unlike the child with congenital limb deficiency whose training of functional motor skills and acceptance of limitations was initiated in infancy, the child with amputation postmalignancy will generally have to adapt to a profound change in functional performance (Pizzutilo 1989).

Juvenile Chronic Arthritis (JCA)/ Juvenile Rheumatoid Arthritis

As suggested above, there are numerous conditions, such as infectious diseases, childhood malignancies and non-inflammatory musculoskeletal lesions, which must be excluded before a diagnosis of JCA is made (Schaller 1984). Furthermore, in view of the heterogeneous nature of JCA the physiotherapist managing a child with chronic synovitis must initially consider the specific type of this disease with which the child presents. The distinct subgroups of JCA – systemic onset disease, rheumatoid factor-negative polyarthritis, rheumatoid factor-positive polyarthritis, pauciarthritis associated with chronic iridiocyclitis (type I), pauciarthritis associated with sacroilitis (type II) – are made on clinical, epidemiological and immunogenetic grounds (Schaller 1984).

SYSTEMIC ONSET JCA

This form of JCA affects boys and girls equally and can occur at any age during childhood. The child presents with high intermittent fevers for a number of consecutive weeks and an evanescent rash, occurring anywhere on their body commonly becoming evident during the febrile periods (Schaller 1984). Pericarditis, hepatosplenomegaly and lymphadenopathy can also develop in this systemic onset disease (Rhodes 1991). These systemic manifestations are dramatic, but rarely fatal. Nearly all children with this systemic onset JCA also have accompanying musculoskeletal complaints which are particularly pronounced during febrile periods (Schaller 1984).

Within the first few months of the disease, a polyarthritis develops in nearly all patients and 25% of such children will develop an unremitting destructive polyarthritis (Schaller 1984). Systemic onset JCA is associated with significant hip involvement which eventually results in poor functional capacity (Jacobsen *et al.* 1992).

RHEUMATOID FACTOR-NEGATIVE POLYARTICULAR JCA

This symmetric polyarthritis affects predominantly girls and, although it may begin at any age during childhood, it often occurs in young children. The small joints of the hands are the most characteristic joint involvement, but knees, ankles, elbows and feet are affected in the majority of children and severe hip disease is a major cause of late disability. The majority of patients ultimately do well, as severe destructive arthritis occurs in only 10–15% of patients (Schaller 1984).

RHEUMATOID FACTOR-POSITIVE POLYARTICULAR JCA

There is a preponderance of females with this form of JCA, and the symptoms present almost always in late childhood. Subcutaneous rheumatoid nodules are frequently present. It is often described as the childhood equivalent of classic adult rheumatoid arthritis, as severe destructive arthritis occurs in the majority of children with this particular subgroup of JCA (Schaller 1984).

PAUCIARTICULAR JCA (TYPE I)

The child needs to have arthritic involvement of four or fewer joints to be assigned the classification of a pauciarticular JCA. There is a preponderance of girls in pauciarticular JCA (type I) and the children are usually young at onset (5 years or younger). These patients rarely have hip or back involvement and, although arthritis may be long-lasting, the prognosis for ultimate joint function is good. During the first 10 years of the disease a number of children (30–35%) will develop chronic iridocyclitis (chronic eye inflammation). Early recognition and treatment of this complication is essential to the preservation of vision (Schaller 1984).

PAUCIARTICULAR JCA (TYPE II)

This type of JCA generally begins later in childhood and there is a predominance of boys. The disease often only affects the lower limb joints. Radiographic sacroilitis is often present either at disease onset or at follow-up evaluation (Schaller 1984).

Physiotherapy Management / JCA

The physiotherapist plays a significant role in the team management of the child with JCA. Indeed, Rhodes (1991) highlights this role, by suggesting that the physiotherapist's assessment of the child's pain, swelling, range of movement (ROM), muscle strength and mobility are critical in determining the overall benefits of team management and are essential in goal setting and treatment planning. The physiotherapy intervention for a child with JCA will address both acute and long-term issues and will focus on educating child and parents as to the most appropriate care of involved joints.

During an acute stage of this disease process, the physiotherapist will assess the child's musculoskeletal system and identify the child's major problems. Symptomatic relief of joint pain, stiffness and swelling is achieved in a vast majority of children through anti-inflammatory medication, which include salicylates and other non-steroidal anti-inflammatory drugs (Schaller 1984). There are second-line drugs (remitting agents or slow-acting or disease-modifying anti-rheumatic drugs) to control synovitis in those children who do not respond to salicylates or non-steroidal agents (Rhodes 1991).

Through the use of various techniques, such as positioning, splinting and active-assistive, active and gentle passive functional ranging of joints, the physiotherapist will also attempt to relieve pain, prevent loss of ROM and maintain muscle strength and functional joint positioning and the most optimal level of function. At all times, the physiotherapist will monitor the child during these exercises and watch for any signs of the child fatiguing or the child's symptoms increasing (Rhodes 1991). These exercises should not

Figure 2 Limited Range of Motion of Joints in a Child with JCA (Systemic Onset)

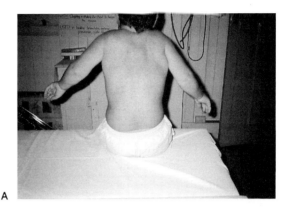

A

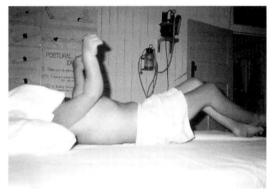

B

be painful (Rhodes 1991). Figure 2 shows the limited ROM of joints in a child with JCA.

Short hydrotherapy sessions are very effective treatments for the child in an acute stage of JCA. The warmth and buoyancy can assist in the relief of pain and facilitate relaxation of protective muscle spasm. The child can also maintain flexibility of joints, as the environment is conducive to gentle ranging of joints. Furthermore, the child's functional performance can often be sustained as the gentle active exercises can maintain the child's muscle strength and fitness. Giannini and Protas (1992) note that results of their study indicate that deconditioning occurs in children with JCA regardless of the severity of the disease. These investigators suggest that aerobic conditioning programmes are indicated for children with JCA in order to improve their exercise capacity and that intervention should occur soon after diagnosis to prevent the cycle of hypoactivity and deconditioning that commonly occurs.

Once the acute stage of the disease process is resolved, the physiotherapist will reassess the child and most likely reprioritize the child's problems. The child's gait will be particularly closely evaluated. Significantly, Lechner et al. (1987) describe a number of gait deviations in populations of children with JCA. Their findings suggest that subjects with JCA walk with significantly decreased velocity, cadence and stride length. They note that reduced velocity and cadence may be due to stiff sluggish joints and that the decreased stride length may relate to decreased hip extension and decreased plantarflexion at the end of stance phase. Undoubtedly, the physiotherapist should address these gait anomalies within the child's exercise programme. Often hydrotherapy is an effective medium to address such problems as the warmth facilitates relaxation of muscle spasm and flexibility of soft tissues and the buoyancy of the water will assist in encouraging greater velocity of movement.

Lechner et al. (1987) also note that many children with JCA consistently appear to demonstrate an increased anterior pelvic tilt postural deviation. They suggest that hip flexor tightness and abdominal muscle weakness are contributing factors to this postural deviation. The physiotherapist therefore needs to incorporate in the long-term management of the child with JCA, functional joint positioning (such as prone lying for periods each day) and introduce into the child's rehabilitation a strengthening programme, such as upper and lower abdominal muscle strengthening. During the chronic stage of the disease, progressive resistive exercises should be included so as to improve the child's functional mobility and fitness. The physiotherapist will also encourage a child to participate in recreational activities, such as general swimming and bicycling, to improve functional performance and socialization.

The physiotherapist will not only play a significant role in educating the child and family about the long-term management of JCA, but should also consult with the child's school-teacher and emphasize the importance of supporting the child's rehabilitation. The physiotherapist should particularly suggest that the child with JCA be included in physical education classes, even if his / her activities are slightly modified, so as to prevent social isolation.

Haemophilia

The physiotherapist involved in the management of children with musculoskeletal problems should be aware that the child with haemophilia may present with significant musculoskeletal morbidity. In recent decades significant advancements have been made in the management of the X-linked recessive bleeding disorders, haemophilia A and B. For example, Smith et al. (1989) note that modern substitution treatment / home therapy (the intravenous infusion of factor replacement) which temporarily replaces the missing clotting factor and thereby converts the haemophiliac's clotting status to normal and allows a functional blood clot to form, has improved the quality and length of life of such individuals. There are boys with severe haemophilia (particularly those children with an inhibitor to factor replacement), however, who still do not reach adulthood with normal joints (Matsuda and Duthie 1984).

Kim et al. (1984) describe acute haemarthrosis as the most constant feature in patients with haemophilia. Recurrent bleeds into the same joint often progress to a chronic arthropathy characterized by persistent joint effusion, chronic synovitis, cartilage destruction, arthritic pain and impaired function. Haemophilic arthropathy occurs most frequently in the knee, elbow, ankle, shoulder, hip and wrist (Kim et al. 1984). See Figure 3.

Synovial hypertrophy is often associated with recurrent joint bleeds in some haemophiliacs (Wiedel 1984), but, Greenan-Fowler et al. (1987) suggest that atrophy of supporting musculature causes further susceptibility to joint haemorrhage. Koch et al. (1982) similarly note that quadriceps muscle atrophy, which often accompanies haemophilic arthropathy, causes instability of the knee joint and hastens the development of joint destruction.

MacDonald et al. (1990) describe soft tissue involvement in haemophilic arthropathy, by suggesting that rotator cuff tears and impingement symptoms are an important manifestation of haemophilic arthropathy of the shoulder.

The musculoskeletal problems associated with haemophilia are also complicated by recurrent bleeds

Figure 3 A Child with Haemophilic Arthropathy of Elbow (A) and Knee (B)

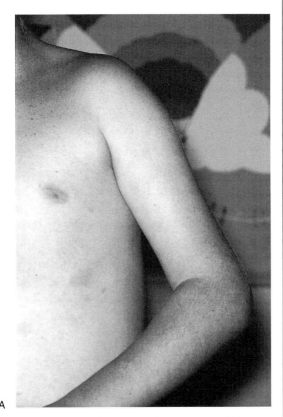

A

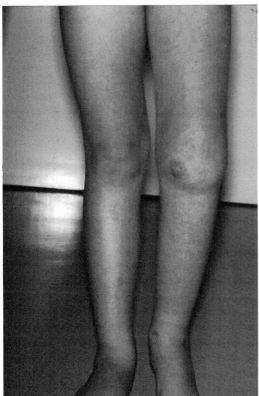

B

into muscle which can develop into muscle haematomas. If such muscle haematomas occur within a confined space (iliacus sheath) a compression or traction injury to nerves may ensue (for example, femoral palsy). This chapter will later discuss the necessary physiotherapy management of such neuropathy.

Not surprisingly, the child with severe haemophilia will often present with a complex history of pain. Such complexity is due to the fact that he will experience both a recurrent acute pain associated with specific bleeding episodes and chronic arthritic and varying soft tissue pains due to haemophilic arthropathy and muscle atrophy. Most importantly, the acute pain of haemorrhage provides a functional signal indicating the necessity for an intravenous infusion of factor replacement. The chronic pain represents a potentially debilitating condition which may result in impaired life functioning and analgesic dependence (Varni et al. 1989).

Haemophilia is not only associated with significant physical problems. Psychological and social difficulties are also often apparent with this condition (Matsuda and Duthie 1984). Mattisson (1984) suggest that considerable psychosocial stress factors accompany haemophilia and notes that boys with haemophilia run a higher than average risk of developing adjustment problems.

The physiotherapist must be sensitive to the psychosocial stresses of the young child and his family, particularly as the physiotherapist plays a significant role in the team management of the child with haemophilia. For example, the physiotherapist must be aware that children and their parents may be very anxious when physiotherapy is commenced after a period of immobilization due to haemorrhagic episode. The child and parents may perceive that exercise will trigger further bleeds. It is extremely important for the therapist to inspire confidence and enthusiasm in their patients and their family and this can only be achieved if the therapist is fully congnizant of the nature of the disease and the varied problems associated with this condition.

Physiotherapy Management of Musculoskeletal Problems associated with Haemophilia

PHYSIOTHERAPY AFTER ACUTE BLEEDING EPISODES

As noted previously, an acute pain will signal to the child a bleeding episode. Immediate substitution therapy and rest should resolve this bleed quickly. The physiotherapist would instruct child and parents to use ice if an involved joint is swollen and tender. Once the joint has settled, isometric exercises of surrounding musculature can be commenced so as to decrease the potential for muscle atrophy.

Hydrotherapy can be an effective medium to encourage active movement of affected joint / limb and assist in reducing fear-related muscle spasm. Furthermore, this buoyant environment is an excellent medium in which to recommence weight-bearing. Passive range of movement exercises should be avoided in this population of children as recurrent bleeding may occur. Greenan-Fowler et al. (1987) suggest that the physiotherapist should not have any difficulties in gaining patient and parents compliance to this treatment regimen after acute bleed as the relatively immediate improvement in function which occurs after an acute bleed serves as a powerful intrinsic reinforcer for both the child and family.

PHYSIOTHERAPY FOR LONG-TERM MANAGEMENT

The physiotherapist's management of the child with haemophilia must include a comprehensive home exercise programme. Several studies highlight why such a home exercise programme for the haemophilic child is essential. For example, Strickler and Greene (1984) demonstrated a profound decrease in strength of knee extensor and flexor musculature in patients with severe haemophilia. Their findings emphasized the need to maintain full knee extension and optimal muscle strength in patients with haemophilic arthropathy as muscle weakness may perpetuate a cycle of vulnerability to stress and progressive joint destruction. Greene and Strickler (1983) suggest that significant strengthening of knee extensors and flexors can

be accomplished by a home programme of modified isokinetic strengthening exercises.

Furthermore, Koch et al. (1984) suggest that the physical fitness / exercise performance of haemophilic children is subnormal due to a lack of physical conditioning. These investigators suggest that physical fitness is not only important for a haemophiliac child's physical well-being, but is also important for his emotional development. Hence, they recommend individual exercise prescriptions to improve fitness of children with haemophilia.

Greenan-Fowler et al. (1987) note that simply prescribing a routine exercise regimen for children with haemophilia is not sufficient to obtain a high level of long-term adherence, particularly as the exercise regimen may be required primarily to prevent further morbidity and may not have immediate beneficial results. These investigators suggest that one approach for programming long-term maintenance of home exercise regimen may involve a greater emphasis upon parental participation and social reinforcement during mutual exercise in a convenient setting.

The physiotherapist should also encourage the child with haemophilia to participate in recreational activities, such as swimming, bicycling and non-contact sports. These activities are important for strengthening as well as maintaining physical endurance and flexibility. Most importantly, such recreational activites are fun and promote a more positive attitude to physical activity.

Other Childhood Musculoskeletal Conditions

Peripheral Neuropathy

Peripheral neuropathy is a relatively uncommon condition during childhood (Lagos 1971). The physiotherapist plays a significant role both in the education of the care of the paralysed / weak and / or anaesthetic / paraesthetic limb and in the active rehabilitation. For example, the physiotherapist highlights to the patient and their parents the importance of preventing the development of pressure areas, maintaining the extensibility of soft tissues and preventing joint malalignment. If and when the neuropathy resolves, the physiotherapist will instigate an appropriate active exercise regimen for the individual child and assist in the reacquisition of their movement skills and functional ability. The child may present with a slowly progressive neuropathy such as peroneal muscular atrophy (Charcot–Marie–Tooth disease/hereditary motor and sensory neuropathy). In this instance, the physiotherapist will be involved in assessing the value of supportive othotics for the feet in order to improve postural alignment and gait pattern, addressing pain issues and assisting the child to participate in activities which will maintain their fitness and facilitate their sense of well-being. Hence, although peripheral neuropathy does not commonly occur during childhood, the potential problems associated with this condition make it imperative that the physiotherapist is familiar with various forms of neuropathy in children.

Guillain–Barré syndrome (GBS)

Lagos (1971) describes GBS as the most common form of neuropathy affecting children. This inflammatory peripheral neuropathy is generally viewed as a post-infectious neuronitis, as approximately two-thirds of cases follow a viral infection (Ropper 1992). This acute disease generally results in progressive symmetrical paralysis beginning in the lower limbs and ascending to and sometimes including the cranial nerves (Pitetti et al. 1993). Paraesthesias in the toes and fingertips and pain, such as aching in the large muscles of the legs or back is commonly associated with this polyneuropathy. Conduction block in motor nerves is responsible for the weakness associated with this syndrome and spontaneous discharges in demyelinated sensory nerves probably cause the paraesthesias and pain (Ropper 1992).

In severe cases this neuropathy can cause respiratory and autonomic difficulties. The physiotherapist often initally becomes involved with the child with GBS because of his/her poor cough and the accumulation of secretions. Although the illness may be less severe in children than in adults, the child may require full ventilation if his/her vital capacity declines dramatically. Medical treatment now includes plasma exchange and infusion of gamma globulin (Ropper 1992).

The weakness associated with this neuropathy generally stops advancing in 1–3 weeks and slowly improves after a plateau phase lasting several weeks. The physiotherapy management goals for such children therefore include: (1) maintaining respiratory status through the removal of excess secretions and facilitation of greater air entry, (2) prevention of pressure areas, (3) relief of musculoskeletal pains (through the use of splint/positioning to achieve the most functional joint position, (4) preservation of joint motion, and (5) graduated active strengthening of affected musculature once the child enters the plateau stage of the disease. Hydrotherapy is useful for gait retraining and aerobic conditioning.

Polyneuropathy

Polyneuropathy in childhood may result from metabolic, toxic or degenerative disorders (Lagos 1971). For example, Swaiman and Flagler (1971) describe central and peripheral nervous system involvement in a child due to mercury poisoning. The presentation was one of diffuse weakness, particularly proximally, absent tendon reflexes and unsteady gait. The child with a thiamine deficiency may similarly present with a polyneuropathy. Hence, although such polyneuropathies during childhood are rare, the physiotherapist should be aware of their existence and the need to prevent secondary complications as listed above.

Peroneal Muscular Atrophy/ Hereditary Motor and Sensory Neuropathy (HSMN)

As noted earlier, peroneal muscular atrophy/hereditary motor and sensory neuropathy (HSMN) is a slowly progressive degenerative familial peripheral neuropathy, primarily affecting the peripheral nerves, posterior root ganglia and the axons of the anterior horn cell. Unlike motor neurone disease or Werdnig–Hoffman disease, the muscle spindles of affected muscle groups in peroneal muscular atrophy are abnormal, suggesting that there is both afferent and efferent denervation of the spindle fibres (Hughes and Brownell 1972). HSMN is clinically divided into types I and II due to differing areas of degeneration of the peripheral nervous system. HSMN type I is the most commonly observed in the young paediatric population. The child with HSMN type I is often initially detected because of foot deformity such as an abnormally high instep (pes cavus), toe walking or clumsiness with frequent falls, and difficulty walking on heels (Ouvrier et al. 1990). The physiotherapist should consider the possibility of such a peripheral neuropathy when assessing the clumsy child.

The child with HSMN type I generally demonstrates much weaker ankle dorsiflexors and evertors than plantarflexors initially, but the plantarflexors gradually weaken and the child subsequently finds it difficult to undertake any propulsive activities or to maintain static standing balance. Undoubtedly, the child's diminished tactile, proprioceptive and kinaesthetic appreciation in the foot and the ankle joint complex further compromises balance reactions. The physiotherapist must therefore undertake a comprehensive neurological and musculoskeletal assessment of the child with HSMN type I, particularly addressing gait anomalies. Shoe inserts may be helpful in providing a more functional alignment of the foot, but one must consider that the ankle musculature is weak and that the added weight of an orthotic may further compromise their gait pattern.

The physiotherapist may introduce the child to hydrotherapy, particularly if the child is complaining of painful feet, as the warmth and buoyancy of the water may provide some relief. Hydrotherapy is very beneficial for the psychosocial development as the buoyancy will often enable the child to undertake functional activities of walking and skipping and running much more freely in the pool. Swimming activities can assist in developing aerobic fitness and increasing/maintaining the muscle strength of unaffected muscle groups.

The child with HSMN type I may also demonstrate wasting and weakness of the small muscles of the hands (Hughes and Brownell 1972). Such weakness may become a functional problem when the child is spending a lot of time at school writing and cannot keep up with peers. The physiotherapist may become involved by providing child, parents and teacher with advice on the most efficient sitting posture and by making various adaptations to the pencil/pen so as to provide greater sensory input to the fingers and thumb. Furthermore, the child should be advised to take short rests when undertaking prolonged hand tasks.

Hereditary Neuralgic Amyotrophy with Brachial Predilection/Idiopathic Brachial Plexus Neuropathy

The physiotherapist should be aware of a familial form of brachial neuropathy which has a tendency to present during childhood. For example, Dunn et al. (1978) describe three young children (age range 4 years to 7 years 10 months) who presented with recurrent episodes of pain in shoulders and arms followed by weakness and wasting of affected muscles. Intervention included analgesics and physiotherapy and there was a gradual recovery.

The individual with idiopathic brachial plexus neuropathy similarly presents with a sudden onset of pain around the shoulder and the development of weakness and wasting of pericapsular muscles. There may also be areas of cutaneous sensory loss. The prognosis is generally good, but recovery may be protracted (Schott 1983). In view of the protracted time span for recovery it is essential that the physiotherapist instigate care of the affected limb, particularly maintaining the extensibility of soft tissues.

Schott (1983) also reports of an atypical form of brachial plexus neuropathy, whereby affected individuals may present with weakness and wasting of musculature, but with no evidence of pain. Serious conditions, such as poliomyelitis and motor neurone disease, should always be considered in a patient with muscle weakness without sensory impairment (Schott 1983).

Mononeuropathy Secondary to Compression/Trauma

Compression neuropathy occurs infrequently in children, but because of the superficial locations of the peroneal, radial, median and ulnar nerves, these particular nerves are susceptible to injury (Lagos 1971). For example, Weiss *et al.* (1992) report on a number of children with peroneal nerve palsy following early hip spica cast treatment for femoral shaft fractures. All palsies resolved on removal of casts. Crossed-leg sitting has also been involved in compression injury to the common peroneal nerve. Lagos (1971) reports of a child presenting with sudden onset of an inability to dorsiflex her (L) foot. Needle electrode examination indicated a block to motor conduction of the peroneal nerve at the level of the head of the fibula. The child sat for long periods of time with her (L) leg crossed over the (R) leg. This sitting posture was discouraged and the muscle weakness disappeared within 4 months. Berry and Richardson (1976) similarly note that the prognosis is generally very good once compression of the common peroneal nerve is relieved.

Carpal tunnel syndrome is the most common of entrapment neuropathies, but it appears to be an uncommon condition during childhood. Sainio *et al.* 1987 report on three teenage girls who presented with pain and numbness in third and fourth fingers and paraesthesia which woke them at night. Electrodiagnostic findings indicated a blocking of the median nerve at the carpal tunnel and they responded well to surgical decompression. Furthermore, Hartz *et al.* (1981) report on a group of people, including children, with pronator teres syndrome, a compressive neuropathy of the median nerve in the arm and forearm. Symptoms of such a neuropathy included aching discomfort in the forearm, weakness in the hand and numbness in the thumb and index finger. Surgical decompression of the median nerve relieved these symptoms in the majority of patients (Hartz *et al.* 1981).

Nerve lesions in children can also occur as a complication of fractures, such as supracondylar fractures of the humerus. Spinner and Schreiber (1969) suggest that in addition to the median nerve being traumatized at the fracture site, a traction injury of the anterior interosseous nerve may occur. The patients with such a traction injury display loss of flexion power of the index finger and distal phalanx of the thumb. These investigators report that spontaneous recovery in all their patients occurred within 6–8 weeks.

As noted earlier, particular muscle haematomas in the haemophilic child may cause a type of entrapment/compression/traction injury to various peripheral nerves. The child will receive substitution therapy which will rapidly resolve pain and bleeding, but the peripheral nerve may have been damaged because of the sudden increasing tension within the sheath of muscle. Neural recovery may take up to several months depending on the severity of the damage, so the physiotherapist must instigate a specific treatment regimen to care for the denervated joints and muscles. Furthermore, in view of this child's potential for significant chronic arthropathy, the physiotherapist will organize frequent hydrotherapy sessions and emphasize to the child and parents the absolute necessity for a daily home exercise programme.

Hence, the physiotherapist who often assesses children because of symptoms of pain and weakness should be ever alert to the possibility of neuropathy in children. Furthermore, s/he must be aware that neuropathy during childhood can have deleterious effects upon the developing musculoskeletal system. Indeed, appropriate treatment measures must be quickly instigated to prevent or at least decrease the potential for these musculoskeletal problems to occur. The physiotherapist is also an essential health worker in the rehabilitation and management of the child with long-term (for example, degenerative) neuropathy.

The Young Child with Limb Deficiencies

As noted in the previous chapter, the greater proportion of paediatric limb reductions are due to perinatal events. For example, Krebs and Fishman (1984) describe congenital limb deficiencies outnumbering acquired losses by a ratio of 2:1. However, these investigators note that among unilateral cases, there are greater numbers of lower limb amputations acquired postpartum than congenitally. A prosthetic clinic, which is supported by a team of workers, such as a paediatrician, surgeon, prosthetist, physiotherapist, occupational therapist and social worker, can

Figure 4 An Adolescent Girl with Lower Limb Deficiency (Acquired Amputation) with Prosthesis Off (A) and On (B)

Figure 5 A Young Schoolgirl with Multiple Congenital Limb Deficiencies Mobilizing with Prostheses

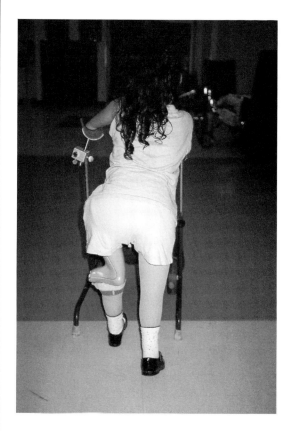

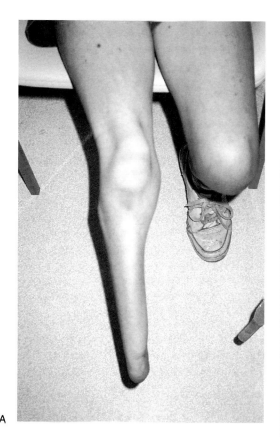

A

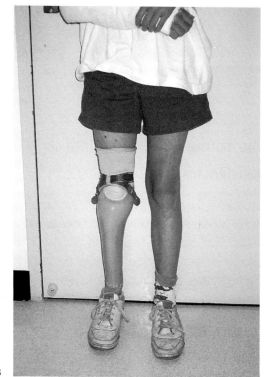

B

provide a most effective and comprehensive rehabilitation for a child with limb deficiency.

An extremely important role of the physiotherapist involved in the rehabilitation programme of a child with limb deficiency is that of educator. For example, children and their parents often ask about the amount of functional ability they will be able to achieve (particularly those children and parents with an acquired amputation). A most effective way for the physiotherapist to provide answers to such questions is to arrange for the child and parents to visit the clinic to meet and talk with other children with a similar deficiency who are mobilizing effectively with their prosthesis and participating in recreational activities. See Figures 4–6.

The previous chapter concentrated particularly on the neurodevelopmental preprosthetic physiotherapy goals for the neonate and young child with congenital limb deficiency. The physiotherapist will continue to facilitate postural and balance reactions

Figure 6 A Schoolgirl with a Congenital Upper Limb Deficiency

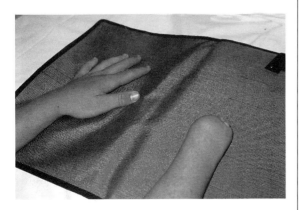

Figure 7 Parents and Child Must Inspect Residuum for Skin Breakdown

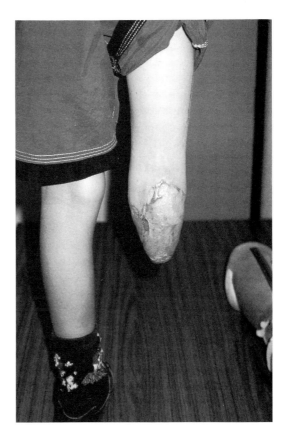

and encourage developmental and age-appropriate sensorimotor experiences for the older child with an acquired or congenital limb deficiency. The physiotherapy regimen for such children will also consider biomechanical issues so as to ensure that the child's functional abilities are most efficiently executed.

Acquired Amputation

The physiotherapist participates in the total management of the child with an acquired amputation. For example, he/she will initially instruct the child (if old enough) and parents on effective stump bandaging. The parents and child are also taught to regularly inspect the residuum (stump) for skin healing/pressure areas (Figure 7).

Furthermore, the physiotherapist will emphasize the importance of preventing various joint contractures and optimizing muscle function. For example, to prevent hip and/or knee flexion contractures prone lying is encouraged and prolonged sitting is discouraged. The child with above-knee amputation (AKA) is specifically instructed to avoid positions of hip flexion, abduction and external rotation as this posture aggravates the amputation-induced muscle imbalance and thereby places the hip extensors and adductors at an even greater disadvantage (Peoples 1989).

Once wound healing is achieved, the child with an acquired amputation can be fitted with a temporary prosthesis which allows for earlier gait acquisition/reacquisition (Krebs et al. 1991). Indeed, the physiotherapist plays an extremely important role in the

gait reeducation of the child with a prosthesis. The child generally acquires functional gait mobility quickly. It must be remembered that the prosthetic leg of the child with a BKA/AKA does not have any tactile, proprioceptive or kinaesthetic sense in the foot or a functioning ankle joint complex (Tedford et al. 1994). It is perhaps not surprising that the child with a lower limb prosthesis may have a less efficient gait pattern than the able-bodied child without limb deficiency.

The Gait Pattern of the Child with a Prosthesis

The physiotherapist should be aware of the potential for asymmetry to develop in the gait pattern of children with lower limb prostheses. Engsberg et al. (1991) highlight, for example, that within their population of children with BKA, the prosthetic limb generally displayed a subordinate role in external loading when compared to the non-prosthetic limb. These investigators suggest that such asymmetry may be due not only to the imposed morphology of the prosthesis, but also to abnormal muscular forces in the residual limb.

Engsberg et al. (1992) similarly emphasize significant differences in the gait pattern between able-bodied children and children with a BKA prosthesis. For example, these investigators note that the centre of mass (COM) in the sagittal plane was lower and more anterior for the children with a prosthesis when compared to that of AB children. Furthermore, the COM in the frontal plane tended to remain on the non-prosthetic side of the body for the children with a prosthesis during the entire gait cycle, whereas COM location of the able-bodied children moved from one side to the other. They suggest that such COM location differences between these populations of children are primarily due to the greater forward flexion of the trunk in the children with BKA and because the child with BKA leans the trunk towards the non-prosthetic side of the body.

The physiotherapist should be aware that gait deviations in the child with a lower limb prosthesis could be due to growth. Krebs et al. (1991) emphasize that maintaining the prosthesis equal to the length of the sound limb is extremely important to prevent the child from walking with excessive lateral trunk bending. A poor fit and malalignment of the prosthesis can affect the child's functional gait pattern.

Tedford et al. (1994) found that children with BKA in comparison to able-bodied children demonstrated significant differences in style of lower limb performance and static balance tests. They suggest that such differences may be due to the lack of function of the prosthesis and strength variations between the non-prosthetic and prosthetic legs. The physiotherapist who is rehabilitating the child with lower limb deficiency is challenged by findings that the lower limb prosthesis does not function in the same way as the leg of an able-bodied child.

The child with a lower limb deficiency will want to undertake the same functional abilities as their peers. The physiotherapist must attempt to provide the child with a rehabilitation programme that will include strength development and balance training.

Tedford et al. (1994) suggest that a physiotherapist should explore better methods to improve the child's prosthetic limb's proprioception and postural reactions. They note that leaning situations could be created to force the prosthetic side to become accustomed to balancing. The child will then have to make the required postural adjustments at more proximal joints (hip and knee).

The physiotherapist could introduce riding therapy into the rehabilitation regimen for the child with limb deficiency who demonstrates asymmetry within functional activities. In riding therapy, the child not only lets herself/himself be passively influenced by the movements of the horse's back (as in hippotherapy), but also actively performs individually prescribed physiotherapeutic exercises on the horse (Kuprian 1981). Heipertz (1981a) suggests that riding therapy particularly assists in the correction of the asymmetrical postural responses associated with the child with limb deficiency because the multidimensional movements of the horse's back facilitate symmetrical trunk movements through gentle alternate torsion forces acting upon the spine and encourage uniform pelvic tilts to both sides. The physiotherapist could further reinforce weight shift on to the side of the child's limb deficiency through various activities on the horse. Exercises can also be designed to strengthen weak musculature in the residuum (stump).

Riding therapy which can relax and stretch tight soft tissues, strengthen muscles, improve posture and coordination and confidence is an excellent complement to other physiotherapeutic treatment techniques. Riding therapy, however, must be individually prescribed so as to ensure the most appropriate intervention for the specific problems for each child. For example, the question of whether or not the child should wear a prosthesis during treatment on the horse must be judged on an individual basis (Heipertz 1981a). After 1 or 2 years of successful riding therapy some limb-deficient children can progress to riding as a sport. Such a sport can promote social integration and psychological development, particularly as the handicapped rider can be as good and in some cases even better than the non-handicapped rider (Heipertz 1981b).

Upper Limb Prostheses

The physiotherapist works in particularly close consultation with the prosthetist and occupational therapist when dealing with the child with upper limb deficiency. A major aim of the physiotherapy programme for such a child is to improve the muscle strength and endurance in the musculature of both the unaffected and affected upper limbs. Shaperman et al. (1992) and Leblanc et al. (1992) suggest that terminal devices (TD) demand adequate upper limb muscle strength to ensure their operating efficiency and functional use. The initial training of TD activation is a complex process and the physiotherapist, as an essential member of the rehabilitation team, will assist in encouraging the child to perform functional upper limb activities with the TD.

Limb Lengthening

The young child with a limb deficiency, such as a congenital deficiency of the fibula, may be managed by leg lengthening techniques (for example, Ilizarov technique) rather than amputation (Miller and Bell 1992). This technique will not only address the marked shortening, but also correct angular deformity of the affected extremity. There are a number of potential complications of Ilizarov method such as knee flexion contractures, and a physiotherapy programme is therefore essential for children undergoing leg lengthening.

The preoperative physiotherapy programme for the child undergoing Ilizarov leg lengthening includes the necessary baseline recording of ROM, muscle strength and functional mobility training. Postoperatively, the physiotherapist will introduce functional positioning and active exercises so as to maintain ROM of joints and muscle strength (Simard et al. 1992). Furthermore, it is essential for the physiotherapist to be aware that there is a prolongation of pain throughout the entire Ilizarov treatment of limb lengthening (Young et al. 1994). Indeed, Simard et al. (1992) similarly note that children who undergo the Ilizarov procedure require support in adjusting to the discomfort and change of lifestyle associated with this procedure.

Summary

This chapter addresses numerous issues which confront the physiotherapist managing the child with musculoskeletal problems. As suggested at the outset, a number of problems which are treated briefly will be explored more fully in the following chapter. There are other topics which have not been introduced, such as the physiotherapy management of soft tissue contractures following burns and post-surgical retraining following surgery in children with chronic conditions such as spina bifida and cerebral palsy. It is hoped that the problem-solving theme of this chapter will encourage the reader to address the child's problems rather than merely treat a musculoskeletal condition. Such an approach will enable the physiotherapist to instigate a much more competent treatment regimen for a child rather than for a condition.

Thought Provokers

- A 6-year-old boy was referred by his school teacher to a community-based physiotherapist because of his considerable clumsiness in the playground. This boy and his family have only recently moved to this city and have relocated many times during the last 2 years. Consider what actions the physiotherapist should instigate after establishing that the child has extensive burn scar contractures of the dorsum of his feet which are causing skeletal and functional deformities. It is now 4 years since this boy's burn injury, and the parents have not attended any follow-up burn clinics for 2 years, nor explored any medical advice. They do think that their son's scarring is more pronounced than it was one year ago (refer to Alison et al. 1993). After referring the child to the burn's unit for medical consultation, the physiotherapist emphasized to the parents and child that once relevant intervention for the musculoskeletal contracture had been addressed, she would be willing to reassess the child's functional performance and establish if there are any other problems which may be contributing to his difficulties in playground activities.

- A 10-year-old girl with spastic diplegia who mobilizes with assistance had bilateral hamstring muscle releases one month ago. The physiotherapist at this child's special school has been undertaking a gait retraining programme for this child. Consider what activities may be incorporated into this child's school programme so as to ensure that the newly gained range of motion at her knees is maintained.

REFERENCES

Alison, WE, Moore, ML, Reilly, A et al. (1993) Reconstruction of foot burn contractures in children. *Journal of Burn Care and Rehabilitation* 14: 34–38.

Alpar, EK, Owen, R (1988) General considerations and principles of management. In: Alpar, EK, Owen, R (eds) *Paediatric Trauma*, pp. 1–17. Kent: Castle House Publications.

Aronson, DD, Carlson, WE (1992) Slipped capital femoral epiphysis: a prospective study of fixation with a single screw. *Journal of Bone and Joint Surgery* 74A: 810–819.

Aronson, J, Tursky, EA (1992) External fixation of femur fractures in children. *Journal of Pediatric Orthopedics* 12: 157–163.

Barry, RJ, Scranton (1983) Flat feet in children. *Clinical Orthopaedics and Related Research* 181: 68–74.

Beck, CL, Burke, SW, Roberts, JM et al. (1987) Physeal bridge resection in infantile Blount disease. *Journal of Pediatric Orthopedics* 7: 161–163.

Bernhardt, DB (1988) Prenatal and postnatal growth and development of the foot and ankle. *Physical Therapy* 68(12): 1831–1839.

Berry, H, Richardson, PM (1976) Common peroneal nerve palsy: a clinical and electrophysiological review. *Journal of Neurology, Neurosurgery and Psychiatry* 39: 1162–1171.

Bickerstaf,f DR, Neal, LM, Booth, AJ et al. (1990) Ultrasound examination of the irritable hip. *Journal of Bone and Joint Surgery* 72B: 549–553.

Blanco, JS, Taylor, B, Johnston, CE (1992) Comparison of single pin versus multiple pin fixation treatment of slipped capital femoral epiphysis. *Journal of Pediatric Orthopedics* 12: 384–389.

Bleck, EE (1982) Developmental orthopaedics. III: Toddlers. *Developmental Medicine and Child Neurology* 24: 533–555.

Bordelon, RL (1983) Hypermobile flatfoot in children: comprehension, evaluation, and treatment. *Clinical Orthopaedics and Related Research* 181: 7–14.

Bowen, JR, Torres, RR, Forlin, E (1992) Partial epiphysiodesis to address genu varum or genu valgum. *Journal of Pediatric Orthopedics* 12: 359–364.

Boyer, DW, Mickelson, MR, Ponsetti, IV (1981) Slipped capital femoral epiphysis: long-term follow-up study of one hundred and twenty-one patients. *Journal of Bone and Joint Surgery* 63-A: 85–95.

Cheng, JCY, Chan, PS, Chiang, SC (1991a) Angular and rotational profile of the lower limb in 2,630 Chinese children. *Journal of Pediatric Orthopedics* 11: 154–161.

Cheng, JCY, Chan, PS, Hui, PW (1991b) Joint laxity in children. *Journal of Pediatric Orthopedics* 11: 752–756.

Coates, CJ, Paterson, JMH, Woods, KR et al. (1990) Femoral osteotomy in Perthes' disease: results at maturity. *Journal of Bone and Joint Surgery* 72B: 581–585.

Cooperman, DR, Charles, LM, Pathria, M et al. (1992) Post-mortem description of slipped capital femoral epiphysis. *Journal of Bone and Joint Surgery* 74b: 595–599.

Corradi-Scalise, D, Ling, W (1990) Normal development of gait. In: Donatelli R (ed.) *The Biomechanics of the Foot and Ankle*, pp. 66–81. Philadelphia: FA Davis Co.

Crutcher, JP, Staheli, LT (1992) Combined osteotomy as a salvage procedure for severe Legg–Calve–Perthes disease. *Journal of Pediatric Orthopedics* 12: 151–156.

Cusick, BD, Stuberg, WA (1992) Assessment of lower-extremity alignment in the transverse plane: implications for management of children with neuromotor dysfunction. *Physical Therapy* 72: 3–15.

Cusick, BD (1990) *Progressive Casting and Splinting for Lower Extremity Deformities in Children with Neuromotor Dysfunction*, 410 pp. Bellevue: Therapy Skill Builders.

D'souza, S, Vaishya, R, Klenerman, L (1993) Management of radial neck fractures in children: a retrospective analysis of one hundred patients. *Journal of Pediatric Orthopedics* 13: 232–238.

Dunn, HG, Daube, JR, Gomez, MR (1978) Heredofamilial brachial plexus neuropathy (heriditary neuralgic amyotrophy with brachial predilection) in childhood. *Developmental Medicine and Child Neurology* 20: 28–46.

Engsberg, JR, Lee, AG, Patterson, JL et al. (1991) External loading comparisons between able-bodied and below-knee-amputee children during walking. *Archives of Physical Medicine and Rehabilitation* 72: 657–661.

Engsberg, JR, Tedford, KG, Harder, JA (1992) Centre of mass location and segment angular orientation of below-knee-amputee and able-bodied children during walking. *Archives of Physical Medicine and Rehabilitation* 73: 1163–1168.

Forlin, E, Guille, JT, Kumar, SJ et al. (1992) Complications associated with fracture of the neck of the femur in children. *Journal of Pediatric Orthopedics* 12: 503–509.

Gebhardt, MC, Ready, JE, Mankin, HJ (1990) Tumors about the knee in children. *Clinical Orthopaedics and Related Research* 255: 86–109.

Giannini, MJ, Protas, EJ (1992) Exercise response in children with and without juvenile rheumatoid arthritis: a case comparison-study. *Physical Therapy* 72: 365–372.

Greene, WB, Strickler, E (1983) A modified isokinetic strengthening programme for patients with severe haemophilia. *Developmental Medicine and Child Neurology* 25: 189–196.

Greenan-Fowler, E, Powell, C, Varni, JW (1987) Behavioural treatment of adherence to therapeutic exercise by children with haemophilia. *Archives of Physical Medicine and Rehabilitation* 68: 846–849.

Haley, SM, Coster, WJ, Binda-Sundberg, K (1994) Measuring physical disablement: the contextual challenge. *Physical Therapy* 74: 443–451.

Hartz, CR, Linscheid, RL, Gramse, RR et al. (1981) The pronator teres syndrome: compressive neuropathy of the median nerve. *Journal of Bone and Joint Surgery* 63A: 885–890.

Heath, CH, Staheli, LT (1993) Normal limits of knee angle in white children — genu varum and genu valgum. *Journal of Pediatric Orthopedics* 13: 259–262.

Heipertz, W (1981a) Riding therapy for orthopaedic cases. In: Heipert, W, Heipertz-Hengst, C, Kroger, A, Kuprian, W (eds) *Therapeutic Riding: Medicine, Education, Sports*, trans. Marion Takeuchi, pp. 55–66. Ottawa: Greenbelt Riding Association for the Disabled (Ottawa) Inc.

Heipertz, W (1981b) Riding as a sport for the handicapped. In: Heipert, W, Heipertz-Hengst, C, Kroger, A, Kuprian, W (eds) *Therapeutic Riding: Medicine, Education, Sports*, trans. Marion Takeuchi, pp. 67–90. Ottawa: Greenbelt Riding Association for the Disabled (Ottawa) Inc.

Hughes, JT, Brownell, B (1972) Pathology of peroneal muscular atrophy (Charcot–Marie–Tooth disease). *Journal of Neurology, Neurosurgery and Psychiatry* 35: 648–657.

Jacobsen, FS, Crawford, AH, Broste, S (1992) Hip involvement in juvenile rheumatoid arthritis. *Journal of Pediatric Orthopedics* 12: 45–53.

Kamegaya, M, Shinada, Y, Moriya, H *et al.* (1992) Acetabular remodelling in Perthes' disease after primary healing. *Journal of Pediatric Orthopedics* 12: 308–314.

Katz, K, Rosenthal, A, Yosipovitch, Z (1992) Normal ranges of popliteal angle in children. *Journal of Pediatric Orthopedics* 12: 229–231.

Kim, HC, Klein, K, Hirsch, S *et al.* (1984) Arthroscopic synovectomy in the treatment of hemophilic synovitis. *Scandinavian Journal of Haematology* (suppl. 40) 33: 271–279.

Koch, BK, Cohen, S, Luban, NS *et al.* (1982) Haemophiliac knee: rehabilitation techniques. *Archives of Physical Medicine and Rehabilitation* 63: 379–382.

Koch, BK, Galioto, FM, Kelleher, J *et al.* (1984) Physical fitness in children with haemophilia. *Archives of Physical Medicine and Rehabilitation* 65: 324–326.

Krebs, DE, Edelstein, JE, Thornby, MA (1991) Prosthetic management of children with limb deficiencies. *Physical Therapy* 71: 920–934.

Krebs, DE, Fishamn, S (1984) Characteriscics of the child amputee population. *Journal of Pediatric Orthopaedics* 4: 89–95.

Kuprian, W (1981) Hippotherapy and riding therapy as physiotherapeutic treatment methods. In: Heipert, W, Heipertz-Hengst, C, Kroger, A, Kuprian, W (eds) *Therapeutic Riding: Medicine, Education, Sports*, trans. by Marion Takeuchi, pp. 14–39. Ottawa: Greenbelt Riding Association for the Disabled (Ottawa) Inc.

Lagos, JC (1971) Compression neuropathy in childhood. *Developmental Medicine and Child Neurology* 13: 531–532.

Landin, LA, Danielsson, LG, Wattsgard, C (1987) Transient synovitis of the hip: its incidence, epidemiology and relation to Perthes' disease. *Journal of Bone and Joint Surgery* 69-B: 238–242.

Lane, JM, Boland, PJ (1986) Osteogenic sarcoma. *Clinical Orthopaedics and Related Research* 204: 93–110.

Leblanc, M, Setoguchi, Y, Shaperman, J *et al.* (1992) Mechanical work efficiencies of body-powered prehensors for young children. *Journal of the Association of Children's Prosthetic Orthotic Clinics* 27: 70–75.

Lechner, DE, McCarthy, CF, Holden, MK (1987) Gait deviations in patients with juvenile rheumatoid arthritis. *Physical Therapy* 67(9): 1335–1341.

Le Veau, BF, Bernhardt, DB (1984) Developmental biomechanics: effect of forces on the growth, development, and maintenance of the human body. *Physical Therapy* 64: 1874–1882.

MacDonald, PB, Locht, RC, Lindsay, D *et al.* (1990) Haemophilic arthropathy of the shoulder. *Journal of Bone and Joint Surgery* 72-B: 470–471.

Margulies, JY, Simkin, A, Leichter, I *et al.* (1986) Effect of intense physical activity on the bone-mineral content in the lower limbs of young adults. *Journal of Bone and Joint Surgery* 68a: 1090–1093.

Matsen, FA, Veith, RG (1981) Compartment syndromes in children. *Journal of Pediatric Orthopedics* 1: 33–41.

Matsuda, Y, Duthie, RB (1984) Surgical synovectomy for haemophilic arthropathy of the knee joint long-term follow-up. *Scandinavian Journal of Haematology* (suppl. 40) 33: 237–247.

Mattison, A (1984) Haemophilia and the family: life-long challenges and adaptation. *Scandinavian Journal of Haematology* (suppl. 40) 33: 65–74.

McGrath, PA, Hillier, LM (1989) The enigma of pain in children: an overview. *Pediatrician* 16: 6–15.

Miller, LS, Bell, DF (1992) Management of congenital fibular deficiency by Ilizarov technique. *Journal of Pediatric Orthopedics* 12: 651–657.

Nafei, A, Teichert, G, Mikkelsen, SS *et al.* (1992) Femoral shaft fractures in children: an epidemiological study in a Danish urban population, 1977–86. *Journal of Pediatric Orthopedics* 12: 499–502.

Ouvrier, RA, McLeod, JG, Pollard, JD (1990) *Peripheral Neuropathy in Childhood*, 242 pp. New York: Raven Press.

Peoples, A (1989) The juvenile amputee: physical therapy and sports partici-pation. In: Kalamachi A (ed.) *Congenital Lower Limb Deficiencies*, pp. 242–249. New York: Springer-Verlag.

Pitetti, KH, Barrett, PJ, Abbas, D (1993) Endurance exercise training in Guillain–Barré syndrome. *Archives of Physical Medicine and Rehabilitation* 74: 761–765

Pizzutillo, PD (1989) Sports medicine in the congenital lower-limb amputee. In: Kalamachi A (ed.) *Congenital Lower Limb Deficiencies*, pp. 236–241. New York: Springer-Verlag.

Rao, UB, Joseph, B (1992) The influence of footwear on the prevalence of flat foot: a survey of 2300 children. *Journal of Bone and Joint Surgery* 74B: 525–533.

Rhodes, VJ (1991) Physical therapy management of patients with juvenile rheumatoid arthritis. *Physical Therapy* 71: 910–919.

Robertson, WM (1987) Distal tibial deformity in bowlegs. *Journal of Pediatric Orthopedics* 7: 324–327.

Ropper, AH (1992) The Guillain–Barré syndrome. *New England Journal of Medicine* 326: 1130–1136.

Rose, GK, Welton, EA, Marshall, T (1985) The diagnosis of flat foot in the child. *Journal of Bone and Joint Surgery* 67B: 71–78.

Royle, SG (1992) Investigation of the irritable hip. *Journal of Pediatric Orthopedics* 12: 396–397.

Sainio, K, Merikanto, J, Larsen, TA (1987) Carpal tunnel syndrome in child-hood. *Developmental Medicine and Child Neurology* 29: 794–796.

Savedra, MC, Tesler, MD (1989) Assessing children's and adolescents' pain. *Pediatrician* 16: 24–29.

Schaller, JG (1984) Chronic arthritis in children: juvenile rheumatoid arthritis. *Clinical Orthopaedics and Related Research* 182: 79–89.

Schott, GD (1983) A chronic and painless form of idiopathic brachial plexus neuropathy. *Journal of Neurology, Neurosurgery and Psychiatry* 46: 555–557.

Shaperman, J, Setoguchi, Y, Leblanc, M (1992) Upper limb strength of young limb deficient children as a factor in using body powered terminal devices – a pilot study. *Journal of the Association of Children's Prosthetic Orthotic Clinics* 27: 89–96.

Simard S, Marchant, M, Mencio, G (1992) The Ilizarov procedure: limb lengthening and its implications. *Physical Therapy* 72: 25–34.

Smith, C, Rosendaal, FR, Varekamp, I *et al.* (1989) Physical condition, long-evity, and social performance of Dutch haemophiliacs, 1972–85. *British Medical Journal* 298: 235–238.

Smoot, EC, Graham, DR, Fisk, JR *et al.* (1993) Development of septic arthritis by hematogenous seeding in a pediatric patient with burns. *Journal of Burn Care and Rehabilitation* 14(1): 55–57.

Spinner, M, Schreiber, SN (1969) Anterior interosseous-nerve paralysis as a complication of supracondylar fractures of the humerus in children. *Journal of Bone and Joint Surgery* 51A: 1584–1590.

Staheli, LT, Chew, DE, Corbett, M (1987) The longitudinal arch: a survey of eight hundred and eighty-two feet in normal children and adults. *Journal of Bone and Joint Surgery* 69A: 426–428.

Strickler, E,, Greene, WB (1984) Isokinetic torque level in haemophiliac knee musculature. *Archives of Physical Medicine and Rehabilitation* 65: 766–770.

Sutherland, DH (1984) *Gait Disorders in Childhood and Adolescence*, pp. 201. Baltimore: Williams and Wilkins.

Swaiman, KF, Flagler, DG (1971) Mercury poisoning with central and periph-eral nervous system involvement treated with penicillamine. *Pediatrics* 48: 639–641.

Tedford, KG, Engsberg, JR, Patterson, JL (1994) A comparison of lower limb performance and balance scores between below-knee amputee and able-bodied children. *Physiotherapy Canada* 46: 190–195.

Theologis, TN, Gordon, C, Benson, MKD (1994) Heel seats and shoe wear. *Journal of Pediatric Orthopedics* 14: 760–762.

Varni, JW, Walco, GA, Katz, ER (1989) Assessment and management of chronic and recurrent pain in children with chronic diseases. *Pediatrician* **16**: 56–63.

Ward, T, Stefko, J, Wood, KB *et al.* (1992) Fixation with a single screw for slipped capital femoral epiphysis. *Journal of Bone and Joint Surgery* **74A**: 799–809

Weiss, APC, Schenck, RC, Sponseller, PD *et al.* (1992) Peroneal nerve palsy after early cast application for femoral fractures in children. *Journal of Pediatric Orthopedics* **12**: 25–28.

Wenger, DR, Mauldin, D, Speck, G *et al.* (1989) Corrective shoes and inserts as treatment for flexible flatfoot in infants and children. *Journal of Bone and Joint Surgery* **71A**: 800–810.

Wiedel, JD (1984) Arthroscopic synovectomy in hemophilic arthropathy of the knee. *Scandinavian Journal of Haematology* (Suppl. 40) **33**: 263–270.

Willett, K, Hudson, I, Catterall, A (1992) Lateral shelf acetabuloplasty: an operation for older children with Perthes' disease. *Journal of Pediatric Orthopaedics* **12**: 563–568.

Young, N, Bell, DF, Anthony, A (1994) Pediatric pain patterns during Ilizarov treatment of limb length discrepancy and angular deformity. *Journal of Pediatric Orthopedics* **14**: 352–357.

Zeltzer, LK, Zeltzer, PM (1989) Clinical assessment and pharmacologic treatment of pain in children: cancer as a model for the management of chronic or persistent pain. *Pediatrician* **16**: 64–70.

FURTHER READING

Atkins, RM, Henderson, NJ, Duthie, RB (1987) Joint contractures in the haemophilia. *Clinical Orthopaedics and Related Research* **219**: 97–106.

Blakeney, P, Moore, P, Broemeling, L *et al.* (1993) Parental stress as a cause and effect of pediatric burn injury. *Journal of Burn Care and Rehabilitation* **14**: 73–79.

Bleck, EE (1971) The shoeing of children: sham or science? *Developmental Medicine and Child Neurology* **13**: 188–195.

Brettler, DB, Levine, PH (1989) Factor concentrates for treatment of hemophilia: which one to choose? *Blood* **73**: 2067–2073.

Butler-Manuel, PA, Smith, MA, Savidge, GF (1990) Silastic interposition for haemophilic arthropathy of the elbow. *Journal of Bone and Joint Surgery* **72-B**: 472–474.

Buzzard, BM, Jones, PM (1988) Physiotherapy management of haemophilia: an update. *Physiotherapy* **74**: 221–226.

Cusick, BD (1988) Splints and casts: managing foot deformity in children with neuromotor disorders. *Physical Therapy* **68**: 1903–1912.

Darby, SC, Rizza, CR, Doll, R *et al.* (1989) Incidence of AIDS and excess of mortality associated with HIV in haemophiliacs in the United Kingdom: report on behalf of the directors of haemophilia centres in the United Kingdom. *British Medical Journal* **298**: 1064–1068.

Desmarres, CH, Laurian, Y (1984) From top to toe: an alternative approach to physiotherapy for haemophiliacs. *Scandinavian Journal of Haematology* Supplement 40, **33**: 469–470.

Dolgin, MJ, Phipps S (1989) Pediatric pain: the parent's role. *Pediatrician* **16**: 103–109.

Engsberg, JR, Lee, AG, Tedford, KG *et al.* (1993) Normative ground reaction force data for able-bodied and below-knee-amputee children during walking. *Journal of Pediatric Orthopedics* **13**: 169–173.

Ganzhorn, RW, Hocker, JT, Horowitz, M *et al.* (1981) Suprascapular-nerve entrapment: a case report. *Journal of Bone and Joint Surgery* **63A**: 492–494.

Garcia, G, McQueen, D (1981) Bilateral suprascapular-nerve entrapment syndrome: case report and review of the literature. *Journal of Bone and Joint Surgery* **63A**: 491–492.

George, A, Hancock, J (1993) Reducing pediatric burn pain with parent participation. *Journal of Burn Care and Rehabilitation* **14**: 104–107.

Herndon, DN, Rutan, RL, Rutan, TC (1993) Management of the pediatric patient with burns. *Journal of Burn Care and Rehabilitation* **14**: 3–7.

Herring, JA, Neustadt, JB, Williams, JJ *et al.* (1992) The lateral pillar classification of Legg-Calve-Perthes disease. *Journal of Pediatric Orthopedics* **12**: 143–150.

Hesenger, RN, Jones, ET (1982) Developmental orthopaedics. II: The spine, trauma and infection. *Developmental Medicine and Child Neurology* **24**: 202–218.

Hurov, JR (1986) Soft-tissue bone interface: how do attachments of muscles, tendons and ligaments change during growth? A light microscopic study. *Journal of Morphology* **189**: 313–325.

Jacquemier, M, Jouve, JL, Bollini, G *et al.* (1992) Acetabular anteversion in children. *Journal of Pediatric Orthopedics* **12**: 373–375.

Kahle, WK, Coleman, SS (1992) The value of the acetabular teardrop figure in assessing pediatric hip disorders. *Journal of Pediatric Orthopedics* **12**: 586–591.

Siegel, LJ, Smith, KE (1989) Children's strategies for coping with pain. *Pediatrician* **16**: 110–118.

Staheli, LT, Corbett, M, Wyss, C *et al.* (1985) Lower-extremity rotational problems in children. *Journal of Bone and Joint Surgery* **67A**: 39–47.

Strong, M, Lejman, T, Michno, P *et al.* (1994) Sequelae from septic arthritis of the knee during the first two years of life. *Journal of Pediatric Orthopedics* **14**: 745–751.

Stuberg, WA (1992) Considerations related to weight-bearing programs in children with developmental disabilities. *Physical Therapy* **72**: 35–40.

Thompson, GH, Leimkuehler, JP (1989) Prosthetic management. In Kalamachi, A (ed) *Congenital Lower Limb Deficiencies*, pp. 211–235. New York: Springer-Verlag.

Yiannikas, C, Walsh, JC (1983) Somatosensory evoked responses in the diagnosis of thoracic outlet syndrome. *Journal of Neurology, Neurosurgery, and Psychiatry* **46**: 234–240.

Zeltzer, LK, Barr, RG, McGrath, PA (1992) Pediatric pain: interacting behavioural and physical factors. *Pediatrics* **90** Supplement 816–821.

19

Sport Related Problems and Other Conditions of Adolescence

MELISSA HEWITT

Injuries to the Growing Skeleton
•
Acute Injuries in the Skeletally Immature Athlete
•
Overuse Injuries in the Skeletally Immature Athlete
•
Growing Pains

The past decade has seen adolescents being introduced to an increasing variety of sports and participating competitively at higher levels. The benefits of participating in sport are well documented – improved well-being, cardiovascular endurance, muscular strength, development of sportsmanship, camaraderie and social skills (Harvey 1982). However, there are inherent risks associated with adolescents training and playing sport at a competitive level.

Both acute and overuse injuries are increasingly common (Harvey 1982, Wojtys 1987, Elliott 1991). Knee injuries in running and jumping sports (Schmidt and Henry 1989, Busch 1990), the occurrence of back pain and injuries in impact and weight-bearing sports (Letts *et al.* 1986, Harvey and Tanner 1991) and upper limb overuse injuries in swimming, throwing and gymnastics (Priest and Weise 1981, Andrish 1990, Micheli and Fehlandt 1992) are commonly reported.

It is argued that the involvement of adults in organizing children's sport has led to an increase in the incidence of musculoskeletal injuries (Wojtys 1987).

Certainly, children self-regulate their level of activity if left to their own devices when playing sport. It is not uncommon to see children stop for 'a breather' when they are cardiovascularly or muscularly fatigued (Lincoln 1984). The imposition of rules including fixed time periods for matches and grading of teams according to age rather than physical maturation and ability increase the susceptibility of the growing child to injury.

The process of growth and the presence of growth cartilage also predisposes the adolescent athlete to injury (Anderson 1991a, Watson 1992). Throughout puberty there are stages when bone growth outstrips muscular growth which can subsequently result in muscular imbalances (Anderson 1991b). The risk of acute and chronic musculoskeletal injuries due to these muscular imbalances is increased (Karlin 1986). The articular cartilage is seen as the 'weak link' in the growing skeleton. Apophyseal avulsions and growth plate and metaphyseal fractures are a more likely acute injury whilst chronic changes in the articular surface and traction apophysitis are commonly seen in teenagers with overuse injuries.

In this chapter how and why children's sporting injuries differ from those of adults will be addressed together with differential diagnosis and physiotherapy management of specific injuries. Risk factors will be highlighted to enhance the reader's understanding of why adolescent injuries occur and the means of minimizing and preventing specific injuries in individual sports. Furthermore, in view of the recent emphasis being placed on weight training for adolescents who compete at high levels in their designated sport, the risks and benefits of gym programmes for muscular strengthening and endurance will be discussed. Whilst this chapter looks mainly at adolescent sporting injuries, the physiotherapy care of the growing child with idiopathic scoliosis and postural kyphosis will also be reviewed, particularly noting the benefits of exercise and postural correction as a means of treatment in conjunction with bracing to improve these deformities.

Injuries to the Growing Skeleton

How do Adolescent Injuries differ from Adult Injuries?

Watson (1992) reports that the incidence of injury in children's sport is 3 per 100 children per year. Less than 1% of these injuries are serious. In many cases the type of injuries children sustain are similar to those of adults (Anderson 1991a). There are some unique differences, however, because of the presence of growth cartilage (Andrish 1990), the process of growth (Meyers 1988), and the activity levels and behaviour of children at play (Elliott 1991).

The growing skeleton has flexible bone, soft cartilaginous structures and ligaments that are proportionately stronger than the adjacent areas of bone growth (Strizak and Stroberg 1986). Whilst the plasticity of developing bone enhances its remodelling capacity and allows speedy resolution of injury, it creates zones of inherent weakness in the skeletally immature athlete (Wojtys 1987, Andrish 1990).

The epiphyseal plates located at both ends of bones allow longitudinal growth and are the site for formation of joint surfaces (Wojtys 1987). The growth plate has undulations in its surface that offer resistance to shearing and tensile forces, but little to torsional stresses (Andrish 1990).

The periosteum is a thick fibrous structure that inserts into the epiphysis and perichondrium. It plays an important role in stabilizing the growth plate biomechanically (Andrish 1990). Ligaments and tendons attach at the perichondrial zone and the tension that these structures receive is then transferred to the growth plate. The ligaments that surround the growth plates are three to five times stronger than the epiphyseal plate. This results in injuries of the growth plate occurring more frequently in adolescents than the ligamentous damage that occurs in adults (Strizak and Stroberg 1986). In view of the vulnerability of the adolescent's growth plate it is essential that any injury to this region is accurately diagnosed and effectively treated to minimize the risk of growth disturbances (Anderson 1991a).

Bony apophyses are also growth sites and are therefore susceptible to injury. Major tendon and ligamentous groups attach at these sites, e.g. the tibial tubercle for the patellar tendon. Acute avulsion of an apophyseal centre can occur. The forces that lead to an apophyseal avulsion in adolescents usually result in a musculotendinous or muscle tear in the adult population (Anderson 1991a). Repetitive loading of the apophysis via tensile forces may result in a traction apophysitis in young athletes (Schmidt and Henry 1989). Tendonitis is the common complaint when an adult is exposed to similar traction forces.

The apophyseal sites are more likely to sustain overuse injuries during periods of rapid skeletal growth (Micheli and Fehlandt 1992). The metaphysis of growing bone has a relatively thin cortex and, as a consequence of this, greenstick and normal fractures are more common in adolescents (Wojtys 1987). Acute injuries normally resolve with little physiotherapy intervention. More chronic injuries often require physiotherapy input in their management to ensure prevention of recurrence. The knee joint is illustrated in Figure 1.

Figure 1 The Apophyseal, Epiphyseal and Metaphyseal Areas of the Knee Joint.

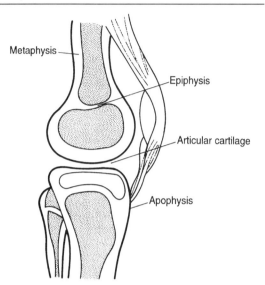

Why do Adolescent Injuries differ from Adult Injuries?

Whilst it is well documented that weight-bearing activity is necessary for the development of normal bone and connective tissue (Wotjys 1987, Maffulli and Pintore 1990), the safe range of loading the skeletally immature musculoskeletal system is hotly debated. Since bones grow faster than associated musculotendinous structures, alterations in flexibility and a propensity for muscular imbalances can occur (Karlin 1986). These imbalances can lead to alterations in limb alignment (Elliott 1991). In the lower limb this can result in gait pattern disturbances that may predispose the growing athlete to chronic injury (Strizak and Stroberg 1986).

Individual children may take variable lengths of time to adjust to these changes in flexibility and it can lead to alterations and deficits in motor coordination (Wojtys 1987). The reacquisition of speed, strength and finally skill in their chosen sport may also be delayed. In this period, the young athlete is at risk of acute injury.

Maturational assessment – via the attainment of sexual characteristics, e.g. development of genitalia, presence of pubic hair – measures an adolescent's progression towards physical maturity (Caine and Broekhoff 1987). This assessment is important as a marker of physical ability and potential compared to chronological age. Its usefulness is highlighted when considering injuries caused by loss of flexibility and muscle–tendon imbalances. Furthermore, pre- and post-pubertal growth spurts can be predicted via maturational assessment. Biomechanical changes can be monitored during these growth spurts and individual training programmes and sport participation can then be appropriately modified and stretching activities highlighted. When this does not occur the skeletally immature athlete is at risk of injury.

As with any sportsperson insufficient warm-up and cool-down, as well as inappropriate conditioning increases the risk of sustaining either an acute or chronic injury. Alterations in flexibility are magnified in the young athlete when combined with these factors. Combine these tendencies with inadequate skill and often minimal supervision at training and playing sessions (Elliott 1991), short attention spans and slower reaction times (Wojtys 1987), and it becomes more obvious why children sustain sporting injuries.

Whilst children tend to play a variety of sports, they often choose ones that have similar biomechanical stresses (Harvey 1982) and therefore the likelihood of repetitive microtrauma to selected structures is increased. If preparticipation screening does not occur, children may choose a competitive sport for which their body type is unsuited. In an attempt to perform at an adequate level they may excessively try to improve a specific technique, e.g. baseball pitching. As children's sport often has inadequate equipment, playing surfaces and coaching input, there is a risk of overuse injuries. It is important that growing athletes participating in sports that require a high level of skill, such as gymnastics, practise difficult manoeuvres under supervision to minimize the likelihood of injury (Micheli and Fehlandt 1992).

Elliott (1991) reports that injuries are more common when there is an increase in sport participation before skeletal maturity. When the child moves into the elite arena more skill and speed are required. Greater forces at impact may result in more acute injuries. As competition intensifies, training demands and the length of sessions increase. Overuse injuries are more common. Elite sport participants, however, are more likely to be aware of the risks of playing with an injury and will usually notify parents and coaches of any injuries sustained (Meyers 1988).

Common Injury Sites

Sites of injury in the skeletally immature athlete are dependent on four factors:

1. whether the injury is acute or chronic
2. the sport in which the adolescent/child is participating
3. the age of the athlete
4. whether the child is currently in an active growth spurt or quiescent period of growth

Nature of the Injury

Fractures are a common acute injury in the skeletally immature athlete. These may include fractures of long bones (Watson 1992); apophyseal avulsion fractures (Karlin 1986); and growth plate fractures – commonly seen about the knee and elbow joints (Carter and Aldridge 1988, DeLee and Pearce 1990).

Ligamentous sprains are also frequently seen with the ankle joint being commonly affected (Turco and Spinella 1986). It was previously thought that ligamentous injuries in the growing athlete were rare, due to the greater comparative strength of ligaments to bone.

In the knee joint especially, with improved diagnostic techniques such as investigative arthroscopy, ligament and meniscal injuries are more frequently reported (Busch 1990, Kellenberger and von Laer 1990). Furthermore, muscular strains are, as in the adult population, frequently confined to those of the back or muscles that cross two joints.

Disc herniation has been reported in the adolescent athlete (Weinert and Rizzo 1992) and the possibility must not be ignored when treating the young sportsperson involved in high-impact sports who presents with a sudden onset of back or leg pain. Dislocations of the shoulder, patella and less commonly the hip, are injuries also seen in the growing population (Karlin 1986, Strizak and Stroberg 1986, Marans et al. 1992).

Chronic or overuse injuries include stress fractures which can be seen in long or short bones that sustain compressive forces (Jackson and Ciullo 1986, Harvey 1992). Osteochondritis dissecans is sometimes seen at a joint surface following an acute injury and requires specific attention. The elbow and knee joint are commonly affected (Andrish 1986, Watson 1992).

Apophysitis can occur at many sites. Conditions such as Osgood–Schlatter disease and Sinding–Larsen Johansson syndrome, which involve the patellar tendon and tibial tubercle are common in the adolescent population (Schmidt and Henry 1989, Anderson 1991b).

Calcaneal apophysitis can occur at the insertion of the Achilles' tendon (Micheli and Ireland 1987). The occurrence of traction apophysites around the pelvis in adolescent runners and footballers is also reported (Karlin 1986). Poor biomechanics is thought to exacerbate lower limb apophysites. Apophysitis at the elbow joint is seen in young gymnasts and throwing athletes (Meyers 1988).

Symptoms of impingement in the presence of anterior shoulder instability cannot be ignored in young swimmers, throwing athletes and tennis players (Andrish 1986, Ryu et al. 1988).

Sports Played

Prediction of injury site according to the sport played is a useful prophylactic measure. Classification is via the number of repetitions of an action performed and the force exerted in a manoeuvre. Sports that exert a moderate amount of force through a body part on impact and require a high repetition of actions include cricket fast-bowling, baseball pitching, selected activities in gymnastic routines and running sports, e.g. netball and football (Elliott 1991). Swimming also can be included in this category, for although the participant is non-weight-bearing, a high number of shoulder revolutions and a moderate amount of force is exerted via the resistance of the water. It is these high repetition/moderate impact sports that predispose the growing skeleton to overuse injuries previously mentioned.

Whilst sports that involve high forces and moderate repetition of activities may predispose the athlete to overuse injuries, they also increase the likelihood of acute trauma (Elliott 1991). Examples include: jumping activities such as basketball, triple and high jumps; the throwing sports of javelin and baseball/softball out-fielding; and take-off and landing manoeuvres in gymnastics.

Athlete's Age

Watson (1992) reports a relatively low incidence of sporting injuries in children less than 12 years old. There is a peak incidence of injury at 14 years for males and 15 years for females. It is hypothesized that this is a result of increased levels of participation and competition, increased weight with a concomitant increase in the forces sustained at impact, decreased muscular flexibility resulting in more sprains and strains, and the gradual closure of epiphyseal plates resulting in an increase in ligamentous injuries.

In children under 12 years, 80% of injuries sustained are chondral fractures, osseous avulsions or peri-osteal in nature (Kellenberger and von Laer 1990). In childhood, ligaments are more likely to stretch and hence injury to the growth plate is more common.

Avulsion fractures are more commonly seen in ado-lescents than children. By this age the growth plate involved has closed but not fused. Combine this with greater muscle strength seen in teenagers and the reason is clear (Meyers 1988). These injuries require accurate diagnosis to prevent long-term sequelae through appropriate and essential medical and physiotherapy input.

The Effect of Growth Spurts

It is reported that in periods of rapid growth the skeletally immature athlete is more prone to apo-physites due to the pull of shortened muscles on the apophyseal growth sites. In periods of quiescent growth the adolescent is more prone to tendonitis type pain (Micheli and Fehlandt 1992).

At the knee joint, where the physeal growth plates contribute greatest to adult lower limb length and are the fastest growing in the body (Strizak and Stroberg 1986), it is purported that the rapid change in the length of the femur may alter the balance of the quadriceps mechanism. This can result in tightness of the iliotibial band and an associated loss of mechanical advantage of the vastus medialis obliquus.

Such factors can cause the patella to move laterally and proximally and thereby may contribute to patellofemoral stress syndrome (Strizak and Stroberg 1986, O'Neill et al. 1992).

Acute Injuries in the Skeletally Immature Athlete

Primary Care

With physiotherapists being first-contact practi-tioners in many parts of the world and becoming more involved in sporting club training and playing sessions, it is not uncommon to be present as an acute injury occurs. At times the child/adolescent may present for physiotherapy care before seeking medical advice. It is therefore essential that physio-therapists have a good working knowledge of the anatomy of the immature musculoskeletal system, to ensure accurate diagnosis of a child's injury. Current first-aid skills are also essential.

Children are notoriously poor historians. They are unused to experiencing pain and, therefore, poorly define its location, intensity or behaviour. They are often frightened and observation is always the best initial indicator of damage sustained. Normal proce-dures of assessing bony alignment, the presence and degree of swelling and/or vascular changes are imperative.

It is important to ask the child first to move the unaffected limb in order to assess their normal range and quality of movement. It must not be forgotten that children have a muscular flexibility that becomes less as they mature. They also have alterations in limb flexibility associated with growth spurts.

The child should then actively move the injured limb as able, starting with the least painful movement and moving on to those that are more painful. It is rare that the health-care provider need move the limb throughout this initial examination. At this stage, palpation to assess the tenseness of any effusion or alterations in skin temperature may occur. Maintain-ing the young athlete's confidence is paramount. In the acute situation, moving the limb should only be undertaken in order to support it in a position that will prevent further injury.

The most common acute injuries sustained by the skeletally immature athlete will be presented now with case histories highlighting physiotherapy involvement. As the physiotherapy management of acute sporting injuries is quite similar for most conditions, rehabilitation and return to sport will be considered together.

Fractures

As young bone is more pliable, greenstick fractures of long bones are more common in children than adults (Andrish 1986). Healing of any fracture usually occurs quickly and with minimal complications as growing bone has a good blood supply. Treatment is via immobilization in a plaster cast unless a rotational or angular deformity with displacement is present. In this instance, open reduction and internal fixation followed by a period of immobilization occurs. As immature bone has a great potential for remodelling, a degree of latitude in the healing position is allowed.

Case Study 1

An 11-year-old boy (AC) was tackled by an opposition rugby union player. He sustained a fracture of his right tibia and was managed in a long leg cast. There was an angulation deformity and 3 weeks following injury, his tibia was openly reduced and internally fixated. He was mobilized non-weight-bearing on crutches.

Six weeks later he began physiotherapy. Whilst knee range of motion was full, there was gross restriction of ankle movement, especially dorsiflexion. Non-weight-bearing ankle ranging was started. Strengthening work via isometric exercises and gait re-education, concentrating on rhythm and equal strides, was commenced with partial weight-bearing on crutches. Swimming in his home pool and gait work in the water was also started.

One week later weight-bearing stretches and strengthening work started: ski squats, lunges, toe raises with support were included. AC began to ride his mountain bike around the neighbourhood before doing his exercises. Balance and proprioceptive work on a minitramp and balance board was introduced. As he was a keen gymnast he returned to training and commenced pain-free manoeuvres.

Six weeks after starting physiotherapy AC was walking normally with full ankle range and good muscle strength and length. Muscle bulk was less. He was beginning to run and could do all gymnastic activities except landings.

Small bones can also be fractured. Vertical fractures of the navicular can occur in adolescents who participate in jumping and landing sports such as basketball and gymnastics. These fractures are prone to non-union. Non-weight-bearing is essential for up to 6 weeks to minimize this likelihood. Open reduction is essential if the fracture is displaced (Turco and Spinella 1986).

Following removal of any form of immobilization children usually self-regulate their recovery. Most rehabilitation of fractures occurs via the child gradually pushing into the limited range of movement as pain allows and building strength via play. As a physiotherapist it is important to ensure that the child has full muscle strength and range of movement before returning to competitive sport. This will then reduce the likelihood of recurrent or associated injuries.

Gymnastics is a sport that produces a high number of elbow fractures and dislocations (Priest and Weise 1981). The mechanism is most commonly that of falling on an outstretched arm resulting in violent hyperextension, with or without a valgus stress (Andrish 1986). Priest and Weise (1981) report that double the injuries occur when there are no spotters to control landings and inadequate thickness of landing mats. In children's sport adequate supervision is imperative.

The distal radius is most commonly fractured in

young gymnasts (Andrish 1986). This is caused by an hyperextension and twisting manoeuvre of the wrist with associated ulnar deviation. It is commonly seen in weight-bearing activities such as the twisting vault or a fall on to the outstretched hand. Again appropriate mats, supervision and instruction in safe landing and falling techniques must be in place to minimize the likelihood of injury.

AVULSION FRACTURES

These are most commonly sustained by adolescents and are seen in high-velocity activities. The elbow, pelvis and the knee are common injury sites.

Throwing sports such as baseball, softball and javelin exert different forces on the elbow at different phases of the throwing action (Andrish 1986, Meyers 1988). The throw includes three phases: winding up or cocking phase, acceleration phase and follow-through. Towards the end of the cocking phase, medial distraction of the elbow joint occurs with lateral compression and translational forces across the olecranon and humeral surfaces. During the acceleration phase these forces neutralize. As follow-through occurs the triceps brachii exert a strong posterior force that results in compression and shearing forces through the radiocapitellar joint as the forearm forcefully pronates to release the ball at full speed. These varying forces can result in fragmentation of the trochlea, olecranon and/or medial epicondyle (Andrish 1986, Meyers 1988). Associated widening between the humeral metaphysis and medial epicondyle may be demonstrated on X-ray. The elbow joint is illustrated in Figure 2.

Treatment involves cast immobilization for 3 weeks. Open reduction and internal fixation is necessary if there is displacement. Physiotherapy involves maintenance of range of movement of the unaffected joints above and below the fracture site and full return of function is required before competing.

In caring for avulsion fractures about the elbow, assessment of paraesthesia in the forearm and hand must be routine as ulnar nerve involvement is not uncommon. The elbow is a joint that responds poorly to passive input and regaining lost range should be achieved via active movement.

Figure 2 Anatomical Outline of the Elbow Joint

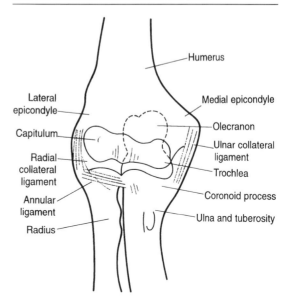

Adolescents often respond well to hydrotherapy activities combined with throwing games, e.g. water polo, to restore full range of movement. As previously mentioned, the involvement of the radial head in any elbow injury often results in an early loss of forearm pronation and supination. If these areas are not quickly targeted stiffness into these ranges is permanent.

Avulsion fractures of the tibial tuberosity are thought to be often associated with Osgood–Schlatter disease (Anderson 1991a). The mechanism of injury can be either a strong quadriceps contraction when the knee is flexed and the foot fixed or a violent passive flexion of the knee when the quadriceps are contracted maximally. Commonly these occur in contact sports such as football. An example of the first mechanism is seen in the player who has someone standing on his foot as he goes to push off from a tackle. The second mechanism is seen when the running player is tackled around the shins from front on and the leg is passively flexed. The adolescent between 12 and 16 years of age is most susceptible to this injury as this is just before the time when the apophysis fuses with the tibia.

When the injury occurs the athlete is unable to extend his knee actively and reports significant localized pain over the anterior inferior surface of

Figure 3 Proprioceptive Facilitation via Balance Board

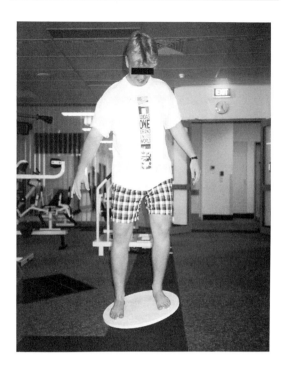

assessment of high-level agility skills is necessary to ensure safe return to sport.

Avulsion fractures about the pelvis occur rarely at the anterior inferior iliac spine (AIIS). The anterior superior iliac spine (ASIS) is more commonly affected as the sartorius, tensor fascia lata muscles and the inguinal ligament — the insertion of the external and internal oblique abdominal muscles — originate and insert here. Sartorius also initiates explosive hip flexion in the sprinter (Karlin 1986). Avulsion usually occurs as the athlete takes off. On examination he will experience pain on the sit-up manoeuvre, hip flexion, hip abduction and prone knee flexion in combination with hip extension. Ischial avulsion can also occur

Initial management includes rest and partial- to non-weight-bearing as pain allows. Isometric exercises, and subsequently range of motion exercises, are commenced as pain allows. Stretching regimes are instituted. Hydrotherapy, especially pool running, is a useful interim activity prior to dry land running. Rigorous warm up is essential prior to competition to minimize the likelihood of injury recurrence. Again high-level agility skills must be assessed prior to return to sport.

GROWTH PLATE FRACTURES

Growth plate fractures are seen at many joints in the young athlete, but commonly occur at the knee joint. In the skeletally immature athlete who suffers an acute knee injury epiphyseal/growth plate disruption should always be suspected. As the distal femoral epiphysis contributes to 70% of the total mature length of the femur, it is important that any disruption be immediately diagnosed. If there is an interruption to growth in early childhood, lower limb length, joint function and leg alignment may be altered (Anderson 1991a).

The Salter–Harris system of classification is used for growth plate fractures (Salter and Harris 1963). Figure 4 outlines the degree of growth plate injury.

If an adolescent or child presents with an acutely swollen and tense joint and/or instability, a growth plate fracture must be uppermost in the clinician's mind. Tenderness on palpation of the growth plate is a good indicator of its involvement. Diagnosis is confirmed by X-ray. In the acute growth plate fracture with an undisplaced fragment, an X-ray

the knee. There is often localized swelling and the patella heights may vary with the patella of the affected leg being higher. If there is no displacement of the tuberosity, the patient's leg is immobilized in a cylinder cast or knee immobilizer in extension (1 month). Open reduction is necessary in the presence of displaced fragments. The physiotherapist must ensure full return of knee flexion as well as quadricep and hamstring strength. Eccentric quadriceps control, for example stepping down from a stair, is a vital prerequisite to return to contact sport. Proprioception is commonly lost and balance board and one-legged standing activities with vision occluded are important parts of treatment (see Figure 3).

Tightness of the rectus femoris is often present. It is unclear as to whether this is a predisposing factor or develops as a result of the avulsion injury. Either being the cause, effective stretching in the prone position initially and then in standing is an important part of treatment. Posterior pelvic tilt is essential to ensure a good length of rectus femoris muscle. Furthermore,

Figure 4 The Different Types of Injuries Involving the Epiphyseal Plate (Salter and Harris 1963). Type I and II Salter–Harris injuries are horizontal fractures to the growth plate. Type III and IV fractures are vertical in nature and will result in degenerative changes to the joint and/or growth disturbances if poorly treated. Type V injuries are compression fractures. Type II and IV fractures have higher complications because of the involvement of the joint surface.

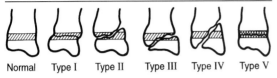

Normal   Type I   Type II   Type III   Type IV   Type V

may be reported as normal for 10–14 days until the periosteal reaction becomes apparent (Andrish 1986).

Associated loose bodies may be cartilaginous and therefore radiolucent on X-ray. It is not until they calcify at a later stage that they will be seen on X-ray. If symptoms persist it is important to repeat X-ray the affected joint.

In the presence of instability in the acutely injured young athlete's knee, it is important to determine also if ligamentous and/or meniscal damage has occurred. The medial collateral ligament attaches to both the distal femoral and proximal tibial epiphyses. The anatomy is such that the distal femoral epiphysis is more likely to be disrupted by a force that will stress the medial collateral ligament in a skeletally mature knee.

Avulsion of the anterior cruciate ligament and fracture to the proximal tibial epiphysis occurs most commonly in the acceleration phase of jumping activities. A high jumper's take-off or a basketball lay-up is the common sporting activity involved. The injury occurs as the body weight is exerted through the take-off leg. Usually occurring between 7 and 15 years of age, the child presents with a swollen tense knee upon which it is painful to weight-bear, some anterior and medial instability on ligament examination, and a reduction in joint range of movement (Meyers and McKeever 1970).

In the absence of displacement there is a closed reduction and immobilization in a cast cylinder/knee immobilizer in full extension (4–6 weeks). Physiotherapy management includes restoration of joint range of movement, muscle strengthening and treatment of any associated ligamentous injuries.

In the young athlete who presents with knee joint line

tenderness, decreased joint movement, persistent swelling and joint locking, meniscal integrity must be ensured. As in the adult the meniscii provide stability to the knee joint and are the shock absorbers that transmit force across the joint surfaces.

If a meniscal tear is untreated in a young patient, not only is function limited via a mechanical blocking but also altered mechanics can lead to joint wear and tear and compensatory movement patterns. Both meniscii are equally involved in knee injuries in the young population (Busch 1990) and are often in association with ligament sprains. Longitudinal tears and peripheral damage are most common and these types of tears are often amenable to conservative management as they can heal spontaneously. A discoid meniscus is a congenital anomaly that is often asymptomatic, but in the adolescent may become a problem following trauma. It involves a lateral meniscus with poor posterior fixation. This results in the hypermobile meniscus moving forwards and backwards over the tibial plateau and continual occurrence results in disc hypertrophying. An audible click on knee movements is a characteristic of discoid meniscus.

Joint Dislocations

The patellofemoral joint can commonly dislocate in young athletes (Strizak and Stroberg 1986). The direction of dislocation is lateral and may be the result of a direct blow to the patella or a sudden contraction of the quadriceps as there is a loading of the knee in a twisting and extended action.

The adolescent has marked tenderness medially as a result of the stretch imposed on the medial retinaculum. Apprehension when the patella is glided laterally is present but ligamentous examination of the knee joint is normal. An X-ray should be performed to exclude concomitant osteochondral fractures. Immobilization (3–6 weeks) in a knee brace is advocated with early rehabilitation to minimize muscle wasting and joint stiffening.

Case Study 2

A 13-year-old boy (JR) sustained a knee injury whilst playing basketball. As he 'layed up' his weight-bearing leg gave way. Intense pain was experienced infer-

> *iorly and medially to the patella. He was carried from the court and his knee swelled immediately. X-rays were normal.*
>
> *He presented at physiotherapy 2 days later, being unable to weight-bear with a swollen hot knee. Palpation detected exquisite tenderness medially to the patella with apprehension to any patellofemoral glides. Knee range of movement was 40–80°.*
>
> *Dislocation of the patella was the provisional diagnosis. Initial treatment was immobilization in a knee brace and the use of crutches to ensure pain-free walking. Reduction of swelling via ice and static muscle contractions was initiated. Early regaining of knee range was achieved by the use of the removable knee brace.*

Traumatic anterior dislocation of the glenohumeral joint in children is another common complaint (Marans *et al.* 1992). Interestingly, a retrospective study by Marans *et al.* (1992) suggests that although immobilization in a sling and binder in internal rotation (6 weeks) was the method of treatment, it did not affect the rate of recurrence as all patients sustained one or more recurrent dislocations. Meyers (1988) similarly reports that there is an 82% recurrence rate for anterior shoulder dislocation in growing athletes. Physiotherapy is not routinely requested, but strengthening work of the shoulder rotators may be of value.

Muscular Strains and Ligament Sprains

The ankle is the most commonly sprained joint in the skeletally immature athlete (Turco and Spinella 1986). This is most likely due to the high number of contact sports played by youngsters and the high energy levels they transmit to the game. Muscular strains are normally confined to the two joint muscles and the hamstrings are most commonly involved.

These conditions are similarly treated in both the immature and mature athlete and therefore do not require specific mention. As in all management of acute sporting injuries reduction of pain, swelling

and inflammation is the first treatment regimen. Rest, judicious application of ice upon young skin, compression via bandaging and elevation are the principal modes of treatment.

Restoration of joint range of movement and muscle length and strength are the next consideration. Children are good self-regulators and controlled play and relative rest allow them to pursue safe sporting activities — such as riding their mountain bike around home or playing in the swimming pool — within pain limits, are often effective means of gaining range.

As always, before returning to competitive sport they must have full muscle strength and have successfully completed sport-related drills. The importance of warm-up must be emphasized to the injured athlete, their parents and the coach. Education plays an important part in injury prevention for the young athlete returning to competitive sport.

Overuse Injuries in the Skeletally Immature Athlete

Children are involved in competitive sport at an earlier age and train longer and harder than in previous generations. Many sports rely on very young participants, for example swimming and gymnastics, where loads are placed on the musculoskeletal system when it is at its most vulnerable. Overuse injuries are therefore increasingly prevalent in the adolescent sporting population (Harvey 1982, Elliott 1991, Micheli and Fehlandt 1992).

The common thread through overuse injuries is repetitive microtrauma. Harvey (1982) reports that overuse is a result of repetitive friction, traction or cyclical loading on an anatomical structure. Elliott (1991) believes that this subacute repetitive loading ultimately leads to fatigue in the stressed tissue. Over time this is manifested by pain, swelling or loss of function to varying degrees. The continuous repetitive injury to the structure involved outstrips the tissue's ability to repair itself (Micheli and Fehlandt 1992).

Training error plays a big part in the occurrence of overuse injuries, characterized by excessive training, poor physical fitness and inadequate skill levels to perform a desired task (Harvey 1982, Elliott 1991). It is claimed that growth is a significant predisposing factor (Micheli and Fehlandt 1992).

In this section, swimmer's shoulder, little leaguer's elbow, osteochondritis diseccans, lower limb apophysitis and tendonitis and the impact of bio-mechanics on these conditions will be addressed.

The knee joint is the most commonly affected joint in terms of sustaining injuries that result in chronic pain. Bipartite patella, stress fractures, patello-femoral pain, referred pain and the issue of neoplasms as a cause of chronic pain are discussed. Whilst growing pains are not related to overuse, they are chronic and therefore will be covered in this section.

Swimmer's Shoulder

Shoulder pain is a common complaint in elite swim-mers. The incidence is said to increase proportio-nately with ability, with 57% of championship swimmers complaining of shoulder pain (Meyers 1988). The pain is often associated with impingement of the supraspinatus tendon below the coracoacro-mial arch. Occasionally, the tendon of the long head of biceps brachii is involved (Andrish 1986). Predis-posing sports are swimming, throwing events and racquet sports (Meyers 1988, Ryu et al. 1988, Micheli and Fehlandt 1992). It has been suggested that a more prominent acromion anteriorly and an increase in the amount of inferior angulation of the acromion may be predisposing factors (Neer, 1972).

Micheli (1983) hypothesizes that impingement is a result of anterior shoulder instability. Weakened stretched anterior structures allow a traction injury of the rotator cuff tendons to occur and inflamma-tion results. Meanwhile, Nirschl (1986) suggests that swimmer's shoulder is the result of excessive internal loading of the tendons associated with pre-existing pathology and an associated muscular weakness results. This causes a muscular imbalance about the shoulder joint which results in the humeral head moving superiorly in the glenoid. Impingement results.

Whatever the cause of swimmers' shoulder, practi-tioners agree that effective results are achieved via assessment of tight and weak structures and the instigation of appropriate stretching and subse-quently strengthening techniques. If non-steroidal

Figure 5 Therapist Stretching a Tight Right Pectoralis Minor Muscle of a Patient with Swimmer's Shoulder

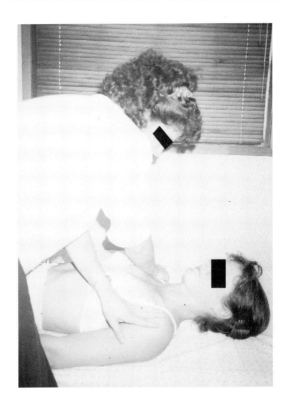

anti-inflammatory agents are required they should be judiciously administered to the young athlete. The pectoralis minor is often tight and is most effectively stretched by another person in the supine position (Figure 5).

Whilst initial strengthening activities are always isometric, as inflammation subsides through range-of-movement strengthening using light weights or elastic exercise tubing is also appropriate. This is important to restore anterior stability of the gleno-humeral joint. The shoulder internal rotators – sub-scapularis, teres major, anterior deltoid, latissimus dorsi and pectoralis major – are often weak as are the external rotators – infraspinatus, teres minor and posterior deltoid. These are initially strengthened below 90° abduction to prevent impingement pain. Hand weights or elastic exercising equipment may be used (see Figure 6). General shoulder strengthening is also important. As pain subsides and strength improves, exercises above 90° are incorporated into the rehabilitation programme.

Figure 6 A Patient with Swimmer's Shoulder Undertaking a Muscle Strengthening Programme

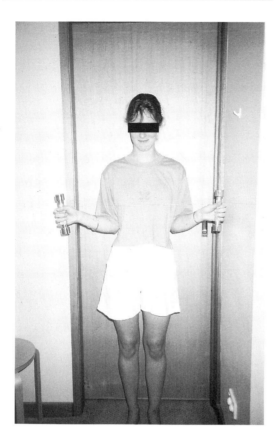

Figure 7 A Patient with Swimmer's Shoulder Undertaking Controlled Scapular Stabilization Exercises

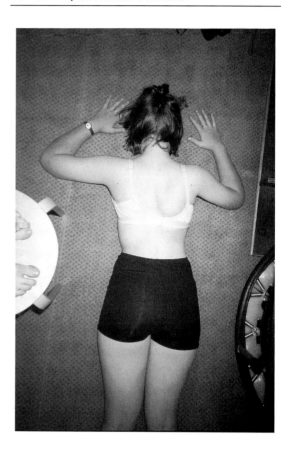

Maltracking of the scapula is not uncommon in these patients and weakness is evident in the lower and middle trapezii, rhomboids major and minor. Retraining of scapular rhythm is essential. Lower trapezius strength is particularly important in this group of patients to minimize elevation and upward rotation of the inferior angle of the scapula as the arm is elevated. Shoulder blade pull-downs, described as drawing a 'J' or reversed 'J' with your shoulder blade (according to the side involved) are extremely effective. Exercises often start in the prone position (see Figure 7), progressing to controlled elevation exercises, such as sliding the hand up the door jam whilst the scapula is actively depressed.

Specific strengthening of serratus anterior can be achieved via extended arm supine punches. Rhomboids and middle trapezius can be strengthened and activated via prone retraction activities. As strength improves, exercises can be incorporated into a supervized weight training programme.

Taping is extremely valuable as it provides proprioceptive input to the athlete regarding scapular position. A porous sports tape is commonly used and remains in place for up to 3 days. Care with skin sensitivity is important and gradual weaning is necessary to allow recruitment of shoulder-stabilizing muscles. Training regimens and technique must be assessed as these are common causes of shoulder pain and its tendency to recur. Gradual return to training and competitive levels is required.

Little Leaguer's Elbow

This is described as pain that occurs in the throwing arm of skeletally immature athletes. Incidence of elbow pain is related to age and sporting level (Andrish 1986, Meyers 1988), with 11–12-year-old baseballers demonstrating a 20% incidence of elbow pain with X-ray changes apparent.

The athletes frequently complain of medial rather than lateral elbow pain. X-ray hypertrophy of the medial epicondyle, flexion contractures, triceps brachii weakness, an increase in the valgus angulation of the elbow, tight anterior structures of the glenohumeral joint, and a rapid growth spurt (Andrish 1986, Meyers 1988, Micheli and Fehlandt 1992) are commonly associated with little leaguer's elbow.

Treatment consists of relative rest: throwing activities should be ceased or restricted until pain subsides. Ice and non-steroidal anti-inflammatories are sometimes used. Stretching of the tight anterior structures of the elbow and shoulder with special attention to the biceps brachii is important.

Progressive strengthening of the triceps brachii is essential. Surgical removal of loose bodies is necessary. Training contributes to this and other overuse injuries, therefore any errors must be examined. Little leaguer's elbow is usually self-limiting unless avascular necrosis or osteochondritis dissecans result (Andrish 1986).

Chronic Knee Pain

There are many causes of chronic knee pain in the skeletally immature athlete. Patellofemoral stress syndrome, Osgood–Schlatter disease, Sinding–Larsen Johansson syndrome, symptomatic bipartite patella and stress fractures can be included as more common causes of persistent pain about the knee joint. Patellar tendonitis and tibial tuberosity apophysitis must also be included. Referred pain from the lumbar spine or hip should always be considered when a child presents with unremitting low-grade knee pain. Neoplasms must also be considered when differentially diagnosing knee pain.

Patellofemoral Stress Syndrome

The patella is a sesamoid bone that provides protection to the anterior aspect of the knee joint. It gives some mechanical advantage to the quadriceps muscle group during knee extension and moves between the femoral condyles as the knee joint flexes and extends. The path that the patella takes as the knee flexes and extends is determined by the bony contours of the patella and the intercondylar notch, the length of the patellofemoral retinaculum and the contraction of the vastus medialis obliquus (Strizak and Stroberg 1986).

Commonly, young athletes complain of retropatellar pain during certain physical activities. The pain may be unilateral or bilateral and often follows a rapid growth spurt. The adolescent may experience this pain on running, ascending or descending stairs and hills, squatting, jumping and/or after prolonged sitting. Occasionally, lateral patellar knee pain will be felt superficially. Crepitus is sometimes evident on knee flexion and extension. At times a softening and fissuring of the articular cartilage of the patella occurs and this is described as chondromalacia patella (Strizak and Stroberg 1986).

A case history highlights common presenting symptoms and appropriate management. Progressive strengthening of the quadriceps and associated iliotibial band and hamstring stretching have been shown to be effective in the treatment of this condition (O'Neill et al. 1992). McConnell (1986) advocates the use of taping to promote a better tracking of the patella and eccentric quadriceps strengthening to reduce pain and restore function.

Case Study 3

A 10½-year-old girl (KC) presented with medial knee and tibial tubercle pain. Both knees were equally affected and pain was evident when participating in sport, but was tolerable once warmed up. Pain was also present when ascending and descending stairs. She reported stiffness upon waking, but no night pain. Pain was relieved by cessation of activity and ice. Her mother reported a significant growth spurt 2–3 months prior to onset of pain.

The pain began after KC high jumped using the scissor manoeuvre for 4 hours without a rest. She was unable to walk the following day because of knee pain. The pain settled with rest, but did not abate.

Training and sports participation included 2.5 kilometres of swimming training/day and four sessions of netball/week. Recently, KC had started cross-country running.

A full physiotherapy assessment demonstrated tightness of the gluteals, hamstrings *and calves, a very mobile lumbar spine and weak lower abdominal muscles, a restriction of hip external rotation, pain on patello-femoral glides and overpronation of both feet. During assessment it was noted that, although KC had chosen a variety of sports to play, she was not allowing time for her knee pain to resolve.*

In treatment the biomechanical factors were addressed, new shoes were purchased to counteract her overpronation, instruction in appropriate warm-up and cool-down activities was given and input regarding appropriate training levels and intensities was included.

Pain resolved within 6 weeks. A strengthening programme concentrating on lower abdominals, gluteals, quadriceps and calves was incorporated into her exercise programme in combination with daily stretching.

Osgood–Schlatter Disease (OSD)

This disease affects the apophyseal cartilage of the tibial tubercle. It is the most common disorder of the adolescent extensor mechanism (Schmidt and Henry 1989, Anderson 1991b) and is related to a repetitive stretch of the apophysis via the patellar tendon as the quadriceps contracts. The osteochondral structure may separate. On X-ray the junction between the tibial tubercle and the tibial epiphysis appears irregular.

The symptoms are associated with a growth spurt and cease once full growth is achieved. Males are more frequently affected than females and the 11–15-year-old age group is particularly susceptible. This is thought to be due both to rapid growth and an increase in sports participation. Both legs are commonly involved and the tibial tubercle may become quite prominent, making kneeling painful. Soft tissue swelling often occurs. There is a reduction of both knee flexion and extension. Resisted quadriceps contraction reproduces local pain. There is a tightness in the hip flexors and rectus femoris. Hamstrings and

calf muscles are commonly tight. By stretching these posterior structures there is a decrease in the resistance offered to the quadriceps as they contract. This in turn lowers the tensile forces exerted on the tibial tubercle (Anderson 1991b).

Lower limb alignment must be assessed as these children commonly have some femoral internal torsion and a restriction of hip external rotation. Marked foot pronation is common in these athletes. A case history looks at the treatment of this condition in a young boy who swims and dances.

Case Study 4

A 12-year-old boy (CD) presented with bilateral inferior patellar pain, with the left knee more affected than the right. Pain was constant but exacerbated on walking up and down hills, descending stairs, kneeling, squatting and lunging.

His two sports were classical ballet and swimming which both reproduced his pain. He suffered the pain for one year before treatment and had no rapid growth spurts in this time. His older brother suffered the same condition when he was in his early teens.

A full muscle imbalance assessment demonstrated marked tightness of his iliotibial bands, rectus femoris and hamstrings. A restriction of hip external rotation was demonstrated bilaterally with reduced gluteal strength. A markedly pronated foot position associated with a valgus heel position was also noted.

Following a month of exercises, CD had significantly less knee pain. He was swimming and dancing more freely, but still complained of pain when squatting and kneeling. A gym programme was set up with his sports teacher to continue at school. One month later an increase in knee pain was triggered by a growth spurt. More pronation was evident and the use of orthotics in ballet and sports shoes was commenced. Lower limb alignment improved. Exercises and orthotics kept the pain at a manageable level.

Sinding–Larsen–Johansson Disease

This is similar to OSD in that it involves the patellar tendon. However, it affects the superior rather than the inferior end in the 10–12-year-old population (Anderson 1991b). It is less common than OSD, but still causes significant pain in the anterior knee. Causes of these two conditions are similar. Lower limb malalignment and muscular tightness are predisposing factors. Management is along similar lines to that of Osgood–Schlatter disease.

Bipartite Patella

Bipartite patella is a congenital anomaly that is a result of the superolateral ossification centre of the patella failing to fuse (Strizak and Stroberg 1986). It is a condition that more commonly affects males than females (9:1) and is frequently bilateral. It is often found incidental to another complaint or injury. It is generally asymptomatic, but may become painful following a direct blow to the knee or after repetitive microtrauma (Anderson 1991b). Pain is experienced in the superolateral aspect of the patella and it is hypothesized that this is due to increased mobility at the join of the normal patella and extrapatellar portion. Treatment is via relative rest, judicious strengthening of quadriceps and hamstrings and stretching of the iliotibial band and lateral retinaculum. In extreme cases immobilization for 3 weeks is recommended (Anderson 1991b). If pain becomes chronic, the accessory patella piece can be excised in conjunction with a lateral release of the patellar retinaculum (Strizak and Stroberg 1986).

Accurate diagnosis is essential in these chronic cases to ensure that the pain is not a result of a stress fracture of the patella. Whilst these are more commonly seen in the tibial plateau of the adolescent athlete, they may occur in the patella (Schmidt and Henry 1989). A bone scan will confirm the presence or absence of a stress fracture. Uptake of the radioactive isotope will occur with a stress fracture but not a bipartite patella. Stress fractures are rarely seen bilaterally.

Lower Limb Tendonitis and Apophysitis

There is much debate as to whether this exists in the growing athlete. As previously mentioned in this chapter, Micheli and Fehlandt (1992) postulate that apophysitis is more common during periods of growth whilst tendonitis is a complaint of quiescent growth periods.

Patellar and achilles' tendonitis, tibial tubercle and calcaneal apophysitis are reported in the skeletally immature population (Micheli and Ireland 1987, Schmidt and Henry 1989). Lower limb alignment is a frequent predisposing factor in combination with tightness of the two joint muscles and a concomitant weakness of opposing muscles.

Orthotics are frequently prescribed to correct foot pronation and heel valgus in patients with calcaneal apophysitis (Sever's disease). Tendoachilles' and hamstring stretching are implemented. Strengthening of the intrinsic muscles of the foot and tibialis posterior are also beneficial in the management of these patients. For patellar tendonitis and tibial tubercle apophysitis, stretching of hip flexors, quadriceps, hamstrings and calf muscles reduces pain.

Local application of ice and ultrasound is appropriate. Great care should be taken with the application of ultrasound over the growth plate. Sporting activity within pain limits is encouraged. Appropriate warm-up and cool-down sessions prior to competition and training are essential. Supervised stretching is a vital part of these sessions. It is important to remember that apophysitis and tendonitis commonly occur in two areas concurrently (Carter and Aldridge 1988) as they are linked with growth.

Osteochondritis Dissecans

This can occur with or without a traumatic injury. It is often discovered on close questioning that an injury occurred many months previously and is now the site of pain. In the knee for example, the child complains of pain and/or dull aches that are made worse by exercise and activity. Swelling is occasionally evident. The knee may catch as it is flexed but rarely locks in a position. There is obvious wasting of the quadriceps and adductor muscles. Pain is elicited on objective examination via palpation of the intercondylar notch with the knee flexed. Sometimes pain can be reproduced with knee flexion as the tibia is held in internal rotation.

A plain X-ray demonstrates an area of lucency in the subchondral bone that is disc shaped. This is usually seen on the medial femoral condyle near the intercondylar notch. The lateral condyle and patella are less commonly involved. A more recent injury as the causative factor results in a better outcome (Strizak and Stroberg 1986).

Treatment is dependent upon the acuteness and severity of the injury. Rest from activity and immobilization followed by progressive strengthening and a gradual increase in activity levels is the preferred management. If locking or pain persists, investigative surgery is warranted to ensure that secondary damage does not occur (Strizak and Stroberg 1986).

Less Common Causes of Knee Pain

Conditions of the hip can refer pain to the anterior aspect of the knee. Slipped capital femoral epiphysis is such a condition. Lumbar spine injuries and disorders can irritate the lumbosacral nerve roots and refer pain to the knee joint. Whilst this is less common in the adolescent than the adult, it has been reported and will be discussed in more depth in the section on the adolescent spine.

Neoplasms may cause persistent knee pain. These should not be disregarded in the differential diagnosis in the adolescent who responds poorly to treatment or has an unusual presentation of pain, for example shifting or diffuse pain or discomfort at rest. Infection and rheumatological causes should also be considered.

Growing Pains

Although growing pains cannot be classified as an overuse injury, because of their chronicity they are described in this section. There is little consensus on the subject of growing pains. Peterson (1986) describes them as a diffuse ache that is limited to the lower limbs. The quadriceps, posterior knee and calf muscles are most commonly affected. The child reports a diffuse ache that is difficult to localize. It does not occur daily and the child does not alter their gait or patterns of activity to accommodate the pain. It is commonly experienced bilaterally and is generally felt following activity. The child may awaken in the night complaining of pain.

Most investigators believe that growing pains are a result of muscle strain and fatigue. It is important that the adolescent/child is thoroughly examined to exclude any underlying pathology that may be a cause of pain. Treatment is usually symptomatic via the use of heat (warm bath), massage and muscle stretching. When growth stops the pains cease, adding weight to the theory that they are linked with musculoskeletal changes associated with the growth process (Peterson 1986).

The Adolescent Spine

BACK PAIN

Persistent back pain should never be ignored in the child or adolescent. Those who participate in sport are less likely to suffer from back pain. Indeed, Harvey and Tanner (1991) report that 85% of the population suffer from low back pain as compared to 5–8% in the athletic population.

Acute pain is usually traumatic in origin whilst chronic pain tends to result from overuse and repetitive microtrauma. Certain sports predispose the athlete to injury. Contact sports (e.g. football) have a high incidence of acute back injuries while overuse injuries are common in cricket fast-bowling, gymnastics, volleyball, rowing and long-distance running (Elliott 1991, Harvey and Tanner 1991).

The trunk links the upper and lower extremities. In all sports one or all limbs are involved in transmitting energy to achieve the requirements of the sport. If the muscles of the trunk and abdominals are weak, poor support is offered to the spine. A normal strength ratio is important. Hamstring and hip flexor length must also be considered. If these muscles are tight the lumbar spine loses its natural dynamic lordosis and its ability to transfer forces associated with the sport played.

Growth is considered a major cause of back injuries (Jackson and Ciullo 1986). The hamstrings and lumbodorsal fascia become tight in periods of rapid growth. Tightening of these structures results in an alteration in the position of the spine. Alterations in proprioception – the automatic knowledge of the spine's position – whilst performing a sports-related activity may result in an acute injury.

Training error, specifically an increase in intensity and frequency, may increase the incidence of back injury. Poor technique is another reported cause. Elliott (1991) reports that high-level cricket fast-bowlers who change from a front to side-on delivery position have a high occurrence of back pain.

Adolescents performing weight training require specific guidance with squats. Incorrect lifting techniques in this position can result in back injuries. Poor modification of equipment is another causative factor. Young cyclists, for example, who are constantly growing require regular adjustment of their bicycle to prevent injury.

Case Study 5

A national mountain biker in his late teens suffered recurrent iliotibial band friction syndrome and low back pain. Having been in the sport since his mid-teenage years he had grown enormously in that time. Despite temporary relief from physiotherapy and massage, full relief of pain was not achieved until his bike set-up had been adjusted to deal with his change in height and associated lower limb levers.

In the adolescent athlete most acute back injuries are those of muscular strains and sprains (Jackson and Ciullo 1986, Harvey and Tanner 1991). The mechanism of injury is usually one of lifting and/or twisting. The adolescent may present with marked tenderness directly over the spinous processes or over the paraspinal muscles while restriction of all movements is common. Treatment includes rest or restricted activity within pain limits, the use of pas-

sive physiological intervertebral movements and the application of ice and appropriate electrotherapy. Ranging exercises such as pelvic tilting and supine rotations may be instigated. Strengthening and stretching exercises can then be introduced as pain eases.

Sprains and strains respond quickly to effective treatment and the athlete usually returns to sport within 2 weeks of sustaining the injury. By 6 weeks, virtually all have returned to previous activity levels. Conditioning is important to prevent injury recurrence.

Whilst not helpful in the child under 10 years it has been found that resistance training/conditioning can improve muscular strength in near-pubescent and pubescent children (Maffulli and Pintore 1990). Muscular power and endurance of adolescents can also be improved by training (Bar-Or 1988), as can aerobic fitness (Shephard 1992). This has important implications for performance and rehabilitation.

It is important to use any training judiciously. Overtraining can lead to 'staleness' in the young athlete and excessive efforts can lead to injury to the joint surfaces of the skeletally immature athlete (Maffulli and Pintore 1990). Strength training should always be submaximal and adequate supervision is always required (Bar-Or 1988). Debate continues on its make-up, but most trainers advocate two sets of 10 submaximal repetitions. Same muscle groups should never be exercised on consecutive days. Effects of training are normally seen after 6–8 weeks.

Compression fractures are another acute injury and may occur when a vertical force is transmitted through the shoulders (Harvey and Tanner 1991). A football tackle is the common mechanism of injury, but in adolescents the nucleus pulposus is almost incompressible (Jackson and Ciullo 1986), so a longitudinal force is more likely to cause a growth plate fracture and herniation of the nucleus pulposus into the adjacent vertebral body. This is a more common occurrence than a disc protrusion.

A fracture of the transverse process of a vertebra may occur as a consequence of a direct blow to the back or via a forceful contraction of the psoas or quadratus lumborum muscles (Harvey and Tanner 1991). If the treating physiotherapist suspects that there is a bony injury then referral to a medical practitioner for further investigations is advisable.

Stress fractures of the pars interarticularis can also occur (Letts *et al.* 1986). Gymnasts and divers are most commonly affected and the injury may be unilateral or bilateral, resulting from repetitive lumbar spine flexion and extension. The loading does not need to be great as it is the cyclical behaviour of this movement that creates the stress. It is believed that one side fractures and then, as more load is placed on the opposite pars, an associated microfracture results (Letts *et al.* 1986). Management is via immobilization, usually in a thoracolumbar spine orthosis.

Back care and education in good posture and safe lifting techniques are essential for these patients (Robertson and Lee 1990). Advice on prevention of injury when playing sport is important. Athletes with unilateral fractures often return to their chosen sports and those with bilateral involvement may also do so with care. However, they are advised to avoid contact sports and seek medical attention if a recurrence of symptoms occurs (Letts *et al.* 1986).

Jackson and Ciullo (1986) report that lumbar facet syndrome can result in acute back pain. It is the result of repetitive hyperextension of the lumbar spine as seen in sports such as diving, golf and gymnastics. Pain is associated with this condition as the spinal nerves run close to the facet joints. Inflammation around these joints results in referred neural pain.

Straight leg raise manoeuvres are always restricted and reproduce pain for this reason. Movement from the forwardly flexed position to neutral also reproduces pain. Rest is the initial treatment regimen. As previously mentioned, appropriate strengthening of the lumbar / abdominal stabilizing muscles and stretching of tight musculature is required.

Hydrotherapy is extremely beneficial while occasionally the use of a back support / brace is required to allow pain-free daily activity.

Another condition that is caused by repetitive hyperextension movements is a spondylolysis. The fifth lumbar vertebra is most commonly affected (Letts *et al.* 1986). A defect through the pars interarticularis of this vertebra occurs. It may be unilateral as seen in the throwing sports such as javelin, and also occurs in

judo and diving. These involve rotation to one side as the spine is hyperextended. In gymnastics where back walkovers and dismounts involve pure hyperextension bilateral defects occur. The child complains of a chronic ache in the region that is exacerbated by hyperextension and rotation. Extension of the hip also reproduces their pain. Characteristically, these young athletes have tight hip flexors and hamstrings and weak abdominal muscles.

Cessation of the painful activity and rest is required to alleviate the symptoms. As for lumbar facet syndrome, bracing or support is often required and hydrotherapy is useful for pain relief. Strengthening and stretching programmes are begun as pain settles.

Whilst intervertebral disc herniations are not common in the adolescent athlete, they have been reported (Weinert and Rizzo 1992) and should not be ignored as a source of acute pain. The athlete is commonly involved in football or basketball and presents with low back pain with or without leg pain. There is a lack of forward flexion and ipsilateral lateral flexion as a result of the disc herniating posterolaterally. A flattening of the lumbar lordosis is apparent and a contralateral list may be evident. Straight leg raise is always reduced even if leg pain is not present. Risk factors are rapid growth spurts and adolescents who are in a high percentile for weight and height (Weinert and Rizzo 1992).

Treatment is with anti-inflammatory medication, rest, passive extension exercises and the wearing of a back brace to stabilize the region. Self-traction and prone mechanical traction as well as passive physiological intervertebral mobilizations are used. Stabilizing and stretching exercises are then begun with pain limits. An increase in activity and a gradual return to sport can then be achieved. Surgical intervention has been reported (Weinert and Rizzo 1992).

SCOLIOSIS

Much research has been done on juvenile and adolescent idiopathic scoliosis. In scoliosis the spine rotates about its longitudinal axis and deviates laterally (Miyaski 1980). This curvature of the spine occurs more frequently in females than males with figures of 10–20 / 1000 children screened reported. Only 1– 2 / 1000 have progressive scoliosis that requires inter-

Figure 8 An Adolescent with Scoliosis

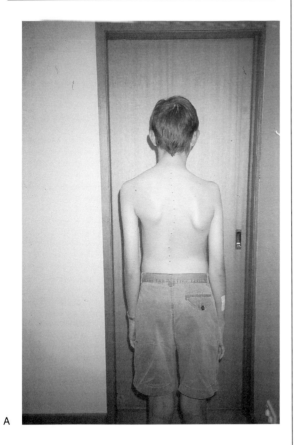

A

B

vention in the form of bracing, electrical stimulation or surgery (Emans 1984). The aetiology of scoliosis is unknown (Byrd 1988), but various hypotheses, such as asymmetrical proprioceptive and tactile responses (Barrack *et al.* 1984), abnormal postural equilibrium reactions (Yekutiel *et al.* 1981) and multifidus muscle asymmetry, have been proposed (Kennelly and Stokes 1993). See Figure 8.

Back pain is not commonly experienced by the adolescents with a lumbar or thoracolumbar scoliosis, but this population are more inclined to suffer back pain in later life (Farady 1983). Many researchers believe that early screening is essential to detect this at-risk group and monitor accordingly. Whilst Focarile *et al.* (1991) question the value of screening, they agree that early treatment is essential to provide a better outcome. They report that curves detected and treated at <30° have a better outcome than those ≥30°.

Treatment of curves greater than or equal to 30° is often initially via bracing. Examples are the Milwaukee (Farady 1983), Boston (Wynarsky and Schulz 1989, Ylikoski *et al.* 1989) and Charleston bending (Price *et al.* 1990) braces. They rely on a three-point process of correction. Wynarsky and Schultz (1989) claim that the Boston brace provides a passive correction of the curve and the brace is worn 23 hours per day to achieve maximum correction (Miyaski 1980).

Researchers (Farady 1983, Wynarsky and Schultz 1989, Focarile *et al.* 1991) agree that early detection and treatment are not the only factors influencing success of bracing. For example, Ylikoski *et al.* (1989) state that results are better if treatment starts before menarche and if a rapid growth spurt occurs before or during treatment. Once a brace is removed, Montgomery *et al.* (1990) report that adolescent idiopathic scoliosis curves will progress an average of 5.1°. This progression usually occurs within the first 2 years following cessation of brace wearing.

If the curve is not held by bracing, surgery is the next mode of treatment. Segmental spinal instrumentation is being used more commonly. Bergoin (1993) advocates its use as opposed to rod instrumentation, as it affords a three-dimensional correction of the deformity. No postoperative immobilization is required unless the scoliosis is particularly severe.

Physiotherapy care postoperatively is to prevent respiratory complications and assist in attainment of independent transfers and mobility. Upon discharge, the adolescent often returns for back care advice.

Lateral electrical surface stimulation (LESS) has been used in the treatment of adolescent idiopathic scoliosis (AIS) since 1977 (Swank *et al.* 1989). Many researchers advocate its use and claim its efficacy. Swank *et al.* (1989) report that curves progressed less than 10° in 65% of patients studied. After 3 years of follow-up only 51% of patients in a study by Bertrand *et al.* (1992) had a curve that progressed 5° or more with treatment via LESS whereas 36% of patients progressed 10° or more, resulting in a change of method of management.

Some researchers believe that LESS is an effective means of treating AIS curves >30°, but report that it has problems in its application (Bertrand *et al.* 1992). Physiotherapists using this as a treatment technique must be proficient in the selection of appropriate patients, correct on/off times, and intensity of stimulating current and electrode placement. Electrodes are placed at the apex of the curve on the convex side. If positioning is incorrect, the risk of curve progression may be increased. Compliance is essential for good results, but with some adolescents this can be a problem. It is claimed by Bertrand *et al.* (1992) that LESS has a good psychological effect on the adolescents treated, but Swank *et al.* (1989) report that skin rashes, sleep disturbances and patient concern regarding correct electrode placement affect compliance.

Exercise is not used in isolation for treatment of AIS ≥30°. Stone *et al.* (1979) reported using exercises in a group of adolescents with minimal scoliosis (5–20°) to attempt to correct the deformity, but a lack of control of variables affecting outcome negates the validity of the results. Routinely, adolescents braced for scoliosis carry out an exercise programme. Swimming is encouraged as a principle means of fitness, as the buoyancy of the water relieves pressure on the spine. Any non-contact sport is encouraged. Specific exercises to improve muscle strength and length are instigated, but these are not designed to correct the curvature. Improvement in posture is a byproduct of performing the exercise programme.

Figure 9 Lateral Flexion Exercises in the Adolescent with Scoliosis

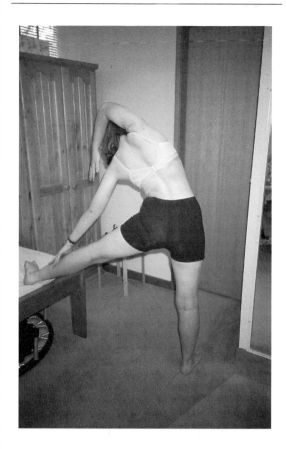

After 1–2 months of wearing the brace, the adolescent attends for an exercise programme. The exercises are performed 5–7 times per week initially out of the brace. Pelvic tilting and hollowing to initiate lower abdominal strength and stretch the back extensor muscles is begun. In supine, the knees are flexed and extended. Active back extension in prone and push-ups are commenced to facilitate back muscle strength. Exercises in standing to correct the dorsal rib hump and lateral flexion of the spine are included. Furthermore, hamstring flexibility exercises and a gluteal muscle strengthening programme is started.

As the adolescent improves, exercises are performed in the brace. More difficult abdominal exercises are introduced. Lateral flexion activities to stretch the trunk are encouraged (Figure 9). Most adolescents enjoy weight training or aerobics and an exercise programme incorporating these activities assists compliance. Adequate instruction and supervision of these programmes is essential. As muscle length and strength improve the programme must be mod-

Figure 10 An Adolescent with Kyphosis

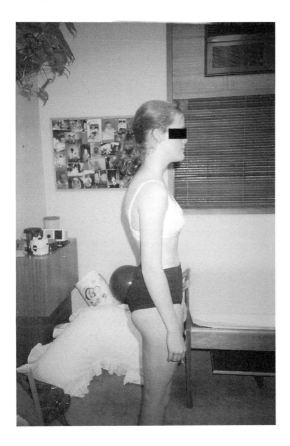

ified. Physiotherapists are ideally placed to advise on back care, posture and brace wearing and should include these areas in their treatment regimen.

KYPHOSIS

Normal values for the thoracic kyphosis are between 20° and 40° of angulation (Sachs *et al.* 1987). When the forward curve of the thoracic spine exceeds this, it is described as a postural kyphosis or Scheuermann's thoracic kyphosis. The two conditions are not the same. The postural condition is a result of various tight and weak muscles acting on the thoracic spine. This type responds well to exercise and postural correction. See Figure 10.

Scheuermann's kyphosis or spinal osteochondritis has a genetic component and is thought to be an autosomal dominant inherited condition (Baker 1988). It is not confined to the thoracic spine and is seen in 20–30% of the population. Males equal females in incidence, but males are usually more

symptomatic than females, suffering back pain and stiffness.

Scheuermann's kyphosis is classified as follows: more than three vertebrae must be wedge-shaped by more than 5°, vertebral endplate irregularity occurs anteriorly and Schmorl's nodes (herniations of the nucleus pulposus into the vertebral bodies) are present (Baker 1988).

Sachs *et al.* (1987) reports good results with exercise for curves <60°. If a curve is greater than this value and progressive, respiratory function may be impaired. Pain is an associated problem and spinal fusion is the treatment of choice. These investigators note in their retrospective study that although surgical correction was initially up to 50% of the measured curve, follow-up 2 years postoperatively showed a progressive loss of correction.

In curves <60° but >40°, treatment is often via a thoracolumbar spinal orthosis. Occasionally, a breast plate will be added if the curve is high in the thoracic spine. The brace is worn 23 hours per day until growth ceases and exercises are instructed to improve muscle strength, length and postural control. If the curve is relatively small, exercise alone may be the choice of treatment.

Exercises are directed towards stretching the hamstrings, gluteals, hip flexors, back extensors and pectoral muscles At the same time strengthening activities specifically target the deep neck flexors, scapular stabilizing muscles, abdominal groups and

Figure 11 An Adolescent with Kyphosis Undertaking Strengthening of Abdominal Muscles

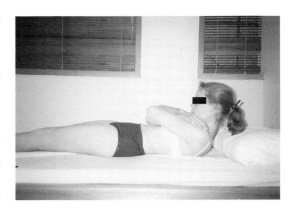

gluteals. Postural correction using feedback is useful. See Figure 11.

Occasionally strapping of the scapulae in a retracted position provides proprioceptive and sensory feedback to the adolescent to promote a more extended thoracic spine. Sports underlay is used and can be left in place for up to 3 days. It is a useful way of facilitating postural correction. Care with sensitive skin is essential and gradual weaning from the strapping is important to allow the muscles reflexly to correct the adolescents' flexed posture.

Summary

Highlighted in this chapter have been the more common injuries unique to the skeletally immature athlete and their aetiology. The presence of growth cartilage and the process of growth itself are important factors. It is essential to be aware of the different methods of managing acute and chronic injuries in adolescents. By so doing, the physiotherapist ensures accurate diagnosis and treatment of the initial problem and prevention of subsequent injuries.

REFERENCES

Anderson, SJ (1991a) Acute knee injuries in young athletes. *Physician and Sportsmedicine* 19: 69–76.

Anderson, SJ (1991b) Overuse knee injuries in young athletes. *Physician and Sportsmedicine* 19: 77–80.

Andrish, JT (1986) Upper extremity injuries in the skeletally immature athlete. In: Nicholas, JA, Hershman, EB (eds) *Upper Extremity in Sports Medicine*, pp. 673–688. St Louis: CV Mosby.

Baker, KG (1988) Scheurmann's disease: a review. *Australian Journal of Physiotherapy* 34: 165–169.

Bar-Or, O (1988) Adaptability of the musculoskeletal, cardiovascular and respiratory systems. In: Dirix, A, Knuttgen, HG, Tittel, K (eds) *The Olympic Book of Sports Medicine*, pp. 269–275. Oxford: Blackwell Scientific.

Barrack, RL, Whitecloud, TS, Burke, SW et al. (1984) Proprioception in idiopathic scoliosis. *Spine* 9: 681–685.

Bergoin, M (1993) Management of idiopathic scoliosis in children. *Annales de Pediatrie* (Paris) 40: 259–269.

Bertrand, SL, Drvaric, DM, Lange, N (1992) Electrical stimulation for idiopathic scoliosis. *Clinical Orthopaedics and Related Research* 276: 176–181.

Busch, MT (1990) Meniscal injuries in children and adolescents. *Clinics in Sports Medicine* 9: 661–680.

Byrd, JA (1988) Current theories on the etiology of idiopathic scoliosis. *Clinical Orthopaedics and Related Research* 229: 114–119.

Caine, DJ, Broekhoff, J (1987) Maturity assessment: a viable preventive measure against physical and psychological insult to the young athlete? *Physician and Sportsmedicine* 15: 67–80.

Carter, SR, Aldridge, MJ (1988) Stress injury of the distal radial growth plate. *Journal of Bone and Joint Surgery* 70B: 834–836.

DeLee, JC, Pearce, JC (1990) Knee ligament injuries in children. *Advances in Sports Medicine and Fitness* 3: 169–196.

Elliott, B (1991) *Adolescent Overuse Sporting Injuries: A Biomechanical Review.* Australian Council for Health, Physical Education and Recreation. National Conference Proceedings.

Emans, JB (1984) Scoliosis: diagnosis and current treatment. *Womens Health* 9: 81–102.

Farady, JA (1983) Current principles in the nonoperative management of structural adolescent idiopathic scoliosis. *Physical Therapy* 63: 512–522.

Focarile, FA, Bonaldi, A, Giarolo, M et al. (1991) Effectiveness of nonsurgical treatment for idiopathic scoliosis. Overview of available evidence. *Spine* 16: 395–401.

Foster, DN, Fulton, MN (1991) Back pain and the exercise prescription. *Clinics in Sports Medicine* 10: 197–209.

Harvey, JS (1982) Overuse syndromes in young athletes. *Pediatric Clinics of North America* 29: 1369–1381.

Harvey, J, Tanner, S (1991) Low back pain in young athletes: a practical approach. *Sports Medicine* 12: 394–406.

Jackson, DW, Ciullo, JV (1986) Injuries of the spine in the skeletally immature athlete. In: Nicholas JA and Hershman EB (eds) *The Lower Extremity and Spine in Sports Medicine*, pp. 1333–1374. St Louis: CV Mosby.

Karlin, LI (1986) Injuries to the hip and pelvis in the skeletally immature athlete. In: Nicholas, JA, Hershman, EB (eds) *The Lower Extremity and Spine in Sports Medicine*, pp. 1292–1332. St Louis: CV Mosby.

Kellenberger, R, von Laer, L (1990) Nonosseous lesions of the anterior cruciate ligaments in childhood and adolescence. *Progress in Pediatric Surgery* 25: 123–131.

Kennelly, K, Stokes, MJ (1993) Pattern of assymetry of paraspinal muscle size in adolescent idiopathic scoliosis examined by real-time ultrasound imaging. A preliminary study. *Spine* 18: 913–917.

King, HA (1986) Evaluating the child with back pain. *Pediatric Clinics of North America* 33: 1489–1493.

Letts, M, Smallman, T, Afanasiev, R et al. (1986) Fracture of the pars interarticularis in adolescent athletes. A clinical–biomechanical analysis. *Journal of Pediatric Orthopedics* 6: 40–46.

Lincoln, E (1984) Sports in childhood: a round table. *Sport Health* 2: 14–19.

Maffulli, N, Pintore, E (1990) Intensive training in young athletes. *British Journal of Sports Medicine* 24: 237–239.

Marans, HJ, Angel, KR, Schemitsch, EH et al. (1992) The fate of traumatic anterior dislocation of the shoulder in children. *Journal of Bone and Joint Surgery* 74A(8): 1242–1244.

McConnell, J (1986) The management of chondromalacia patellae. A long term solution. *Australian Journal of Physiotherapy* 32: 215–223.

Meyers, JF (1988) Injuries to the shoulder girdle and elbow. In: Sullivan JA, Hershman, WB (eds) *The Paediatric Athlete*, pp. 145–153. Baltimore: Port City Press.

Meyers, MH, McKeever, FM (1970) Fracture of the intercondylar eminence of the tibia. *Journal of Bone and Joint Surgery* 52A: 1677–1684.

Micheli, LJ (1983) Overuse injuries in children's sports: the growth factor. *Orthopedic Clinics of North America* 14: 337–360.

Micheli, LJ, Fehlandt, AF (1992) Overuse injuries to tendons and apophyses in children and adolescents. *Clinics in Sports Medicine* 11: 713–726.

Micheli, LJ, Ireland, ML (1987) Prevention and management of calcaneal apophysitis in children: an overuse syndrome. *Journal of Pediatric Orthopedics* 7: 34–38.

Miyasaki, AA (1980) Immediate influence of the thoracic flexion exercise on vertebral position in Milwaukee brace wearers. *Physical Therapy* 60: 1005–1009.

Montgomery, F, Willner, S, Appelgren, G (1990) Long-term follow-up of patients with adolescent idiopathic scoliosis treated conservatively: an analysis of the clinical value of progression. *Journal of Pediatric Orthopedics* 10: 48–52.

Neer, CS II (1972) Anterior impingement for the chronic impingement syndrome in the shoulder: a preliminary report. *Journal of Bone and Joint Surgery* 54(A): 41–50.

Nirschl, RP (1986) Shoulder tendinitis. In: Pettrone, FA (ed.) *Symposium on Upper Extremity Injuries.* St Louis: CV Mosby.

O'Neill, DB, Micheli, LJ, Warner, JP (1992) Patellofemoral stress: a prospective analysis of exercise treatment in adolescents and adults. *American Journal of Sports Medicine* 20: 151–155.

Peterson, H (1986) Growing pains. *Pediatric Clinics of North America* 33: 1365–1371

Price, CT, Scott, DS, Reed Jr, FE *et al.* (1990) Nighttime bracing for adolescent idiopathic scoliosis with the Charleston bending brace. Preliminary report. *Spine* 15: 1294–1299.

Priest, JD, Weise, DJ (1981) Elbow injury in women's gymnastics. *American Journal of Sports Medicine* 9: 288–295.

Robertson, HC, Lee, VL (1990) Effects of back care lessons on sitting and lifting by primary students. *Australian Journal of Physiotherapy* 36: 245–248.

Ryu, RK, McCormick, J, Jobe, FW *et al.* (1988). An electromyographic analysis of shoulder function in tennis players. *American Journal of Sports Medicine* 16: 481–485.

Sachs, B, Bradford, D, Winter, R *et al.* (1987) Scheuermann kyphosis. Follow-up of Milwaukee brace treatment. *Journal of Bone and Joint Surgery* 69A: 50–57.

Salter, RB, Harris, WR (1963) Injuries involving the epiphyseal plate. *Journal of Bone and Joint Surgery* 45A: 587–622.

Schmidt, DR, Henry, JH (1989) Stress injuries of the adolescent extensor mechanism. *Clinics in Sports Medicine* 8: 343–355.

Shephard, RJ (1992) Effectiveness of training programmes for prepubescent children. *Sports Medicine* 13: 194–214.

Stone, B, Beekman, C, Hall, V *et al.* (1979) The effect of an exercise program on change in curve in adolescents with minimal idiopathic scoliosis: a preliminary study. *Physical Therapy* 59: 759–763.

Strizak, AM, Stroberg, AJ (1986) Knee injuries in the skeletally immature athlete. In: Nicholas, JA, Hershman, EB (eds) *The Lower Extremity and Spine in Sports Medicine*, pp. 1261–1291. St Louis: CV Mosby.

Swank, SM, Brown, JC, Jennings, MV *et al.* (1989) Lateral electrical surface stimulation in idiopathic scoliosis. Experience in two private practices. *Spine* 14: 1293–1295.

Turco, VJ, Spinella, AJ (1986) Injuries to the foot and ankle in the skeletally immature athlete. In: Nicholas, JA, Hershman, EB (eds) *The Lower Extremity and Spine in Sports Medicine*, pp. 1233–1261. St Louis: CV Mosby.

Watson, AS (1992) Children in sport. In: Bloomfield, J, Fricker, PA, Fitch, KD (eds) *Textbook of Science and Medicine in Sport*, pp. 436–466. Melbourne: Blackwell Scientific.

Weinert, AM, Rizzo, TD (1992) Nonoperative management of multilevel lumbar disk herniations in the adolescent athlete. *Mayo Clinic Proceedings* 67: 137–141.

Wojtys, EM (1987) Sports injuries in the immature athlete. *Orthopedic Clinics of North America* 18: 689–694.

Wynarsky, GT, Schultz, AB (1989) Trunk muscle activity in braced scoliosis patients. *Spine* 14: 1283–1286.

Yekutiel, M, Robin, GC, Yarom, R (1981) Proprioceptive function in children with adolexscent idiopathic scoliosis. *Spine* 6: 560–566

Ylikoski, M, Peltonen, J, Poussa, M (1989) Biological factors and predictability of bracing in adolescent idiopathic scoliosis. *Journal of Pediatric Orthopedics* 9: 680–683.

Section G:

Physiotherapy Practice in Neurological, Neuromuscular and Developmental Conditions from Infancy to Adolescence

PROLOGUE: YVONNE BURNS

Prologue

YVONNE BURNS

Infants, children and adolescents with a movement disorder due to damage to or dysfunction of the central nervous system (brain and/or spinal cord) form one of the largest groups, and often present with the most complex set of problems requiring physiotherapy services.

In no other group of conditions is the knowledge of child development and interaction of the various aspects of the whole child more important or pertinent. Furthermore, the issue of maturation and environment has a number of implications for programme development in so far as an understanding of the variations accepted to be within normal limits and those considered to be outside the normal range is essential. Consider how some children within a family have advanced physical and motor attainments while others may develop early in the area of manipulation of objects or language. We do not know how much family or inborn traits influence response to intervention, but we do know that some children, despite the apparent severity of their impairment, have a functionally better outcome than others who appear to have a much lesser degree of impairment.

Assessment provides the basis for programme planning, but repeated re-evaluation of progress and outcome of intervention is essential. Careful interpretation of assessment findings is necessary as it is often not the approach or technique which is at fault, but the appropriateness of the intervention to the particular child and the problem being addressed. Physiotherapists working in this area of paediatrics need to be flexible; that is they must have the ability to change, adapt and modify together with a patient and family. An open, friendly personality and an ability to engage the child in play which will achieve therapeutic goals are additional helpful attributes.

Just as there are different ways of teaching the same or different subjects at school, there are different approaches to intervention which can be used as alternatives, or for different purposes at different times. Over the last two decades much has been written regarding various approaches to the assessment and treatment of infants and children with central nervous system impairments, particularly cerebral palsy. The aim of this section therefore is not to describe in detail these various techniques and approaches, but to provide some basic principles for decision-making and a range of options which may be suitable for different types of problems and in different age groups. In this section much use is made of typical case scenarios and stories.

It is important that we do not try to place our own perceptions and expectations on to the child. A lesson learnt from experience was as follows:

> *Having worked for several years with a young girl with quite severe cerebral palsy and much determination to achieve independent walking, I found that she seemed to lose interest in using this new achievement. She seemed surprised when I asked about this and said 'I have more exciting things to do with my time and energy'. She went on to say 'if you learnt to ski it would not mean that you would want to ski for the rest of your life, but you would be satisfied that you had achieved your goal and go on to seek further challenges.'*

We must always be ready to listen and to learn!

Before and during the reading of this section it may be helpful to refer back to Chapter 9, 'Principles of Physiotherapy Management'. Section G opens with a chapter on the physiotherapy management of the preterm and high-risk term infant, while case scenarios are used to illustrate some typical situations involving developmental movement dysfunction and physiotherapy management of infants 4 and 8 months of age.

Chapter 21 follows the child from initial physiotherapy contact until commencing school. The story of Joe addresses some important aspects and principles of treatment of cerebral palsy. Down's syndrome has been used to highlight some developmental and other problems, such as low muscle tone, experienced by children with a chromosome abnormality and similar conditions. Following this, the story of Alex highlights the problems faced by a child with spina bifida and some of the management strategies and issues that need to be addressed in the treatment of a child with this complex congenital anomaly. Physiotherapists need to be aware of possible reasons for loss of ability in some older children and adolescents with spina bifida. The scenario portrayed in the story of Tess will help to understand some of the issues involved. Many aspects of management of the child with spina bifida will be applicable also to the child with spinal cord injuries.

Damage to the more mature brain through trauma brings another perspective to the type of problems encountered, in particular the loss of previous skills and some of the behavioural/emotional implications. Jack sustained a head injury when his bike collided with a motor vehicle. He was not wearing a safety helmet. Acquired brain injury due to near drowning is frequently a preventable tragedy as it usually involves the briefly unsupervised 2-year-old toddler near unprotected areas of water such as private swimming pools. Some special features of care are included in this section.

Tumour in the form of medulloblastoma opens the issues of the primary lesion and secondary or associated problems. At the age of 13 years Tom was diagnosed with a tumour which was surgically removed. Although prognosis and early recovery were good, at the age of 14 he was facing a number of frustrating problems.

The final chapter in this section addresses the assessment and management of minor coordination difficulties, 'clumsiness' or minimal cerebral dysfunction which are terms used to describe a group of problems which adversely affect the quality of motor performance of preschool and school-aged children. Although seemingly mild or almost insignificant in terms of clinical presentation and therefore often overlooked, this group of problems can be a major handicap for the individual child and family.

20

Physiotherapy Management of the Neonate and Infant – Developmental Problems

KYM MORRIS

Development of Muscle Tone, Posture and Movement
•
Movement and Muscle Activity
•
The Neonatal Intensive Care Unit (NICU)
•
Gastro-oesophageal Reflux (GOR)
•
Cerebral Insult
•
Chronic Neonatal Lung Disease (CNLD) and Motor Development
•
Management of the Developmentally Delayed Infant

One of the first experiences a newborn infant must deal with is the organization of posture in the extra-uterine environment. A full-term newborn has a small, but definite degree of postural control. The infant has appropriate muscle control to achieve some postural adjustments and body position changes.

Babies who are born a number of weeks early and with a very low birth weight often require special life-supporting care. Immaturities in development at birth, and consequent reduction of time spent in the optimal environment provided by the uterus, together with the procedures associated with sustaining this very fragile life in the neonatal intensive care unit, and within the confines of an incubator may limit the baby's development of muscle strength, movement and body control. In contrast to the newborn full-term neonate, the newborn premature neonate is unable to achieve postural adjustments due to low muscle tone and immature organizational systems.

Before discussing how environmental constraints may influence the premature infant's movement and postural control, it is necessary to understand some aspects of this very early development. Although infants born as young as 24 weeks of gestation move their limbs spontaneously and in an isolated or disorganized way, very little resistance to passive movement can be felt. This is described as hypotonia (Campbell 1974).

Development of Muscle Tone, Posture and Movement

Muscle tone appears to develop in a caudocephalic direction from about 28 weeks of gestation to term (Campbell 1974). In infants of 28 weeks or younger gestation there is marked hypotonia with the legs lying in extension and the arms in whatever position they are placed. Movements are jerky and brief. In general by 30 weeks of gestation the preterm infant's basic tone is developing in the distal segments of the lower limbs. The infant may display more spontaneous bursts of activity, which are wide and swiping. The posture and movement of the infant at 32 weeks of gestation demonstrates evidence of more tone in the infant's hips and knees resulting in a flexion and abduction posture. By 34–35 weeks of gestation the upper limbs tend to be less hypotonic, exhibiting smoother movements and more overall flexion, particularly as term approaches.

Posturally, in the newborn term infant flexor tone predominates over extension, and they adopt a curled position. This means their shoulders are forward, the bottom is tucked under with hips and knees curled up and the chin is tucked in. Arms and legs tend to be close in to the body. At term the preterm born infant usually has less-developed 'physiologic flexion' in the limbs, trunk and pelvis than the full-term newborn (Campbell 1984, Sweeney 1986, Allen and Capute 1990). Although the postural characteristics of the preterm infant tend to be related to gestational age these infants are also under the influence of gravitational forces and are further affected by the nature and degree of acute illness.

Movement and Muscle Activity

The cyclic repetition of movements evident both in-utero during the later stage of pregnancy and in the newborn term infant are not apparent in infants of less than 32 weeks gestation of age. Although fetal movements have been observed by real-time ultrasonography before 12 weeks of gestation (Mastaglia 1981, Cintas 1987), it is in the last few weeks before term that babies very actively push against the elastic sides of the womb and meet with gentle resistance thus building up their muscle strength. If born prematurely, an infant nursed in an incubator has considerable air space around them, with nothing to push against.

The third trimester is important in the development of muscle fibre differentiation and it has been suggested that resisted muscular activity is a major factor responsible for the final differentiation and hypertrophy of the muscle fibre types (Goldspink 1980,

Mastaglia 1981, Cintas 1987). It is proposed that, in the hypotonic and hypokinetic sick preterm neonate, changes in the viscoelastic properties of the muscles and tendons may result from prolonged inactivity of movement (Casaer 1979, Mastaglia 1981). Consequently, it is possible that the setting of the muscle receptors may be imbalanced and in turn may affect the neonate's later postural and movement behaviour.

The consequence of poor muscle tone, little spontaneous activity, lack of appropriate resistance, positioning for care procedures and the continuing influence of gravity can result in a 'flattening' of the sick preterm neonate's body against the supporting surface (Campbell 1984, Sweeney 1986, Fay 1988). The characteristic features of this 'flattening' are:

- lower limbs — flexed, externally rotated and abducted with feet abducted and dorsiflexed (may affect later weight bearing)
- upper limbs — retracted with shoulders abducted and externally rotated, arms flexed (may delay development of midline orientation)
- lateral head flattening – (dolichocephaly) with head positioned from one side to the other and remaining on the side (may result in difficulties in controlling head turning and holding in the midline)
- palatal narrowing – interplay of compressive forces between gravity and the supporting mattress surface (Morris and Burns 1994), and possible effects of endotracheal tube (may contribute to aberrant feeding patterns)

Positioning

PRONE VERSUS SUPINE
Whilst this body 'flattening' may result from either prone or supine lying, supine lying has been reported to cause more asymmetries. An asymmetrical tonic neck reflex to the side the head is turned may be reinforced (Burns and Bullock 1980). Hand preference to the side the head is turned has been reported (Konishi et al. 1986). Trunk and continued skull asymmetries have been noted also to result (Desmond 1980).

Perhaps this difference may be explained by the earlier development of head control observed in prone-lying infants (Holt 1960). It has been reported also that prone-lying infants lift their head more frequently than supine-lying infants, hence reducing the effect of a prolonged head position (Casaer 1979).

Prone positioning in the acutely ill preterm infant has been shown to have other benefits over supine positioning (as described in Chapter 13). Clinically, it has been observed that infants positioned a $\frac{1}{4}$ turn away from full supine or prone move more freely.

PROLONGED POSITIONING

As the premature infant's medical condition stabilizes and overall improvement occurs, then active muscle tone appears to improve allowing movement within the 'flattened posture'. Continued activity in this pattern may lead to an imbalance in motor function and may result in the infant adopting a 'flying' or 'startle' posture with a predominance of an extensor/retracted pattern of movement activity.

Consequently, at term gestation very prematurely born babies may have an extended posture rather than being curled in or flexed. The flexor muscle groups may remain weak due to decreased motor activity. This functional imbalance may lead to deviations in the quality of feeding patterns and motor milestones, such as head control in midline, pelvic control in sitting, shoulder and trunk stability with hands to midline/reaching, and weight-bearing in prone and later in standing.

When more active, infants have often been observed attempting to achieve postural stability and orientation within their environment. The infant may do this by seeking out a stable surface, such as the side wall of the isolette, to rest against or rhythmically push against. Therefore, boundaries and supports for containment, security and encouragement of flexion are important for these infants.

Development of Behavioural Stability

Along with the development of postural control is the differentiation and stability of attentional behaviours (Casaer 1979, Campbell 1984). It has been reported that babies who lie on their tummies spend more time in quiet sleep and display less disturbed sleep (Masterton 1987). Soothing through natural care-giving of stroking or resting a hand on body parts, and the infant's own natural self-comforting such as non-nutritive sucking on a pacifier, help develop the ability to cope better with stressful situations. Gaining stability of motor and behavioural states is likely to facilitate social responsiveness, which is fundamental for the initiation of early bonding and attachment with parents (Sweeney 1986).

The Neonatal Intensive Care Unit (NICU)

Apart from the infant's degree of illness and physical limitations due to prematurity, the environment of a NICU may itself be unfavourable for the integration and stability of motor and behavioural function. By astutely interpreting the individual infant's behavioural signals (Als et al. 1982), the physical environment and care-giving activities may be used to enhance the infant's attempts to gain postural and behavioural stability.

Positive Infant Behaviours

- pink, stable colour
- smooth respiration
- hand clasping, foot clasping, finger holding
- hand-to-mouth manoeuvres
- tucking in
- suck searching and suckling
- clearly defined sleep states
- rhythmical robust crying
- effective self-quieting
- intent or animated facial expression

Negative or Stress Behaviours

- averting gaze, stare or roving eye movements
- fussing, crying or drowsy state
- pale or mottled skin colour
- hiccoughing, sneezing
- straining as if or actually producing bowel motion
- frowning and other facial grimaces
- frequent twitching, tremoring, startling

- 'flat' body and facial expression
- body and facial hyperresponsiveness through:
  - extensor movements, finger splaying or arching
  - over-strong flexor postures or fisting

Effects on Parents

It has been reported that it is not so much the extent of early separation of infant and parent that influences later behaviours, but rather the quality of parental intervention during the infant's hospital stay (Field 1977). Research has shown that parents of preterm babies react differently and they tend to handle the babies less (Anderson and Auster-Liebhaber 1984).

Parents may go through many emotional states which will affect how 'close' they get to their infant. These anxieties can interfere with the normal process of getting to know their infant during care-giving. Therefore support and education of parents in the needs of their infant may facilitate early positive interactions and enhance the process of attachment. It would appear critical that parents play an active role in managing their infant in relation to handling, positioning and stimulation, in order to facilitate bonding and confidence in preparation for caring for their infant at home (Piper et al. 1986).

Developmental Intervention

Numerous studies have been undertaken to investigate effects of various supplemental stimulation programmes on the growth and development of premature infants (Lieb et al. 1980, Rausch 1981, Field et al. 1986, Field 1986, Piper et al. 1986, Lester and Tronick 1990, Parker 1990). Though results have been variable there has been a consensus on three points for any form of developmental intervention:

- All intervention should suit the needs of the individual infant with respect to their medical, motor and behavioural states.
- Any intervention should involve the parents to facilitate bonding and confidence in preparation for caring for their infant at home.
- The development of motor and behavioural responses in the preterm infant may be enhanced by appropriate positioning and handling techniques. This is not considered as something extra being done to or for the infant, but, rather a 'special way' of performing the everyday care-giving activities.

The physiotherapist with a knowledge of the development of posture, movement and motor control has much to contribute to the early and ongoing care of the very premature and very sick infant. A thorough assessment of the infant's neurodevelopmental and behavioural status is the initial step in establishing an intervention programme.

Assessment of Neurodevelopment

A number of assessments (Als et al. 1982, Brazelton 1984, Dubowitz 1985), have been developed to provide a profile of neonatal behaviours and neurological progress. Some of these tests require training before to use or involve considerable handling. As frail infants do not tolerate much handling or long periods of testing much of the assessment should be through observation. It is important to include in an assessment consistent/spontaneous postures and movement patterns and muscle responsiveness as well as autonomic and behavioural status.

When instituting a developmental handling programme the physiotherapist's goals should include:

- enhance physiological flexion and flexor movement patterns
- encourage midline orientation
- promote stability of behavioural state
- promote parent–infant interaction
- enhance early functional abilities such as feeding
- prevent secondary posture and movement problems

Routine Care and Procedures

During the baby's stay in hospital parents/caregivers are educated in the 'special way' of handling and providing comfort for the infant through the use of neurosensory and motor techniques. Initially, parents are instructed on how to look for behavioural cues from their baby when being handled for routine care

Figure 1 Nursing Positions: A, prone with rolls and supports; B, $\frac{1}{4}$ from prone with supports; C, $\frac{1}{2}$ turn with supports; D, $\frac{1}{4}$ from supine.

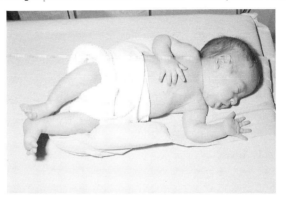

D

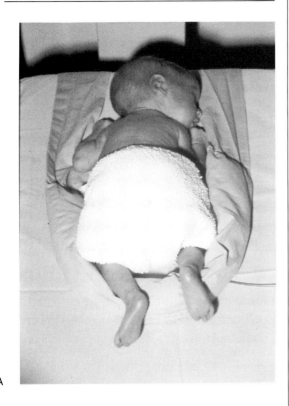

A

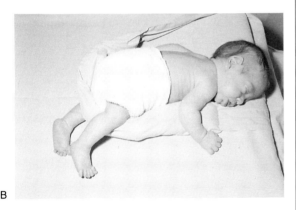

B

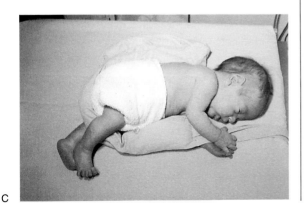

C

or procedures. Suggestions are then given to encourage self-comforting by the infant along with the use of touch/stroking, voice, movement and eye contact to comfort and promote behavioural stability.

Emphasis is made on the need to ensure that touch is a definite contact — not feather-light touch or tickling as many babies are tactile hypersensitive. When talking to the infant it is important to try to establish eye contact (i.e. the face should always be at the infant's eye level). Input should be provided near to the infant's midline to encourage centralization. It should be stressed that inputs may need to be introduced to the baby one at a time whilst watching the baby's responses for signs of needing time out. Rolled towelling and later wrapping are used to provide postural stability and offer definite boundaries for the infant to push against, whilst promoting behavioural stability through containment and security.

The needs of the prematurely born infant during their hospital stay may be addressed more specifically in three phases, as outlined next.

PHASE I: THE ACUTELY ILL AND VENTILATED NEONATE

This phase includes the ventilated neonate who may be receiving respiratory physiotherapy intervention. The infant may be nursed on a radiant heat table or in an isolette. Aims of positioning and handling at this stage are as follows:

- to maintain and promote respiratory function
- to reduce effect of immobility and peripheral oedema

- to alleviate possible risks of gastro-oesophageal reflux (GOR)
- to facilitate the positive use of major and minor handling times
- to reduce unfavourable and unnecessary auditory, visual and tactile stimulation and enhance positive and rewarding stimulation
- to encourage stability of behavioural states.

Some ways of achieving these aims are summarized next.

- The use of sheepskin (covered by a sheet), to provide comforting tactile experiences and to reduce the effect of immobility and pressure-bearing surfaces.
- The use of prone and $\frac{1}{4}$ turn from prone positioning regimens with 4–6 hourly position changes. The $\frac{1}{4}$ turn from prone position reduces the weight-bearing pressure on the zygomatic arch and associated bony structures which contributes to lateral craniofacial flattening and palatal narrowing (Morris and Burns 1994). During this phase, supports such as the 'pressure dispersing pads' may be introduced to provide relief of such pressures (Morris and Burns 1994). The $\frac{1}{2}$ turn (side-lying) is incorporated into the positioning regimen as soon as respiratory function is stable [see Figure 1A–C].

A rolled or folded nappy and small narrow rolls are essential to support the infant in the above-mentioned positions. These supports provide a source of containment and alleviate the effects of gravity. Facilitation of flexion at the hips, knees, trunk and shoulders is encouraged where possible to minimize positional moulding and promote physiological flexion.

Although the benefits of prone outweigh the benefits of supine (a more settled behavioural state, stability of postural state, improved ventilation and respiratory patterns and improved gastric emptying with reduced risk of GOR), supine positioning does allow easier infant access, easier observation of chest movement, and umbilical catheter integrity. Supine and $\frac{1}{4}$ turn from supine positioning (Figure 1D) may be selected while the infant is critically unstable.

- Routine nursing of infants with the head of the bed elevated to alleviate possible risks of:
  - abdominal contents interfering with diaphragmatic movement
  - spontaneous and often clinically non-apparent GOR due to immature sphincter control.
- Coordinating all intervention to allow major handling times and minor or (no) handling times.
- Encouraging parents to hold their infant's hand, cup their hand around their infant's head or bottom, or gently stroke their infant in times of infant stress and when the infant is well rested. Also encouraging the infant to suck on a finger or pacifier provides a source of self-comfort during times of stress or pain. Depending on the infant's physiological stability a brief 'cuddle' has many benefits to parent and infant.
- The sick ventilated neonate should be positioned to avoid high traffic areas. Parents are encouraged to talk or read to their infant in soft tones or provide a cassette for them to listen to.

PHASE 2: THE CONVALESCING INFANT

This phase includes those infants who are not on mechanical ventilation and not requiring respiratory physiotherapy intervention.

The preterm infant may still require an isolette for temperature control and close observation. Gastric feeds are gradually being increased to full quota for the infant and the aims of positioning and handling at this stage include:

- facilitation of feed tolerance and hence promotion of weight gain
- alternating pressure-bearing surfaces
- reduction of positional moulding
- reinforcement of major and minor handling times to facilitate stability of behavioural states
- promotion of coordinated motor activity
- provision of favourable tactile, auditory and visual environment
- promotion of bonding and the process of attachment

Positioning at this stage may involve avoidance of lying left side down to prevent pooling of milk in the fundus of the stomach as volume of gastric feeds are increased. Pooling of milk in the stomach increases the risk of GOR. Use of the position (R)$\frac{1}{4}$ turn from prone is ideal until the infant has enough postural stability to maintain (R)$\frac{1}{2}$ turn (i.e. side-lying) while the infant remains in an isolette. Once the infant graduates to an open crib and may be swaddled (and full gastric feeds are tolerated), then side-lying positions are normally used.

Once the infant's physiological state tolerates handling better, the parents are encouraged to have their infant out for a 5 minute cuddle regularly and more definite responses to sensory inputs can be expected. In an attempt to represent a day and night pattern, lighting, noise and handling should be controlled. Sucking on a pacifier during gastric tube feeds is used to promote food digestion and during times of stress to calm the infant's behavioural and motor state.

From about 34 weeks of gestation, once the protective oral reflexes are present (Burns *et al.* 1987) oral feeds may be introduced gradually. Parents are encouraged to be involved in this care-giving activity. Instruction to the parent on positioning the infant may be provided to facilitate oral motor function and interaction of the infant with the parent. It is important to be aware of the vital connection between 'physiological flexion' (as in a term neonate) and sucking (i.e. sucking is a flexor skill) (Morris and Klein 1987). Thus the preterm infant with poor muscle tone and strength may present with:

- decreased tongue mobility
- increased jaw opening
- decreased lip seal
- decreased strength in sucking pads

In some infants the prolonged use of oral endotracheal intubation and ventilation may increase the amount of head and neck extension, leave their mouth hypersensitive, and disorganize their early suck/swallow patterns.

Some aspects to consider in achieving trouble-free functional feeding are:

- use of walking or rocking beforehand to promote better sensory organization
- adjusting the environment to ensure the infant is not too warm, the background noise not distracting, and lighting not too bright

- firm swaddling of the infant to provide a constant, firm, tactile input and promote motor and behavioural stability
- positioning of the infant with the chin tucked and neck elongated which brings the tongue and lips into a more forward position (not head flexed forward); neck aligned with the spine; shoulders depressed and forward (not retracted); hips flexed and whole body elevated to at least a 45° angle to eliminate the effect of gravity on oral musculature.

PHASE 3: POSITIONING AND HANDLING IN PREPARATION FOR DISCHARGE

By this time infants are in an open crib and the aims are extended to increase support to the parents in developing their skills and confidence in handling and caring for their preterm infant at home. Regular developmental follow-up (such as at 1, 4, 8 and 12 months corrected age) may be advisable depending on age at birth, subsequent progress and presence of risk factors.

Instruction and advice to parents on handling their infant during care-giving activities may include small group educational sessions, demonstrations and the use of a small booklet which they take home with them (Morris 1993). The booklet is not an intervention programme, but designed to help parents, other family members and friends in the daily care and handling of their infant. For example see Figure 2.

The guidelines set out in the booklet aim to boost the parents' confidence and skills in handling their infant in those often anxious first 1–3 months at home. This will facilitate the attachment process and promote the premature infant's motor and behavioural development. Ideas for providing appropriate tactile, proprioceptive, visual, auditory and vestibular input, the importance of the infant spending short periods of time (5–10 minutes) daily on their stomach during their wakeful time is stressed and caution is given regarding the use of some common baby equipment. There are certainly some reported concerns regarding the use of baby walkers (Crouchman 1986).

The general principles as just described may be adapted for term neonates or very young infants with conditions where there may be a deviation/impairment in their neurosensory motor development such as a cerebral insult, chronic neonatal lung

Figure 2 Picking Up: A, rolling to side; B, lifting up sideways and tilting forward.

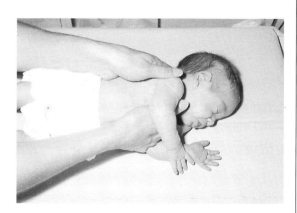

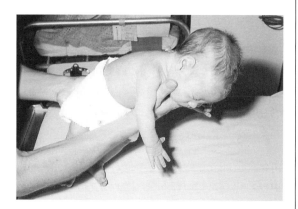

disease or clinical GOR. There are, however, some specific needs that should be addressed in each of these conditions.

Gastro-Oesophageal Reflux (GOR)

The baby with GOR whether term, preterm or during the first 6–8 months, is often very irritable with poor sleep patterns, restless during and/or shortly after feeds, exhibits periods of discomfort and pain by back arching and may vomit often or demand frequent short feeds. Conservative management of these infants is addressed largely through the use of specific handling and positioning which optimizes the influence of gravity.

Physiotherapists with skills in educating on handling techniques have much to offer the parents of infants with suspected or proven GOR. Some of these techniques include the following:

Figure 3 Carrying in Crook of Arm

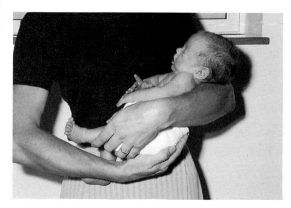

- Keeping the infant elevated (with the chest higher than the bottom) at all times; that is with carrying (Figure 3), sleeping, bathing, with nappy change (Figure 4) (use of a wedge on the change table and never lifting infant by the ankles), and during and after feeding (Figure 5).
- Keeping the infant tilted forward for carrying, especially after feeds to prevent pooling of milk in the fundus of the stomach. Examples of achieving this are over forearm, over knee, over shoulder, on chest when semireclined, in a sling/pouch (Figure 6). For this reason some infants with GOR do not like car travel as in their car seat safety restraint they are tilted backwards.

In some cases the elevated and tilted forward posture (i.e. prone) is the only position that pain may be abated and sleep achieved. There is certainly well-documented evidence for this (Meyers and Herbst 1982, Orenstein and Whitington 1983,

Figure 4 Changing a Nappy — maintaining elevation

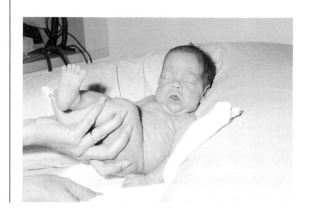

Figure 5 Breastfeeding an Infant with GOR

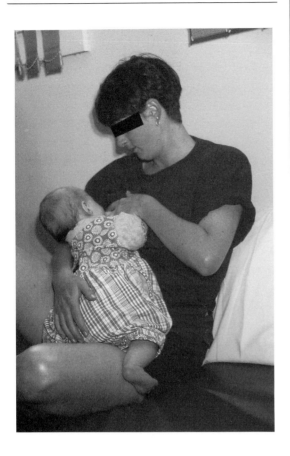

Newell *et al.* 1989). This may appear incongruous with the risk factors attributed to sudden infant death syndrome (SIDS), however, the National SIDS Council of Australia (1993) acknowledge that these infants do not come under the 'healthy full-term baby' category.

- Providing rocking and swaying in the elevated and tilted forward posture to soothe baby and ease into sleep. This may be achieved with pushing the baby in the pram, holding as shown in Figure 6A, or walking with the baby properly positioned in a sling.
- Avoiding vigorous movements such as bouncing and jigging or anything that provides pressure to the balls of the feet. These movements reinforce the extensor pattern and may aggravate GOR.
- When burping keep the baby flexed at the hips with trunk erect and slightly tilted forward. Avoid vigorous patting, but instead use circular massage/rubbing in a clockwise direction. Do not allow the baby's feet to push against the carer's body as this

may trigger the extensor thrust reflex and augment the symptoms of GOR.

The physiotherapist may need to continue to monitor the developmental progress of some babies with GOR as symptoms may reoccur with new developmental milestones such as rolling and crawling.

Cerebral Insult

The baby with cerebral haemorrhage, hydrocephalus or hypoxic ischaemic encephalopathy may present initially as lethargic, 'floppy' and with slow/poor feeding abilities. Later the infant may become irritable, tense, jittery and extensor in movement and posture. Functional feeding may certainly still be a problem.

It is important that parents understand the different handling needs of their infant at these times and the importance of positive emotional interaction with their baby. The aims of specific activities and handling include optimizing the baby's potential for postural control and efficient movement patterns, functional feeding and behavioural stability. It is vital to ensure parents are confident in handling their baby during all care-giving activities, including feeding, bathing, dressing, playing and sleeping; and that they understand the principles of such handling.

Some suggested techniques/approaches include the following:

- the use of massage either to stimulate the 'floppy' baby or to calm/relax the 'tense' baby
- prone bathing to relax the 'tense' baby and allow the 'floppy' baby to initiate motor activity more easily
- firm swaddling of the 'tense' baby to give confinement to their movements and loose swaddling of the 'floppy' baby to allow movement with slight resistance
- controlled rocking/swaying/swinging movements to mature the vestibular system and promote organization of movement and behavioural states
- using the technique of rolling the infant forward on to the side for picking up and lying down (see Figure 2), to promote head and postural control

Figure 6 Carrying Positions for Infant with GOR: A, over forearm; B, up over shoulder; C, in pouch.

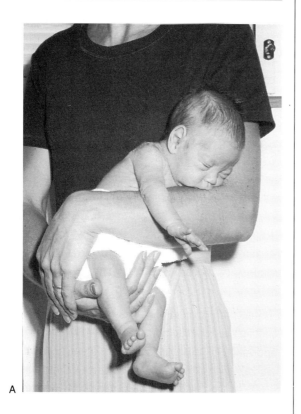

A

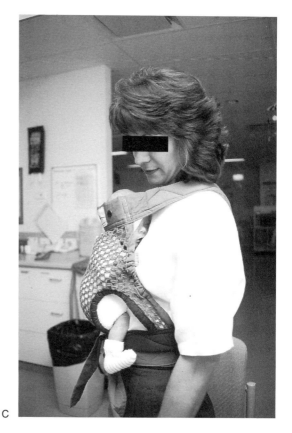

C

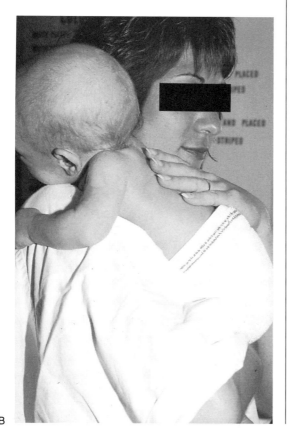

B

- for feeding, the 'floppy' baby may be sat almost upright to alleviate the influence of gravity, whereas the 'tense' baby may be in an elevated prone position to alleviate the influence of extensor patterns of movement and reflex activity.

It is essential to be aware of the family home environment and ensure that all treatment guidelines given to parents are incorporated as part of their daily routines. Parents at this time may have many mixed feelings and the physiotherapist should reassure, support and continue to educate the family on their baby's changing neurodevelopmental needs.

Chronic Neonatal Lung Disease (CNLD) and Motor Development

The chronic lack of oxygen in CNLD babies often impairs their neuromotor development (see Chapter 13). Muscle weakness and rapid onset of fatigue are common findings in the infant with CNLD. It is necessary therefore to plan handling and positioning which not only leads to positive gains, but also is cost-effective in terms of energy expenditure and respiratory demands. These infants often exhibit short bursts of activity rather than sustained postural control.

Sometimes a number of positions need to be tried to determine which is the most beneficial in terms of both breathing and postural and motor development. For example, positioning the infant on a wedge (using elevation to improve oxygenation, Dellagrammaticas *et al.* 1991) and then providing short bursts of visual/auditory/tactile/proprioceptive input while in prone with a rolled towel under the chest and side-lying with rolled towels front and back of infant's trunk. Short periods of time in a well-constructed hammock which provides elevated support to the infant's trunk without slumping may be useful to initiate some postural responses. When involved in the management of these infants, it is important to remember the close relationship between 'stability of posture and the regularity of respiration' (Casaer 1979, p. 86).

Management of the Developmentally Delayed Infant

Term to 6 Months

Normally this is a period of rapid change in the posture and movement of infants. For the very weak, sick or neurologically impaired infant, however, assessment may reveal slow or inconsistent patterns of development. Furthermore, the infant may demonstrate a poor ability to interact positively and consistently.

Parents may or may not express concerns about their baby at this stage, depending on their knowledge and experience of infant development. It is important therefore to be sensitive in the way special handling, positioning and activities are introduced. If they know their baby is/has been very sick then diagnosis of definitive delay or abnormality is usually delayed until about 8–12 months and instruction in handling is taught as an extension of care procedures for frail infants. It can be more difficult when the parents are not aware or deny that there may be a problem.

Assessment should commence with observation of spontaneous movement, adjustment of posture and awareness/interaction with the environment before any special handling or testing. It is often advisable to then observe the infant's response to specific visual, auditory and tactile input before testing stereotyped or reflex reactions in various positions. It is important to understand how to interpret infant responses as well as the testing procedures. For example, a number of testing proformas include a pull-to-sit manoeuvre to evaluate head control. The usefulness of this procedure is questioned as it does not differentiate between flexor muscle weakness, low postural tone, lack of interest or increased extensor tone. As an alternative it is suggested that the infant is supported in sitting and gently lowered backwards. The baby will attempt to maintain the head-up position and loss of control due to weakness will be a head drop only while increased extensor tone can usually be felt through the retraction of the shoulders and extension of the trunk.

On the basis of expected development of the first 6 months the aims would generally include the following:

- enabling day-to-day activities of feeding, bathing, changing/dressing, carrying, socially interacting and sleeping to be as enjoyable and functionally near to normal as possible
- achieving head and body alignment (supine and prone)
- stability on elbows in prone
- sitting with support with appropriate hip flexion
- postural alignment to rotation as in facilitated roll
- reach to grasp and hold (note tactile grasp usually precedes eye/hand)

and then graduating to:

- hands and feet to the midline in supine
- push-up and/or pivot in prone
- head and body 'righting' to gravity
- initiating independent rolling

The type and plan of intervention will be specific to each infant depending on their abilities, background medical status and presenting problems or aspects of delay. The following story illustrates some useful strategies.

Case Study 1

Angelica was a frail baby of 4 months corrected age. She was 26 weeks of gestation and 540 grams at birth. She subsequently developed necrotizing enterocolitis (NEC), a grade III intraventricular haemorrhage (IVH) and CNLD. At the time of her assessment she still required 0.25 l of continuous supplemental oxygen administered via subnasal prongs. Her mother used a portable oxygen supply for Angelica when she attended physiotherapy. Although generally weak she tended to shoulder retraction and trunk extension. In supine she could not hold her head in the midline and in prone she could lift her head only momentarily. Angelica had accommodated well for her limited energy reserves in that she was a social baby with lots of smiles and visual interaction. Functional feeding was slow with Angelica receiving continuous nasogastric tube feeding at night.

The aims of Angelica's intervention programme at this stage were: (1) to improve the strength and endurance of her oromotor function; (2) to promote midline orientation; (3) to enhance proximal stability around limb girdles; and (4) to stimulate head and body postural responses.

Before oral feeding it was important to achieve an optimal behavioural state with attention to temperature, lighting and background noise. Facilitatory exercises to stimulate tongue movement and lip closure were then given with Angelica held in a supported sitting position on her mother's lap and facing her to achieve good eye contact. Angelica's mother then gave her the bottle in this position while providing jaw support. The feed was interrupted regularly to avoid fatigue. A 'peanut pillow' was placed behind Angelica's head whenever in a supported sitting position or in supine to allow her head to rest in the midline. Elevation was also used to reduce the influence of gravity on respiratory and activity efforts. The use of elevation enhanced Angelica's opportunities for bringing her hands forward to swipe at toys. Side-lying in elevation was another position that promoted midline orientation and upper limb function without taxing Angelica's limited energy reserves. At nappy change and change of clothing times with arms supported in a reaching-forward posture, gentle compressions were given to enhance muscle co-contraction proximally. In elevated prone positions, the use of the 'peanut pillow' under the chest and axilla provided some supported weight-bearing through elbows. In order to promote postural responses her mother made up a game with a singing rhyme during change of clothing to facilitate rolling. A similar game was played with Angelica sitting supported by her mother's thighs in crook lying and being gently rocked side-to-side and back-and-forth. It was essential that all handling and activities were of short duration to avoid fatigue and subsequent increased demand on respiratory efforts.

By 6 months Angelica could prop on elbows in prone for very short periods and hold her head steady in the midline when held in supported sitting. In supported sitting she was able to reach for her favourite toy and bring it to her mouth. In supine, however, there was still the tendency to retract her shoulders and anteriorly tilt her pelvis. Ongoing re-evaluation of home programme and education of parents regarding the progress and indications of difficulty was vital to reduce deviations in developing movement and postural patterns.

6 TO 12 MONTHS

It is usually during this period that infants become increasingly able to move around their immediate environment by rolling, creeping, crawling and cruising or even walking independently. Posturally they can maintain antigravity positions, weight-shift and support and attain the ability to move fluently from one position to another such as rotating from sit to side and then on to hands and knees or vice versa. Sitting becomes stable allowing freedom to use both hands and lumbopelvic control is developing.

The infant with motor delay may present with poor or virtually absent antigravity postural control, persistence of immature or sometimes primitive patterns of movement, inability to weight-shift or support, or sit independently and delayed development of the ability to move around their immediate environment.

At this stage detailed assessment and history are likely to identify more clearly the main contributing factors causing a delay or abnormality of motor development. The same basic principles already mentioned continue to apply, but the increasing developmental needs should be considered in any programme of intervention. For example, the need to experience their immediate environment from different positions, to feel with their hands and to be talked with face to face. It is important, therefore, to support the child in sitting while communicating, rather than talking over a recumbent child.

Some general aims may include the following:

- facilitation/stimulation of improved antigravity postural control
- encouragement of more functional movement patterns
- facilitation of weight-shift to encourage one side stabilization while allowing the movement of the other and progressing to dynamic body rotation
- use of appropriate patterns of weight-bearing
- maturation of prehension and manipulative ability

The following story of a child with a varying increase in muscle tone throughout all limbs and trunk will be used to illustrate some practical ideas for management.

Case Study 2

Jacob born at term and weighing 3840 grams had a difficult delivery and suffered moderate hypoxic ischaemic encephalopathy (HIE). Initially after birth he was very lethargic and was slow to establish functional oral feeding. By 2 weeks of age he was visually alert and his movement patterns were becoming more vigorous with some evidence of increasing muscle tone. At this stage feeding was coming ahead with bursts of a coordinated suck–swallow pattern. There were, however, some symptoms of GOR with frequent small vomits and irritability after feeds. The question being asked was, therefore, 'was the evidence of increased muscle tone and the tendency to irritability due to HIE or the GOR or both?' While this was being medically appraised the parents were shown appropriate quiet handling and positions which were suitable for both problems, for example, with the head elevated and pressure away from the tummy. The baby was discharged from the hospital and his parents took him home to the country. Regular medical follow-up was arranged with the nearest paediatrician. The local physiotherapist was contacted, but she transferred to another area about a month later. Jacob was nearly 8 months of age when next seen by a physiotherapist in paediatrics. Presenting problems included an inability to sit unsupported, rolling over from prone to supine only, a tendency to mainly use the right hand to grasp objects using fingers and the palm and to drop objects placed in the left hand, some head control, but very poor trunk postural control and reports of occasional choking during feeding. He had one bout of pneumonia due to food aspiration. He enjoyed being held upright in standing, but when excited he tended to extend/adduct both lower limbs and flex the upper limbs, particularly the left. He was socially alert and responsive and liked being entertained.

355

On assessment it was found that a number of the problems were being reinforced by inappropriate handling. He was sitting in a position of trunk flexion and hip extension so his weight was being taken over the sacrum rather than the ischial tuberosities. In this semirecline position there was quite strong shoulder retraction, especially on the left, and during feeds he sometimes tended to arch back; on these occasions he was fed while his neck was in extension. When visually interested he had quite good voluntary neck flexion associated with strong rectus abdominus muscles, but when supported in sitting with hips flexed appropriately he had no lumbopelvic control.

You may like to list Jacob's presenting problems at 8 months; try to identify the possible reasons for these and plan what you might do.

Problems identified and appropriate action for the case of Jacob should include the following:

- Parent education: teach parents why (aims), what and how to correct and assist, but also open up opportunities for their son.
- Sitting: correct sitting during all activities (i.e. feeding, communication, playing, watching, being carried, nursed or in 'stroller').
- Mobility: teach / facilitate rolling, weight-shift to move to one side or other, and assess possibility of reciprocal creep.
- Weight-bearing: use elbow and hand to shoulder girdle weight-bearing, hands and knees position and controlled supported weight-bearing on feet.
- Use of hands: position shoulders forward of hip alignment, encourage left hand support while using the right and vice versa; give support to allow two hands free for use and encourage transfer to left from right, and use of gross pincer grasp.
- Postural control: establish stability in sitting, integrated use of abdominal (especially transversus) and deep lower trunk muscles for lumbopelvic

stability; facilitate body-on-body postural adjustment, increase functional head control and postural hold during activity.
- Learning experiences: introduce age-related movements, sensations, language, social interactions and expectations / responsibilities.

Summary

Management of the developing and young infant offers a great challenge to the physiotherapist. It is essential in treating this age group to be aware of the specific needs of the baby as they develop, but equally as important is the education and support of the parents. The aims and examples given within this chapter are guidelines only and the needs of each individual baby and their parents must be addressed.

REFERENCES

Allen, MC, Capute, AJ (1990) Tone and reflex development before term. *Pediatrics* 85: 393–399.

Als, H, Lester, BM, Tronick, EZ et al. (1982) Manual for the assessment of preterm infants' theory and behaviour (APIB). In: Fitzgerald, H et al. (eds) *Theory and Research in Behavioural Pediatrics*, vol. I, pp. 65–132. New York: Plenum.

Anderson, J, Auster-Liebhaber, J (1984) Developmental therapy in the neonatal intensive care unit. *Physical and Occupational Therapy in Pediatrics* 4: 89–106.

Brazelton, TB (1984) *Neonatal Behavioural Assessment Scale*, pp. 125, 2nd edn. Philadelphia: JB Lippincott.

Burns, YR, Bullock, MI (1980) Sensory and motor development of preterm infants. *Australian Journal of Physiotherapy* 26: 229–243.

Burns, YR, Rogers, Y, Neil, M et al. (1987) Development of oral function in pre-term infants. *Physiotherapy Practice* 3: 168–178.

Campbell, SK (1974) The developing infant: neuromuscular maturation. *Proceedings from The Comprehensive Management of Infants at Risk for CNS Deficits*, North Carolina, pp. 65–73.

Campbell, SK (ed) (1984) *Pediatric Neurologic Physical Therapy, Clinics in Physical Therapy*, vol. V, 430 pp. New York: Churchill Livingston.

Casaer, P (1979) *Postural Behaviour in Newborn Infants, Clinics in Developmental Medicine*, no. 72, 112 pp. London: Spastics International Medical Publications.

Cintas, HM (1987) Foetal movements: an overview. *Physical and Occupational Therapy in Pediatrics* 7(3): 1–15.

Crouchman, M (1986) The effects of babywalkers on early locomotor development. *Developmental Medicine and Child Neurology* 28: 757–761.

Dellagrammaticas, HD, Kapetanakis, J, Papadimitriou, M et al. (1991) Effect of body tilting on physiological functions in stable very low birthweight neonates. *Archives of Disease in Childhood* 66: 429–432.

Desmond, MM, Wilson, GS, Alt, EJ et al. (1980) The very low birth weight infant after discharge from intensive care, anticipatory health care and developmental course. *Current Problems in Pediatrics* 10: 5–59.

Dubowitz, L (1985) Neurological assessment of the full-term and preterm newborn infant. In: Harel S and Anastasiow N (eds) *The At-risk Infant*, pp. 185–196. Baltimore: Paul H. Brooks.

Fay, MJ (1988) The positive effects of positioning. *Neonatal Network* April: 23–28.

Field, TM (1977) Effects of early separation interactive deficits and experimental manipulations on infant-mother face to face interaction. *Child Development* 48: 763–771.

Field, TM (1986) Intervention for premature infants. *Journal of Pediatrics* 109: 183–191.

Field, TM, Schanberg, SM, Scafidi, F et al. (1986) Tactile/kinesthetic stimulation – effects on preterm neonates. *Pediatrics* 77(5): 654–658.

Goldspink, DF (1980) *Development and Specialisation of Skeletal Muscle*, 155 pp. Cambridge: Cambridge University Press.

Holt, KS (1960) Early motor development. *Journal of Pediatrics* 57(4): 571–575.

Konishi, Y, Mikawa, H, Suzuki, J (1986) Asymmetrical head-turning of preterm infants: some effects on later postural and functional lateralities. *Developmental Medicine and Child Neurology* 28: 450–457.

Lester, BM, Tronick, EZ (1990) (eds) *Stimulation and the Preterm Infant: The Limits of Plasticity, Clinics in Perinatology,* vol 17:1, 244 pp. Philadelphia: WB Saunders.

Lieb, SA, Benfield, G, Guidubaldi, J (1980) Effects of early intervention and stimulation of the preterm infant. *Pediatrics* 66(1): 83–90.

Mastaglia, F (1981) Growth and development of the skeletal muscles. In: Davis JA and Dobbing J (eds) *Scientific Foundations of Paediatrics*, pp. 590–620. London: Heinemann Medical Books.

Masterton, J, Zucher, C, Schulze, K (1987) Prone and supine positioning effects on energy expenditure and behaviour of low birthweight neonates. *Paediatrics* 80: 689–692.

Meyers, WF, Herbst, JJ (1982) Effectiveness of positioning therapy for gastroesophageal reflux. *Pediatrics* 69: 768–772.

Morris, KM (1993) *Handling your Prematurely Born Baby: A Guide for Parents*, 28 pp. Brisbane: Copyright Publishing.

Morris, KM, Burns, YR (1994) Reduction of craniofacial and palatal narrowing in very low birthweight infants. *Journal of Paediatrics and Child Health* 30: 518–522.

Morris, SE, Klein, MD (1987) *Pre-feeding Skills*. Tuscon: Therapy Skill Builders.

National SIDS Council of Australia (1993) Help Reduce the Risks of Cot Death (leaflet).

Newell, SJ, Booth, IW, Morga, MEI et al. (1989) Gastroesophageal reflux in preterm infants. *Archives of Disease in Childhood* 64: 780–786.

Orenstein, SR, Whitington, PF (1983) Positioning for prevention of infant gastroesophageal reflux. *Journal of Pediatrics* 103: 524–537.

Parker, A (1990) Expert handling. *Nursing Times* 86: 35–37.

Piper, MC, Kunos, VI, Willis, DM et al. (1986) Early physical therapy effects on the high-risk infant: a randomised controlled trial. *Pediatrics* 78(2): 216–224.

Rausch, PB (1981) Effects of tactile and kinesthetic stimulation on premature infants. *Journal of Obstetric Gynecological and Neonatal Nursing* Jan/Feb: 34–37.

Sweeney, JK (ed.) (1986) *The High-risk Neonate: Development Therapy Perspectives*, 388 pp. New York: Haworth Press.

21

Physiotherapy Management of Children with Neurological, Neuromuscular and Neurodevelopmental problems

YVONNE BURNS, JOHN GILMOUR, MEGAN KENTISH
AND JULIE MACDONALD

Cerebral Palsy
•
Down's Syndrome
•
Spina Bifida
•
Acquired Brain Injury (ABI)
•
Immersion
•
Medulloblastoma

A number of representative 'case scenarios' are explored in this chapter with relevant background information on both the condition and treatment approaches. Undoubtedly, these case studies will not address all of the neurological, neuromuscular and neurodevelopmental problems which may occur during childhood. This chapter is designed, however, to provide the reader with a basis for using a problem-solving and individualized approach in their physiotherapy management of children. Lists of references and recommended reading are included and the reader is encouraged to access further information to enhance their knowledge and understanding of the many varied paediatric neurological, neuromuscular and neurodevelopmental conditions.

Cerebral Palsy

Case Study 1

Joe first presented to physiotherapy with his parents when he was about 8 months of age. They had just learned from the doctor that Joe had cerebral palsy. They were keen to learn about the condition, what it meant for Joe, for them and the other members of the family now and in the future. Joe is now 8 years of age so we have the advantage of looking back over that time and learning from the experiences of Joe and his family.

Cerebral palsy is defined as a persistent, but not unchanging disorder of movement due to

Yvonne Burns, John Gilmour, Megan Kentish and Julie MacDonald

Figure 1   Meet Joe!

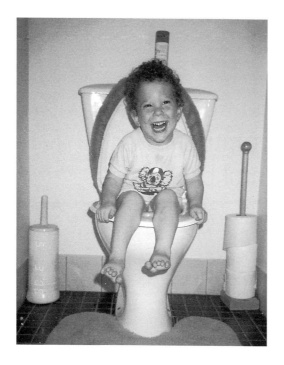

non-progressive damage to the brain occurring before the age of 3 years. There are multiple causes and the damage to the brain varies considerably, resulting in a unique pattern of disability in each child. The disorder may originate from problems before (prenatal), during (perinatal) or after (postnatal) the time of birth due to abnormal development of the brain, hypoxia, intracranial haemorrhage, excessive neonatal jaundice, trauma or infection. Cerebral palsy is frequently found within a population of surviving very/extremely premature and high-risk infants (Stanley *et al.* 1993). The incidence is very high among those who have cystic periventricular leukomalacia (Rogers *et al.* 1993).

The cerebral palsies present as a heterogeneous group of conditions, but the primary disorder is faulty control of posture and movement resulting in delayed development of motor abilities, abnormalities of muscle tone and patterns of movement and functional difficulties. Many children with cerebral palsy have associated problems. These may be part of the movement dysfunction such as difficulties controlling the muscles of the mouth (affecting feeding, swallowing and speech), muscles of the eye (causing strabismus or problems of eye follow), or directly associated with the brain lesion itself such as

cognitive dysfunction, sensory impairments of vision or hearing, seizures (epilepsy), problems of praxis, perception or learning and/or social/emotional disorders.

Joe was born several weeks early; his mother had hypertension during pregnancy and there were some difficulties during the birth process. At the time of birth Joe was 'flat' and required resuscitation. His apgars were 2 at 1 min, 5 at 5 min and 9 at 10 min. He was lethargic and hypotonic for a few days, but appeared to pick up, began to feed and was discharged 12 days later. His mother reported to the doctor at the 1 month visit that Joe was slow to feed, often irritable and had irregular sleep patterns. On examination of the baby the doctor did not identify any aspects of particular concern and as the mother was obviously tired and tense the doctor felt that the baby may have been reflecting his mother's tension. At 3 months the baby was definitely irritable, tense and tending to extend his back when held. Gastro-oesophageal reflux and oesophagitis was diagnosed. It was felt that the irritability and arching were associated with abdominal pain. Medication and additives to the feed were prescribed. A physiotherapy friend recommended positioning Joe with head and trunk raised during sleep and demonstrated some holding, nursing and carrying positions. By 6 months Joe was feeding and sleeping better, but the parents were concerned that he was not reaching for toys. The delays in motor development and some stiffness in his legs were attributed to the arching and tension due to abdominal pain. At the 8 month visit Joe was not able to roll, he was difficult to place in sitting, when excited his legs extended and adducted and when lying supine he tended to turn his head to the side resulting in extension of the arm on the face side and flexion of the other elbow. When sitting on his mother's knee he was much more relaxed, but his deep tendon reflexes were very brisk.

Diagnosis and Classification of Cerebral Palsy

Early diagnosis of cerebral palsy is not clear-cut and there is no test which in itself is confirmatory (Scherzer and Tscharnuter 1982). Burns *et al.* (1989) found that identification does not depend on the presence of isolated abnormal signs, but on a combination of neurological signs, delayed postural reactions and motor dysfunction. In hindsight it is often easy to identify the presenting signs, but particularly in children who have been very sick, very premature or have other problems as with Joe, the significance of various signs may be masked. In children with very mild cerebral palsy it may not be recognized and diagnosed until the child is walking. When parents have concerns, motor delays are present or functional problems exist, intervention should not be delayed while awaiting definitive diagnosis. Incorrect labelling must be avoided, but advice on appropriate handling and positioning can be helpful to most parents with a young infant, particularly if the infant responds differently from the average baby.

Cerebral palsy is classified according to :

- the area of the body affected; for example, a hemiplegia if involving one side, diplegia if it is mostly the lower limbs affected and quadriplegia if all limbs and trunk are affected
- the type of movement disorder such as spastic or rigid determined by the type of hypertonicity in the muscles, athetoid when involuntary and varying (often twisting/writhing movements interrupt the flow and sequence of movement), or ataxic if there are problems of balance and coordination
- the severity of the disability in terms of function, i.e. mild, moderate or severe

When Joe presented at 8 months the physiotherapist completed a full assessment and identified the following. While sitting on his father's knee Joe was observed inter-

acting with his mother and some brightly coloured rings and a bell toy. He was alert, attentive and responsive. He grasped the toy well with his left hand, but his right grasp was hesitant and involved the whole palm. He controlled the position of his head and followed objects with his eyes. When placed on the floor in sitting he became anxious and extended his trunk. Assessment of tone and patterns of movement revealed increase in tone, especially during quiet activity. In supine an asymmetrical tonic neck reflex was easily elicited, he had difficulty in moving his legs into flexion and his ability to open his hands and reach was reduced. The influence of the tonic labyrinthine reflex (TLR) was tested by sitting him up and then gently lowering him back to supine by supporting under the arms and with hands over the scapulae. Joe maintained head control until the last 20–30 degrees when his head pulled back into extension and his shoulders retracted. An influence of TLR in supine was confirmed. Joe was also found to have a strong extensor thrust in both feet and easily elicited plantar grasp. In prone he could maintain support on his elbows, but could not weight-shift and support on one elbow to enable him to reach for and play with a toy. Testing of head righting indicated good responses when supported in the vertical position, but when supported horizontally his side-to-side responses were below the midline and in supine he could not flex forward. Held prone he lifted his head, but had no Landau reaction. Some body-on-body righting was found to be present in the upper trunk and neck, but none in lower trunk and legs. Held in standing, his legs adducted and feet plantarflexed with weight taken on the toes.

Assessment of Cerebral Palsy

Comprehensive assessment, as explained in Chapter 7, is the first essential step in the physiotherapy management of a child. The initial assessment, before the treatment/intervention, is important for identifying and diagnosing the movement problems which need to be addressed by the physiotherapist, as well as providing a baseline of the main posture and movement characteristics, abilities and disabilities for that particular child. Cerebral palsy has the potential to affect adversely all aspects of normal development and control of movement described in Chapters 2 and 3.

> *It was decided that Joe's level of disability was moderate, the muscle tone was hypertonic and the distribution diplegic as the problems mainly concerned the lower limbs. It was important also to acknowledge the difficulties evident in his right upper limb. In addition, postural control was delayed and some infant reflex and immature patterns of movement persisted. Positive aspects included alertness and responsiveness, head righting (vertical), head control in prone and upright, and while sitting with mild support an ability to reach and grasp. No deformities or contractures limited the range of movement.*

At each visit further understanding of the problems being faced by the child is gained through observation, questioning/listening, use of specific input and encouragement. This forms an essential part of the treatment programme. This more detailed knowledge about the child as well as the positive and negative aspects of development and movement is important for determining the necessary modifications and changes to treatment needed to ensure the most appropriate approach is used to meet the needs of the individual child and family. Regular review assessments of postural control and patterns of movement being used by the child in a variety of positions and under different conditions of play and daily functional activities record progress as well as the results of intervention strategies which have been applied. From time to time, for example, after one year, a full formal review assessment should be carried out to ensure that some aspects of progress or dysfunction are not being overlooked.

> *For Joe the selected approach to treatment at this stage involved teaching his parents the use of positions where tone and patterns of movement were near to normal. Then, while keeping the child's interest and cooperation, to move him into positions of more difficulty. By using facilitation and specific handling to limit build-up of tone or undesirable patterns of movement it was possible to help Joe into a reasonably stable sitting position which he could maintain for a short while alone. Joe was obviously very pleased with himself. His parents had been following the assessment carefully and gained some understanding of Joe's difficulties, but it had been a long session of 45 minutes. Therefore, on the first visit three aims were agreed upon as the basis of the home programme. The three aims for Joe were to improve independent sitting, quality and quantity of rolling, and weight-shift/support to one side to allow better use of the other arm/hand. The methods of achieving each were demonstrated and the parents were encouraged to try these before leaving the session. Joe's father was too shy but his mother did try and was pleased with the result.*
>
> *Within a week both parents were handling Joe more confidently and were keen to add to their list of aims, activities for the right hand and how to relax the strong patterns in his feet. Very soon the parents were noting an improvement in the way Joe was moving and an increase in his attempts to reach for and play with toys using his right hand. By 12 months, Joe was mainly rolling for mobility, but he could creep on his tummy when encouraged and with assistance hold the hands and knees position. He was keen to be on his feet and preparation for this had been included in a number of aspects of his programme (e.g. squat-to-stand, foot-to-opposite knee, weight-shift and support with the hip, knee and ankle in various positions). Now he was ready for a more active role in the control of his own patterns of movement. Play and task activities which*

Figure 2   Watching my favourite show on television (20 months of age)

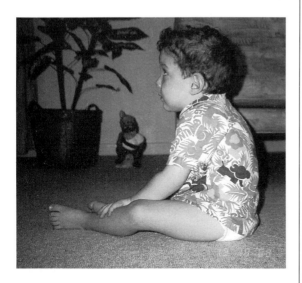

involved an element of planning and challenge were introduced so he could gain a sense of achievement when successful.

Management of Cerebral Palsy

When formulating a plan of home management and physiotherapy intervention it is essential to address the child's needs in terms of age, health, family, their social, cultural and environmental background as well as the specific primary and secondary problems relating to the cerebral palsy condition. Other interventions or treatments are often necessary and need to be incorporated into the one programme. It is not possible in the early stages to predict the likely long-term outcome, but most parents seek this and will tend to ask for positive reassurance that the child will 'get better'. The chronic and permanent nature of the injury to the brain is difficult for many to comprehend. It is first necessary to set short-term aims which can be understood and achieved and then to establish medium-term goals. It is essential also that all those involved in the care of the child work together to ensure that parents and child are not given conflicting advice or direction. Parents, medical consultants in paediatrics and perhaps orthopaedics, neurology and ophthalmology as well as physiotherapists, speech therapists, occupational therapists,

teachers, social workers and psychologists in addition to the family doctor are some of those likely to be involved in the team. When feasible, combined assessments and treatments may avoid confusion, but when this is not feasible each carer / therapist / teacher should consider all of the child's special strengths and needs as well as allowing the child to be themselves.

The immediate environment of an infant is usually at home with the family. Either or both parents provide the necessary input during daily care and interaction with their baby. Movement is an integral part of living so movement therapy cannot be separated from what is happening every day. There is a two-way interaction between infant and family, one reflecting the responses in the other so an unresponsive or 'good' baby often elicits less response in the family (Scherzer and Tscharnuter 1982). Other members of the family such as grandparents, siblings and/or carers are also involved, so all must understand not only the aims, techniques and expected outcome of the physical handling, but also the need for social interaction and a variety of learning experiences.

Development and maturity mean change. It is important for the plan of management, techniques and approaches to treatment to be sensitive to that change because as the child develops, new needs, movements, cognition, communication and functional abilities should be incorporated. It is essential to be constantly aware of family needs and social pressures or expectations. In the early stages and when management is on a fairly regular basis there is considerable contact and communication between parents and therapists, but it is important to recognize the ongoing need to reassure parents from time to time and to reconfirm positive changes, continuing or new problems and the features of the condition affecting their child. In all matters it is important not to usurp the role of the parents.

Joe walked independently at the age of 33 months. At the age of 24 months he became very frustrated and started to pull to stand at every opportunity. The effort and strong flexion of his arms in this activity led to overall

Figure 3   Look what I can do now!

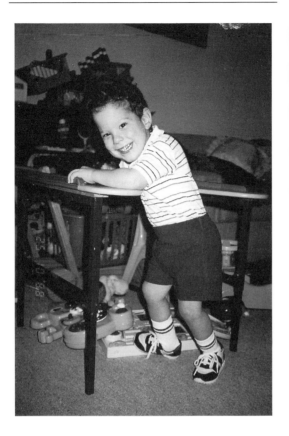

Figure 4   Here I am at the football

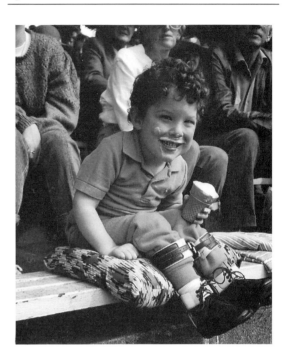

Figure 5   Now I can walk with 10 legs!

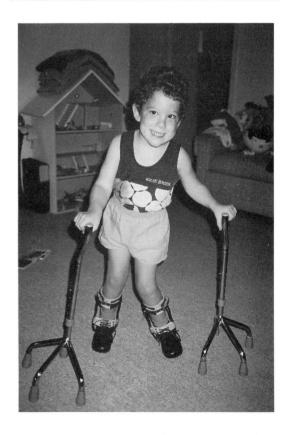

postural flexion. In addition to holding on to the furniture he soon learned to lean on and push chairs and other objects. It was very important to retain his motivation to walk, but at the same time to avoid overuse of abnormal movement patterns. He was given a weighted trolley with an upright handle which kept his centre of gravity back over his feet, but he tended to develop overactivity in calf musculature. He was measured and fitted bilaterally with below-knee callipers with an anterior strap to limit plantarflexion but encourage dorsiflexion (see Figures 4 and 5).

It was noted that he was lacking postural control in both sitting and standing and gained stability by flexing at the hips. The length and action through range of his hip flexor and extensor muscles was checked and found to compare favourably with previous assessments; however, further assess-

ment revealed poor transversus and oblique abdominal muscle action. Specific sensory input was used to stimulate the muscles while activities using diagonal movement patterns were used to improve the strength of the abdominal muscles. It was a challenge to find activities of interest to a 2-year-old which then incorporated all the desired postural and movement patterns. For some time Joe had been a member of the local toy library. He looked forward to having fun when he went to get a new toy or activity and his mother enjoyed the informal and more formal group contact with other parents. One day they met Amelia and her mother at the toy library. Amelia had cerebral palsy, but her head and body seemed to move a lot especially when she tried to talk. It soon became clear that Amelia had athetosis. She had a specially designed insert in her chair to give her stability, but her mother told Joe's mother how much Amelia's sitting had improved since attending a conductive education group for preschool children. Joe was very happy when a place became vacant for him just after his third birthday. He enjoyed the challenge of the group and after a few months seemed to gain more self-confidence in his ability to solve problems.

Approaches to Treatment of Cerebral Palsy

There is no one technique or system of treatment/intervention for cerebral palsy. Each child has individual needs which change with age and although some problems are more specific to particular types of cerebral palsy it is inadvisable to conclude that a technique that works for some will be suitable for others. Assessment must guide treatment decisions. Usually a number of techniques will be employed concurrently and or successively to achieve a goal or task. There are a number of different philosophical approaches which have contributed much to the

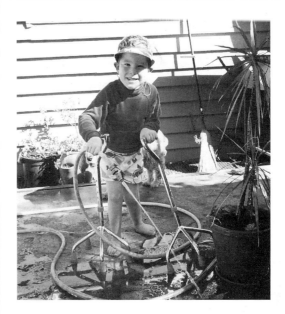

Figure 6   I'm pleased I can now help Dad in the garden

development of programmes and techniques (Eckersley and King 1993).

A number of techniques and approaches have been mentioned throughout the story of Joe, but there are many other possible clinical presentations of cerebral palsy. In the early stages techniques which elicit an automatic response such as positioning, facilitation and or stimulation tend to predominate, but as the infant is able to be more actively involved there is usually an increasing use of goal-orientated tasks to encourage and motivate action. The child may be independent for part of the movement or task, but require input to complete or correct it. At other times it may be necessary to provide initial input and then allow the child to take over. The goal is for the child to initiate control and modify or adapt their own movement. A study by Campos et al. (1994) indicates that the extent to which a child may achieve functional independence in walking will depend to a certain degree on their achievements in the first 2–3 years in terms of head control by 9 months, sitting by 24 months and crawling by 30 months. Trahan and Marcoux (1994) reported that failure to achieve walking was due to the topography and severity of the motor problem. In a study of independence in daily activities, Bairstow (1994) found no strong relationship between gross motor variables and those concerned with the achievement of daily activities, but rather an association between fine motor variables and independence in daily living activities.

THE NEURODEVELOPMENTAL APPROACH

The technique of facilitation of movement and automatic postural responses while at the same time controlling the influence of abnormal tone (particularly increased tone) and abnormal patterns of movement was largely developed by Berta and Karl Bobath (1964, 1967, 1972). In their approach they recognize the importance of the changes which occur normally in the development of posture and movement and the interrelationship between various automatic reflexes or reactions and the performance of volitional movement. The various handling, positioning and movement techniques of this approach have the advantage of using, wherever possible, the child's own automatic responses. Facilitation provides a very useful initial technique for use with the young infant and parents soon learn the key points to handling and controlling movement, the most appropriate positions for daily activities and the best movement patterns for assisting development of their child (Scherzer and Tscharnuter 1982). The techniques of facilitation also have application in association with other techniques in ongoing treatment programmes.

SENSORIMOTOR APPROACHES

Sensation is essential for the development and modification of functional movement and balance. Tactile, proprioceptive, vestibular, visual and auditory input all play a part and can be used specifically or generally to help elicit automatically a desired response or to increase awareness and thus assist the child to improved performance (Stockmeyer 1972). Rood (1962) not only emphasized the importance of sensation in the control and development of movement, but also drew attention to different types of muscle fibres (slow twitch type 1 and fast twitch type 2) and their contribution to the control of posture and movement. Understanding muscle action is important in the selection of appropriate treatment approaches as some techniques will enhance particularly the fast twitch type muscle action to the detriment of slow twitch muscle fibres.

CONDUCTIVE EDUCATION

In the 1940s a Hungarian neurologist, Andras Peto began to develop a system of special education for children and adults with motor disorders known as 'conductive education' (Bairstow and Cochrane 1993, p. 84). The last 25 years have seen an increasing interest world-wide in this approach. Cognitive, communication, motor, social and daily living skills are all addressed in a comprehensive programme which aims to achieve in each individual a way of overcoming their various difficulties to function as a member of society with minimal special aids or adaptations. The programme is led by a 'conductor' or conductors who are responsible for directing most aspects of the child's development and everyday care. Children with cerebral palsy are considered to have a learning disorder so intervention is viewed as education rather than treatment (Hari and Tillemans 1984) and the conductor uses every daily activity as a learning situation. The children work in groups which are specifically designed to develop particular attributes. All members of the group have the same schedule of activities, but the way they achieve or perform the activity may vary. A series of activities or tasks is designed to teach the children basic control of movement in particular positions. Each is practised through rhythmically verbalizing the intention of the activity or task. All children are expected to participate in and complete all parts of the programme set for the group. Facilitation is used if and when necessary to ensure completion of the activity. Introduction and value of conductive education in other countries has been evaluated (Bairstow et al. 1993, Dowrick 1993).

OTHER APPROACHES

Overaction of specific muscle groups particularly in the children with spasticity can lead to deterioration of patterns of movement, contractures and deformity if left unchecked (Levitt 1984). In all approaches to treatment it is important that activities which ensure muscles work through the whole range are included. Weight-bearing is a useful technique in upper as well as lower limbs to control the development of contractures (Chakerian and Larson 1993). Weight-bearing plasters or casts (Sussman 1983 and Watt et al. 1986), orthotics and callipers (Knutson and Clark 1991,

Figure 7 Who is coming for a swim?

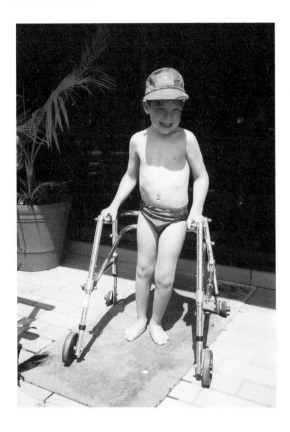

Figure 8 Don't you think I'm good-looking!

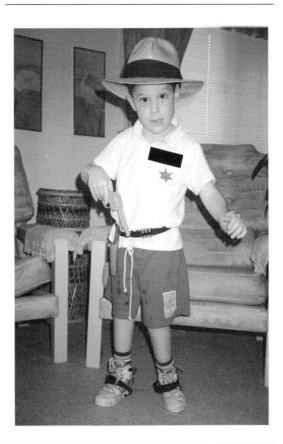

Cusick 1988), seating and special chairs (Seeger *et al.* 1984, Myhr and von Wendt 1990, 1993), standing (Levitt 1982) and surgery (Bleck 1979, Jones and Knapp 1987) all contribute to the prevention, control and treatment of these problems. Hydrotherapy and riding therapy are useful avenues for treatment, while swimming and horse riding provide enjoyable recreational ways of gaining some more control over posture, balance and movement.

When Joe was 4 years 6 months of age he started at the local preschool with the little boy next door. He was using a posterior walker (see Chapter 11) for outside in the garden or playground and becoming more and more mobile and active, but increasingly walking on his toes. Walking slowly at home or with the physiotherapist he could get his heels down, but not during everyday activities and his dorsiflexion range was only to a right angle. It was decided that a series of

plasters to increase his dorsiflexion range and improve his heel-bearing gait pattern was warranted. The reason for this was explained to Joe who was also given a chance to ask questions. He had a series of four bilateral plasters over a period of 6 weeks applied by a special team of physiotherapists. During this time he walked in the plasters once dry, and practised a specific set of exercises which aimed to improve strength and control of other lower limb and trunk muscles. The result was pleasing with a definite improvement in his gait pattern.

He was just 6 years old when he started at the local school. He participated in all the same activities as the other children. Once a week they went swimming and on Saturdays on Joe's request his father took him to a special horse riding club for children with disabilities.

At 7 years of age Joe was having a problem with very tight hamstring muscles and surgery was suggested. Joe was present in the discussions so he could be involved and understand that it would mean extra effort and work to improve his gait and abilities after the surgery. Tendons of Joe's hamstring musculature were lengthened and postoperatively the importance of early weight-bearing and mobilizing was recognized. He was casted for 3 weeks and then commenced standing and mobilizing in callipers.

Joe is now 8 years of age and continuing to cope well at normal primary school. He tends to use elbow crutches for mobility at school and a wheelchair for long outings (due to fatigue), but walks without aids around the home and schoolroom. Recently he was watching the disabled athletes compete at an international meet and Joe expressed an interest in joining a local 'sporting wheelies' group.

Typical Clinical Features of Cerebral Palsy

Most children with cerebral palsy have a mixture of different symptoms, distribution and types of muscle tone and movement dysfunctions. Although the lesion is non-progressive, the manifestations are likely to change with musculoskeletal growth and maturity of the nervous system. Some symptoms such as athetosis may not appear until 2–3 years of age, spasticity may increase particularly with growth spurts and ataxia may not be diagnosed until there is concern over delay in independent walking. The common features are abnormalities of posture, movement and muscle tone and in most there is a delay in achievement of motor milestones. Although abnormalities of muscle tone have both diagnostic and therapeutic significance, difficulties in characterizing and accurately measuring tone persist (Katz and Rymer 1989).

Hypertonicity may be spastic (clasp-knife) or rigid (lead-pipe or slowly 'giving' through range). In spasticity there is an exaggerated response to quick stretch which may occur at the beginning, middle or end of range. Because of this feature there is usually a limitation of range of movement and a tendency to contracture. Overactivity of spastic muscles may tend to inhibit antagonist muscle groups resulting in weakness. Spastic muscles themselves also may be weaker than expected. Change in position is likely to alter the level of tone in different muscle groups. These changes may be associated with retention of primitive (reflex) patterns of movement normally present only in the first few months after term. The distribution of spasticity may be hemiplegia, diplegia or quadriplegia. In the case of quadriplegia there is often an asymmetrical presentation. Treatment programmes should place importance on working all muscles through their full range and limit overuse of activities involving only a limited range rather than trying to stretch against an already overactive stretch reflex.

Hypertonicity of the rigid type sometimes described as 'plastic' is not often seen without spasticity or athetosis, but it is important to recognize its presence early. The slow 'giving' or 'plastic' feel to passive movement is due largely to muscle cocontraction. When present there is usually a marked delay or absence of development of automatic postural reactions and when hypertonicity is actively inhibited the child can appear to be 'floppy' or posturally hypotonic. There is less likelihood of contracture developing and too much emphasis on inhibition of tone may be detrimental. The emphasis in treatment needs to be on the establishment, as early as possible, of active functional movement.

The infant with athetosis may present early as 'floppy' (low tone) or with increased tone and many display strong primitive (reflex) patterns. These particularly include the asymmetrical tonic neck, Moro and Galant reflexes (Yokochi et al. 1993) which may dominate or adversely influence posture and movement patterns. Later there is a tendency to fluctuations or variations in tone which may occur as quite sudden large-amplitude movements or small slow or fast writhing or jerking involuntary movements called athetosis. These involuntary movements increase with excitement, insecurity and effort, but decrease at rest and in stable positions. Some children with athetosis are very tense often referred to as tension type while others tend to have more relaxed patterns of movement. Usually the distribution is quadriplegic, but occasionally a hemiplegic presentation occurs. Emphasis in treatment may need to be on the establishment of stable postural positions (prone, supine, sitting and standing) and voluntary control of basic patterns of movement.

The main features of ataxia are generalized hypotonia, postural instability, incoordination and dysmetria. Some children present with intention tremor and nystagmus of the eyes. Emphasis in treatment will be on proximal stability, coordination and balance. Additional information regarding some of the more typical clinical presentations of cerebral palsy and more detailed explanations of a number of treatment techniques can be found in Levitt (1995).

Thought Provokers

1. Consider your management of a child with a right hemiplegia who is now 28 months of age. He received physiotherapy from the age of 3 months when his parents noted a lack of movement in his right arm and leg. He walked independently at the age of 16 months. He used a toe—heel pattern of weight-bearing on the right and was shifting weight towards the right during some supervised activities. He was using his right hand, with fingers semi-flexed as an assistive for jobs requiring two hands. He was considered to be making steady improvement.

Now at 2 years and 4 months he does not want to be touched by any therapists and pulls away or gets angry with his parents when he realizes they are encouraging 'therapy-like' activities. His gait has deteriorated as he leads with the left, weight-bears on the ball of his right foot with the knee and hip in a few degrees of flexion and his weight shift is always to the left. When walking or trying to run his right arm flexes at the elbow and

wrist, abducts at the shoulder and is retracted. He refuses to use this hand.

- What factors may have contributed to this change?
- How could you manage this situation?
- What techniques or approaches to treatment may be useful at this stage in the management of his asymmetry, abnormal movement patterns and increased muscle tone?

2. You are working as a physiotherapist with a group of preschool children who have various developmental delays and problems of movement. One little girl who is just 4 years of age has a diagnosis of mild to moderate cerebral palsy with athetosis being the major component of the motor disability. She can walk slowly across the room using a ladder-backed chair and seat herself with supervision on an appropriately sized chair at a table. She is very alert and keen to do all of the preschool activities such as drawing, paper collage, threading and puzzles. You note she is putting her legs behind the legs of the chair then sitting sideways to the table. She faces the right and uses her extended right arm in an attempt to control her grasp and hold objects. Occasionally she links her left arm over the back of the chair.

- List the features of athetoid cerebral palsy which may be contributing to the above.
- How could you improve her posture, but also assist her ability to perform these activities?
- What approach could you use to assist this intelligent little girl to be more aware of self?

Down's Syndrome

Case Study 2
Libby is now 5 years of age and enjoys attending preschool. At birth, characteristics of Down's syndrome were observed and the

Yvonne Burns, John Gilmour, Megan Kentish and Julie MacDonald

diagnosis was confirmed by genetic karyo-
typing.

Down's syndrome occurs in children in all parts of the world and is not restricted to any culture, race or social class (Gunn 1993). It is due to an abnormality of chromosome 21. This is usually in the form of an extra chromosome 21 (trisomy) giving a total of 47, but in 5% the abnormality may be of mosaic or transloca-tion type. Although the children have specific fea-tures of the syndrome due to the extra genetic material it is important to recognize that they also carry other normal genetic or inherited characteris-tics and have their own individual personalities and attributes. Some physical features which affect motor development may include shorter than normal length of long bones, joint laxity, hypotonia, immature hand, wide space between first and second toes and delayed postural control and balance. It is important for the physiotherapist to be aware that congenital heart defects occur in about one-third of children with Down's syndrome and they are vulnerable also to upper respiratory tract infections and many exhibit one or more biomechanical (joint) problems. Recur-rent dislocations particularly of the patella and occa-sionally the hip, mild to moderate scoliosis, atlanto-axial instability and metatarsus varus with hallux valgus are those most commonly encountered. Atlanto-axial instability has been found in 14—22% of children (Pueschel and Scola 1987), but only a small number become symptomatic, show cord compres-sion signs and require surgical stabilization (Pueschel and Scola 1987). Posterior atlanto-occipital instability also has been reported (Hungerford et al. 1981, Colla-cott et al. 1989). Opinions differ concerning the need for screening, but radiographic assessment is defi-nitely advised for children with Down's syndrome who participate in sports (e.g. contact sports) which may place stress on the head and neck (Committee on Sports Medicine 1984). While recurrent dislocation of the hip will usually require surgical intervention for relief of pain and maintenance of function, recurrent subluxation of the patella usually does not have a marked effect on function and appears to cause little pain (Dugdale and Renshaw 1986). Subtalar and fore-

foot displacements, if severe, can lead subsequently to painful foot conditions, therefore regular assessment and implementation of management strategies should be included in intervention programmes.

Hearing and visual problems may also be present while cognitive and developmental problems are generally aspects which require specific attention.

Libby was born to older parents 12 years after their previous child. Marked hypotonia was noted at the time of birth. From the outset feeding was a major problem due to inability of the baby to sustain lip closure around the nipple. There was a physiotherapist working at the hospital where Libby was born so she was asked to advise and assist with handling and feeding this very frail infant. During initial assessment excessive joint laxity and a tendency to subluxation, particularly of the shoulders, was noted. As soon as Libby's fluid intake was satisfactory she was dis-charged home. Her parents were managing all care procedures.

Parents of an infant with a disability need emotional support as well as advice on care and intervention and information about the condition (Cunningham and Glenn 1987). Commencement of practices which assist with the care and handling of their infant often helps parents cope with some early anxieties and during parent–infant interaction it is possible to draw attention to the positive aspects of the baby's development while at the same time identifying spe-cial needs. Gradually more specific positioning, hand-ling and stimulation will be introduced to enhance normal automatic postural and movement responses during daily caring activities (Lydic and Steele 1979, Harris 1981, 1988). A number of ideas on handling, feeding, carrying and facilitating mobility in the infant and young child with Down's syndrome have been provided by Price and Kelso (1993).

The initial aims of the programme devised for Libby were: (1) to establish an effective pat-

tern of feeding; (2) to give stability, but allow movement by providing support to neck, trunk and major joints when handling; (3) to stimulate muscle cocontraction around major joints. To feed Libby her mother had to support her neck, just beneath the occiput, on her forearm then hold the bottle while at the same time supporting the chin with her middle finger and the cheeks with her other fingers. Libby soon learned to cope without the cheek support, but continued to require chin support for a couple of months. Lip, tongue and oral control continued to be part of her programme for many months. When resting, Libby could not be left lying in prone as she was too weak to lift the head and clear the face. She was supported on either side during the day and for sleeping was positioned ¼ turn off supine. In prone, support on elbows was only possible with hand support under her chin and use of a towel rolled (bone-shaped i.e. thicker at the ends under the shoulders and a depression for chest) under her chest and axilla. While in supine very gentle compressions through each supported joint were used to try to stimulate some muscle cocontraction.

Aims of home programme were gradually increased and modified as she gained some control with: (1) introduction of supported sitting; (2) use of specific stimulation techniques to gain postural control and movement; and (3) encouragement of interaction with people and toys. By about 4 months Libby had brief head control when supported in upright sitting, but, there was no evidence of head or body righting reactions. Owing to the very low muscle tone and joint laxity, tactile, proprioceptive, vestibular and visual input were used to stimulate desired postural control and motor responses. Social interaction between Libby and her family also played a very important role gaining her cooperation and desire to achieve. By 8 months while sitting with support she was reaching for and playing with toys suspended on a bar in front of her. In prone

she could support on both elbows and control her head, but she could not weight shift or support on one elbow to allow her to reach with the other.

Delay in development of head and body righting in infants with Down's syndrome has been noted by several authors (Cowie 1970, Haley 1987), also a lack of rotation around the central axis of the body (Lydic and Steele 1979, Harris 1984). It was thought that the delay in development of these reactions and also the poor balance frequently seen in these children may have been due to the low muscle tone, but a study by Shumway-Cook and Woollacott (1985) suggests that there are defects or differences within the higher level postural control mechanisms. These authors suggest that intervention programmes should concentrate on improving coordination and planning mechanisms which demand postural adaptation in response to changing tasks and activities.

Libby learnt to roll over by 12 months, but preferred to sit. Sitting with her legs in W position or widely abducted to about 160° were her preferred options. She could attain this position from prone by abducting her legs and then pushing on her arms until her buttocks were behind her hips. To improve postural control, whenever possible the family encouraged long sitting with the legs as close as possible or side sitting. She often placed her free hand onto her thigh for support as her arms were too short to reach the floor. Weight-bearing on hands and knees and shifting weight forwards and back were incorporated also into play activities, but at this stage she could not maintain her legs together or bear full weight on her arms without assistance. Later two tennis arm bands sewn together and placed around each thigh did provide some stability, but crawling was not achieved until after walking.

Children with very low tone frequently have difficulty adopting various sitting positions particularly those involving trunk rotation (Kelso and Price 1993) and tend to prefer positions of stability with wide hip abduction and knee extension (Akerstrom and Sanner 1993). The hip acetabulum in the child with Down's syndrome tends to be deep and face distally (Shaw and Beals 1992) so congenital dislocation is rare. It needs to be kept in mind therefore that soft tissue differences, for example, ligamentous laxity, muscle tone and patterns of movement may be the main factors contributing to later problems of hip stability.

At 18 months Libby could pull to stand at a low table when starting from sitting. She lacked confidence and would not weight-shift. Her programme included techniques to encourage sideways weight-shift and limit her tendency to hyperextend her knees. Step standing, reaching for objects, turning to retrieve a fallen toy, and climbing over a roll were all included in her programme. She sat at the table with the family at mealtimes and self-feeding was encouraged. The occupational therapist and speech therapist provided advice and ideas on play and language development. All three aspects of motor control, play and communication were integrated into the same activity whenever possible. She had to work hard to maintain control of her body posture and fatigue was still a problem despite successful heart surgery. She started cruising along a support by 2 years and took her first stiff wide-based steps just before her third birthday.

Note that only a few infants and young children with Down's syndrome have such excessively low muscle tone as the child in the story above and with encouragement many achieve motor milestones much closer to the average age. Sometimes independent walking may be achieved between 15 and 24 months, but frequently it is much later. A persistent immaturity and inefficiency of the gait pattern is a commonly recognized feature. A number of contributing factors are likely, such as poor control of weight-shift and postural stability (Shepherd 1979), slow onset latency of postural muscles in response to disturbance to balance (Shumway-Cook and Woolacott 1985) and joint laxity and low tone. In the older child or adult, forefoot abnormalities, scoliosis, knee and hip problems may interfere with physical abilities.

Exploration of the environment is a very important component of development, but this activity may be limited in children with Down's syndrome due to their physical inability to move freely, sensory defects of vision or hearing, poor general health and tendency to fatigue or a delay in development of interactional skills. It is important for programmes designed to encourage development, to provide an environment which encourages self-motivation to explore and not just contrived 'play' activities which focus on skills for their own sake (Jobling 1993).

Libby attended a small combined play group one morning a week to allow and encourage interaction and play with children of her own age. Intervention goals were achieved incidentally as part of the interactions not as a focus. At home and during more formal sessions with the therapists, play activities were specifically designed to achieve desired goals in the areas of communication and function as well as improved trunk posture, gait (central rotation and forward step), pincer grip, fine and gross motor skills and endurance. She commenced attending preschool each morning a few months before her fifth birthday.

Down's syndrome has been used as an example of infants and young children with motor and general delay due to a syndrome affecting overall developmental progress. Other chromosomal abnormalities may lead to similar types of problems (e.g. Prader Willi and Fragile X syndromes), while endocrine and metabolic disturbances (e.g. hypothroidism and mucopolysaccharidoses), disruption to the process of neural migration or conditions of early childhood such as Rett's syndrome may also often present as either weak or low tone infants/young children. It is important to be alert to the possibility that weak or apparently low tone infants and young children may have a disorder of muscle or peripheral nerves such as spinal muscular atrophy or one of the dystrophies or, of connective tissue as in Ehlers–Danlos syndrome. Careful assessment, keen observation and a readiness to request further specialist paediatric neurological investigation should avoid incorrect management.

Thought Provoker

Margaret is a little girl now 3 years of age. She has recently come with her family to live in your district. Although she has been receiving physiotherapy since the age of 9 months because of extremely low muscle tone and developmental delay, it is only recently that magnetic resonance imaging (MRI) brain scans have shown the most likely cause of her problems is an interruption to neural migration during early fetal development.

The initial physiotherapy assessment report indicates that at 9 months she had very poor head control and no ability to roll, sit or take weight. She took little interest in toys and did not sustain grasp of even light objects. She liked to follow people visually and obviously enjoyed watching the antics of her two sisters. At the age of 2 years when she was not attempting to vocalize or speak, a hearing impairment was suspected, but tests indicated normal hearing.

Now at the age of 3 years she is walking independently with an unsteady, irregular, wide-based gait, is starting to use some simple sign language and vocalize some simple commonly used words. Play involves uncomplicated cause–effect toys (press the top and up pops a little man), but she comprehends and follows clear verbal instruction. She is unable, however, to plan a task or deduce a solution for even a simple problem such as, find the toy hidden from view or a ball which rolled under her dress. Through repetition she is starting to assist with some daily tasks such as dressing and feeding, but a solution learned in one situation is not transferred to another. For example, she has learnt to get on to a low chair at home, but is unable to do it at kindergarten even though the chair is similar in height and shape. She knows what she wants to do and says 'Margie it air' (Margie sit chair), but has difficulty turning her body around so her bottom faces the chair.

- What assessment techniques would identify a problem of motor planning?
- What principles of management would guide your approach to treatment of this problem?
- How could you lessen the impact of her movement and motor planning problems on other aspects of her development?

Spina Bifida

Case Study 3

Alex is 6 years old and beginning his first year of school. He has recently seen the physiotherapist for an assessment, and review of his equipment. He will also be reviewed by the various consultants (paediatrician, orthopaedic surgeon, neurosurgeon, urologist), attached to the specialized clinic held in the large paediatric hospital

Alex was initially seen by a physiotherapist when 16 hours old. Alex had spina bifida and the physiotherapist had been notified that this baby would require an assessment prior to attending theatre for closure of a large thoracolumbar myelomeningocoele lesion. He had been delivered by elective caesarean section in a major metropolitan centre even though his family lived 500 km away. Alex's mother had an ultrasound scan during her pregnancy, that identified an abnormality at the level of the brainstem. Further investigation indicated that the baby had spina bifida. The family were referred both to specialists and the support group for parents and families of children with spina bifida where they were provided with information

Figure 9   Categories of Spina Bifida Cystica: A, lipomeningocoele – vertebral defect with lipoma or fatty mass merging with the spinal cord in the lumbosacral area; B, meningocoele – protrusion of the meninges and cerebrospinal fluid into a sac that is covered with epithelium; C, myelomeningocoele – protrusion of both meninges and elements of the spinal cord

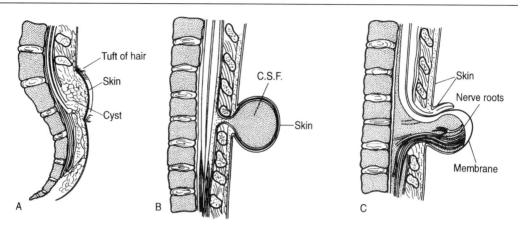

about spina bifida and its management. Alex's parents decided that they wanted Alex to be offered care through a centre specializing in the management of children with spina bifida. An elective caesarean section allowed for planned and immediate care of their first baby.

Vertebral and Neural Tube Defects

Spina bifida occulta and spina bifida cystica both are vertebral defects characterized by non-closure of the posterior elements of the vertebral arch. The latter is accompanied by a cystic protrusion of meninges, or the spinal cord and meninges. Defects include meningocoele, myelomeningocoele and lipomeningocoele (Figure 9).

Myelomeningocoele (commonly termed spina bifida) is the most common and serious defect. The cystic protrusion may present in any size or form, and occur at any location. It is most commonly covered by a transparent membrane that may have neural tissue attached to its inner surface, or may be open with neural tissue exposed (see Figure 10). Other neural tube defects include encephalocoele where there is protrusion of cerebrospinal fluid (CSF) and meninges through a bony defect in the skull, and anencephaly where the cranial end of the neural tube has failed to fuse, resulting in an exposed malformed brain not compatible with life.

Figure 10   Newborn Infant with Large Intact Thoracolumbar Lesion – prior to surgical repair

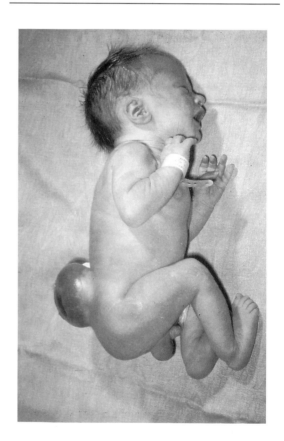

Clinical Manifestations of Spina Bifida

Spina bifida is the most complex treatable congenital anomaly of the CNS that is consistent with life (Bunch 1976), and is characterized by impaired mobility

(Liptak *et al.* 1992). The child with spina bifida faces potential health problems in four areas: the central nervous system (CNS), the genitourinary tract, the musculoskeletal system and the skin (Morrissy 1978). Clinical manifestations vary in severity from mild distal sensory and motor deficits and neurogenic sphincter dysfunction, to complete paralysis, severe skeletal malformation, and a range of accompanying developmental and neurological abnormalities. These may include upper extremity dysfunction or cognitive, perceptual or attentional deficits that affect ambulation, independence in activities of daily living, school performance and quality of life (Sand *et al.* 1974).

Pathogenesis and Aetiology of Spina Bifida

Although investigated for many years, the pathogenesis and aetiology of myelomeningocoele continue to be the subject of debate, and are still not clearly understood. Embryological studies indicate that spina bifida may result from a failure of neural tube closure during the process of neurulation (Osaka *et al.* 1978). This process is complete by the 28th day of gestation. These authors also report that the malformation may occur after 28 days, when neurulation has already occurred. Regardless of the mechanism and timing of defect formation, the neural tube in spina bifida is open, with what was meant to be the central canal lying open on the dorsal surface of the sac (McLone 1980). Spina bifida is believed to have multiple aetiologies, with studies implicating genetic, environmental and dietary factors, or the interaction of these factors (multifactorial), as possible causes (Smithells *et al.* 1980).

Incidence of Spina Bifida

Incidence of neural tube defects (NTD) ranges from very low to 6 per 1000 live births depending on geography and ethnic background of the parents. The highest incidence occurs in the British Isles, mainly Ireland and Wales, where it ranges from 3 to 6 per 1000 births (Alexander and Steg 1989). Women who have had a pregnancy resulting in an infant or fetus with a NTD have an increased risk of recurrence in subsequent pregnancies (Little and Elwood 1991). Daily oral supplementation with folic acid before

conception and during early pregnancy substantially reduces the risk for NTDs in subsequent pregnancies and is recommended (MRC Vitamin Study Research Group 1991). The use of folate supplements for women taking some anticonvulsant drugs (associated with an increased risk of NTDs) is also recommended, but only under the close supervision of their physician (Bower 1994). Debate about the use of folic acid supplementation to prevent first occurrences of NTDs is ongoing with current evidence suggesting benefits (Elwood 1991).

Prenatal Diagnosis of Spina Bifida

One area of development in research has been the discovery of a means of prenatal diagnosis of open spina bifida defects. Elevated levels of α-fetoprotein within the amniotic fluid, as well as maternal serum, between 16 and 18 weeks of pregnancy, have been found to be predictive of open neural tube defects (Brock and Sutcliffe 1972). Elevated amniotic fluid acetylcholinesterase, a CNS enzyme, can be used more specifically to diagnose open neural tube defects after the 20th week of gestation (Brock *et al.* 1985). Ultrasonography has also been advocated as a useful prenatal diagnostic tool (Brock *et al.* 1985).

An initial assessment of Alex allowed baseline information to be gathered and documented, as well as initial contact made with the family. The physiotherapist who assessed Alex worked within a specialized clinic caring for children with spinal disabilities. This initial contact was continued with long-term follow-up and monitoring which allowed for consistent support for the family. Alex was assessed when awake and active. The lesion was covered with sterile dressing. Care was taken during the assessment not to cause any trauma to the lesion or introduce any infection.

Care of Neural Tissue

Many authors, including McLone (1983), emphasize that exposed neural tissue in open myelomeningocoele is viable, and potentially capable of conducting motor and sensory impulses. This has been substantiated by the presence of function below the level of the myelomeningocoele, and postoperative recovery of motor function. This highlights the need for care of exposed neural tissue before surgery, ensuring that it does not become dry, or traumatized by clothing, tight bandages, or the baby lying and putting pressure on the lesion. Assessment of the infant's lower limb movement before surgery must be performed with utmost care in terms of positioning and handling to prevent trauma to the lesion, and the introduction of infection.

Careful observation and palpation to evaluate both the available range of motion and motor function was performed with Alex positioned in alternate side-lying to protect the back lesion. No significant deformities of the hips or knees were noted, with 30° flexion contracture at the hips and 10° at the knees considered to be within the range of physiological flexion normally seen in neonates. Both ankles were in a position of equinovarus but were easily corrected to a square plantigrade position.

Despite obvious active movement of arms during stimulation around the face and upper body, and when Alex was crying, no active lower limb movement was observed. A flicker of activity was palpated in both iliopsoas muscles and graded as 'grade one' under the muscle-grading scale of Daniels and Worthingham (1980). The abdominals were noted to be active. Flickers of toe movements and activity in the tendoachilles were also noted but only on tickling the lower legs. This movement was determined to be reflexive rather than useful voluntary movement. Holding the baby in an upright position did not result in any ability to take weight through his legs.

Following preoperative evaluation by the paediatrician, neurosurgeon and physiotherapist, Alex's myelomeningocoele

lesion was repaired. No significant kyphosis or scoliosis were present and adequate skin coverage was not a significant problem.

Determination of Motor Level

Evaluation of motor function in patients with spina bifida conventionally involves manual muscle testing and grading of all muscles of the lower extremities (Hoffer *et al.* 1973, Huff and Ramsey 1978). The neurosegmental level of lesion is determined on the basis of these findings and classified according to the most caudal intact nerve root (Huff and Ramsey 1978, Samuelsson and Skoog 1988). The term 'neurosegmental level of lesion' has been used throughout the literature, as a means of classifying patients with myelomeningocoele into groups, for the purposes of communication, so comparisons, predictions and management practices could be discussed. In particular, when discussing ambulatory function, many authors refer to the neurosegmental level of lesion, as the level of lesion determined by motor function (Huff and Ramsey 1978). This is because of the generally held view that lower limb muscle strengths, which form the basis for the widely accepted motor levels described by Sharrard (1964a), are important to ambulatory outcome (DeSouza and Carroll 1976, Huff and Ramsey 1978, Samuelsson and Skoog 1988). It has been noted, however, that children assigned the same motor level will vary significantly in their muscle function (Asher and Olson 1983, McDonald *et al.* 1991), making it preferable to grade muscle strengths individually as this will provide far more useful and accurate information.

Manual Muscle Testing

A patient's ability to contract actively a muscle or group of muscles against gravity or manual resistance is assessed during manual muscle testing (Daniels and Worthingham 1980). Lovett in 1912 initially used these assessment techniques to determine the degree of paralysis in children with poliomyelitis and graded muscle strength as totally paralysed, trace, poor, fair, good or normal (Daniels and Worthingham 1980). Numerical 0–5 grading was introduced some 30 years later.

The accuracy and predictive value of manual muscle testing, especially in infants and younger children has been questioned (Kendall *et al.* 1971, Murdoch 1980, McDonald *et al.* 1986, Schopler and Menelaus 1987). Murdoch (1980) reported that the correlation between early muscle strength determined by manual muscle testing and subsequent mobility was poor and recommended that muscle strength be graded full, weak and absent during infancy. McDonald *et al.* (1986) noted that the ability of manual muscle testing to predict precisely future muscle strength varies according to the muscle evaluated and the age of the child.

Accuracy of manual muscle tests increase from birth to 5–6 years when peak accuracy is reached (McDonald *et al.* 1986). Physiotherapists' confidence in the accuracy of their assessments matches this. Age-related factors that contribute to these findings were identified as an inability of infants and young children to contract voluntarily a muscle fully against resistance, problems understanding instructions, and behaviours in some children preventing accurate testing. The quadriceps are the easiest muscles to evaluate accurately and reliably, and the hip abductors the most difficult (McDonald *et al.* 1986).

VOLUNTARY VERSUS REFLEX MOVEMENT

Duckworth and Brown (1970) noted that movement that is not cortically initiated, seldom has any functional value, and may be mistakenly interpreted as useful motion. Stimulation for lower limb movements should be above the waist as this helps to avoid reflex reactions to sensory stimulus to the lower leg or foot. Voluntary movement is more likely to be observed in the lower extremities when the infant is alert or crying and actively moving the arms. Stark and Baker (1967) note that the reflexive character and stimulus dependency of involuntary muscle responses help distinguish them from voluntary movement.

Despite the limitations of manual muscle testing when applied to newborn and young children with spina bifida, quantifying muscle strength by use of grades remains the principle means by which clinicians evaluate muscle function and paralysis (McDonald *et al.* 1986, Shurtleff 1986). Assessment of muscle power by

manual muscle testing can be used to: establish a baseline analysis for use in long-term follow-up so neurological stability can be monitored; assess remaining muscle function; evaluate the extent of muscle imbalance at each joint; assist in the evaluation of existing deformity; predict the potential for development of deformity; assist in determination of need for splinting, orthoses and surgery; and assist with realistic aims in management (Mazur and Menelaus 1991).

ALTERNATE METHODS OF STRENGTH ASSESSMENT

Because the subjective nature of manual muscle testing was recognized, alternatives have been advocated in the past to evaluate motor function in children. Somatosensory evoked potentials have been reported to be of some value in evaluation of children with varying degrees of paralysis, and for following patients for early signs of deterioration (Duckworth *et al.* 1976).

Various isometric and isokinetic devices (Molner *et al.* 1979, Agre *et al.* 1987) have been used to quantify the amount of force generated by particular muscles or muscle groups in children. Agre *et al.* (1987) noted that quantitative isometric assessment of patients, with no motor deficit detected on manual muscle testing, revealed significant decreases from normal values for hip and knee extensors. This emphasizes the importance of quantitative assessment of strength. These studies, however, have only involved children of 5 years and over.

Ingberg and Johnson (1963) found electromyography (EMG) helpful in accurate evaluation of the infant by indicating motor function at and below the level of the sac. Clinical assessments were found to correspond with EMG findings (Duckworth and Brown 1970) leading to the conclusion that manual muscle testing by experienced clinicians can be a reasonably accurate means of assessing muscle function in patients with spina bifida.

Closure of the Lesion

The most important reasons for early closure of an open myelomeningocoele are to prevent infection and to preserve existing or potential nerve function

(McLone 1980, Guthkelch *et al.* 1981, McLone *et al.* 1982). Many techniques for closure of the open myelomeningocoele have been discussed and debated in the literature. Irrespective of the technique used, McLone and Dias (1991) and Shurtleff and Stuntz (1986) advocate that operative intervention should be directed towards preserving neurological function, minimizing the risk of tethering, and optimizing subsequent repair of a tethered cord, should this become necessary.

> *During the early postoperative period, Alex's parents were both nervous and emotional, requiring support and appropriate information. Alex's grandparents frequently visited the ward and while very concerned about their small grandson's problems were also willing and in a position to offer support and assistance to the family. Alex's parents were keen to understand more about his condition and how they would be best able to assist him. Communication between team members occurred regularly so all members were aware of findings and able to deliver consistent, accurate and appropriate information. Information delivered sensitively and in a positive and caring way helped to prevent the family becoming confused and frustrated. Potential problems such as tethering, learning difficulties and latex sensitivity were introduced. These discussions allowed Alex's parents to understand their baby's condition and gain insight into current and future management.*

Latex Sensitivity in Children with Spina Bifida

Children with spina bifida are at risk of developing sensitivity to latex. Reduced exposure to latex products may prevent this sensitivity developing. Family, health professionals and teachers need to be aware of individual children's allergies. If allergic reactions occur, stop the exposure. If this reaction includes any difficulties with breathing, seek medical attention.

Some common latex/rubber products and the likely reactions are as follows:

Products

- examination gloves
- rubber catheters
- enema devices
- operative devices
- condoms
- balloons

Reactions

- skin redness and rash
- swelling
- itchiness
- wheeze or coughing
- breathing difficulties
- life-threatening anaphylaxis

> *The physiotherapist assisted and encouraged Alex's parents to handle and interact with him confidently whilst taking care not to jeopardize the healing of the lesion. This became easier after the initial postoperative period. Such education was very important as Alex was their first child and neither parent was confident handling their small baby.*
>
> *The physiotherapist demonstrated different methods of positioning Alex ensuring protection of the newly repaired lesion and appro-*

Figure 11   Baby Prone on Lap Demonstrating 'Opening Out' of Flexed Hips

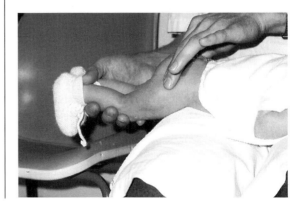

priate alignment of lower limbs, and care of skin. Alex settled happily when positioned prone over his parents' knees and rocked. This allowed for opening out of flexed hips (see Figure 11).

Gentle passive range of movement exercises for the lower limbs were practised with Alex's parents and they were then able to continue with these themselves.

A variety of different positions for carrying, playing and interaction were demonstrated. These allowed Alex the opportunity to practice various skills such as visual fixing and following, holding his own head and adjusting to various positions and to movement. Encouraging Alex's parents to gradually take responsibility for these activities (positioning, handling, passive movements, skin care) assisted their relaxed interaction with Alex and enabled them to be more confident about their ability to cope when discharged home. Alex's parents were keen to understand the background to the physiotherapy programme and how it fitted in with longer term management.

During the period following repair of the back lesion, Alex was closely monitored for signs of increasing intracranial pressure. Alex had no clinical evidence of hydrocephalus at birth and this was confirmed with head ultrasound (US). As with the majority of babies with spina bifida, however, Alex's head circumference increased, his cranial sutures separated and his anterior fontanelle bulged and became increasingly tense. Repeat US and computerized axial tomography (CAT) scan clearly demonstrated dilatation of the lateral ventricles and a (R) lateral ventriculoperitoneal shunt was inserted to control hydrocephalus when Alex was 10 days old. Although expected, this represented another major stress for Alex's parents and information and close support for the family was provided by various team members. Because the physiotherapist had spent a considerable amount of time with the family by this stage, she became a valuable part of this support team.

Figure 12   Position of Ventriculoperitoneal (VP) Shunt

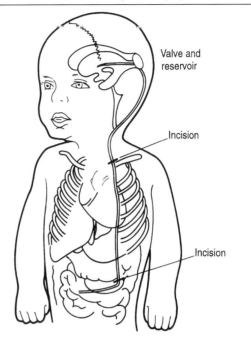

Valve and reservoir

Incision

Incision

Hydrocephalus in Spina Bifida

Both hydrocephalus and the Arnold–Chiari malformation are commonly associated with spina bifida. Hydrocephalus in children with spina bifida is generally considered to be due to obstruction of cerebrospinal fluid (CSF) flow by the Arnold–Chiari malformation and results in increased intracranial pressure (ICP) and an enlarged ventricular system (Stein and Schut 1979). If untreated or poorly controlled, signs and symptoms of hydrocephalus in infants may include bulging and tense fontanelles, separation of sutures, increasing head circumference, vomiting, somnolence, irritability, 'sunsetting' eyes, onset of or increased spasticity in the lower extremities, onset or worsening of scoliosis, reduced vital signs and opisthotonos. In older children headaches, subtle personality changes, lethargy, decreased eye–hand coordination and decreases in school performances may be seen (Stein and Schut 1979, Shurtleff et al. 1986).

In most centres, hydrocephalus is currently managed by the surgical insertion of a ventriculoperitoneal (VP) shunt which diverts CSF away from the lateral ventricles (see Figure 12). While about 98% of children born with myelomeningocoele will have or

Figure 13 MRI Demonstrating Arnold–Chiari Malformation

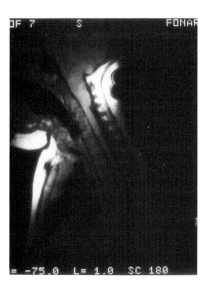

develop an enlarged ventricular system, hydrocephalus requiring shunting occurs in 80–90% of children with myelomeningocoele (McLone *et al.* 1985).

Hydrocephalus has been reported by many authors to be a limiting factor in the intellectual functioning of children with myelomeningocoele (Tew and Laurence 1975). This has been disputed by McLone *et al.* (1982, 1985) who suggest that mental retardation in children with myelomeningocoele and hydrocephalus is not an associated trait, but rather an acquired deficit related primarily to the onset of CNS infection – ventriculitis and / or meningitis.

Arnold–Chiari Malformation in Spina Bifida

The constellation of hindbrain anomalies that accompany spina bifida are known as the Arnold–Chiari or Chiari II malformation. The essential features of this anomaly include an elongated small cerebellum and brainstem, with caudal displacement of the medulla, parts of the cerebellum and pons through an enlarged foramen magnum into the cervical spine canal (Gilbert *et al.* 1986). Magnetic resonance imaging (MRI) clearly demonstrates this anomaly (Figure 13).

The roots of cranial and cervical nerves are crowded together, and often take off below their respective foramina. In patients who have spina bifida, the prevalence is believed to be at least 90% (Gilbert *et al.* 1986). Onset of brainstem dysfunction caused by compression of the Arnold–Chiari malformation, is often insidious in infants. Symptoms may include stridor, impaired vocal cord and palatal movement, swallowing difficulties, apnoea and cyanosis (Venes *et al.* 1986, Barnet *et al.* 1993). Older children may also present with nystagmus, opisthotonos (Venes *et al.* 1986), increasing weakness, spasticity, upper limb dysfunction (Park *et al.* 1985, Venes *et al.* 1986, Samuelsson and Skoog 1988), scoliosis (Park *et al.* 1985) and changes in urodynamics (Lais *et al.* 1993). Although older children, adolescents and young adults respond consistently to cervical laminectomy and posterior decompression of their Arnold–Chiari malformation (Park *et al.* 1985, Bell *et al.* 1987), infants frequently have persistent postoperative symptoms (Bell *et al.* 1987). Arnold–Chiari malformation is the principle cause of mortality in both infants (McLone *et al.* 1985, Bell *et al.* 1987) and older children and adolescents (McLone *et al.* 1985).

It is well-recognized that a malfunctioning shunt exacerbates or causes signs and symptoms (McLone *et al.* 1985, Park *et al.* 1985, Bell *et al.* 1987) of brainstem compression. The mechanism for this effect is unknown. Bell *et al.* (1987) suggest that the combination of the caudal brainstem compression and the abnormal brainstem architecture, result in the clinical signs and symptoms seen. Most authors (Park et al. 1985, McLone *et al.* 1990) emphasize the importance of ensuring that hydrocephalus is well controlled, and the shunt functioning before other causes for neurological deterioration are sought.

Children with spina bifida, Chiari II malformations and hydrocephalus may have a spectrum of difficulties including delayed development of gross motor milestones (Wolf and McLaughlin 1992), learning difficulties (McLone *et al.* 1985), visual perceptual problems (Tew and Laurence 1975), upper limb dysfunction (Sand *et al.* 1974) and reduced goal-directed behaviour (Landrey *et al.* 1990).

Alex was seen daily by his physiotherapist to monitor his progress. He was fully assessed and the findings documented 14 days after back closure. By this stage, Alex had recovered well from his shunt insertion and his back lesion was healing (an uncomplicated postoperative period is the primary goal of management). He was breastfeeding with-

out difficulties, was easy to settle between feeds, seemed to enjoy handling and inter-action, and was visually fixing on faces and just beginning to follow if held in a stable position. During the limited supine periods now allowed because the back wound was healing well, he was unable to hold his head in the midline unless a peanut roll (folded nappy) was used. In prone he was beginning to lift and turn his head to lie on the (R) side (in this case the shunt side), and showed a definite preference for this position. This necessitated the use of a small gel pad under the shunt to disperse the pressure over this area during this early postoperative stage and (L) side-lying was encouraged. This early preference for head position led to discus-sions about the importance of promoting symmetry and alignment, as continuous use of one position may lead to asymmetry in all positions and result in soft tissue tightness and cranial and facial asymmetries.

Activity in the lower limbs was noted and close evaluation showed a little activity in iliopsoas, palpable on the (L) and producing slight movement on the (R). No other lower limb activity could be detected apart from the flickers of reflex activity in the toes and calf muscles. The possibility of this activity contributing to loss of extensibility and range of motion at the ankle and foot was noted. The presence of weak hip flexion was also noted to have the potential to contribute to fixed flexion contracture and/or hip subluxa-tion or dislocation due to muscle imbalance and lack of stability around the hip.

Sensory testing, while difficult to interpret accurately, was attempted when Alex was quietly awake. He responded to light touch and tickling along the groin area and over the abdomen. Other areas of his lower limbs appeared to be insensitive to this touch and this served to remind Alex's parents of the need for care of the skin and protection against pressure, rubbing, scrapes and burns.

The assessment findings and their signifi-cance were shared with the parents. The reasons for regular monitoring of progress and neurological status were explained. A simple written programme for home man-agement was provided so the parents could refer to this as necessary. As the parents were already confident with much of this pro-gramme, discussion and demonstrations were able to focus on the benefits of hand-ling, positioning and play, allowing Alex a greater opportunity to practice and develop movement control, especially mature head control. The importance of movement and normal experiences were emphasized. Encouraging the development of visual motor skills at this early stage was also given emphasis, particularly in view of the high incidence of visual problems (nystagmus, strabismus, poor conjugate gaze, etc.) in this population.

Like many parents of children with spina bifida, one of the first questions Alex's par-ents asked was 'will Alex walk?'. They initi-ally focused very much on his paralysed legs and wanted to know what this would mean for him in terms of future walking potential. Ongoing discussions throughout the period of hospitalization allowed this issue to be explored and better understood.

Ambulation/Myelomeningocoele Gait

The term 'ambulation' is commonly used in the litera-ture when referring to myelomeningocoele gait, and means upright mobility, both with and without assis-tive devices such as orthoses and crutches. This terminology allows for a variety of gait patterns to be grouped together, as 'walking' may conjure up a vision of reciprocal stepping, rather than the swivel-ling or swing-through gait pattern used by some patients.

To be able to make valid comparisons of ambulatory outcome from the literature, ambulatory function needs to be clearly defined. Functional levels of ambulation have been classified to give a means of knowing how well patients are able to walk (Hoffer *et al.* 1973) as follows:

- Community ambulation: Walks indoors and outdoors for most activities; may use crutches or orthoses or both; wheelchair only used for long trips.
- Household ambulation: Walks only indoors using assistive devices; gets in and out of chair with little if any assistance; wheelchair used indoors for some activities; wheelchair used for all community activities.
- Non-functioning ambulation: walking for therapy; wheelchair used for all transportation.
- Non-ambulation: wheelchair bound; usually can transfer from chair to bed.

Investigators have repeatedly found the neurosegmental level of lesion as determined by motor function, to be the most important factor in determining ambulatory outcome in patients with myelomeningocoele (Hoffer *et al.* 1973, DeSouza and Carroll 1976, Feiwell *et al.* 1978, Asher and Olson 1983, Stillwell and Menelaus 1983, Gaff *et al.* 1984, Samuelsson and Skoog 1988). Other important factors influencing ambulatory outcome in children with spina bifida include:

- treatment philosophies and early ambulation (Mazur *et al.* 1989)
- physiotherapy focused on walking (Charney *et al.* 1991)
- parental compliance (Charney *et al.* 1991)
- achievement of motor milestones (Findley *et al.* 1987)
- severity of sitting balance deficit (Swank and Dias 1992)
- level of ambulation by 4–5 years (Charney *et al.* 1991, Swank and Dias 1992)
- spasticity in both upper and lower limbs (Mazur *et al.* 1986a)

Evaluation of ambulatory outcome by various investigators has also identified factors that frequently contribute to the loss of ambulatory function with increasing age of this population:

- increasing energy cost of walking for older children and adolescents (Hoffer *et al.* 1973, DeSouza and Carroll 1976, Asher and Olson 1983, Mazur *et al.* 1989)
- neurological loss (Samuelsson and Skoog 1988, Swank and Dias 1992)
- spasticity, in lower and / or upper limbs (Mazur *et al.* 1986a)
- increased body weight with age and obesity (Asher and Olson 1983)
- recurrent skin breakdown (Harris and Banta 1990, Taylor and McNamara 1990)
- poor design of orthoses (Taylor and McNamara 1990)
- inability to get new orthoses (Taylor and McNamara 1990)
- toileting issues (Taylor and McNamara 1990)
- prolonged immobilization following orthopaedic intervention (Taylor and McNamara 1990)
- scoliosis and other musculoskeletal deformity especially hip flexion deformity (Asher and Olson 1983, Samuelsson and Skoog 1988)
- knee pain and medial / anteromedial instability (Williams *et al.* 1993)
- lack of motivation (Asher and Olson 1983)
- psychosocial reasons – not always measurable by physical factors (Dudgeon *et al.* 1991)

Provided the clinician has an understanding of the factors that influence ambulatory outcome, it is possible to determine the potential of a child with spina bifida to walk.

Table 1 summarizes the features to consider for ambulatory outcome.

It is important to note that children with spina bifida who show no motor deficit (strength losses were not apparent on manual muscle testing) may have less than normal usual walking and running speeds (Agre *et al.* 1987). Quantitative isometric strength of hip and knee extensors in a small group of these children was found to be reduced when compared with normal values.

The adult population of myelomeningocoele patients cited in the literature is still relatively young and few

Table 1
Ambulatory Outcome

Neuroseg-mental level	Critical motor function	Muscles innervated	Common deformities	Preambulation orthosis[a]	Ambulation orthosis[a]	Assistive devices	Ambulatory potential[b]
Thoracic	Lower limb paralysis	± Abdominals	Spinal deformity	Standing frame	RGO or ParaWalker or HKAFO or parapodium or swivel walker[c]	Walking frame or elbow crutches	**Children:** therapy or household ambulation; community ambulation more likely if good sitting balance and ambulating by age 4 **Adolescents/Adults:** reliant upon wheelchair for independent mobility
Upper lumbar	Hip flexion ± hip adduction	Muscles above ± iliopsoas ± sartorius ± adductors	Spinal deformity Hip flexion contracture	Standing frame	RGO or ParaWalker or HKAFO or parapodium	Walking frame or elbow crutches	**Children:** household or community ambulation **Adolescents/Adults:** small percentage therapy or household ambulation; majority reliant upon wheelchair for independent mobility
Mid lumbar L3	Knee extension	Muscles above + quadriceps	Hip dislocation/subluxation Hip flexion contracture Tibial torsion	Standing frame	RGO or ParaWalker or HKAFO or KAFO or AFO ± twister cables	Walking frame or elbow crutches	**Children:** household or community ambulation **Adolescents/Adults:** variable outcome – household or community ambulation more likely if quadriceps grade 4 or 5
L4	Knee flexion	+ medial hamstrings ± tibialis anterior					
Low lumbar	Ankle dorsiflexion Ankle inversion ± ankle eversion ± hip abduction	Muscles above + lateral hamstrings + peronei ± tibialis posterior ± gluteus medius ± toe flex/ext	Hip flexion contracture Ankle/foot deformity	Standing frame or AFO or no orthosis	KAFO or AFO	Walking frame or elbow crutches or no aids	**Children:** household or community ambulation **Adolescents/Adults:** majority household or community ambulation – independent gait may be possible with moderate deviations
Sacral S1 S2–3	Hip extension Ankle plantarflexion	Muscles above + gluteus maximus + gastroc/soleus + foot intrinsics	Toe clawing	Standing frame[c] or AFO[c] no orthosis	AFO or UCBL or no orthosis	Walking frame[c] progressing to no aids	**Children:** community ambulation **Adolescents/Adults:** community ambulation – independent gait with moderate to minimal deviations

[a] RGO = reciprocating gait orthosis; HKAFO = hip–knee–ankle–foot orthosis; KAFO = knee–ankle–foot orthosis; AFO = ankle–foot orthosis; UCBL = University of California Biomechanics Laboratory shoe inserts.

[b] Functional levels of ambulation [Hoffer et al. 1973].

[c] Reduced motor control as a result of CNS anomalies.

data are yet available on middle- and old-aged patients. The cumulative data that exists on adults is limited, with most studies involving individuals with complications that may now be avoided. The problems of these adult patients will not be the same as the adult patients in 10–15 years, as there have been major changes in back closure, shunt management, infection control, recognition and management of CNS anomalies and orthopaedic treatments.

Spasticity in Spina Bifida

A significant percentage of patients with spina bifida will demonstrate spasticity in the lower extremities because of the nature of the lesion (Stark and Baker 1967, Stark and Drummond 1971, Mazur *et al.* 1986a) or because of associated CNS anomalies (Park *et al.* 1985, McLone *et al.* 1990, Petersen 1992, Rabb *et al.* 1992, Herman *et al.* 1993). Traditionally, patients with myelomeningocoele have only been classified according to the neurosegmental level of the lesion. Mazur *et al.* (1986a) demonstrated that classifying the type of paralysis, spastic or flaccid, is equally important.

Spasticity in the upper limbs may occur because of associated CNS anomalies (Park *et al.* 1985, McLone *et al.* 1990, Petersen 1992, Rabb *et al.* 1992, Herman *et al.* 1993) and/or may be related to the number of shunt operations done for hydrocephalus (Mazur *et al.* 1986a). Patients with spasticity in their upper limbs were less likely to be independent in activities of daily living with upper limbs not only weaker, but poorly coordinated making control of crutches difficult (Mazur *et al.* 1986a). It was noted that patients with flaccid lower limbs below the level of the lesion and normal upper limbs had the best prognosis, functioned best in activities of daily living and had the most potential in terms of ambulation.

As Alex's parents became more confident they were keen to be shown some of the equipment he might use to assist him in achieving upright stance and ambulation, and other mobility equipment such as scooter boards and wheelchairs. They also felt that they could cope with meeting other parents and the team social worker introduced them to a family with a 5-year-old

child with spina bifida. While recognizing that no two children would be the same, Alex's parents found it very helpful to be able to share and discuss concerns. These included issues such as how to recognize shunt dysfunction, how to manage incontinence as Alex grew older, would Alex be as mobile as this 5 year old child in a reciprocating gait orthosis (RGO) and so on. Prior to discharge the physiotherapist summarized management goals and encouraged Alex's parents when they returned home to enjoy their baby, to move and play with him, to fit the home programme into the normal activities of the day and to feel comfortable about ringing to discuss any concerns or questions that may arise.

Physiotherapy Goals for Spina Bifida

These goals are as follows:

- educate parents in ways of handling, positioning, playing and interacting to assist in reducing the effects of both the spinal defect and associated CNS anomalies on the baby's development (gross motor, fine motor, cognitive and perceptual development)
- educate parents to improve/maintain passive range of motion and prevent joint contracture
- increase parental awareness for the need for skin care and thus prevent skin breakdown
- assist in the prescription of appropriate orthosis and equipment which will assist in meeting the longer term goals of independent mobility and ambulation
- monitor for neurological deterioration by performing regular assessments to include functional assessment, musculoskeletal review, muscle testing, assessment of tone
- record and communicate assessment findings appropriately with other professionals within the team and with parents

Alex returned to the paediatric hospital for physiotherapy and specialist medical review

Figure 14   Frog-leg Posturing of Lower Limbs

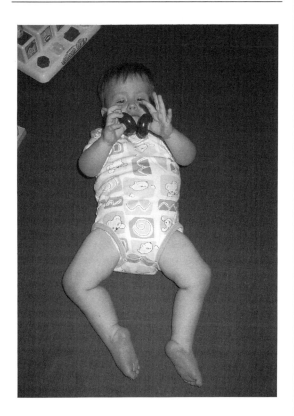

at frequent intervals during his first year of life.

4-month review

When reviewed at 4 months, Alex was alert, smiling and interactive. He showed no signs of the initial asymmetry with positioning of his head and although head stability and control had improved in all positions, this activity still required much effort and was quite immature. Alex tended to use marked shoulder elevation with the upper limbs held stiffly to assist in stabilizing the head. These compensatory patterns interfere with the development of righting reactions and free use of the arms. This pattern was particularly evident in prone, where Alex could only maintain his head up for short periods. Alex's parents had followed an early suggestion and set up a wedge for prone play and this assisted Alex to tolerate the position

more easily and spend increasing periods of time in this position. His parents also reported that Alex enjoyed sitting in a small seat watching a mobile. The physiotherapist cautioned against the child spending prolonged periods in a seat and again emphasized the importance of movement and floor play. It was reassuring for the physiotherapist to see how confident and relaxed both parents were in handling Alex and also that he showed no signs of being nervous of movement and handling.

In all positions Alex's hips tended to be in flexion, abduction and external rotation (commonly termed frog-leg position, see Figure 14). The (R) ankle was in a position of plantarflexion/inversion with resistance to correction to plantigrade because of increased calf tone. A small splint moulded out of thermoplastic material was made to assist in maintaining (R) foot/ankle range.

This was initially only worn for short periods until both the physiotherapist and Alex's parents were confident that no pressure areas would develop, especially over vulnerable bony prominences such as the lateral malleolus. As Alex's parents understood the need for care and regular monitoring of the skin for marks, the physiotherapist encouraged them to increase Alex's time in the splint and to work out a schedule of use that suited both them and Alex. They quickly developed the pattern of the splint on during sleeping time and off at other times allowing them to mobilize the ankle gently. Alex's parents were shown how to make minor adjustments to the splint if it were to mark the skin. The possibility of outgrowing the splint before the next review was discussed and the family were aware that they could manage this by increasing the passive ranging for the ankle. This approach was suggested as there was no local physiotherapy service available for Alex and his family.

Alex's home programme was updated with

more emphasis placed on assisting Alex to develop improved head control in all positions. The physiotherapist provided more treatment and handling ideas, e.g. ways of picking Alex up to give him the opportunity to right his head, carrying positions, gently rocking and moving Alex in supported sitting, facilitating rolling and positioning in prone. These activities were noted in Alex's homework book and a number of photographs were also taken to act as visual reminders.

8-month review

Alex could assist in pushing up to sitting with facilitation by his 8-month review. He was able to sit independently propping with one or both hands. Reaching was limited as weight-shift and equilibrium reactions in this position were poorly developed and Alex had difficulty freeing his arms and moving them away from his trunk. Two-handed play/bilateral hand skills was not possible. Earlier compensatory patterns of shoulder elevation and stiffly held arms were still evident. Protective reactions to the side were emerging but still slow, inconsistent, and not yet functional. In both sitting and prone Alex still demonstrated an immature pattern of upper cervical extension (poke chin) rather than actively using his neck flexors to appropriately align his head on body.

Alex showed poorly developed weight-shift in prone, making reaching in this position limited. Pivoting in prone was slow at this stage. Some pushing up on to stiffly extended arms occurred causing Alex to slide backwards. If his legs were not widely abducted he would use this extension to initiate rolling to supine. During the 8-month review the emphasis of treatment centred around assisting Alex with more dynamic postural control and being able to change position on the floor to prepare better for activities such as reaching, pivoting, rolling, creeping and

moving in and out of sitting allowing greater exploration and learning. In the meantime Alex's parents positioned Alex in various places around the house to allow him to explore these areas, introduced movement on a scooter board and he also had regular short times sitting in the high-chair using rolled towels to give added stability and allowing for two-handed play and further development of fine motor skills.

Alex was measured for a standing frame and this was fitted on his next visit. Alex's parents found the prospect of the standing frame a little daunting as well as an exciting step. On the whole, Alex had been able to be treated very much like any baby since his discharge from hospital. The prospect of standing equipment was a very obvious reminder that Alex did have a significant disability and this invoked some of the grief and sorrow that these parents had initially felt.

Innervated lower limb musculature and normal tone are necessary for the development of pelvic and trunk stability. Delayed motor development and compensatory and immature movement patterns are commonly seen in children with spina bifida, including those with minimal paralysis, because of the abnormal muscle tone (commonly hypotonia), delayed development of automatic reactions and delayed integration of primary reflexes (Wolf and McLaughlin 1992). Muscle paralysis and reduced proprioceptive and tactile discrimination play varying roles depending on the level of lesion. The impact of these deficits may result in movement difficulties which affect exploration, motivation and ultimately learning. Movement difficulties contribute to and are compounded by perceptual difficulties and reduced goal-directed behaviour, both commonly occurring in children with spina bifida (Tew and Laurence 1975, Landry et al. 1990). It is important that the physiotherapist continue the earlier work to ensure families have an appropriate understanding of these potential problems and are

Figure 15   Standing and Enjoying Having Hands Free to Play

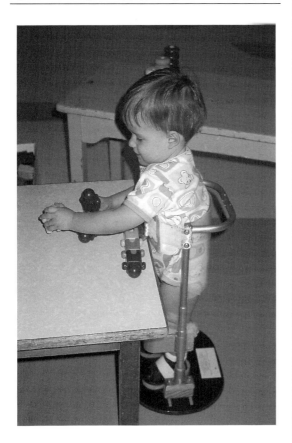

encouraged to continue a home programme of activities to help lessen the impact of these problems on their baby's development.

12-month review

The delight that Alex displayed once upright in the standing frame and the obvious freedom of his arms for play when wearing this orthosis quickly reassured his parents that this was going to be a useful piece of equipment (Figure 15).

The benefits of standing and being upright were discussed and included orthopaedic, developmental, physiological and personal–social benefits. Much emphasis was given to the philosophy that a standing frame should not be considered as purely a static device and that moving in the frame was integral to the use of this orthosis.

AMBULATION VERSUS WHEELED MOBILITY

To be able to walk, or achieve upright ambulation, even with the use of assistive devices such as orthoses and crutches, is an important objective for many patients who have spina bifida (Mazur *et al.* 1989). Although the ability to walk independently is not the goal for every child with spina bifida (Stillwell and Menelaus 1983), many authors strongly promote ambulation. This includes those authors who acknowledge that some children, particularly those with thoracic and high-lumbar lesions, will use a wheelchair for mobility later in life (Hoffer et al. 1973, Carroll 1974, DeSouza and Carroll 1976, Mazur *et al.* 1986a, Charney *et al.* 1991, Swank and Dias 1992). These authors strongly recommend ambulation for children with myelomeningocoele because of the potential benefits of standing and walking for the child's development (Carroll 1974, DeSouza and Carroll 1976, Charney *et al.* 1991). Alternatively, those who advocate the early use of wheelchairs for children with high lesions (Shurtleff 1986, Liptak *et al.* 1988) postulate that children with myelomeningocoele who use wheelchairs exclusively, become more skilled in activities of daily living at an earlier age, move faster and can compete better in sports, and are more likely to be continent and independent in bowel and bladder function. Controversy and uncertainty still exist about the merit of wheelchair use versus assistive devices for ambulation, and further research in this area is necessary.

STANDING FRAME

The timing for introduction of the first standing orthosis has caused some debate in the literature (Carroll 1974, Taylor and Sand 1975, Drennon 1976). The standing frame is generally introduced at 10–12 months when children are normally weight-bearing through the lower limbs, and the child has developed adequate head control. Independent sitting may not yet be achieved. Postural extension may be promoted through standing and facilitate the development of sitting control.

Dynamic use of the standing frame must be encouraged, as development of head and trunk righting and dynamic control can be facilitated through tilting and

Figure 16   Confident with Movement

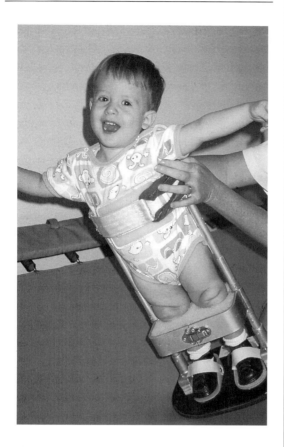

rocking the child in all directions in the frame. See Figure 16.

The movements can become more challenging to the child as their balance responses improve. Play on the trampoline, with action songs and dance is usually thoroughly enjoyed. Protective reactions can also be encouraged with controlled falling on the trampoline or on a soft mat. From this position the child is encouraged to push up to assist in getting back up into the upright position. As the child becomes more confident and trunk control increases, the bracing around the trunk may be reduced to provide pelvic support only. Not only do these activities assist in the development of balance and postural reactions, but they also help to make the child very confident in the upright position. In addition, the free-standing allowed by these devices gives the child an opportunity to play in a well-supported position, with hands free from the need to prop.

Increasing independent mobility – 18 months onwards

A castor cart was introduced when Alex was 18 months and allowed for safe (no grazes/scrapes on insensitive skin), efficient independent mobility outside. At this stage and with assistance, he was beginning to weight-shift and swivel in the standing frame using parallel bars or holding someone's hands. He then progressed to a walking frame and became increasingly mobile and independent with this over the next 12–18 months. The size and shape of the baseplate was modified with these progressions. Because Alex had sufficient upper limb strength and function, he was also able to jump and progress to a swing-through pattern. A lightweight manual wheelchair was prescribed for Alex when he was 3 years old and this was used for outside mobility at kindergarten/in the community. It was not used inside as Alex was very mobile creeping and the exercise and upper limb strengthening which resulted from this was seen as extremely valuable. Alex was supplied with a parapodium at this stage, so he would have the added function of being able to sit while still wearing his orthosis. Alex was able to use these various methods of mobility at kindergarten and this not only allowed him choice and a variety, but also allowed him to participate in the many activities offered and to relate appropriately with his peers.

It was noted that Alex had a leg length discrepancy and further investigation revealed that his (R) hip was dislocated. His orthopaedic surgeon discussed this with Alex's parents and it was decided that no surgical intervention was necessary; however, maintaining the range of movement at that hip was given particular emphasis with specific positioning and passive range of movement exercises reviewed and reinforced. A shoe build-up was used to accommodate the leg length discrepancy.

Figure 17   Fracture Following Surgery to Relocate Hip – (R) leg presented as hot, red and very swollen.

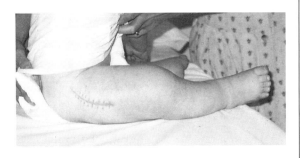

Hip Dislocation in Spina Bifida

Hip subluxations and dislocations in children with spina bifida are common and may be present at birth or develop, usually due to muscle imbalance around the hip (Samuelsson and Eklof 1990, Swank and Dias 1992). In the past these hips were aggressively treated with open reduction, femoral and/or pelvic osteotomies and various procedures used to transfer muscles in an effort to balance musculature and prevent redislocation (Sharrard 1964b, Lee and Carroll 1985). There was much discussion and debate among orthopaedic surgeons and in the literature about methods of intervention; however, more recently this has centred around whether relocation of hips is necessary (Samuelsson and Skoog 1988, Fraser *et al.* 1992, Swank and Dias 1992). Procedures to relocate hips in children, especially those without a high possibility of community ambulation, has become much less common. This has occurred for the following reasons: stiffness or immobility of the hip, fractures (Figure 17) and redislocations are common post-operative complications (Weisl *et al.* 1988); dislocation of the hip in children spina bifida is generally not associated with pain (Samuelsson and Skoog 1988); and studies have shown little correlation between the level of ambulation and status of hips (Samuelsson and Skoog 1988, Fraser *et al.* 1992). Maintenance of a mobile flexible joint and prevention of contractures are noted to be more important than dislocation or subluxation of the hip (Ryan *et al.* 1991).

Fracture warning signs are as follows:

- swelling of a limb
- deformity of a limb
- local heat or redness and a limb
- fever

Alex was fitted for an RGO at 4 years and with a short period of intensive training, became mobile using a posterior walking frame. His parents and Alex were particularly pleased to have this orthosis, as the reciprocal pattern of stepping was more acceptable from an aesthetic viewpoint and Alex was able to ambulate longer distances without tiring. The only disadvantage noted was that Alex was no longer able easily to free-stand as he had been able to in both the standing frame and parapodium. This was a safety problem initially requiring close supervision; however, Alex and his family quickly adjusted. A video of Alex using the RGO (donning, walking, sitting down, standing up and doffing) and also showing his other forms of mobility (wheelchair use, transfers, creeping, bottom shuffling) was made. This was found to be very useful to the local physiotherapist and teachers. It also ensured that Alex was able to use various equipment items at school to increase his independent mobility and function and improve his opportunities to interact with school friends.

Case Study 4

Tess is 12 years old and has spina bifida and hydrocephalus. Tess's physiotherapy contact in the last 12 months has been limited:

- *to a review of ankle–foot orthoses (AFOs) because of redness on the medial aspect of one foot*
- *to visiting Tess in burns unit (Tess sustained friction/heat burns to her buttocks while sliding on the giant slides at an adventure park)*

Tess has presented for her yearly review. It was noted that Tess has had a significant growth spurt in the last 12 months, increasing significantly in height and showing signs of the onset of puberty. Discussions revealed that there has been some problem with back pain in the last month, although no triggering incident could be identified. No deterioration in gait or other changes in function have been noted. On questioning, both Tess and her mother feel that there may have been a slight reduction in walking endurance, with Tess tiring more easily when walking up the hill to the library at school. Because it is only the second week back at school after 7 weeks of holidays, and not a great deal of hill or stair walking had occurred during the holidays, it is difficult to determine whether this change is as a result of reduction in fitness levels, changes in weight and height reducing mechanical advantage, a loss of range of motion, or because of deterioration in neurological status. Comprehensive evaluation and comparisons with previous assessment findings are necessary to assist in interpreting these changes.

Ongoing Evaluation of Spina Bifida

Older children and adolescents with spina bifida often have less regular contact with physiotherapists than infants and young children. This is generally appropriate as most of the major mobility issues will have been addressed in preschool and early school years to allow the child to be independently mobile so they can actively partake in the activities of their peers. Regular assessments are necessary, however, to monitor neurological function, as well as to identify and address issues directly relating to physiotherapy management.

MONITORING NEUROLOGICAL FUNCTION

Cord pathology and other CNS anomalies can produce neurological deterioration, with early symptoms commonly noted as loss of muscle power (Park *et al.* 1985, Peterson 1992). Regular and accurate monitoring of the neurological status of the patient is necessary (Rabb *et al.* 1992, Lais *et al.* 1993). The diagnosis of CNS anomalies is based on clinical findings indicating a deterioration in neurological signs (Rabb *et al.* 1992). For example, many children with spina bifida have

Figure 18   A, Tethering of the Spinal Cord — MRI, note the bowstring appearance of the cord above the tethering (main clinical finding was increasing spasticity and loss of isolated muscle function in the lower limbs). B, Standing with Increasing Flexion and Adduction — note ankle/foot deformity (same child)

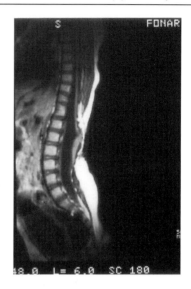

cord tethering on MRI (McCullough *et al.* 1990), but treatment is indicated only when one can demonstrate loss in muscle power, increasing spasticity, progressive scoliosis or changes in urodynamics (Begeer *et al.* 1986). Results show that the earlier neurological deterioration is detected and surgery is performed, the better the outcome (Begeer et al. 1986, Lais et al. 1993).

CNS ANOMALIES IN SPINA BIFIDA

In addition to the spinal cord defect, the patient with spina bifida may be affected by associated CNS anomalies such as Arnold–Chiari malformation, hydrocephalus and syringohydromyelia. These anomalies are now thought to be part of a spectrum of CNS malformations, rather than secondary to myelomeningocoele (Gilbert et al. 1986). Together with tethering of the spinal cord and cyst formation, these CNS anomalies have been found to contribute to further neurological dysfunction in these children.

TETHERING OF THE SPINAL CORD

Tethering of the spinal cord occurs as a delayed consequence of the repair of the spinal cord lesion (Balasubramaniam et al. 1990) with scarring or adhesion of the spinal cord at the level of repair. MRIs show a low-lying and often enlarged conus fixed at the site of previous repair (Tamaki et al. 1988) inhibiting normal spinal cord movement which usually occurs with activity and with growth. The spinal cord appears taut within the spinal canal (Balasubramaniam et al. 1990). See Figure 18.

Tethering in patients with spina bifida is characterized by progressive neurological deterioration, with worsening of the existing neurological deficit, or a new deficit superimposed on the existing one (Balasubramaniam et al. 1990, O'Neill and Stack 1991). In most cases deterioration occurs in a slow progessive way (Begeer et al. 1986, Petersen 1992, Herman et al. 1993). The clinical presentation of tethered cord includes symptoms such as:

- spasticity
- muscle weakness or muscle atrophy
- deterioration in gait patterns
- decreased sensation and changes in sensory level
- back pain or stiffness, progressive scoliosis
- progressive foot deformities
- changes in bladder or bowel function
  (McLone et al. 1990, Petersen 1992, Herman et al. 1993).

Other CNS anomalies can produce similar progressive symptoms and include syringohydromyelia, Arnold- Chiari malformation and spinal arachnoid cysts (Petersen 1992).

Tethering has been noted to occur in 11–27% of the population with myelomeningocoele (Begeer et al. 1986, Tamaki et al. 1988, McLone 1992, Petersen 1992), the percentage varying according to the criteria for diagnosis and recognition of symptoms during regular clinical assessment. It is possible that the diagnosis will become more common as a result of increased long-term survival, increased awareness, regular monitoring and better imaging modalities (Balasubramaniam et al. 1990).

It is necessary to distinguish between asymptomatic and symptomatic patients (Petersen 1992). MRI studies of asymptomatic patients with spina bifida and those with tethering recently released, all have the anatomical appearance of tethering. There appears to be no way yet of predicting which patients will go on to have symptoms (McLone et al. 1990, Petersen 1992) and which will not.

Tethering is likely in the presence of diastematomyelia, a longitudinal division or cleft in the spinal cord associated with a linear cartilaginous or bony septum (O'Neill and Stack 1991). Excision of the bony spur is recommended (Begeer et al. 1986, O'Neill and Stack 1991). Tumours of fat (lipomas) may adhere to or invade the cord or meninges, and represent a potential cause of tethering (Tamaki et al., 1988). Begeer et al. (1986), McLone (1980) and others note the need to continue searching for a technique of initial myelomeningocoele repair that may prevent the tethering of the spinal cord at the site of repair.

SYRINGOHYDROMYELIA

Syringohydromyelia (also termed hydromyelia or syrinx) is defined as a dilated spinal cord central canal (usually an elongated cavity) filled with CSF, that may be continuous with the fourth ventricle (Park et al. 1985). See Figure 19.

This CNS anomaly may cause slow relentless neurological deterioration, with progressive spasticity and/ or weakness in the upper and/or lower limbs and

Figure 19   A, Longitudinal Fluid-filled Cavity in the Cord at Thoracic Level – MRI, main findings were rapid loss of motor function and changes in bladder function. B, 10-year-old Boy with Syrinx Requiring Shunting – presented with rapidly progressing scoliosis

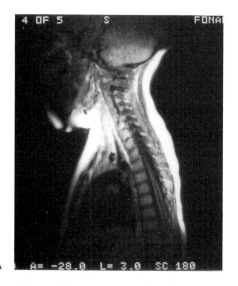

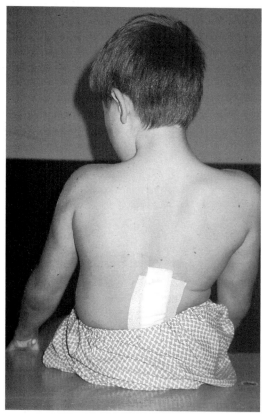

B

Figure 20   A, Marked Wasting of Upper Limbs – this child's MRI showed AC malformation, arachnoid cyst and syrinx in the cervical cord and tethering of the spinal cord in the lumbar region. B, Loss of Fine Motor Function – due to marked weakness

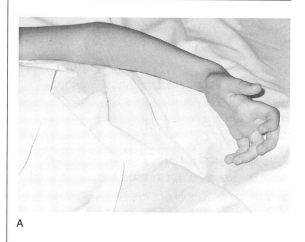

A

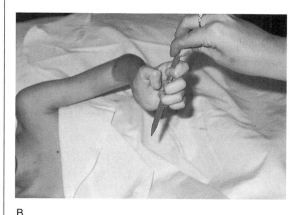

B

scoliosis in children with spina bifida (Park *et al.* 1985). Changes in urodynamic function may also occur (Lais *et al.* 1993). Syringohydromyelia may occur in up to 50% of patients with myelomeningocoele (Gilbert *et al.* 1986).

SPINAL ARACHNOID CYSTS

Spinal arachnoid cysts develop as a result of abnormal CSF flow and the extensive arachnoid adhesions that are found in many patients with myelomeningocoele (Rabb *et al.* 1992). These fluid-filled cysts usually communicate with the subarachnoid space, enlarge, and become symptomatic, with the symptoms of neurological deterioration mostly arising from spinal cord compression (Rabb *et al.* 1992). See Figure 20.

The Adolescent with Spina Bifida

Adjusting to adolescence for the individual with lack of voluntary bladder and bowel control, lack of protective sensation and paralysis of the lower limbs requiring bracing or wheelchairs for mobility is understandably difficult. Problems such as renal complications, complications with hydrocephalus management, learning difficulties, subtle intellectual impairment, loss of function due to secondary neurological deterioration, obesity, arthritis, low self-esteem, family attitudes, delayed or abnormal psychosocial behaviour and lack of independence in activities of daily living may compound to further impede adjustment to adolescence (Hayden 1985). Furthermore, societal attitudes and opportunities may not always be appropriately geared towards catering for the needs of these individuals as they move towards adulthood.

PHYSIOTHERAPY MANAGEMENT

There are a number of issues physiotherapists often need to address with the adolescent and these may include assisting with changing mobility needs because of changing environmental demands, especially at secondary school. These changes are usually coupled with increasing energy demands for ambulation because of increasing weight and height, changing mechanical advantages making ambulation less efficient and thus leading to more difficulty keeping up with peers. The amount of energy required to ambulate may inhibit the child or adolescent's overall performance and activities and this may offset any mobility advantages (Franks et al. 1991). Wheelchair propulsion has been shown to be faster and more energy efficient than walking (Williams *et al.* 1983). Greater self-awareness contributes to some adolescents preferring the image of themselves in a wheelchair rather than walking 'differently'. Increased body weight and obesity can and often does complicate these issues (Agre *et al.* 1987). Arthritis, particularly of the knees and shoulders and deformities such as scoliosis have been identified as contributing to reduced ambulation. As a result of these and other issues, such as involvement in sports and recreational activities, many adolescents choose a wheelchair for functional mobility.

It is imperative that the seating is inspected to ensure appropriate positioning and cushioning to reduce the risk of skin breakdown. Pressure relief by regular push-ups to unweight the buttocks is necessary even with special pressure-relieving cushions. Transfers need to be performed safely so the skin of the buttocks is not scraped. Compliance with daily skin inspections, skin care, toileting issues, ambulation and independence in activities of daily living may be difficult to maintain in some adolescents.

Skin warning signs are as follows:

- redness / discoloration
- swelling
- local heat
- blistering
- peeling.

Tess wears bilateral solid AFOs and walks independently for all activities. She is able to stand still quite easily when wearing her orthoses, but finds this much more difficult if barefoot. Tess had bilateral tibialis anterior transfers (the tendon is passed through the interosseous membrane to attach to the tendoachilles) when she was 5 years old. Prior to this the marked muscle imbalance at the ankles prevented Tess from standing still and caused cavus deformities and elongated heels. Postoperatively the resultant weak, but active plantarflexion gave Tess much more stability in her stance allowing her to stand still and also enabling a smoother gait pattern. The foot deformity improved over time following the tendon transfers.

Tess stands with an increased lumbar lordosis, anterior pelvic tilt and slight hip and knee flexion on both sides (Figure 21).

A similar pattern is maintained during walking. However, the most striking feature of Tess's walking pattern is the 'waddling' gait pattern (Trendelenburg gait pattern) with increased excursion of the trunk into alternate side flexion. This had been noted previously on assessment and occurs because of weakness of hip abductors (Figure 22).

Figure 21   Tess's Posture

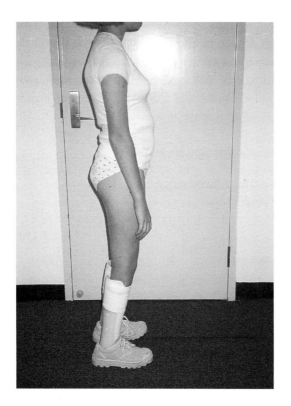

Figure 22   Tess's Walking — Trendelenburg Gait

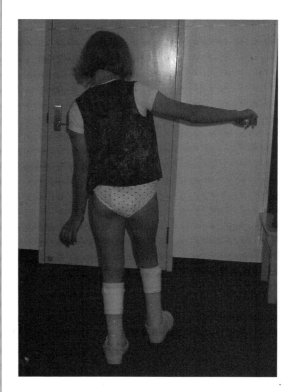

Assessment of gait is, unfortunately, a difficult and subjective process. Even video recordings, with slow-motion and freeze-frame facilities, do not give a really objective measure of the various parameters of gait. The usefulness of computerized gait analysis in detecting deterioration in gait patterns has yet to be fully explored; however, this is not a readily accessible tool for clinical use in most centres. This sort of objective measure may become more readily available and useful in the monitoring of neurological status in the future.

Musculoskeletal assessment found fixed hip flexion contractures of 5° bilaterally. Assessment of Tess in sitting and forward flexion revealed the development of a thoracic scoliosis convex to the (R). Neither of these findings had been present on previous evaluations. Straight leg raise and popliteal angles were also noted and found to have reduced, particularly on the (R) side when compared with the previous assessments.

Muscle strength of upper limbs, trunk and lower limbs was assessed by manual muscle tests as described by Daniels and Worthingham (1980) and Kendall et al. (1971). No changes from previous assessments were noted with either the upper limb or trunk musculature. Tess has always demonstrated some intrinsic and lumbricals weakness in both hands and this, in combination with reduced tone and poor proprioception in the hands, has led to writing difficulties and slowness. Tess was given prewriting activities when she was younger and these had assisted in addressing this issue.

It is well-documented that children with spina bifida experience difficulties performing upper limb functional activities (Sand *et al.* 1973, Anderson 1976, Mazur *et al.* 1986a). These may include handwriting, fine manipulation for dressing, eating (knife and fork), cutting (scissors) and other functional tasks such as use of crutches. Handwriting problems in particular

Table 2
Physiotherapy/Manual Muscle Test

Name: Tess			Reason for MMT:		back pain, ↓ endurance, ↑ scoliosis
Muscles	*	Left	Right	*	Comment
Quadratus lumborum T12–L1		5	5		
Abdominals T8–T12		5	5		
Iliopsoas L1–2		4	4	↓	(R) previously stronger than (L)
Sartorious L1–3		4	3	↓	(R) previously grade 4
Hip adductors L2–4		4	4		
Quadriceps L2–4		4	4	↓	(R) previously stronger than (L)
Medial hamstrings L4–S2		4	4		
Lateral hamstrings L4–S1		2	2		
Gluteus medius L4–S1		4	4		
Gluteus maximus L5–S1	↓	1	4		(L) previously grade 3
Tibialis anterior L4–L5		–	–		transferred (L) + (R) to tendo-achilles
Tibialis posterior L4–L5		1	1		
Peroneus longus/brevis L5–S1	↓	1	1		⎫ previously grade 3 on (L)
Peroneus tertius L5–S1	↓	1	1		⎭
Ext. hallucis longus L5–S1		1	0		
Toe extensors L5–S1		1	0		
Flex. hallucis longus S1–S2		1	0		
Toe flexors S1–S2		1	1		
Gastroc.–soleus S1–S2		–	–	*	tib. ant. transfers assisting PF

Indicate   ↓   or   ↑   in strength in comparison to previous test dated   11 months previously.
Indicate   *   if possible inaccuracy of muscle grading.

have caused concern as difficulties and dysfunction in this area impedes schooling. Handwriting speed in these children has been shown to be consistently reduced and legibility reduced (Ziviani *et al.* 1990). Studies to determine possible reasons for functional upper limb difficulties so commonly experienced by this population have identified multiple factors which may contribute to this problem. These include:

- frequency of shunt revisions (Mazur *et al.* 1986)
- level of spinal lesion (Mazur *et al.* 1986)
- inattention and distractibility (Tew *et al.* 1980)
- reduced goal-directed behaviour (Landrey *et al.* 1990)
- poor sequencing ability (Landrey *et al.* 1990)
- poor visual perception (Anderson 1976)

- early postural abnormalities and delayed motor development (Wolf and McLaughlin 1992)
- reduced sensory hand function including light touch, position sense, two-point discrimination, stereognosis, graphesthesia (Hamilton 1991)
- decreased strength, coordination and motor control (Minns *et al.* 1977)

Lower limb muscle strength was carefully assessed and recorded on a muscle chart (see Table 2). These findings were compared with previous evaluations and loss of strength of one or more grade noted.

Resting tone was assessed by moving the limbs with Tess lying relaxed in supine. Upper limb tone was found to be slightly hypotonic and this matched previous findings. Tone in the lower limbs on passive movements was felt to have increased with catches of resistance felt during passive movement of the limbs. This did not match previous assessment findings. Deep tendon reflexes were only just elicitable in the upper limbs and not able to be elicited at the ankles. The knee jerk was brisk bilaterally – a new finding.

Findings which may indicate some change in CNS function for Tess were summarized:

- *possible increase in fatigue during walking*
- *development of slight fixed flexion contractures at hips*
- *development of mild thoracic scoliosis*
- *loss of muscle strength of more than one grade*
- *spasticity in the LLs where tone had previously been within normal range*
- *brisk reflexes at knees (R) > (L)*

These findings were recorded and discussed with the medical team during the next clinic meeting. It was decided that these findings represented a deterioration in CNS function that needed to be fully investigated. This led to medical reviews and investigations including urodynamics, to look for changes in bladder function, CT scan to check that Tess's VP shunt was functioning, spinal X-ray to monitor the scoliosis and a MRI to review brainstem and spinal cord pathology.

Tess's MRI indicated, as most MRIs of children with spina bifida, tethering of the spinal cord. The cord appeared to be under tension and the scoliosis was noted. An Arnold–Chiari malformation was also present. No other cord pathology was present. It was decided that Tess's CNS deterioration could be attributed to tethering of the spinal cord and surgery to release this tethering was discussed. Surgical untethering occurred. The physiotherapist evaluated muscle strength both before and after operation. In

the early postoperative period physiotherapy management included assistance with bed exercises and early mobilization. Tess, like many children following release of tethering of the spinal cord felt unsteady walking initially, as her legs felt 'different and strange' and early mobilization in the ward was assisted by using a walking frame.

Tess quickly discarded this as she became more confident and steady with her mobility. As Tess's discomfort settled, physiotherapy management addressed her posture in both sitting and standing and introduced a graded exercise programme to improve flexibility and strength. Particular attention was directed to the abdominal, back and hip extensors and quadriceps musculature to improve Tess's trunk stability, posture and gait. This programme continued over a period of 6 weeks and Tess cooperated well with her home activities.

Evaluation of Tess's muscle strength, spasticity and scoliosis over the next 2 years indicated that the release of the cord tethering had halted the progression of symptoms.

Ongoing monitoring, however, was still required as symptoms do recur in some patients.

Acquired Brain Injury (ABI)

Case study 5

A child who sustained a severe closed head injury 21 days ago has just been transferred from an intensive care unit (ICU) to a general ward setting. The physiotherapist assigned to this ward is presently reviewing this boy's medical charting and the transfer notes from the ICU physiotherapist. The relevant details she extracted from charting and physiotherapy notes are as follows.

Jack, an 11-year-old bicyclist, who was not wearing a helmet, sustained a closed head injury when hit by a car. He was unconscious and fitting on admission to his local rural hospital, and a Glasgow coma score (GCS) of 6 was recorded. He had extensive bruising and contusions to his face and skull, particularly to the (R) side. He had also sustained closed fractures of his (R) radius and ulna. Immediate medical care included: the control of fitting, nasogastric tube insertion, intubation and mechanical ventilation, and immobilization of (R) radius and ulna. After this initial work-up, Jack and his mother (Sally), were airlifted on the day of injury to the ICU in the provincial city's children's hospital.

Jack's time in the ICU was rigorous. There were problems with a rising intracranial pressure (ICP). CT scan findings indicated significant oedema. On day 4 he developed pneumonia. His ICP was stabilized on day 8 after injury. He continued to be mechanically ventilated for 19 days, for although several attempts were made to extubate, he consistently desaturated. Extubation was successful on day 19 after injury and he has remained medically stable over the last 2 days. His GCS on discharge from ICU was 10.

While in ICU the physiotherapist had assessed and listed Jack's problems in the following order:

- retained mucopurulent secretions
- (R) lower lobe atelectasis
- decreased arousal
- abnormally high muscle tone (L) side > (R) side
- exacerbation of stereotypical patterning of movement such as tonic neck and labyrinthine reflex patterning and marked extensor thrust
- potential for contracture, particularly of the achilles tendons
- hypersensitivity to tactile input – exacerbating stereotypical reflex patterns such as, extensor thrust, asymmetrical tonic neck reflex (ATNR)

The ICU physiotherapist had addressed Jack's problems with the following regimen:

- Frequent adapted positioning, manual clapping and expiratory vibrations and suctioning (hyperinflation procedure) was carefully undertaken for very short periods due to problems with fluctuating ICP during the first 2 weeks. After the pneumonic process resolved this treatment regimen was then reduced to twice a day until extubation. After extubation, the physiotherapist continued positioning Jack and encouraged bibasal expansion through verbal, tactile and proprioceptive facilitation techniques. Jack had a spontaneous cough and the cough was not moist.
- Positioning to inhibit the exacerbation of stereotypical patterns of movement and decrease heightened muscle tone.
- Passive range-of-motion exercises, particularly attempting to maintain the extensibility of the calf musculature. (An inhibitory plaster series was considered, but it was felt it was too soon to consider, as Jack's medical status was too unstable during his ICU stay.)
- Avoidance of tactile input which exacerbates stereotypical patterns of movement (e.g. extensor thrust) and increases the potential for contracture.

The ICU physiotherapist further noted that Jack's mother has been with him most of the time and she has acted on suggestions to talk to Jack about familiar people, such as his four brothers and his classmates.

Before the ward physiotherapist assesses this child and implements a patient-specific treatment programme the therapist should have a background understanding of the problems associated with acquired brain injury and the principles of physiotherapy management of such children.

Problems Associated with Acquired Brain Injury

Acquired brain injury is a significant cause of mortality and morbidity in children. There are difficulties, however, in predicting the short- and long-term functional outcome of children with acquired brain injury. It is generally felt that no one method of assessing the severity of the injury is appropriate in every situation, but noting the duration of coma and post-traumatic amnesia (PTA – considered over, when the child is orientated to time, place and person) are viewed as significant predictive factors of final functional outcome. The prognosis for recovery of motor function is more favourable if the duration of the coma is less than 3 months. Furthermore, complications of injury, such as prolonged hypertension, ventricular enlargement and seizures significantly reduce the potential for functional independence (Brink et al. 1980).

The Glasgow coma scale (GCS), which assesses three aspects of responsiveness – whether the eyes are open, what verbal behaviour occurs and amount/type of motor activity – is a useful and reliable tool to assess the severity of brain injury (Jennett 1976). Investigators often use the GCS as a means of delineating individuals with closed head injury into groupings such as mild head injury (GCS 13 or over), moderate head injury (GCS 8–12), severe head injury (GCS 7 or less) (Knights et al. 1991). Such a numerical classification of head injury has prognostic significance (Fletcher and Ewing-Cobbs 1991).

Children with severe brain injury are mechanically ventilated and have a high incidence of pneumonia occurring in the first week after injury, which prolongs ICU and hospital stay (Hsieh et al. 1992). Not surprisingly, Craven et al. (1986) similarly describe the presence of an ICP monitor as an associated risk factor for hospital-acquired pneumonia. Furthermore, health workers should be aware that in the early rehabilitation stage of traumatic brain injury, the child may not be able to report and/or indicate pain secondary to undetected fractures and soft tissue trauma (Sobus et al. 1993). Mital et al. (1987)

note the presence of ectopic bone formation in children and adolescents in coma following head injury. The sites of heterotopic bone formation In order of decreasing frequency are hips, elbows, shoulders, thighs, finger joints and clavicle. Symptomatology of ectopic bone formation initially includes local signs of acute inflammation and pain on motion which progresses to almost total loss of motion at the involved site (Mital et al. 1987).

The sensorimotor and motor deficits following brain trauma are often quite variable and complex (Duncan 1990). Variations in site, nature and severity of injury undoubtedly explain to a degree the variable sensorimotor and motor deficits associated with brain trauma. The fact, however, that the traumatic brain injury of a child is often diffuse suggests why the children can present with many and varied problems. For example, abnormally heightened muscle tone, and the loss of selective motor control through the exacerbation of stereotypical synergistic movement patterns are often common problems which must be addressed. Weakness, contractures and extracranial complications such as fractures and soft tissue injury can also prolong the rehabilitation of the child with severe brain injury. Furthermore, children who sustain traumatic brain damage often demonstrate deficits in their tactile, proprioceptive, kinaesthetic, vestibular and visual systems which can cause significant coordination, balance and perceptual difficulties. The motor performance of such children may also be disrupted by motor planning difficulties. Hence, children who sustain severe closed head injuries will generally demonstrate some movement skill problems due to some anomalies in the information processing and/or neuromotor systems.

The functional outcome of children with acquired brain injury is variable, and depends on numerous factors. For example, the amount of spontaneous neurologic recovery, normal growth and development and the effect of intensive rehabilitation will affect outcome (Eiben et al. 1984). Undoubtedly, severe brain injury in children can result in significant disability. Cognitive and communication problems, however, can contribute significantly to such disability and dependency (Eiben et al. 1984).

Behavioural problems, irritability, limited attention span and difficulties with social interaction are other difficulties which the child with traumatic brain damage may experience. Indeed, premorbid personality problems are often exacerbated after such an injury (Knights et al. 1991). Perhaps not surprisingly, after a child has sustained a severe traumatic brain injury there can be a significant deterioration in the psychosocial functioning in a number of families, particularly in those families who have poor coping resources (Rivara et al. 1992).

Rivara et al. (1994) highlight the fact that children who sustain traumatic brain damage should be provided with a comprehensive rehabilitation programme which provides long-term support for the child and family. These investigators are particularly concerned that educational plans for such children should be constantly reviewed and renegotiated as they often demonstrate persisting difficulties in school performance. For example, Fay et al. (1994) note that children and adolescents with moderate and severe traumatic brain injury demonstrate persisting and comprehensive neuropsychological deficits 3 years after the resolution of their post-traumatic amnesia (PTA). A 23-year follow-up study of children with head injuries similarly suggests that, although intervening life events are interactive, the severity of the head injury is the primary factor in the prediction of long-term outcomes (Klonoff et al. 1993).

Physiotherapy Management of Severe Closed Head Injury

Ideally, physiotherapy management of the child with severe closed head injury is a comprehensive process. The physiotherapist will play a significant role during both the acute and long-term care of these patients. Most importantly, the physiotherapist should be seen as part of a transdisciplinary team who will attempt to facilitate the child with severe brain injury to achieve as much functional independence as possible and to be ultimately a happy and active participant in the community.

During the acute care of the child with severe brain injury the physiotherapist will be particularly involved in the maintenance of the child's cardiorespiratory system. Common problems such as heightened muscle tonus and undesirable primitive reflex/stereotypical patterns of movement are also addressed with varying techniques so as to avoid secondary problems developing, such as abnormal posturing and contractures. Since the physiotherapist will interact often with the child throughout the day, it is appropriate that he/she should participate in the arousal of the child, particularly through auditory, visual, tactile and proprioceptive means.

Even during this acute stage of recovery the physiotherapist will attempt to involve parents where possible in the treatment regimen. The physiotherapist will explain to parents why he/she is handling and positioning the child in various ways and if possible the parent may participate in the regimen. Such early involvement by the parents in the rehabilitation process of the child can often assist in the coping mechanisms of the family.

Once the child is medically stable, the physiotherapist will undertake a more comprehensive and dynamic assessment of the child in order to establish the primary problems underlying their motor dysfunction. The assessment, therefore, will incorporate various elements such as an evaluation of:

- the quantity and quality of any spontaneous movement
- stereotypical patterns of movement and associated reactions
- muscle tone, joint range of motion, soft tissue extensibility, postural alignment and soft tissue trauma
- postural and balance reactions
- visual, tactile, proprioceptive, kinaesthetic and vestibular responses

The physiotherapy assessment will also consider the child's cognitive, emotional and perceptual abilities, as difficulties in these areas can dramatically affect functional performance.

Accurate problem-solving skills are necessary for the physiotherapist to design an appropriate patient-specific treatment regimen. Undoubtedly, physiotherapy treatment regimens for children with severe brain injury will vary dramatically as there can be quite different underlying causes to movement dysfunction subsequent to acquired brain injury. For example, one child may have primarily sensory feedback problems resulting in poor motor performance, whereas another child may have significant motor planning problems which severely compromise his/her motor performance. The physiotherapist will often use many varied techniques in the management of children with severe brain injury as the techniques must appropriately address the underlying problem of the movement dysfunction.

A major premise underlying physiotherapy intervention for the child with neurological deficits is that neural development is dependent on activity (Leonard 1994). Furthermore, activity is essential for optimum musculoskeletal development. Not surprisingly, the physiotherapist working with the child who sustained traumatic brain damage will attempt through many varied techniques to encourage as much functional spontaneous isolated movement/activity as possible. The facilitation of proficient postural and balance reactions is also a major feature of physiotherapy management of the child with severe brain injury. The facilitation of such reactions enables the patient to move into antigravity positions and thereby provide him/her with a more appropriate perception of the environment.

Recovery from central nervous system insult does not necessarily follow a developmental sequence (Leonard 1994). Hence, early sitting and standing and weight-shifting is generally a major component of the physiotherapy regimen of a child after traumatic brain damage, particularly as it commands extensive sensory participation and thereby assists in the arousal of the child. It also provides an excellent means of decreasing heightened muscle tone, stretching tight soft tissue (especially calf musculature) and encouraging appropriate biomechanical alignment. Unfortunately, extracranial complications, such as fractures and soft tissue trauma, may disrupt this early standing regimen.

The physiotherapy treatment regimen for a child with severe brain injury will inevitably concentrate on addressing patient-specific movement skill problems. The motor relearning process is a complex task and

the physiotherapist will initially address the areas which have been assessed as contributing most to the child's difficulties. For example, for one child it may be his impulsivity and short attention span which interfere significantly with his learning process and reacquisition of movement skills, while in another poor fine motor coordination and in another poor control of posture.

Since the child with severe brain injury will often demonstrate a multiplicity of problems, the physiotherapist works in close consultation with other members of the rehabilitation team. Realistic expectations for the child should be discussed and established by the team members, parents and child (in the most appropriate manner). Such expectations will be constantly renegotiated, as the rehabilitation of such a child is a long-term process. As the child's movement control significantly improves and the child is reintroduced into mainstream schooling, the physiotherapist will encourage the child to participate in leisure/sport activities which will improve self-image and confidence.

After a comprehensive assessment of Jack's motor performance the ward physiotherapist identified the following problems:

- *decreased arousal and marked confusion*
- *limited visual fixation and follow*
- *heightened tone – spasticity (L) side > (R) side*
- *exacerbation of primitive reflexes/stereotypical patterns of movement*
- *hypersensitivity to touch (particularly feet)*
- *tight achilles tendons (L) and (R) ankle equinus*
- *limited spontaneous isolated movement*
- *ineffective head and body righting reactions*
- *limited head control / lack of endurance*
- *ineffective sitting balance / poor weight-shift to (L)*
- *ineffective oromotor control*

The physiotherapist discussed these listed problems and treatment planning with Jack's mother, Sally, and asked if she would be willing to be an active participant in Jack's physiotherapy treatment regimen. Sally was very happy to play an active role in Jack's rehabilitation. The physiotherapist demonstrated to Sally a number of techniques to increase Jack's arousal and how to avoid exacerbating primitive reflexes/stereotypical patterns of movement during daily physiotherapy sessions. Sally then continued to work on these techniques throughout the day.

An inhibitory plaster series (prolonged stretch) for the contracted achilles tendons was commenced as Jack could now be supported in standing. These inhibitory plasters also addressed problems such as Jack's tactile hypersensitivity and extensor thrust. Furthermore, these ankle inhibitory plasters provided more appropriate proprioceptive input and biomechanical alignment through the lower limbs when standing. Although inhibitory plasters can at times shunt tone to other muscle groups, in this instance, the inhibitory plasters assisted in the general reduction of the heightened muscle tone, particularly during the standing programme.

Jack's ineffective head and body righting reactions and limited head control was specifically addressed by a daily mat work programme. The physiotherapist encouraged and facilitated functional activities such as rocking the pelvis (to reduce heightened truncal muscle tone) and rolling (taking due care of Jack's immobilized (R) arm) and moving into and out of sitting through (L) side-lying. Weight-bearing through the extended (L) upper limb decreased Jack's heightened muscle tone and also assisted in developing greater weight-shift on to the (L) side. Sitting balance was further encouraged through tactile facilitation of abdominal muscles. Sally continued to encourage Jack to take weight equally through his buttocks when sitting in bed/wheelchair.

The speech pathologist started her therapy in conjunction with the physiotherapy programme as Jack was most alert during his standing programme. Jack's head and oromotor control was most effective during this time. Sally quickly took advantage of the opportunity to learn techniques to improve Jack's oromotor control.

During the following 6 weeks Jack made considerable improvement. He became fully alert and recorded a GCS of 15. His oromotor control improved significantly, his nasogastric tube was removed and he began to cope with thickened fluids and soft foods. He was able to say a few words, though his breath control and articulation were still poor. He was now able to participate more dynamically during the physiotherapy sessions, but became quite frustrated and irritable at times. His fractured (R) radius and ulna showed signs of consolidation and the immobilizing plaster was removed, he was still very tentative with this arm, indicating that it was painful to move. Stereotypical patterns of movement and heightened tone were decreasing and he was now able to get into sitting from lying independently, though he still lacked dynamic sitting balance. The inhibitory plaster series was completed as the lost ankle range was regained and was maintained with tone reducing orthoses (TRO).

The ward physiotherapist now identified Jack's main problems as:
- pain on movement/weight-bearing (R) upper limb (UL)
- hypersensitivity to touch/compression (R) UL
- frustration/ irritability
- reduced isolated movement, particularly (R) UL and (L) LL
- inefficiency of postural and balance reactions
- decreased weight-shift (L) LL
- potential for tight achilles tendon
- poor eye–hand coordination/decreased fast eye follow

- short-term memory difficulties/short attention span

The physiotherapist felt that hydrotherapy would be an excellent means of addressing Jack's present problems, particularly as Sally reported that Jack was always a keen swimmer. Indeed, the warmth and buoyancy of the water assisted in the reduction of pain and hypersensitivity to touch in his (R) upper limb. (Sally reported that Jack was (R) hand dominant prior to his injury.) The support that the water provided for his (R) arm also enabled Jack to begin to move his (R) wrist and elbow actively. Indeed, this buoyant medium enabled the physiotherapist to facilitate more isolated movements in Jack's (L) lower limb.

Because Jack actually found hydrotherapy fun and was able to stand independently in the water, his frustration and irritability decreased and Jack participated more actively in the learning process. For example, Jack was much more interested in ball-catching activities in the water which thereby encouraged eye–hand coordination and the reacquisition of throwing and catching skills. The physiotherapist also found that Jack's postural and balance reactions were effectively facilitated in the water as this medium gave Jack enough time to react more appropriately.

Jack's morning hydrotherapy programme was complemented by an afternoon gait and mat session. Jack was now walking with assistance of one person. This assistant encouraged Jack to shift his weight on to his (L) side during stance phase and was able to give support through his (L) upper limb when his balance reactions to the (L) were inadequate. The physiotherapist used visual feedback (via a mirror) as well as tactile and proprioceptive input to encourage greater weight-shift on to his (L) side. A very simple biofeedback procedure was instigated as Jack particularly enjoyed the tactile and proprioceptive stimulus he received when he put his body weight through his (L) LL and popped the air bubbles in plastic packaging. Jack continued to wear his TROs for 2 hours a day to maintain stretch on his tendon achilles, particularly (L).

The physiotherapist in conjunction with the occupational therapist and speech pathologist continued to provide Sally and Jack with clues as how to avoid the frustration of his short attention span and short-term memory loss. Jack's treatment sessions were varied, but Jack was encouraged to attend to the task at hand before a more pleasurable task was offered. Excess distractions were also avoided during the treatment sessions by undertaking Jack's programme in a quiet treatment room rather than the gym area among a number of other clients. A notice board was placed beside his bed where relevant details of the day's events could be entered so that Jack could reread them through the day.

Jack continued to make significant improvements and 4 months after admission to the children's hospital, it was felt by all members of the rehabilitation team that Jack's rehabilitation could now be appropriately addressed by the respective health, education and social workers in Jack's provincial township. Jack's mother, Sally, has been particularly anxious during the last 2 weeks to return home to her other children who have been cared for by Sally's mother, as one of the younger children has been unwell with asthma. The team members are aware that, unlike most other acquired brain injury inpatients, Jack had not been home on a weekend trial visit, but, the various team members, particularly the occupational therapist, spent a considerable amount of time with Sally discussing the home and community setting in an attempt to make Jack's return home as safe and positive as possible. Various team members spoke to Jack's school teacher and the visiting school guidance officer and they have sent relevant reports of Jack's abilities and limitations.

Jack's physiotherapist contacted the physiotherapist in his township and discussed Jack's problems and treatment regimen while he was an inpatient. She also prepared a discharge summary for Jack's new physiotherapist. She listed Jack's current problems as follows:

- decreased weight-shift (L) LL
- decreased proximal control of (L) UL and LL
- lack of rhythmicity in movement
- weakness and coordination difficulties (R) UL
- frustration/impulsivity

The physiotherapist also described to Jack's physiotherapist the home programme and emphasized how much Jack's frustration and impulsivity reduced when he was able to do some of his treatment regimen in the pool.

Jack's home programme included:

- Walking on his bottom both forwards and backwards with Sally participating in races. (This activity certainly achieves significant weight-shift on to his (L) side and facilitates rotation of trunk and rhythmicity of movement. Sally noted that his brothers will be able to assist in races at home.)
- Half-kneeling positioning while catching balls and throwing quoits and tug-of-war activities to assist in proximal control of (L) LL and (L) UL and improve strength of (R) UL.
- Walking on heels, running, skipping and jumping activities in the pool to maintain muscle and tendon extensibility and encourage greater rhythmicity and control of movement (Jack's nextdoor neighbours have an inground pool which they said he can use at any time).
- An adapted breaststroke encouraged so as to particularly assist in coordination of (R) UL.

The physiotherapist felt certain that Jack would be very cooperative and willing to participate fully in a treatment programme with a new team and continue to make gains. She also emphasized that she would be willing to be of any assistance in the future, and that she looked forward to seeing Jack in 3 months when he returned for a neurological review.

Thought Provokers

1. A 5-year-old child who sustained a severe brain injury 4 months ago is regaining some functional movement. However, her functional performance is severely limited by a significant (L)-sided 'neglect'. List all possible underlying reasons for this 'neglect' and consider how the physiotherapist may be able to address the underlying problems of 'neglect' in the child's physiotherapy treatment regimen.

2. A 10-year-old child who sustained a closed head injury 1 year ago is now attending a mainstream school, but she is experiencing considerable difficulties sitting still in her chair as she still lacks effective proximal stability. Her ineffectual proximal stability is also causing problems with her functional performance during class, particularly with respect to her handwriting. Consider some treatment ideas which may address this child's problem of proximal stability.

Immersion

Discussions of the management of acquired brain injury in childhood would not be complete without reference to the tragic and emotive issue of drowning/immersion or near-drowning incidents. Though management of the survivors of immersion will be similar to that of the head injured child, there are some specific issues related to immersion which should be noted.

Drowning is the leading cause of injury/death for children 0–4 years of age in Australia and the USA. In Australia from 1976 to 1990, 700 toddlers had died, 200 have measurable brain damage, and at least 40 survived in a persistent vegetative state (Pearn 1991). Australian studies show that 80% of immersion incidents requiring hospitalization occur in swimming pools (Pitt and Balanda 1991).

Early ICU management of the immersion child is similar to that of other ABI patients. The nature of the injury with fluid aspiration (Conn and Barker 1984), however, implicates significant respiratory involvement. Fluid restrictions are often imposed in the ICU setting and whether the child drowned in clean or dirty water may have an influence upon respiratory complications.

TYPES OF DROWNING

Immersion in salt water, fresh water or polluted water can cause similar respiratory problems. Polluted or chemically tainted water is more likely to cause lung irritation/infection complications.

Terms, such as 'wet' and 'dry' drowning are used to describe the differing pathophysiology of immersion. 'Wet drowning' occurs when water is aspirated into the lungs and this is by far the most common type of drowning pathology (occurring in 90% of victims). The primary problem in aspiration of water into the lungs is:

- dilution or destruction of alveolar surfactant with subsequent atelectasis
- varying degrees of pulmonary oedema
- reduction in lung compliance and ventilation
- hypoxaemia due to perfusion of unventilated alveoli, representing right-to-left shunt (Mitchell and Gorman 1994, p. 9).

In contrast to 'wet drowning', the 'dry drowning' victim experiences laryngospasm during immersion which may result in hypoxic brain damage but no water in the lungs. It is reported that 'dry drowning' occurs in 10% of victims (Mitchell and Gorman 1994).

The survivor with severe neurological impairment often presents with flaccid tone initially, but commonly develops severe decerebrate/decorticate or opisthotonic posturing. The extreme global tonal presentation of these children is related to the significant generalized hypoxic insult to the brain due to the drowning episode and is commonly far greater than other acute brain injury aetiologies. Spastic quadriplegic presentation is the most common with ongoing seizure problems evident. The management of these severely neurologically impaired children in the post-ICU period and within the community upon hospital discharge must consider a number of aspects.

Medical management aspects may include nasogastric or gastrostomy feeding, tracheostomy, muscle relaxant and the need for seizure medication. Aspiration pneumonia and respiratory complications are the major cause of death in this population in the first 1 to 4 years following the immersion incident (Abrams and Mubarak 1991). These patients often have impaired swallow, gag and cough reflexes, significant bite reflex and pool secretions in the oropharynx. Therefore, caregivers must be adequately skilled in respiratory management including suctioning techniques via nose/mouth or airway. Education of the family and other caregivers on appropriate positioning and handling to limit abnormal tonal influences is a vital role of the physiotherapist. This is often difficult to achieve due to the excessive tonal presentation.

Provision of wheelchair mobility with adaptive support and tilt in space/recline functions will be required as well as other assistive devices and aids for ongoing management. Contractures and orthopaedic problems are common as routine splinting and inhibitory plastering can fail due to the extent of muscle tone. Physiotherapists need to be aware of the potential for contracture in this group of children. For example, Abrams and Mubarak (1991) report that in a study of 36 postimmersion survivors, 82% of the cohort demonstrated equinus deformity of the feet, 53% hip adductor contractures, 34% hip dislocation, 33% hamstring/quadriceps tightness or contracture and 18% severe scoliosis.

The physiotherapist will have an important role to play in early and long-term management of the immersion survivor with significant neurological disability and a supportive and educative role for carers.

Medulloblastoma

Case Study 6

Tom is 14 years of age and lives in rural Australia, he is attending a review at the rehabilitation clinic at the major children's hospital in the state. It is now 12 months since his surgery for removal of a medulloblastoma.

The classical medulloblastoma is a diffuse cellular tumour consisting of small round cells which usually arise in the vermis or midline of the cerebellum. It is mainly a disease of childhood and in every reported series of medulloblastoma patients there is a preponderance of males (Deutsch 1990).

Prior to diagnosis, Tom was a reasonable student in school, often described as 'a bit of a joker' by teachers. He was captain of the regional representative football team and recently had an increased interest in girls. His mother and the school reported he was becoming a little more disruptive, he was not playing as well at football and he was complaining of headaches. The doctor at the local hospital reviewed Tom and referred him to the major children's hospital for investigations. The tumour was diagnosed and surgically removed and an intraventricular shunt inserted. Tom underwent radiotherapy, as a good prognosis was expected by his neurosurgeon.

The patient with medulloblastoma commonly presents with clinical symptoms in association with raised intracranial pressure, such as headache, vomiting and ataxia (Park *et al.* 1983). The primary tumour may infiltrate adjacent structures, such as brainstem, upper spinal cord, midbrain and cerebellar surface.

There can be further dissemination within the CNS and it can occasionally disseminate beyond the CNS (Deutsch 1990). Generally, surgeons undertake gross total resection of primary medulloblastoma. Shunts are also often undertaken to relieve hydrocephalus. The newly diagnosed medulloblastoma patient is also treated with craniospinal irradiation. Surgery and irradiation offer long-term survival rates of at least 50% for certain good prognosis subsets of medulloblastoma (Deutsch 1990).

At the 12 month review, Tom was walking independently, but was still obviously ataxic, to the extent that he often ran into people or obstacles whilst walking if he didn't concentrate. His shunt was in situ and functioning well. His ataxia was a frustration to Tom as well as other issues which he and his mother discussed with the neurosurgeon and other members of the rehabilitation team:

1. *Would he ever be able to play football again? He was frustrated with not being able to participate in general sports.*
2. *He was having difficulty settling in at school again scholastically and socially and was especially frustrated that girls appeared to be uninterested in him.*
3. *His ataxic gait made him look as if he was 'drunk' and this posturing was one of the factors contributing to his problems of settling back into peer relationships and school life in general.*

In view of the relative success of the medical management of medulloblastoma (>50% of patients can now expect to survive 5 years or longer (Johnson *et al.* 1994)), it is pertinent to examine quality of life issues after medulloblastoma. A study by Johnson *et al.* (1994) of 32 children with greater than 5 years survival after diagnosis found that perceptual motor skills were below average in more than 50% of children, but motor dexterity was more severely affected than perception. Problems in learning and a delay in both

Yvonne Burns, John Gilmour, Megan Kentish and Julie MacDonald

growth and development were seen in a majority of children.

> *The rehabilitation team in consultation with Tom and his mother decided to approach Tom's problems with an intensive 3-week programme to be undertaken by the team during this school holiday period as no local services were available. Initial intervention plans were to include:*
>
> - *physiotherapy for general coordination and stability work to limit his ataxic movements*
> - *specific occupational therapy programme emphasizing fine motor/handwriting skills as a progression on the general work of the physiotherapy programme*
> - *the psychologist would reassess general cognitive abilities and introduce self-esteem awareness and social skills strategies to assist Tom with his scholastic needs and peer interactions*

The Physiotherapy Treatment Plan

The aim of the physiotherapy was to establish a variety of activities Tom could do to improve his general unsteadiness and in turn improve his general motor abilities and skills. A neurodevelopmental assessment was performed and the findings provided the basis of the treatment plan. At rest, Tom was very stable and only upon active movement did his ataxia become evident. He tended to do activities at speed because he found if he went fast he managed to achieve general tasks before falling. He presented with general proprioceptive deficits and vestibular testing showed hypersensitive postural responses to total body rotation. General eye–hand coordination was poor, especially at slow speed, and ball skills were a significant concern to Tom.

The aim of treatment of ataxia centred on a number of key principles. It must be emphasized, however, that achievement of each principle is not in isolation, but in association with other aims. The principles applied to Tom's programme were as follows:

- *improvement of quality and speed of proximal stability to establish a firm background for distal movement; the amount of weight-bearing support is a factor influencing stability*
- *utilization of vestibular, proprioceptive and other sensory stimuli as a preparation to movement or to augment movement*
- *use of muscle cocontraction to aid in stability of proximal joints*
- *application of general coordination activities including gait training*
- *introduction of hydrotherapy as a treatment medium*

As part of the team approach, the physiotherapist and occupational therapist combined to design a number of easy preparatory activities which improved sensory input and utilized muscle cocontraction during the day, especially useful in the classroom. These included:

- *Body lifts off a seat, as a paraplegic person would do for pressure relief, to encourage upper limb weight-bearing and muscle co-contraction.*
- *His chair was to be tilted forward to improve weight-bearing on his feet and forearms in sitting at home and school; this was achieved by adding build-ups to the rear of the chairs.*
- *A variety of finger/hand exercises such as work with exercise putty or a squash ball during the day.*
- *Finger tapping and drumming upon a desk and thumb and finger patterns.*
- *Tom was given a pencil build-up to improve his pencil grip during writing, and was encouraged to hold another item such as a tubular pencil case in his other hand as a bracing technique to improve general stability.*

More specific tasks/skills were designed by the occupational therapist and therapy sessions were timetabled to run in close proximity to each other and occasional combined sessions were planned. Specific therapy activities to address the key principles were designed and tested by Tom and his physiotherapist and are discussed below.

By emphasizing stability in the trunk and proximal joints the physiotherapist was establishing a base of stability on which to build active movements distally. To assist with obtaining proximal stability the therapist provided hands-on support on various body parts to increase awareness of position and offer manual external support. For example, in a four-point kneeling position Tom was required to lift his leg into hip and knee extension. His physiotherapist gave manual support and guidance at his pelvis.

To augment the need for proximal control, the positions which provided maximal support and weight-bearing were used initially in therapy activities. These included lying, four-point kneeling, kneeling and sitting. Active movements and exercises were undertaken in these positions. As stability improved, positions were used providing less external support and requiring more internal control, such as half-kneeling, stride stand and wide-based standing.

Whilst in these positions, specific exercises and movements were undertaken. The emphasis was on general body stability whilst performing specific isolated active movements. Initially, Tom was instructed to think about the movement as it was performed to develop a 'cortical control' component to the movement.

Later the movements were used as part of a more functional activity. Simple arm control movements could be incorporated into ball throw/bowl and catch activities later and leg extension exercises formed the basis of other balance activities. Though Tom's physiotherapist advised him that the initial exercises may be a little boring, his concentration

on tasks allowed progression to introducing general coordination and hand–eye activities in all positions. Games involving quoit activities, skittle/bowling work and bat/ball style activities were used to add interest and skill.

As a further progression on improving stability and proximal control, work in various positions, subtle weight-shift and control of small changes in body position were performed. These activities were to teach Tom movement awareness and balance control work. Again the emphasis was on 'cortical awareness' of body reactions to minor centre-of-gravity variations and the aim was to limit excessive responses in movement. Initially a mirror provided good visual cueing, and hands-on assistance from Tom's physiotherapist was allowed. Later these activities involve an elimination of such cues.

Sensory techniques are a vital aspect of the management of cerebellar ataxia and other neurological conditions (Umphred and McCormack 1985). Emphasis is placed upon the significant role of the cerebellum in the integration of proprioception and vestibular stimuli. The use of compressions by manual application or via the use of weighted cuffs for limbs or belts and vests for the trunk can enhance proprioceptive input and assist in better muscle control. Weight and compressions would be applied proximally and progressed to more distal joints as control improved. Another idea is the use of heavier bats and balls in general games activities as these may achieve a similar result since they require increased muscle effort and control.

Vestibular input can be utilized via controlled trampoline activities initially and progressed to swinging and spinning activities. Simple bounce work on the trampoline combines both proprioceptive and vestibular stimulation, and this provided Tom with a good basis of preparation before undertaking other motor skills. Spinning or whole-body rotation was not useful for Tom, as it provided excessive postural responses which increased his instability. It must be acknowledged that although spinning activities were not effective for Tom, other young people may obtain significant benefits from the use of this modality. A programme of desensitization could be developed at a later date for Tom. Simple tactile input was used also during treatment during tasks with tapping and stroking over specific muscle groups. Various positions were used on the trampoline, e.g. standing, long sit and half-kneeling, whilst undertaking different games and exercises.

Cocontraction of muscle groups as agonists and antagonists act to stabilize a joint in a position, or induce control over the movement of a joint. This can be achieved in a formal exercise process such as rhythmic stabilization in use of PNF patterns (Knott and Voss 1968). It is important, however, not to over-stabilize, so dynamic activities such as push/pull in tug-of-war games can be beneficial.

Tom's physiotherapist sat inside a mobile box whilst Tom had to push it in a straight line, and this was progressed to a winding path around an obstacle course. An activity of Tom maintaining a four-point kneeling position whilst his physiotherapist induced small bounces on the trampoline was also used to achieve cocontraction in activities. This activity was made more demanding by reducing the number of support limbs whilst in this position. Simple isometric activities were designed for use in the classroom to assist in limb stability such as prayer position hand press and bottom lifts before writing activities.

It was apparent to Tom's physiotherapist that sensory and specific formal exercise techniques would not assist Tom, unless these gains were incorporated into general activities. Emphasis was placed on coordination and timing activities, or those involving eye–hand coordination work. These activities were used in various body positions reducing support as stability improved. Tom's therapists used a simple bat/ball skill activity as an example to Tom and his Mum of how to progress with the difficulty of control of an activity.

Tom was seated on a high-backed chair with a large ball in an old stocking suspended

from an overhead grill. He had a light plastic cricket bat with which he had to lightly hit the ball. Initially, he hit the ball in small strokes, all from the one direction. As he improved, various components could be altered to increase demands:

(a) Tom could kneel, half-kneel or stand thus reducing stability and external support.

(b) A smaller ball or smaller bat or both in combination could be used to increase the difficulty of the task.

(c) Alternating the direction in which he hit the ball, e.g. left side then right, could be progressed to various sequences of hits, e.g. 2 (L), 3(R), 2(L).

(d) To make it more difficult he could stab at the suspended ball with the end of the bat/ stick, thus reducing the target and increasing the skill component of the activity.

(e) Then the lever arm of the stick or heaviness of the stick could be increased.

(f) Holding the stick with the hand in various upper limb positions, e.g. with elbow flexed at 90° or in full extension and

(g) with two hands to increase the use of more trunk rotation.

(h) Gradually the back support of the chair could be lowered then removed.

These basic progression ideas were applied to other bat/ball games, hand ball, soccer work, football catch and throw skills. Tom's physiotherapist emphasized again that changes in body position, item size and weight, sequence of activity, speed of activity or distance between objects all could contribute to altering the difficulty of the task and thus improve his movement control.

Basic balance activities were also introduced with the emphasis on progressing the activity to increase the demands on Tom for internal control. Initially, simple one-leg balance work with visual cues was undertaken with a support surface near by for safety. As this skill improved Tom was given a simple task such as throwing a tennis ball into a large box whilst maintaining the one-leg stance position. This addition reduced Tom's concentration on the balance adjustments thus requiring a more automatic balance response. Tom was progressed on to balance board skills using boards with various degrees of balance difficulty, and in turn other skills whilst balancing were introduced. Finally, balance beam work was used and the width of beam was altered. Tom was required to perform forward, sideways and backward gait work as he could manage.

Despite the need for the other treatment principles Tom's physiotherapist was cognisant that improved gait abilities was one of the vital goals of Tom's programme. Weighted leg or pelvic cuffs and pushing weighted boxes were also used in the gait training programme. Activities were designed to incorporate a 'cortical control' component to gait. The physiotherapist laid out footprint shapes on the floor thus setting and varying the gait control required of Tom. Varying the pattern, stride length and width of base were used to alter the difficulty of the task. Hoops in a hopscotch pattern could also be used for both gait and hop/jump patterns.

Other gait skills tasks included Tom walking between the rungs of a ladder lying on the floor. This required control of both swing and stance phases of the gait cycle with limitation of the foot placement area. Varying the steps between the rungs and introducing sideways and backwards walking between the rungs as well as stride walking outside each side or upon the main length pieces of the ladder were all used to progress the skill.

Finally zigzag and figure eight gait/jog patterns were combined to increase the muscle control and balance difficulty of the gait training. Throughout much of the gait activities a rhythmical sequence to enhance consistent timing of the gait strides was

emphasized. This was done with simple counting patterns and clap patterns, or music to set the rhythm and timing of the gait pattern.

The use of hydrotherapy or water as a medium for the management of ataxia and other neurological conditions provides numerous benefits. The water provides a safe environment in relation to stability for the patient to work in as it can be both resistive and supportive to the patient. Water provides balance support and sensory input and warmth to enhance muscle activity. Finally, the medium adds enjoyment, general skills development and general fitness to the rehabilitative programme.

General exercise activities for improved strength and control of movement were designed for Tom to use in the pool. These included general upper limb movements and muscle groups such as hip abductors and extensors and quadriceps in the lower limb. Gait training was also undertaken in the water. The depth of water in which the gait work was done could be gradually decreased to increase the control/balance demands on Tom. Various gait patterns were given, including sideways walk, backwards walk as well as varying speed and effort of the normal gait pattern. Further skills such as jumping, hopping and balance activities were also added.

Floating work was also used as a means of teaching Tom more about balance and control of his body and weight shift. Slow controlled limb movements were undertaken whilst maintaining the floating position. Swimming was successful enough to enable Tom to consider it as a recreation/sports option which was socially appropriate for his peer interactions and for his general fitness and other physical benefits.

This was an important discovery as Tom's neurosurgeon had confirmed that involve-

Yvonne Burns, John Gilmour, Megan Kentish and Julie MacDonald

ment in contact sports was not an option in the future due to the surgery, presence of the shunt and his incoordination increasing his risk of injury. Tom was obviously unhappy with the news, but he at least now had swimming as a sports option. When his physiotherapist noted a drop in enthusiasm in his commitment to the programme, she took the opportunity to introduce Tom to Cathy, who was a 16-year-old girl with cerebral palsy in the form of ataxia. Cathy was involved in the local disabled sports programme and she had started competing in track events. In an informal setting Cathy was able to share with Tom some of the frustrations and difficulties she had encountered in her life and was able to show Tom what she was achieving now at both school and athletics. Cathy sat in on a physiotherapy treatment session and shared some knowledge, sympathy and laughs. Tom admitted later it certainly helped to clear his 'blues'.

From the wide range of the activities undertaken during the visit, based on the key principles, Tom and his Mum videotaped a number of activities they found most successful. His gait and other activities were videoed also as a means of reassessing his skills on his next visit in 6 months time. The improvements acknowledged by Tom and his mother were a strong motivation for continued work at home. It was re-emphasized that many of the programme aspects agreed upon would need to be considered as a long-term management plan of his ataxia. If in future a local physiotherapy service became available the rehabilitation team would be very happy to pass treatment details and programmes on so Tom could be monitored and managed locally; however, in the meantime it was up to him.

REFERENCES

Abrams, RA, Mubarak, S (1991) Musculoskeletal consequences of near-drowning in children. *Journal of Pediatric Orthopedics* 11: 168–175.

Agre, JC, Findley, TW, McNally, MC et al. (1987) Physical activity capacity in children with myelomeningocoele. *Archives of Physical Medicine and Rehabilitation* 68: 372–377.

Akerstrom, Ms, Sanner (1993) Movement patterns in children with Down's syndrome: a pilot study. *Physiotherapy Theory and Practice* 9: 33–41.

Alexander, MA, Steg, NL (1989) Myelomeningocele: comprehensive treatment. *Archives of Physical Medicine and Rehabilitation* 70: 637–641.

Anderson, E (1976) Impairment of a motor (manual) skill in children with spina bifida myelomenigocele and hydrocephalus. *British Journal of Occupational Therapy* 39: 91–92.

Asher, M, Olson, J (1983) Factors affecting the ambulatory status of patients with spina bifida cystica. *Journal of Bone and Joint Surgery* 65: 350–356.

Bairstow, P (1994) Abilities of children with cerebral palsy and rationale for programmes of intervention. In: van Rossum, JHA, Laszlo, J (eds) *Motor Development: Aspects of Normal and Delayed Development*, pp. 127–128. Amsterdam: VU Uitgeverij.

Bairstow, P, Cochrane, R (1993) Is conductive education transplantable? *British Journal of Special Education* 20: 84–88.

Bairstow, P, Cochrane, R, Hur, J (1993) *Evaluation of Conductive Education for Children with Cerebral Palsy. Final Report (Part II)*. 297 pp. London: HMSO.

Balasubramaniam, C, Laurent, JP, McCluggage, C et al. (1990) Tethered-cord syndrome after repair of meningomyelocele. *Child's Nervous System* 6: 208–211.

Barnet, AB, Weiss, IP, Shaer, C (1993) Evoked potentials in infant brainstem syndrome associated with Arnold–Chiari malformation. *Developmental Medicine and Child Neurology* 35: 42–48.

Begeer, JH, Meihuizen de Regt, MJ, HogenEsch, I et al. (1986) Progressive neurological deficit in children with spina bifida aperta. *Zeitschrift für Kinderchirurgie* 41 (suppl.I): 13–15.

Bell, WO, Charney, EB, Bruce, DA et al. (1987) Symptomatic Arnold–Chiari malformation: review of experience with 22 cases. *Journal of Neurosurgery* 66: 812–816.

Bleck, EE (1987) *Orthopaedic Management of Cerebral Palsy*, 497 pp. Oxford: Blackwell Scientifico.

Bobath, B (1967) The very early treatment of cerebral palsy. *Developmental Medicine and Child Neurology* 9: 373–390.

Bobath, B, Bobath K (1964) The facilitation of normal postural reactions and movements in the treatment of cerebral palsy. *Physiotherapy* 54: 3–19.

Bobath, K, Bobath, B (1972) Cerebral palsy. In: Pearson, P, Williams, C (eds) *Physical Therapy in the Developmental Disabilities*, pp. 31–35. Springfield: Charles C Thomas.

Bower, C (1994) Epilepsy in pregnancy: neural tube defects and folate. *Medical Journal of Australia* 160: 56–57.

Brink, JD, Imbus, C, Woo-Sam, J (1980) Physical recovery after severe closed head trauma in children and adolescents. *Journal of Pediatrics* 97: 721–727.

Brock, DJH, Sutcliffe, RG (1972) Alpha-fetaprotein in the antenatal diagnosis of anencephaly and spina bifida. *Lancet* 2: 197.

Brock, DJH, Barron L, Van Heyningen, V (1985) Prenatal diagnosis of neural tube defects with a monoclonal antibody specific for acetylcholinesterase. *Lancet* 1: 5–8.

Bunch, WH (1976) Myelomeningocele: general concepts. *American Academy of Orthopaedic Surgeons: Instructional Course Lectures* 25: 61–65.

Burns, YR, O'Callaghan, M, Tudehope, DI (1989) Early identification of cerebral palsy in high risk infants. *Australian Paediatric Journal* 25: 215–219.

Campos da Paz, A, Burnett, SM, Braga, LW (1994) Walking prognosis in cerebral palsy: a 22 year retrospective analysis. *Developmental Medicine and Child Neurology* 36: 130–134.

Carroll, N (1974) The orthotic management of the spina bifida child. *Clinical Orthotics* 102: 108–114.

Chakerian, DL, Larson, MA (1993) Effects of upper extremity weight bearing

410

on hand opening and prehension patterns in children with cerebral palsy. *Developmental Medicine and Child Neurology* 35: 216–229.

Charney, EB, Melchionni, IB, Smith, DR (1991) Community ambulation by children with myelomeningocoele and high level paralysis. *Journal of Pediatric Orthopedics* 11: 579–582.

Citta-Pietrolungo, TJ, Alexander, MA, Cook, SP et al. (1993) Complications of tracheostomy and decannulation in pediatric and young patients with traumatic brain injury. *Archives of Physical Medicine and Rehabilitation* 74: 905–909.

Collacott, RA, Ellison, D, Harper, W et al. (1989) Atlanto-occipital instability in Down's syndrome. *Journal of Mental Deficiency Research* 33: 499–505.

Committee on Sports Medicine (1984) Atlantoaxial instability in Down syndrome. *Pediatrics* 74: 152–154.

Conn, AW, Barker, GA (1984) Fresh water drowning and near-drowning: an update. *Canadian Anaethetics Society Journal* 3: 538–544.

Cowie, V (1970) *A Study of the Early Development of Mongols*, 110 pp. Oxford: Pergamon Press.

Craven, DE, Kunches, LM, Kilinsky, V et al. (1986) Risk factors for pneumonia and fatality in patients receiving continuous mechanical ventilation. *American Review of Respiratory Disease* 133: 792–796.

Cunningham, DA, Glenn, SM (1987) Parent involvement and early intervention. In: Lane, D, Stratford Cassell, B (eds) *Current Approaches to Down's Syndrome*, pp 347–362. Kent: Gillingham.

Cusick, BD (1988) Splints and casts: managing foot deformity in children with neuromuscular disorders. *Physical Therapy* 68 (12): 1903–1912.

Daniels, L, Worthingham, C (1980) *Muscle Testing: Techniques of Manual Examination*, 191 pp, 4th edn. Philadelphia: Saunders.

DeSouza, L, Carroll, N (1976) Ambulation of the braced myelomeningocoele patient. *Journal of Bone and Joint Surgery* 58A: 1112–1118.

Deutsch, M (1990) Medulloblastoma. In: Deutsch M (ed). *Management of Childhood Brain Tumours*, pp. 411–440. Boston: Kluiver Academic.

Dowrick, M (1993) Conductive education in Australia: an investigation. *Australian Journal of Special Education* 17: 42–50.

Drennan, JC, Banta, JV, Bunch, WH, Lindseth, RE (1989) Symposium: current concepts in the management of myelomeningocele. *Contemporary Orthopaedics* 19: 63–88.

Drennan, JC (1976) Orthotic management of the myelomeningocele spine. *Development Medicine and Child Neurology* 18(suppl 37): 97–103.

Duckworth, T, Brown, BH (1970) Changes in muscle activity following early closure in myelomeningocoele. *Developmental Medicine and Child Neurology* 12 (suppl. 22): 39–45.

Duckworth, T, Yamashita, T, Franks, CI et al. (1976) Somatosensory evoked cortical responses in children with spina bifida. *Developmental Medicine and Child Neurology* 18: 19–24.

Dudgeon, BJ, Jaffe, KM, Shurtleff, DB (1991) Variations in midlumbar myelomeningocele: inplications for ambulation. *Paediatric Physical Therapy* 3: 57–62.

Dugdale, TW, Renshaw, TS (1986) Instability of the patellofemoral joint in Down syndrome. *Journal of Bone and Joint Surgery* 68: 405–413.

Duhaime, AC, Alario, AJ, Lewander, WJ et al. (1992) Head injury in very young children: mechanisms, injury types, and ophthalmologic findings in 100 hospitalized patients younger than 2 years of age. *Pediatrics* 90: 179–185.

Duncan, PW (1990) Physical therapy assessment. In: Rosenthal, M, Griffith, ER, Bond, MR, Miller, JD (eds) *Rehabilitation of the Adult and Child with Traumatic Brain Injury*, pp. 264–283. Philadelphia: FA Davis Co.

Eckersley, PM, King, LM (1993) Treatment systems. In: Eckersley PM (ed.) *Elements of Paediatric Physiotherapy*, 513 pp. Edinburgh: Churchill Living-stone.

Eiben, CF, Anderson, TP, Lockman, L et al. (1984) Functional outcome of closed head injury in children and young adults. *Archives of Physical Medicine and Rehabilitation* 65: 168–170.

Elwood, M (1991) Folic acid prevents neural tube defects. *Medical Journal of Australia* 155: 579–580.

Fay, GC, Jaffe, KM, Polissar, NL et al. (1994) Outcome of pediatric traumatic brain injury at three years: a cohort study. *Archives of Physical Medicine and Rehabilitation* 75: 733–741.

Feiwell, E, Sakai, D, Blatt, T (1978) The effect of hip reduction on function in patients with myelomeningocele. *The Journal of Bone and Joint Surgery* 60A: 169–173.

Findley, TW, Birkebak, RR, Mcnally, NMC (1987) Ambulation in the adolescent with myelomeningocele: early childhood predictors. *Archives of Physical Medicine and Rehabilitation* 68: 518–522.

Fletcher, JM, Ewing-Cobbs (1991) Head injury in children. *Brain Injury* 5: 337–338.

Franks, CA, Palisano, RJ, Darbee, JC (1991) The effect of walking with an assistive device and using a wheelchair on school performance in students with myelomeningocele. *Physical Therapy* 71(8): 570–578.

Fraser, RK, Haffman, EB, Sparks, LT et al. (1992) The unstable hip and mid-lumbar myelomeningocele. *Journal of Bone and Joint Surgery* 74B: 143–146.

Gaff, JE, Robinson, JM, Parker, PM (1984) The walking ability of 14- to 17-year-old teenagers with spina bifida – a physiotherapy study. *Physiotherapy* 70: 473–474.

Gilbert, JN, Jones, KL, Rorke, LB et al. (1986) Central nervous system anomalies associated with meningomyelocele, hydrocephalus, and the Arnold–Chiari malformation: reappraisal of theories regarding the patho-genesis of posterior neural tube closure defects. *Neurosurgery* 18: 559–564.

Gunn, P (1993) Characteristics of Down syndrome. In: Burns, Y, Gunn, P (eds) *Down Syndrome: Moving Through Life*, pp. 1–18. London: Chapman and Hall.

Guthkelch, AN, Pang, D, Vries, JK (1981) Influence of closure technique on results in myelomeningocoele. *Childs Brain* 8: 350–355.

Haley, SM (1987) Sequence of development of postural reactions by infants with Down syndrome. *Developmental Medicine and Child Neurology* 29: 674–679.

Hamilton, AM (1991) Sensory hand function of the child with spina bifida myelomenigocele. *British Journal of Occupational Therapy* 54: 346–349.

Hari, M, Tillemans, T (1984) Conductive education. In: Scrutton D (ed); *Management of the Motor Disorders of Children with Cerebral Palsy*, pp. 19–33. London: Heinemann.

Harris, MB, Banta, JV (1990) Cost of skin care in the myelomeningocele population. *Journal of Padiatric Orthopaedics* 10: 355–361.

Harris, SR (1981) Effects of neurodevelopmental therapy on motor perfor-mance of infants with Down syndrome. *Developmental Medicine and Child Neurology* 23: 477–483.

Harris, SR (1984) Down syndrome. In: Campbell, SK (ed.) *Pediatric Neurologic Physical Therapy*, pp. 169–204. New York: Churchill Livingstone.

Harris, SR (1988) Neuromotor assessment and intervention for infants with Down's syndrome. *Down's Syndrome: Papers and Abstracts for Professionals* 11 (7): 1–4.

Hayden, PW (1985) Adolescents with meningomyelocele. *Paediatrics in Review* 6: 245–252.

Herman, JM, McLone, DG, Storrs, BB et al. (1993) Analysis of 153 patients with myelomeningocoele or spinal lipoma reoperated upon for a tethered cord. *Pediatric Neurosurgery* 19: 243–249.

Hoffer, M, Feiwell, E, Perry, R et al. (1973) Functional ambulation in patients with myelomeningocoele. *The Journal of Bone and Joint Surgery* 55A: 137–148.

Hoffman, HJ, Hendrick, EB, Humphries, RP (1975) Manifestations and management of Arnold–Chiari malformations in patients with myelo-meningocoele. *Childs Brain* 1: 255–259.

Hsieh, AH, Bishop, MJ, Kublis, PS et al. (1992) Pneumonia following closed head injury. *American Review of Respiratory Disease* 146: 290–294.

Huff, CW, Ramsey, PL (1978) Myelodysplasia: the influence of quadriceps and hip abductor muscles on ambulatory function and stability of the hip. *Journal of Bone and Joint Surgery* **60A**: 432–443.

Hungerford, GD, Akkaraju, V, Rawe, SE *et al.* (1981) Atlanto-occipital and atlantoaxial dislocations with spinal cord compression in Down's syndrome: a case report and review of literature. *British Journal of Radiology* **54**: 758–761

Ingberg, HO, Johnson, EW (1963) Electromyographic evaluation of infants with lumbar meningomyelocele. *Archives of Physical Medicine and Rehabilitation* **44**: 86–92.

Jennett, B (1976) Assessment of the severity of head injury. *Journal of Neurology, Neurosurgery and Psychiatry* **39**: 647–655.

Jobling, A (1993) Play and movement education. In: Burns, Y, Gunn, P (eds) *Down Syndrome: Moving Through Life*, pp. 109–135. London: Chapman and Hall.

Johnson, DL, McCabe, MA, Nicholson, HS *et al.* (1994) Quality of long term survival in young children with medulloblastoma. *Journal of Neurosurgery* **80**: 1004–1010.

Jones, ET, Knapp, R (1987) Assessment and management of the lower extremity in cerebral palsy. *Orthopedic Clinics of North America* **18**: 729–738.

Katz, RT, Rymer, WZ (1989) Spastic hypertonia: mechanisms and measurement. *Archives of Physical Medicine and Rehabilitation* **70**: 144–155.

Kelso, R-A, Price, S (1993) Activities during pre-toddler and toddler period. In: Burns, Y, Gunn, P (eds) *Down Syndrome: Moving Through Life*, pp. 65–94. London: Chapman and Hall.

Kendall, HO, Kendall, FP, Wadsworth, GE (1971) *Muscles, Testing and Function*, 284 pp., 2nd edn. Baltimore: Williams and Wilkins.

Klonoff, H, Low, MD, Clark, C (1977) Head injuries in children: a prospective five year follow-up. *Journal of Neurology, Neurosurgery and Psychiatry* **40**: 1211–1219.

Klonoff, H, Clark, C, Klonoff, PS (1993) Long-term outcome of head injuries: a 23 year follow up study of children with head injuries. *Journal of Neurology, Neurosurgery and Psychiatry* **56**: 410–415.

Knights, RM, Ivan, LP, Ventureyra, ECG *et al.* (1991) The effects of head injury in children on neuropsychological and behavioural functioning. *Brain Injury* **5**: 339–351.

Knott, M, Voss, DE (1968) *PNF: Patterns and Techniques*, 2nd edn, 225 pp. New York: Harper and Rowe.

Knutson, LM, Clark, DE (1991) Orthotic devices for ambulation in children with cerebral palsy and myelomeningocele. *Physical Therapy* **71**(12): 947–960

Lais, A, Kasabian, NG, Dyro, FM *et al.* (1993) The neurosurgical implications of continuous neurological surveillance of children with myelodysplasia. *Journal of Urology* **150**: 1879–1883.

Landrey, SH, Copeland, D, Lee, A *et al.* (1990) Goal-directed behaviour in children with spina bifida. *Developmental and Behavioural Pediatrics* **11**: 306–311.

Lee, EH, Carroll, NC (1985) Hip stability and ambulatory status in myelomeningocele. *Journal of Pediatric Orthopedics* **5**: 522–527.

Leonard, CT (1994) Motor behaviour and neural changes following perinatal and adult-onset brain damage: implications for therapeutic interventions. *Physical Therapy* **74**: 753–767.

Levitt, S (1995) *Treatment of Cerebral Palsy and Motor Delay*, 341 pp, 3rd edn. Oxford: Blackwell Science.

Levitt, S (1984) *Paediatric Developmental Therapy*, 265 pp. Oxford: Blackwell Scientific.

Liptak, GS, Bloss, JW, Brisken, H *et al.* (1988) The management of children with spinal dysraphism. *Journal of Child Neurology* **3**: 3–20.

Liptak, GS, Shurtleff, DB, Bloss, JW *et al.* (1992) Mobility aids for children with high level myelomeningocoele: parapodium versus wheelchair. *Developmental Medicine and Child Neurology* **34**: 787–796.

Little, J, Elwood, JM (1991) Epidemiology of neural tube defects. In: Kiley, M (ed.) *Reproductive and Perinatal Epidemiology*, pp. 251–336. Boca Raton, Florida: CRC Press.

Lydic, JS, Steele, C (1979) Assessment of quality of sitting and gait patterns in children with Down's syndrome. *Physical Therapy* **59**: 1489–1494.

Mazur, JM, Stillwell, A, Menelaus, M (1986a) The significance of spasticity in the upper and lower limbs in myelomeningocoele. *Journal of Bone and Joint Surgery* **68B**: 213–217.

Mazur, JM, Menelaus, MB, Hudson, I *et al.* (1986b) Hand function in patients with spina bifida cystica. *Journal of Pediatric Orthopaedics* **6**: 442–447.

Mazur, JM, Shurtleff, D, Menelaus, M *et al.* (1989) Orthopaedic management of high level spina bifida: early walking compared with early use of a wheelchair. *Journal of Bone and Joint Surgery* **71A**: 56–61.

Mazur, JM, Menelaus, MB (1991) Neurological status of spina bifida patients and the orthopedic surgeon. *Clinical Orthopaedics and Related Research* **264**: 54–64.

McCullough, DC, Levy, LM, DiChiro, G *et al.* (1990) Toward the prediction of neurological injury from tethered spinal cord: Investigation of cord motion with magnetic resonance. *Pediatric Neurosurgery* **16**: 3–7.

McDonald, CM, Jaffe, KM, Shurtleff, DB (1986) Assessment of muscle strength in children with myelomeningocoele: accuracy and stability of measurements over time. *Archives of Physical Medicine and Rehabilitation* **67**: 855–861.

McDonald, CM, Jaffe, KM, Mosca, VS *et al.* (1991) Modifications to the traditional description of neurosegmental innervation in myelomeningocoele. *Developmental Medicine and Child Neurology* **33**: 473–481.

McLone, DG (1980) Technique for closure of myelomeningocoele. *Childs Brain* **6**: 65–73.

McLone, DG (1983) Results of treatment of children born with myelomeningocoele. *Clinical Neurosurgery* **30**: 407–412.

McLone, DG (1992) Continuing concepts in the management of spina bifida. *Pediatric Neurosurgery* **18**: 254–256.

McLone, DG, Dias, MS (1991) Complications of myelomeningocoele closure. *Pediatric Neurosurgery* **17**: 267–273.

McLone, DG, Czyzewski, D, Raimondi, AJ *et al.* (1982) Central nervous system infections as a limiting factor in the intelligence of children with myelomeningocoele. *Pediatrics* **70**: 338–342.

McLone, DG, Dias, L, Kaplan, WE *et al.* (1985) Concepts in the management of spina bifida. *Concepts in Pediatric Neurosurgery* **5**: 97–106.

McLone, DG, Herman, JM, Gabrieli, AP *et al.* (1990) Tethered cord as a cause of scoliosis in children with a myelomeningocoele. *Pediatric Neurosurgery* **16**: 8–13.

Minns, RA, Sobkowiah, CA, Skardoutsou, A *et al.* (1977) Upper limb function in spina bifida. *Zeitschrift für Kinderchirurgie* **22**: 493–506.

Mital, MA, Garber, JE, Stinson, JT (1987) Ectopic bone formation in children and adolescents with head injuries: its management. *Journal of Pediatric Orthopedics* **7**: 83–90.

Mitchell, S, Gorman, D (1994) Clinical forum: near drowning. *General Practitioner* **23**: 8–9.

Molner, GE, Alexander, J, Gutfeld, N (1979) Reliability of quantitive strength measurements in children. *Archives of Physical Medicine and Rehabilitation* **60**: 218–221.

Morrissy, RT (1978) Spina bifida: a new rehabilitation problem. *Orthopedic Clinics of North America* **9**: 379–389.

MRC Vitamin Study Research Group (1991) Prevention of neural tube defects: results of the Medical Research Council Vitamin Study. *Lancet* **338**: 131–137.

Murdoch, A (1980) How valuable is muscle charting? A study of the relationship between neonatal assessment of muscle power and later mobility in children with spina bifida defects. *Physiotherapy* **66**: 221–223.

Myhr, U, von Wendt, L (1990) Reducing spasticity and enhancing postural control for the creation of a functional sitting position in children with cerebral palsy: a pilot study. *Physiotherapy Theory and Practice* **6**: 65–76.

Myhr, U, von Wendt (1993) Influences of different sitting positions and abduction orthoses on leg muscle activity in children with cerebral palsy. *Developmental Medicine and Child Neurology* 35: 870–880.

National Perinatal Statistics Unit (1989) *Congenital Malformations Monitoring Report Number 33.* Sydney: University of Sydney.

O'Neill, P, Stack, JP (1991) Magnetic resonance imaging in the pre-operative assessment of closed spinal dysraphism in children. *Pediatric Neurosurgery* 16: 240–246.

Osaka, K, Tanimura, T, Hirayama, A et al. (1978) Myelomeningocele before birth. *Journal of Neurosurgery* 49: 711–724.

Park, TS, Hoffman, HJ, Hendrick, EB et al. (1983) Medulloblastoma: clinical presentation and management – experience at the hospital for sick children, Toronto 1950–1980. *Journal of Neurosurgery* 58: 543–552.

Park, TS, Cail, WS, Maggio, WM et al. (1985) Progressive spasticity and scoliosis in children with myelomeningocoele. *Journal of Neurosurgery* 62: 367–375.

Pearn, J (1991) Safety legislation and child mortality. *Medical Journal of Australia* 154: 155–156.

Petersen, MC (1992) Tethered cord syndrome in myelodysplasia: correlation between level of lesion and height at time of presentation. *Developmental Medicine and Child Neurology* 34: 604–610.

Pitt, WR, Balanda, KP (1991) Childhood drowning and near-drowning in Brisbane: the contribution of domestic pools. *Medical Journal of Australia* 154: 661–665.

Price, S, Kelso, R-A (1993) Activities during infancy. In: Burns, Y, Gunn, P (eds) *Down Syndrome: Moving Through Life*, pp. 37–64. London: Chapman and Hall.

Pueschel, SM, Scola, SH (1987) Atlanto-axial instability in individuals with Down syndrome: epidemiologic radiographic and clinical studies. *Paediatrics* 80(4): 555–560.

Rabb, CH, McComb, JG, Raffel, C et al. (1992) Spinal arachnoid cysts in the pediatric age group: an association with neural tube defects. *Journal of Neurosurgery* 77: 369–372.

Rinehart, MA (1990) Strategies for improving motor performance. In: Rosenthal, M, Griffith, ER, Bond, MR, Miller, JD (eds) *Rehabilitation of the Adult and Child with Traumatic Brain Injury*, pp. 331–350. Philadelphia: FA Davis Co.

Rivara, J'MB, Fay, GC, Jaffe, KM et al. (1992) Predictors of family functioning one year following traumatic brain injury in children. *Archives of Physical Medicine and Rehabilitation* 73: 899–910.

Rivara, J'MB, Jaffe, KM, Pollissar, NL et al. (1994) Family functioning and children's academic performance and behaviour problems in the year following traumatic brain injury. *Archives of Physical Medicine and Rehabilitation* 75: 369–379.

Rogers, B, Msall, M, Owens, T et al. (1993) Cystic periventricular leukomalacia and type of cerebral palsy. Abstract The American Academy for Cerebral Palsy and Developmental Medicine Annual Meeting. *Developmental Medicine and Child Neurology* (suppl. 69) 35: 22.

Rood, MS (1962) The use of sensory receptors to activate, facilitate and inhibit motor response, automatic and somatic developmental sequence. In: Sattely C (ed.) Approaches to treatment of patients with neuromuscular dysfunction. *Third International Congress – World Federation of Occupational Therapists*, Iowa, pp. 26–37.

Ryan, KD, Ploski, C, Emans, JB (1991) Myelodysplasia – the musculoskeletal problem: habilitation from infancy to adulthood. *Physical Therapy* 71(12): 935–946

Samuelsson, L, Eklof, O (1990) Hip instability in myelomeningocele: 158 patients followed for 15 years. *Acta Orthopaedic Scandinavica* 61: 3–6.

Samuelsson, L, Skoog, M (1988) Ambulation in patients with myelomeningocoele: a multivariate statistical analysis. *Journal of Pediatric Orthopedics* 8: 569–574.

Sand, PL, Taylor, N, Rawlings, M et al. (1973) Performance of children with spina bifida manifesta on the Frostig Developmental Test of Visual Perception. *Perceptual and Motor Skills* 37: 539–546.

Sand, PL, Taylor, N, Hill, M et al. (1974) Hand function in children with myelomeningocoele. *American Journal of Occupational Therapy* 28: 87–90.

Scherzer, AL, Tscharnuter, I (1982) *Early Diagnosis and Therapy in Cerebral Palsy*, 289 pp. New York: Dekker.

Schopler, SA, Menelaus, MB (1987) Significance of the strength of the quadriceps muscles in children with myelomeningocoele. *Journal of Pediatric Orthopedics*: 507–512.

Seeger, BR, Caudrey, DJ, O'Mara, NA (1984) Hand function in cerebral palsy: the effect of hip flexion angle. *Developmental Medicine and Child Neurology* 26: 601–606.

Sharrard, WJW (1964a) The segmental innervation of the lower limb muscles of man. *Annals of the Royal College of Surgeons of England* 35: 106–122.

Sharrard, WJW (1964b) Posterior iliopsoas transplantation in the treatment of paralytic dislocation of the hip. *Journal of Bone and Joint Surgery* 46B: 426–444.

Shaw, ED, Beals, RK (1992) The hip joint in Down's syndrome. A study of its structure and associated disease. *Clinical Orthopaedics and Related Research* 278: 101–107.

Shepherd, R (1979) Problem analysis with Down's syndrome infants. *Australian Journal of Physiotherapy Paediatric Monograph* 117–124.

Shumway-Cook, A, Woollacott, MH (1985) Dynamics of postural control in the child with Down syndrome. *Physical Therapy* 65(9): 1315–1322.

Shurtleff, DB (1986) Mobility. In: Shurtleff, DB (ed.) *Myelodysplasias and Extrophies: Significance, Prevention and Treatment*, pp. 313–356. New York: Grune & Stratton.

Shurtleff, DB, Stuntz, JT (1986) Back closure. In: Shurtleff, DB (ed.) *Myelodysplasias and Extrophies: Significance, Prevention and Treatment*, pp. 117–138. New York: Grune & Stratton.

Shurtleff, DB, Stuntz, JT, Hayden, P (1986) Hydrocephalus. In: Shurtleff, DB (ed.) *Myelodysplasias and Extrophies: Significance, Prevention and Treatment*, pp. 139–179. New York: Grune & Stratton.

Smithells, RW, Sheppard, S, Shorah, CJ (1980) Possible prevention of neural tube defects by periconceptual vitamin supplementation. *Lancet* I(8169): 647.

Sobus, KML, Alexander, MA, Harcke, HT (1993) Undetected musculoskeletal trauma in children with traumatic brain injury or spinal cord injury. *Archives of Physical Medicine and Rehabilitation* 74: 902–904.

Stanley, FJ, Blair, E, Hockey, A et al. (1993) Spastic quadriplegia in Western Australia. A genetic epidemiological study I: Case population and perinatal risk factors. *Developmental Neurology and Child Development* 35: 191–201.

Stark, GD, Baker, GCW (1967) Neurological involvement of lower limbs in myelomeningocoele. *Developmental Medicine and Child Neurology* 9: 732–744.

Stark, GD, Drummond, M (1971) The spinal cord lesion in myelomeningocoele. *Developmental Medicine and Child Neurology* 13 (Suppl. 25): 1–15.

Stein, SC, Schut, LA (1979) Hydrocephalus in myelomeningocoele. *Childs Brain* 5: 413–419.

Stillwell, A, Menelaus, M (1983) Walking ability in mature patients with spina bifida. *Journal of Pediatric Orthopedics* 3: 184–190.

Stockmeyer, SA (1972) A sensorimotor approach to treatment. In: Pearson, PH, Williams, CE (eds) *Physical Therapy Services in the Developmental Disabilities*, pp. 186–222. Springfield: CC Thomas.

Sussman, MD (1983) Casting as an adjunct to neurodevelopmental therapy for cerebral palsy. *Developmental Medicine and Child Neurology* 25: 804–805.

Swank, M, Dias, L (1992) Myelomeningocele: a review of the orthopaedic aspects of 206 patients treated from birth with no selection criteria. *Developmental Medicine and Child Neurology* 34: 1047–1052.

Tamaki, N, Shirataki, K, Kojima, N et al. (1988) Tethered cord syndrome of delayed onset following repair of myelomeningocoele. *Journal of Neurosurgery* 69: 393–398.

Taylor, A, McNamara, A (1990) Ambulation status of adults with myelomeningocele. *Zeitschrift fur Kinderchirurgie* 45 (Suppl. 1): 32–33.

Taylor, N, Sand, PL (1975) Verlo orthosis: Experience with different developmental levels in normal children. *Archives of Physical Medicine and Rehabilitation* **54**: 129–135.

Tew, BJ, Laurence, KM (1975) The effects of hydrocephalus on intelligence, visual perception and school attainment. *Developmental Medicine and Child Neurology* **17**: 65.

Tew, B, Laurence, KM, Richards, A (1980) Inattention among children with hydrocephalus and spina bifida. *Zeitschrift für Kinderchirurgie* **31**: 381–386

Trahan, J, Marcoux, S (1994) Factors associated with the mobility of children with cerebral palsy to walk at six years: a retrospective study. *Developmental Medicine and Child Neurology* **36**: 787–795.

Umphred, DA, McCormack GL (1985) Classification of common facilitatory and inhibitory treatment techniques. In: Umphred DA (ed.) *Neurological Rehabilitation*, pp. 72–117. St Louis: CV Mosby Co.

Venes, JL, Black, KL, Latack, JT (1986) Preoperative evaluation and surgical management of the Arnold–Chiari II malformation. *Journal of Neurosurgery* **64**: 363–370.

Watt, J, Sims, Harkham, F et al. (1986) A prospective study of inhibitive casting as an adjunct to physiotherapy for cerebral palsy children. *Developmental Medicine and Child Neurology* **28**: 480–488.

Weisl, H, Fairclough, JA, Jones, DG (1988) Stabilization of the hip in myelomeningocele: comparison of posterior iliopsoas transfer and varus-rotation osteotomy. *Journal of Bone and Joint Surgery* **70B**: 29–33.

Williams, LO, Anderson, AD, Campbell, J et al. (1983) Energy costs of walking and wheelchair propulsion by children with myelodysplasia: comparison with normal children. *Developmental Medicine and Child Neurology* **25**: 617–624.

Williams, JJ, Graham, GP, Dunne, KB, Menelaus, MB (1993) Late knee problems in myelomeningocele. *Journal of Pediatric Orthopedics* **13**: 701–703.

Wolf, LS, McLaughlin, JF (1992) Early motor development in infants with meningomyelocele. *Pediatric Physical Therapy* **4**: 12–17.

Ylvisaker, M, Chorazy, AJL, Cohen, SB et al. (1990) Rehabilitative assessment following head injury in children. In: Rosenthal, M, Griffith, ER, Bond, MR, Miller JD (eds) *Rehabilitation of the Adult and Child with Traumatic Brain Injury*, pp. 558–592. Philadelphia: FA Davis Co.

Yokochi, K, Shimabukuro, S, Kodama, M et al. (1993) Motor function of infants with athetodi cerebral palsy. *Developmental Medicine and Child Neurology* **35**: 909–916.

Ziviani, J, Hayes, A, Chant, D (1990) Hand writing: a perceptual motor disturbance in children with myelomeningocele. *Occupational Therapy Journal of Research* **10**: 12–26.

Recommended Reading

Jennett, B, Teasdale, G (1981) *Management of Head Injuries*, 361 pp. Philadelphia: FA Davis Co.

Rosenthal, M, Griffith, ER, Bond, MR et al. (eds) (1990) *Rehabilitation of the Adult and Child with Traumatic Brain Injury*, 652 pp., 2nd edn. Philadelphia: FA Davis Co.

Montgomery J (ed) (1995) *Clinics in Physical Therapy: Physical Therapy for Traumatic Brain Injury*, 219 pp. New York: Churchill Livingstone.

22

Physiotherapy Management – Minor Coordination Dysfunction

PAULINE WATTER

Neurodevelopmental Assessment
•
Associated Problems of MCD
•
Treatment of MCD

The term which has been used to define the population discussed in this chapter is 'minor coordination dysfunction' or MCD. This label is useful since it describes a heterogeneous group of problems which the patient may experience. Although definitions abound, there is general agreement that affected children experience impaired motor skills without any identifiable intellectual or physical disorder (Hulme and Lord 1986, Henderson 1987). Treatment planning requires an accurate full neurodevelopmental assessment, allowing the physiotherapist to evaluate the specific and unique combination of functional difficulties with which each child presents.

There has been a proliferation of 'umbrella' terms referring to this population of young people who are regarded as having normal intelligence, minor degrees of sensory and/or motor dysfunction, with a certain proportion also experiencing learning problems and/or behavioural difficulties. Such proliferation of descriptive labels is understandable if the broad range of possible symptoms and the unclear aetiology are considered (Bullock and Watter 1987,

Henderson 1987, Smyth 1992, Herrgard *et al.* 1993). In general it can be observed that the terms generated tend to reflect the discipline of the author. Consequently, 'learning disability' tends to be employed by educators, the medical profession may talk of 'minimal neurological impairment' or even 'attention deficit/hyperactive disorder (ADHD)', while psychologists developed terms such as 'perceptual-motor dysfunction'. Periodically, particular terms become popular and are often used inaccurately within the general population, resulting in some terms being applied inappropriately to large groups of children. The overuse of popular labels such as hyperactivity, ADHD and dyslexia are good examples of this.

A problem also arises when parents or teachers think that every child with a learning problem also has motor problems, or vice versa. Smyth (1992) and Hadders-Algra and Touwen (1992) support the overlap between clumsiness and academic difficulties, while Watter (1982) suggests that of all school-aged children with minor motor problems about one-half will also experience significant learning disability (LD). In any population with diagnosed learning problems, between one-third and one-half will also have MCD (Watter 1982, Watter and Bullock 1983, Watter and Bullock 1987). Gillberg and Gillberg (1989) report from their epidemiological study that attention deficit disorder was present in 65% of their clumsy sample. The reasons for this degree of overlap between these conditions are two-fold. Firstly, both MCD and LD involve common aetiological factors, and secondly certain sensorimotor problems may underlie or at least contribute to LD.

There is a growing body of research indicating that MCD children have problems with central processing, recall and storage of information, as well as poor intersensory integration, all of which adversely affect motor skill. Van Dellen and Geuze (1988) and van der Meulen et el. (1991a, b), for example, report that clumsy children have longer reaction times and slower performances than normal children. Williams et el. (1992) concluded that clumsy children had poorer timing control of movements compared with matched normal children, and deduced that this was due to problems in a central time-keeping mechanism. Recent research indicates that clumsy children have delays and differences in the electromyographic (EMG) recordings of feedforward (Steele 1994).

It is reported that at time of initial referral for neurodevelopmental physiotherapy, approximately one-third of the children will already be experiencing some form of behavioural difficulty severe enough that they have sought help on this issue (Bullock and Watter 1987). Behavioural problems in clumsy children are reported by Hadders-Algra et al. (1988), Laszlo et al. (1988) and Smyth (1992). Smyth (1992) also reports severe anxiety in clumsy children, while persisting behavioural difficulties are noted during a long-term study by Gillberg and Gillberg (1989).

The incidence of MCD is broadly accepted as being of the order of 6–10% of the normal population (Watter 1982), but varies depending on the stringency of the definition used (Laszlo et al. 1988, Gillberg and Gillberg 1989). Boys are between 6 and 10 times more likely to be affected than girls (Watter 1982) with local studies consistently reporting at least 3 boys to every

girl affected. First-born boys have a greater likelihood of being affected than later born. While authors support the possibility of a genetic component in LD, there is little direct evidence of familial factors in MCD. It is common, however, for clinicians to report treating several children in the one family and often a parent will comment that s/he experienced similar physical difficulties as a child, even though they consider they currently have no motor problems.

It is important that the nature of the sensorimotor difficulties be understood. These children do not generally have conditions which affect sensory acuity, but rather the deficit is in information processing. That is the child may feel a touch on the finger but be unable to assign location to it, or may not assign the correct emotional connotations to it. These children's reactions may be characterized by immature patterns of response, an inability to inhibit unwanted activity or emotion, or an inability to control the level of activity or impulsivity. While motor patterns used by each child are unique they may follow general population movement patterns. It is important to recognize that the pattern exhibited may vary not only from one child to the next, but also significantly within the one child during the course of the day (better morning than afternoon), with level of health (worse when sick), or indeed from day to day (worse as the week progresses).

It is interesting to observe that as treatment progresses, the variability which is an inherent and frustrating part of the whole problem tends to decrease, and parents report that their child is more even in temperament and has better self-control than previously.

Neurodevelopmental Assessment

This assessment follows that described by Burns and Watter (1974), Burns et al. (1989) and Burns (1992), and was further developed for use with MCD children by Bullock and Watter (1978) and Watter (1982, 1984). The neurosensory motor developmental assessment (NSMDA) of Burns (1992) which outlines the basis of this type of assessment is described in Chapter 7. However, there are some specific features which require clarification as they pertain to the common abnormalities found when assessing children with minor motor dysfunction.

Areas of Neurodevelopmental Assessment

Localizing Signs
tone
reflexes
clonus
associated reactions
tremor

Primitive Movements
extensor thrust
asymmetric tonic neck
symmetric tonic neck
tonic labyrinthine reflex

Postural Reactions
weight shift
positive support
righting reactions
protection reactions
equilibrium reactions

Sensorimotor Aspects
tactile
proprioception
vestibular
occular / motor
praxia (motor planning)
diadochokinesia
crossing midline
auditory sequence
coordination

Musculoskeletal Features
ROM and muscle length
deformity
alignment, e.g. hips / knees

Localizing Signs

In neurodevelopmental physiotherapy assessment, localizing signs must be examined although major problems in this area are not anticipated in the child

with MCD. Multiple abnormal responses in this area indicate that there are likely to be focal or specific lesions and the underlying problem is not MCD. The child should be referred to the appropriate professional, usually via the family doctor.

In MCD, the deep tendon reflexes are usually normal although in some children with very low tone they may be difficult to elicit. Muscle tone should be considered at rest as well as during activity. In children with MCD, problems of tone are a common finding, with about half exhibiting low tone, and the rest fairly evenly divided between normal, high, rigid and fluctuating tone. When examining muscle tone, it is important to remember that in some children the presence of strong persisting primitive or immature movement patterns may affect the tone felt due either to the child's body position or head position. Underlying abnormal tone will be abnormal despite changes in body position. Clonus is only likely to be present when tone is high, and usually only one or two beats will be felt in MCD children.

Associated and synkinetic reactions may be increased in children with MCD, generally in conjunction with effort. In these children relatively little effort is sufficient to produce associated reactions due to inadequate suppression or inhibition of unwanted movements.

The extent to which tremor is seen depends in part on the base from which the treatment population is drawn. In a clinic based outside a hospital where many referrals will come from educational sources and parents as well as from the family doctor and medical specialists, tremor is rarely noted. When tremor is present it is generally a baseline tremor, not affected by intention, but occasionally worse with fatigue. This tremor often responds well to treatment, causing little functional difficulty. Tremor may be familial and its response to treatment is often less satisfactory. If the clinic is operated within a hospital or sees a number of follow-up clients (e.g. head injury or premature babies) there may be a higher incidence of tremor and a greater variety of type. The child with a tremor which does not rapidly respond to treatment should be quickly referred for further opinion.

Primitive or Immature Movement Patterns

These should be assessed by asking the child to perform the eliciting movement. It is easy to facilitate these patterns when passive movement or active/assisted movement is used. Assuming the child is above 3 years of age, those immature patterns which commonly persist in the MCD population include extensor thrust, asymmetric and symmetric tonic neck reflex (ATNR and STNR) and tonic labyrinthine reflex (TLR) patterns.

These primitive patterns are tested in more advanced positions than the classical infant tests, using positions more conducive to revealing the patterns in MCD children. Thus the extensor thrust should be tested with the child in supine lying with the knee slightly flexed, with pressure applied against the base of the hallux. If the pattern is present, extension of the whole leg with plantarflexion of the foot against the stimulating pressure will occur. It may be an asymmetrical response, and often produces a toe-walking gait. The tendoachilles may become shortened. In standing, the extensor thrust may be seen in conjunction with the ATNR pattern. In many children with MCD no extensor thrust is elicited in lying, but once the child walks, then a strong thrust may become functionally apparent.

When evaluating the ATNR pattern the prone kneeling position is a more revealing testing position than the classical test in supine, and should always be used for MCD children. The persistence of this pattern in this position produces elbow flexion on the occipital side in response to head turning, while the trunk also side flexes to that side. The extensor phase is frequently seen as hyperextension of the elbows on the face side. It is not common for the lower limb to demonstrate a similar pattern in this position, but often there is a loss of pelvic stability in conjunction with the trunk side flexion. This may be so strong that the child falls out of the prone kneeling position.

The STNR pattern should also be evaluated in the prone kneeling position. It is common for the MCD child to flex the elbows during the neck flexed phase, and to lose pelvic stability rather than demonstrate a full hip extension as in the classic test with more

neurologically disabled children. Similarly, the neck extension elicits elbow extension as well as a tendency to flex the hips and knees and sit back on the haunches. Sometimes there is a loss of stability rather than hip flexion. Both the ATNR and the STNR patterns may be present in standing and sitting, and like the extensor thrust may be used by the child to reinforce postural stability. In general, MCD children are not confined by these persisting immature patterns, but may tend to use them transiently and in a compensatory manner, to provide functional stability.

The tonic labyrinthine reflex (TLR) pattern should be assessed as described in the NSMDA (Burns 1992) during lowering from sitting to supine. Many children with MCD only have phasic control during this test. It is important to recognize the effects of low tone and muscle weakness when testing for these patterns. For example, if a child has difficulty controlling head position during movement from sitting to supine, it is important to differentiate between the probable causes of low tone, muscle weakness and persisting TLR.

Postural Reactions

Normal postural responses are fast, automatic and relaxed. In children with MCD these responses may be at either end of the spectrum. They may be too fast or jerky, with the child always being 'ready' to fall and maintaining an abnormal degree of readiness, or at the other extreme, the child may be slow to react with resultant clumsiness, poor orientation and ineffective movement.

In the age group being considered, the weight-shift response and positive supporting response should occur together. Thus as the weight shifts to one side, there is pressure through that limb which stimulates the positive support reaction, allowing for the maintenance of antigravity postures. At the same time the limb which is no longer weight-bearing loses cocontraction. In normal children this reaction undergoes further adaptation to allow for dynamic control of the limb through range of motion. This prevents total collapse of the supporting limb once the knee or elbow leaves full extension. In MCD children, the positive support and weight-shift reactions may be exaggerated, not occur together or indeed, not at all.

When righting reactions are assessed, the common abnormality is the persistence of 'en bloc' responses rather than rotation between body segments. The more advanced derotated phase where the child is mature enough to lie at full stretch without obligatory follow, is seen less often than in normal children. In some MCD children, the lack of these reactions affects gait patterns and running style, and may be evident in a lack of generalized body rotation, and may present in poor ability to rotate across the body midline.

Optical head righting is normally fast, symmetrical and relaxed, and is in the direction which corrects the head to gravity. Changes in tone during testing, as well as asymmetry of response, are frequently seen in MCD children. Testing in horizontal suspension is often more discriminating for the MCD child. It is important to remember that this is a dynamic test, not one of static holding. Therefore, the child must be continuously moved through space rather than held still in each position. These reactions generally reflect other patterns of asymmetrical response throughout the sensorimotor systems.

Assessment of protection and equilibrium reactions do not pose any particular difficulties in the MCD population. The MCD child can function at either extreme of range, with a tendency to overuse protective reactions when equilibrium reactions are poor. There is a link between poorly developed weight-shift, positive support and equilibrium reactions.

Sensorimotor Assessment

TACTILE SYSTEM

Tactile localization of light touch on the body and double simultaneous discrimination are assessed, as well as the emotional reactions to being touched. Any tactile avoidance manoeuvres also need to be noted, as well as particular areas of sensitivity or lack thereof. Tactile localization in the hand is particularly important to fine motor function, and any tendency to cue using extra tactile input should be noted. In this area as well as the other sensorimotor areas, it is important to note any asymmetry in responses. A child with

tactile problems might not interpret different levels of input appropriately, may not be able to feel when he is hurt, and may be seen as aggressive because he does not feel how hard he is touching or hugging others. Importantly, since the tactile system is related to level of arousal, input can be used differentially to inhibit as well as to stimulate. This has implications for the use of tactile input during treatment and handling.

PROPRIOCEPTION

Problems in this area are some of the most common in MCD children (Bairstow and Laszlo 1981, Laszlo et al. 1988). It may have isolated effects, such as poor finger kinaesthesia or may have a generalized effect throughout the body. When testing, remember that you are testing the responding hand or limb. This can be evaluated at several levels depending on the age of the child. Younger children use visual guidance to copy a visually demonstrated position, while the most mature response is to use proprioceptive guidance to copy a position demonstrated (but not seen) on their resting hand (Lynch et al. 1992). There is an element of motor planning as well as memory when such responses are required, and these aspects must be evaluated separately.

For tests of limb position awareness and static holding in standing the tests employed are commonly those used for adult testing. Static holding of the body is difficult for many clumsy children, with increased body sway or over stabilization (locking) being seen. The child's proprioception will occasionally be so poor that falls occur, often always in one particular direction.

VESTIBULAR SYSTEM

This system allows the body to adjust to movement through space and controls the orientation of the body to gravity. It includes the head righting response when the vision is occluded, and postrotatory nystagmus. Some authors categorize the latter reaction as proprioceptive because it relies upon the gravitationally induced movement of otolithic particles to displace the cilia. For discussion purposes, both are considered here. The vestibular system has close interactions with many other systems, particularly the visual (vestibulo-ocular reflex), and is intimately involved in the maintenance of postural tone, which has implications for treatment.

The vestibular head righting response (VHR) should be intact in the first month or so after birth, but in many children with MCD the reaction is absent, partial or intermittent. While the normal reaction orients the head so that it is corrected beyond the midline, in clumsy children the head is frequently dropped in the direction of gravity. The tone throughout the whole body may also decrease, making the child very difficult to hold. Usually in MCD the vestibular head righting is less efficient than the optical, but occasionally the reverse will be true. It is common for responses to be asymmetrical and this may reflect patterns of asymmetry noted in other areas of the assessment. The child with problems may also exhibit a fear of heights or being moved suddenly, and may cling or align his body to the examiner's body. If the child has middle ear effusions or nasal discharge, a poor reaction to this test may be misleading.

The postrotatory response has been the subject of considerable discussion and research throughout recent years, and the testing procedure is described in the NSMDA (Burns 1992). The most reliable observations are the degree of postural lean during spinning (per rotatory response) and after (postrotatory), and the quality of the nystagmus beat. It is easy to affect the response by poor testing procedures, such as incorrect head position or insufficient rest between tests, i.e. in opposite direction.

In children with MCD there are frequent adverse reactions to spin, in terms of loss of postural control (falling or excessive lean), loss of orientation, or increased autonomic reactions. The last can render the child nauseous and needs to be inhibited. The response is also frequently asymmetrical as well as irregular, absent or exaggerated.

Testing should not be performed on children with middle ear effusion, and it is advisable to leave this test until the closing stages of the assessment, and certainly until after observation of fine motor skills. Stop testing if the child starts to have a negative (loss of tone, excessive fear, blanching) response.

OCULARMOTOR SYSTEM

This system plays an important role in postural control and balance. The eye positioning assessment involves reflex and functional movement of the extraocular muscles. It is important to remember that these are simply a group of voluntary muscles and can therefore be affected by factors such as abnormal muscle tone, weakness and poor coordination.

When testing visual tracking in children with MCD, poor concentration frequently affects, and is affected by, the quality of the movement. Both visual tracking and convergence movements are commonly uncoordinated, slow (resulting in loss of visual contact with target) or asymmetrical in clumsy children. They may be performed well for part of the range only and fatigue of control is rapid, with subsequent effects on tasks requiring maintenance of visual control. This is particularly relevant for classroom activities. Midline crossing problems are also frequently apparent during visual tasks.

Strabismus is probably no more common in this clinical population than others, and conservative management by an ophthalmologist is common. The child is more likely to have a convergent than divergent squint, and if underlying tone is abnormal this may contribute in part to the degree of squint.

Visual fixation refers to the ability of the child to keep the eyes fixed on a desired object (face, board, book) for the required length of time. It can be considered that it is a proprioceptive function, being literally a static hold of the extraocular muscles. It may therefore be affected by factors which influence function in other muscle groups. For example, 'follow', both affects and is affected by concentration. The child also needs to be able to achieve visual release at will, and this fix–release (or glancing quickly from one object to another) must be assessed. This aspect of fixation and control of visual release is often difficult for children with MCD who may have difficulty maintaining fixation as well as changing the point of fixation. Another aspect which many MCD children find difficult is keeping the head still while following with the eyes. Instead of being able to dissociate these movements, the child continues to move head and eyes together.

Clinical Question

Consider a child with no dissociation of head and eye movement at age 8 years. He also has strong persisting ATNR movement pattern. What are the likely effects on posture when sitting at the desk in the classroom? Consider particularly the effect during reading (e.g. as the eyes sweep the page to the right)?

PRAXIS OR MOTOR PLANNING

Praxis refers to the ability voluntarily to plan or organize movements or sequences of movements. When a child is said to be apraxic, it implies that although he may understand and be able physically to perform a movement, he cannot voluntarily do it on demand. Thus MCD children may not be able to plan or organize movements they are shown, such as letter shapes or body positions. Further, they may not be able to plan in response to a verbal instruction. It is clear this will have a marked effect on classroom behaviour. Such children frequently display frustration when attempting tasks, since they know what they should do, know they have done it before, but cannot do it when asked. It is the 'how to' aspect which causes the difficulty. Motor planning problems are exacerbated by poor memory where the child forgets the task or instruction. Importantly, such memory difficulties can be sense-specific too, affecting either or both of the visual and verbal parameters.

DIADOCHOKINESIA

Diadochokinesia refers to the ability to perform rapidly alternating movements, such as tapping the index finger or pronating and supinating the forearm. As children mature, such movements are performed more easily, smoothly and rapidly, with little overflow of unwanted movements to other body parts. In children with MCD, there is a loss of smoothness in alternating movements, with interruption or loss of the pattern being attempted, as well as increased overflow to other body parts. This becomes more noticeable if the child is required to move faster.

CROSSING THE MIDLINE

When a child with MCD has difficulty crossing his body midline it frequently occurs across systems. Such difficulties may present when attempting to take the hands across the midline to reach for an object, or move his eyes across the mid-point of range. The first has implications for postural rotation, general coordination and development of hand preference, while the second has implications for reading and writing. Poor ability to cross the midline of the body may also be seen in association with poor weight-shift, poor rotation and inadequate postural control.

AUDITORY SEQUENCING

The ability to copy clapped rhythmical and arrhythmical sequences presented auditorily, is a sequential auditory-motor memory task which is not language based. Therefore, it can be described as a short-term verbal sequential memory task, and it is in the NSMDA. Children with MCD often perform poorly in auditory sequence testing. However, often it appears their performance relates to poor overall short-term memory as well as an inability to order or sequence or establish a rhythmical pattern of movement. In many children this translates in the classroom to poor spelling and to a lesser extent poor recall of a number of facts and retention of verbal instructions. Since it is a frequently encountered problem which not many professionals address, it has of necessity become an important focus of physiotherapy programmes, usually with good results. It is one of the areas which continues to cause difficulties if untreated.

COORDINATION

In general terms 'coordinated movement' is an outcome of adequate and efficient functioning of the sensorimotor systems. It is common for children with MCD to exhibit a pattern of dysfunction unique to each child, but with overall commonalities which result in so called 'clumsy' movements. It is, however, important to remember that not all MCD children are clumsy. They may have problems which do not impinge on gross or fine motor skill per se such as apraxia and poor short-term memory. They may have fine motor problems in isolation from gross motor, or vice versa. Usually, however, the effect of common combinations such as low muscle tone, poor postural and orientation reactions and decreased propriception will be reflected in poor gross and fine motor coordination. Sometimes the child may be able to achieve a skill (for example be able to hop), but the level of control or the pattern used will be inappropriate. Thus the movement may be performed too fast with strong associated movements, or it may be slow and require considerable effort which results in excessive fatigue. The quality of movement is such that the child is referred to as immature in his movement, since the method of control is similar to that used by younger children. Very occasionally a child will present with clumsy movement without apparent major underlying abnormalities in tone, proprioception, vestibular or other sensorimotor systems, and this may be due to a central processing deficit.

In a similar way, fine motor incoordination is often the outcome of underlying problems. In particular, tactile and proprioceptive development essential for fast and accurate hand functions may be ineffective. Motor planning also plays a major role, as does background postural control. Ball-catching skills depend in part upon fine motor control, but also upon background body positioning and setting as well as experience, concentration and visual control. A problem at any of these levels will affect the ability to catch a ball.

Musculoskeletal Assessment

The strictly neurological components of assessment are not the only important aspects even when assessing children with a minor neurological condition. Many children with MCD also have musculoskeletal problems which may limit function and have specific implications for management.

At initial presentation, some clumsy children exhibit structural deformity such as scoliosis or foot abnormalities, or more commonly postural problems such as pronounced kyphosis, poked chin or poor sitting posture. These will be exacerbated in many who have limited range of movement due to tight mucles, fascia and joint capsule. It is quite common for children with MCD to have hamstrings

so tight that they cannot long sit (or sometimes even cross leg sit) without discomfort. Clinically this is often associated with tightness of the internal hip rotators and adductors. A compensatory exaggerated thoracic kyphosis may then develop in conjunction with increased lumbar flexion, particularly in sitting. In this position the line of the body weight falls behind the base of support, and there is over reliance on the hip flexors for sitting stability. This can contribute to increased restlessness and fidgeting in sitting, with consequences for classroom concentration. Clumsy children who present with tight hamstrings frequently have positive neural tension tests when the neck is flexed and foot dorsiflexed with the knee extended (Butler 1993). This has marked implications for treatment.

Problems of alignment such as at ankle/knee/hip are frequently seen, especially in conjunction with low or increased muscle tone, or with actual muscle weakness. The neurological picture may be compounded by orthopaedic factors such as differences in leg length, which must be simultaneously managed.

Associated Problems of MCD

VISUAL PROBLEMS

As well as having functional difficulties controlling the extraocular muscles, these children will have their share of intrinsic visual problems such as poor acuity, astigmatism, low vision and impairment. While these need to be managed by the ophthalmologist or in some cases the optometrist, the therapist needs to be aware of how they impinge on the child's physical function as well as on the therapist's treatment demands.

HEALTH

Sometimes MCD children will present with poor general health due to some other condition and the physiotherapy treatment offered will need to take this into account. For example, the child with MCD may also have problems associated with coeliac disease, asthma or pulmonary conditions, all of which will affect management of the MCD. Conditions such as epilepsy and asthma are relatively common, and diagnosis of ADHD is increasing. With the use of medication to control such problems, it is important that the physiotherapist knows what pharmacological therapy the child is undergoing. A common persisting problem which has marked implications for MCD children is middle ear infection. Studies have shown (Bullock and Watter 1987) that 37% of children with MCD have a history of chronic middle ear infection, with its implications for decreasing function throughout the day, poor attention and behavioural difficulties.

BEHAVIOUR

If you consider the problems that have been discussed as typical of children with MCD, and consider further that these children have normal intelligence, are trying to cope within the normal classroom and have normal expectations held for them, it becomes clear that some of them will be frustrated by the difficulties they encounter. Their lack of success whether it be at hopping, remembering or reading and writing, contributes to a lack of feeling of worth and poor self-confidence. These children may attract negative attention, or become reluctant to work and difficult to motivate. Some actually become aggressive, usually more markedly at home with their family members than with their school friends.

Attentional difficulties may be severe enough that the MCD child is classified as having ADHD, with behaviour being impulsive, restless, distractible and disruptive. Many children with MCD also display emotionally immature behaviours, with exaggerated reactions to ordinary situations. They are in general more labile emotionally than others, and this increases the difficulty of their management. Some will require medication to manage some elements of their behaviour, particularly those related to aggression and attention.

SPEECH AND HEARING

The therapist will encounter clumsy children who are also hearing impaired. Some of these impairments may be transient due to the effects of chronic middle ear infection, and will be expected to improve with appropriate management. In about one-third of children with MCD some concerns regarding speech development or speech problems will be expressed and will have had either assessment or treatment in this area at the time of initial physiotherapy assessment (Bullock and Watter 1987). Powell and Bishop (1992) also report on the overlap between speech and hearing problems and motor clumsiness. Difficulties with auditory figure/ground perception, short-term verbal memory and central processing as well as aphasias may all present in conjunction with clumsiness, and require specialized management by speech and language pathologists.

When assessing and treating children presenting with MCD or clumsiness it is important to realize that many progressive conditions involving deteriorating muscle or neurological conditions present initially with mild postural or movement problems.

Treatment of MCD

Objectives of treatment

The overall objective must be to improve the child's consistent function to as near normal as possible. Treatment aims to provide a normal sensory stimulus and at the same time facilitate the expected normal response to that input. Input to different systems occurring simultaneously allows comparison of information across the systems, and the processing of the multiple and sensorily confirmed input enhances the normality of the outcome. There is a progressive moulding of the child's response based on improved quality of experiences and improved intersensory linkages. The motor outcome imposes structure and organization on the incoming information. At the same time there is frequently a need to address the problems of muscle tightness, weakness and postural deformity.

As the processing of the sensory input improves and the quality of the output advances, more demanding activities in conjunction with a greater degree of cortical control and direction results in increasingly normal motor output. That translates for the child to improved functional motor skills. For some children the end-point of treatment is when their function has returned to within normal limits. Some children, however, do not reach normal performance levels, although they may be considered to have made considerable gains in function. They may continue to experience some degree of difficulty with specific types of tasks, or may have difficulties (such as musculoskeletal) which are to some degree growth dependent, and may therefore need more intermittent treatment.

General Principles of Treatment

Treatment requires active involvement of the child and (usually) the family. It may be possible in dysfunctional families to find others to carry out the programme. This could include a neighbour, teenage family friend, aunt or grandmother, or perhaps a school-based teacher aid. None of these may be ideal, but may be the only realistic option for treatment. It is most helpful if the person carrying out the programme has direct contact with the physiotherapist to avoid confusion in relaying of information. In some cases shared responsibility has been successful, but clear division of responsibility for specific aspects of the programme needs to be understood and negotiated between the two people sharing the supervision, and understood by the physiotherapist describing the activities. One of the issues that arises is that the children often develop a strong bond with the person/s carrying out the programme, so if one person is responsible, it is best if that person can be a parent.

In some situations unavailability or unwillingness of parents to carry out home-based programmes has led to schools initiating programmes under the guidance of therapists, but carried out by a variety of school-based personnel. Watter and Bullock (1989) have shown that school-based group treatment programmes produced significant gains for the children involved. In these situations, close direction was provided by the physiotherapist to the persons actually carrying out the programme, with regular review and update of the activities.

The dynamic nature of treatment is also reflected in the way activities are continually tailored to the developing abilities of the child to ensure s/he is optimally challenged and that progress is ongoing. Good communication between the therapist and parents enables the parents to understand the reason for selecting particular activities and the outcome aim. Dynamism and variety in treatment is then assured because the parents will frequently find interesting alternative activities which serve the original treatment goal.

Children with MCD have normal intelligence and have normal expectations held for them, as well as having normal expectations for themselves. Unlike children who are more physically disabled or in hospital for protracted periods, these children are normally active. They need active exciting and appropriately challenging activities in their treatment programme if they are to remain positive about the experience of physiotherapy treatment.

TREATMENT GUIDED BY ASSESSMENT

Carrying out the assessment provides the main information for formulating a treatment plan. Taking an adequate history may explain or highlight certain of the child's difficulties, and reveal how the problems noted during assessment affect the child in his daily life. In addition, the most important aspect of assessment is considering how the various problems interact with each other, and establishing which are the underlying factors and which are the outcomes of combined factors.

Once the problems and their relative importance have been ascertained, it is possible to plan a programme tailored to the specific needs of each child. This planning should be done in consultation with the child and parents, to ensure their needs as well as those of the therapist are met. The child's programme should then be reviewed regularly and updated or progressed so that the child is always optimally challenged.

At the same time it is usually necessary to prioritize activities given to avoid overloading the family or child. A good general guide might be to group exercises or activities under specific aims and list in the order of importance. Parents tend to cope well if activities are limited to no more than three separate aims, and can be completed in 10 minutes. The parents usually carry out the programme on at least 4 days each week, and in most cases appreciable gains are made before returning for review in one month. Plan activities which can take advantage of ordinary daily experiences. Some families need alternative activities listed for them, from which they may select a variety each day. The most important thing is to give clear instructions, demonstrate carefully and allow parents to practice techniques. Recognize the limitations of and pressures on each family group. It does not help a family if the treatment demands are too time-consuming, or if the child dislikes the games you have chosen. Avoid giving a generalized sensorimotor programme unless this is exactly what the child needs. Nonspecific treatment programmes can waste everyone's time and discredit physiotherapy.

FOCUS ON POSITIVE AND ADAPTIVE METHODS

In the management of children with MCD, accurate assessment and well-designed home programmes with patient/family compliance, should yield a good rate of progress. In the management of some specific problems there are considerable differences in approach from treating similar problems in neurologically more affected populations. A good example is the treatment of a child with strong persisting primitive movement patterns. In some children with cerebral palsy (CP) these patterns are frequently very strong and may severely limit the active movement of the child (Yokochi et al. 1993). Children with MCD are less limited by these immature movement patterns which tend to remain strong because the child is using them to provide antigravity stability, particularly in the presence of low postural tone. Rather than being physically limited to a position due to the primitive pattern, the child with MCD may use the pattern for improved function. In comparison to the more affected child with CP, the child with MCD moves more easily and quickly into and out of the immature pattern.

Where a child is using an ATNR or STNR pattern, treatment which just focuses on inhibition of the pattern may simply decrease the child's function. Inhibition is often easy in children with MCD, and the danger is that the inhibition which decreases the immaturely produced dynamic tone leaves the child without adequate postural antigravity extension. It is imperative then that the treatment focus is not on the negative (i.e. inhibit the unwanted), but rather is on the positive (i.e. facilitate the normal positive support with weight-shift reactions). If the resultant tone and supporting reactions are more normal, there will be decreasing reliance on the immature patterns to provide stability.

WORKING OR PLAYING?

The developmental physiotherapist manipulates a situation through tasks or games to expose the child to activities necessary to encourage the development or acquisition of particular skills. Children can be encouraged to compete against their own efforts or those of the therapist to enhance their participation in exercise activities. In general the child should enjoy the treatment programme which should be a positive experience for both child and family. Many parents also enjoy the extra time spent with their child when carrying out the home programme, and feel that they gain as a family through this interaction. If possible, the programme should accommodate the needs of other children in the family who may wish to be involved.

With older children a more cortically directed approach may be useful, as they like to be in charge of their own programme, with the parent helping only as needed. For those children who dislike activity, such as low tone children (who prefer to lie rather than sit, and sit rather than stand) reinforcement appropriate to the age of the child may be useful. In such cases a chart may be used, on which the child can tick off games as he participates, and trade a number of ticks for a negotiable reward after an agreed period of time. The aim here is to complete the activities essential to gain improvements, and with the child succeeding at carefully graded activities, to gradually improve the child's enjoyment of challenging activities. Success breeds success as well as improved behaviour and attitude.

Case Study 1

Ben, aged 5 years 6 months, has low tone posturally and at rest, poor protective and equilibrium reactions, and no vestibular head righting reactions. He is fearful of movement and does not like outdoor play at preschool, and will not climb or swing.

He can perform two hops and can balance on one leg for 3 seconds. How would you treat him and what do you do first?

The temptation for some physiotherapists is to practice what the child cannot do – that is practice hopping and standing on one leg. While this may lead to some initial gains, they are likely to be minimal overall and the gains will not necessarily transfer across to other activities or situations. Practising what Ben cannot do may also lead to considerable frustration and perhaps poor behaviour.

Consider instead what happens if you focus on analysing his problems. They amount to the following:

- Low tone and poor orientation in space (vestibular) and poor coping with displacement (protection and equilibrium). These imply that stability may be poor, meaning that movement does not occur from a stable base and is therefore likely to be poorly controlled.
- Poor weight-shift (and therefore positive support) may be associated with poor hip control (low tone and stability). This would explain the poor position for balancing and for hopping.
- Fear of heights and dislike of challenging movements are quite reasonable given the underlying problems.

The aims of any programme should be to improve confidence, postural tone, weight-shift and head righting. Ben is likely to be reluctant to start with games that challenge his balance, but might be happy to sit on your lap on a balance board or trampoline. In this position compression down through the head/shoulders would increase tone and cocontraction at the joints. Holding him so he is not scared you could gently rock side-to-side, and he could have hands down to facilitate compression through the arms which in turn may improve shoulder stability. The lateral movement would also stimu-

late head righting and weight-shift, as well as changes in postural tone. As he starts to enjoy making you rock – that is he initiates the movement – perhaps the game could develop into a 'boat in a storm' which would increase the range and variety of movement of the support. Ben may then need to change his position to rock the boat harder – for example, on to hands and knees or later, to high kneeling and standing.

Another approach could be needed if Ben was too scared to get on to a tilt board or trampoline. Perhaps he would get on to his hands and knees and pretend to be a rock and you a bulldozer. Then he would have to hold still while you tried to push him over (long slow pushes for stable holding first, little fast pushes for dynamic balance later). You might begin by giving 'heavy rain down on the rock' (compression at shoulders and hips) to improve cocontraction before lateral pushing. Positions can be advanced as gains are made. Having gained proximal postural stability then movement could be introduced against this improved background control.

Often when a child like Ben returns for his next visit, standing balance as well as hopping have improved, although no exercises targeting these specific areas have been included. Because he is more stable and postural control more normal, function begins to advance without specific exercises. An improved ability to cope with movement often means a readiness to try activities previously avoided. Progress next to games involving two feet jumping and stopping, changing directions, galloping and hopping. Ball games involving postural control while directing throwing or bouncing may also be helpful. Activities to help maintain the improved active tone might include trampoline, walking, swimming or water play, or simply increased play activity. Finally, include refinement of age-appropriate activities.

Referral and Treatment

There are some issues to be considered regarding referral and treatment which seem to present therapists with difficulties when they first begin working in this area.

Clinics situated within a hospital or health service tend to receive referrals which include children being followed up for reasons such as premature birth (Weisglas-Kuperus *et al.* 1994), or a head injury. Children with uncertain diagnoses who present clinically as exhibiting signs of MCD (at least initially) or perhaps as developmentally delayed, may also be referred from within the hospital. Such referrals tend to be couched in medical terms and the suspected problem is clearly indicated.

Clinics which operate in a community setting not apparently associated with a health service, receive more referrals from educational personnel, and their framework for referral as well as their terminology are quite different. When providing a service in a community setting, there is a specific responsibility on the physiotherapist to relate the educationally oriented problems causing concern to the likely neurological or musculoskeletal factors which may be involved.

Prioritizing in Treatment Programmes

Once a history has been taken, the referring problems discussed and the neurodevelopmental assessment completed, the physiotherapist should have a clear picture of the specific areas of dysfunction, their interrelationships and how they have produced the presenting problems. The next step is to decide what the most urgent priorities are, and which are underlying or basic difficulties. The age and needs of the child cannot be ignored when prioritizing for treatment programming, since if the older child perceives that his most urgent problem is not addressed he may not be compliant with treatment.

In consultation with both the child and parents and probably with input from the teacher, the physiotherapist needs to develop a clear plan of management which the family understands and agrees to adopt. Usually it is clear what needs to be done first, and this is frequently a combination of the

most basic or fundamental work and some specifically targeted work (such as hand function). If the child has other therapy needs, a joint management plan should be agreed upon by family and therapists to establish priorities, avoid duplication and provide most efficient time usage on home programmes.

Keeping the programme demands to manageable proportions is an important issue for all children. Resist overburdening the child and family, remembering that they have other commitments (possibly other therapy as well as their own occupation) and perhaps other children to organize. Give the family clear and precise instructions, teach them techniques and get them to show you if they are proficient, and explain how each activity will benefit the child. If you have done your job well many parents will return to show you how they have developed a treatment idea, adapted it to make it more difficult as the child progressed, or transferred the requirement to a new game. This is only possible if you have taken the time to ensure that they understand the nature of their child's problems and strengths, and the relevance of each activity.

The professional judgement and experience of the physiotherapist is also called upon in evaluating just how much and what depth of explanation the family can understand. Occasionally programmes have to be very simple due to limited understanding and some families may need more overall support than others. Most families manage to carry out excellent home programmes with good treatment outcomes for their child. Difficulties are regularly encountered when the parents have similar learning problems to their child and therefore cannot read a written programme (so use diagrams and printing rather than cursive writing), or for parents whose first language is not English. Good intentions of therapist and parent, and physical interaction usually help overcome such difficulties.

Case Study 2
Joshua is a 6-year-old boy (grade 1 at school) with low muscle tone (active and at rest), strong persisting primitive ATNR and extensor thrust. He is unstable in all positions even four-foot kneeling, and has poor fine and gross motor skills. The teacher is concerned

that he is not interested in writing and is falling rapidly behind his peers despite progressing well in reading and number concepts. Where do you start?

It is likely that the ATNR and extensor thrust patterns are being used to build up functional tone, and that if you merely focus on inhibiting them it may not help function. It seems likely that the shoulder girdle will be unstable with inconsistent trunk extension and stability, so just working on hands in isolation will not give satisfactory or consistent gains in hand function. Similarly, beginning with gross motor activities would provide limited advantages. Using a variety of techniques to improve functional tone, central and girdle stability, would seem a sensible place to start. As in previous examples, with the child in prone kneeling 'being a hard rock' and you being a 'bulldozer' it is possible to employ rhythmic stabilizations in a variety of directions, focusing on dynamic hip and shoulder control. Graded resistance permits weight-shift to be incorporated. Other techniques such as compression across joints or vertically through shoulder and hip to promote a strong positive supporting reaction may be needed. As control improves, progression to more active control and initiation may involve activities such as active rocking on a balance board or a trampoline, with increasing force and variability of movement demands.

The resultant improved stable holding can then be used in activities such as wheelbarrows and bridging to promote further shoulder girdle stability, and stimulate strong proprioceptive input through the arms. This will provide the background setting for more isolated wrist and finger activity. Similarly, such gains will also allow progression to gross motor activities. An initial home programme could include holding games in prone on elbows or kneeling, progressing to wheelbarrows, and to high and half kneeling positions. Ball games could be incorporated into these positions. The parents could be instructed how to do similar activities if a trampoline was available, and how to progress them. Balance games in sitting would stimulate postural tone and reactions as well as confidence. At the same time it may be appropriate to begin trying basic whole hand movements incorporated in preschool type hand games (tents, caterpillars, finger walks), progressing to games where the hands were hidden. Then encouraging Joshua to play pencil and paper games will be introduced to develop a more positive attitude to pencil activity and lead into prewriting patterns. Specific tactile and proprioceptive stimulation of fingers and wrists may also be needed.

Once he was stable, progression to games including gross motor patterns would be possible. The parents would need to be aware that low tone cannot be 'fixed' but should be addressed long-term by developing an active life style to boost functional tone.

Linking Problem Areas

Clinical experience as well as a sound theoretical knowledge allows the physiotherapist to link problems across areas. Understanding the nature of the links between concurrently developing systems and between early and later developing systems, allows us to appreciate which areas are likely to underlie others in terms of function and clinical significance. In addition, it clarifies how it is possible to affect functioning in one system by activating or stimulating another. For example, a child who has a disorienting reaction to the postrotatory nystagmus test can have the response inhibited by using strong compression to promote orientation of the body, overriding the vestibularly generated loss of postural control.

Progression of Treatment Programmes

Progression of treatment programmes occurs in several ways. If the child is improving then s/he will need increasingly challenging and diverse age-appropriate activities in those specific areas requiring attention, and the addition of further activities aimed at the other areas where problems were identified, but not initially addressed. It is important not to let the home programme simply expand with each treatment session. Achieved activities need to be omitted as more advanced ones are added.

Gains may occur with improvement in quality of performance of already developed but poorly managed skills, as well as in the acquisition of new skills. Progression of the programme is reflected in increasing demands for speed and ease of execution, flow and sequencing of movement as well as in the development of higher level or more complex skills and movement combinations.

CONCENTRATION DIFFICULTIES AND INCREASED ACTIVITY LEVELS

Many children with MCD present with difficulties directing and maintaining concentration, or display excessive levels of activity. This can be so severe that the physiotherapist is unable to carry out an adequate assessment, and the assessment can deteriorate into a 'first catch the child' situation. In such cases it may be necessary to address this issue before accurate sensorimotor assessment is possible. The physiotherapist may employ a range of inhibitory and behavioural techniques, and the child may be referred to a specialist in attentional problems who may employ a range of procedures from behaviour modification to medication.

With reference to inhibitory physiotherapy techniques, there are three main options as described next.

1. A Quietly Directive Approach. Slow inhibitory stroking down the limbs or body using firm whole hand pressure may be dramatically successful in settling the child. (In general, avoid the face and neck since these areas are more likely to evoke defensive or emotional responses, and ensure that the child will tolerate tactile input to distal extremities before moving on to more central and proximal areas.) Occasionally the child may respond to stimulatory tactile input to settle him and in these cases vibration or fast stroking up the limb and brushing may be more useful. Sometimes a combination of stroking and vibration will be particularly effective.

2. Use of Sensory Input. Use of compressive or resisting techniques which facilitate cocontraction around joints and therefore provide stability, are frequently a satisfactory way of reducing activity and aiding concentration. This is quite an unobtrusive method, and can be used in any social situation almost regardless of age. For example, the child could use activities like push-ups in his chair to help himself to settle in class.

3. Slow Rhythmic Movement. This is organizing in nature, and may have a side-effect of improving functional tone, which can further improve stability. The main sensory input involved is vestibular. Both linear and rotatory input can be inhibitory when slow, but are highly excitatory when performed fast.

Some children could be described as functionally underaroused and move excessively to increase their sensory feedback. Improving the processing of the sensory information, or providing increased input by stroking, rotating or compressing, may reduce the child's need to move himself, resulting in less movement and better concentration. When trying these techniques, it is usual to see an immediate effect in terms of better concentration or reduced activity, and the length of time the improvement lasts will vary from minutes to hours. If there is a negative or nil effect from such techniques, then it is wise to seek other alternatives.

Particular Considerations when Treating Adolescents

Teenagers are neither big children nor small adults. They come with their own specific problems, some of which are connected to hormonal and growth-related changes as well as the difficulty confronting ongoing problems in memory, writing, reading and coordination. Emotionally they are affected by their changing bodies. Relationships with their parents and sometimes therapists at times can be delicate.

Unlike treating younger children, a more cognitive approach needs to be adopted, but as far as possible a relaxed atmosphere and an element of fun should be maintained. Adolescents still enjoy competing against themselves, but finding age-appropriate and socially acceptable activities is a challenge. They need to feel in control of their own programme, and it should not be a source of added friction between themselves and their parents. If the teenager has no insight into or is unaccepting of the fact that he has a significant problem, then it may be best to wait for further maturation before offering treatment, since the parents and therapist will be unable to facilitate the programme if the teenager refuses to become involved. It is imperative that a physiotherapy programme does not cause a deterioration in parent/child relationships (important considering the incidence of behavioural problems) and direct negotiation between the teenager and the therapist will usually achieve the best results.

In teenagers the problems are usually much more specific than in younger children. A study of 35 teenagers and adults presenting for initial physiotherapy assessment (Watter and Bullock 1987) reported that these clients were highly specific in the type of problems cited as reasons for referral. Frequently they had entered what they perceived to be a crisis situation precipitating the request for assistance. The main reasons for referral included persisting writing difficulties (62%), poor short-term memory (30%), difficulty reading (41%) and poor gross motor coordination (30%). Interestingly, when assessed nearly all actually exhibited coordination difficulties although they no longer considered it a major issue. It is important to realize that these clients are frequently involved in secondary or tertiary education, and an inability to write fast enough to take lecture notes, or to read the volume of material expected has marked implications. It seems that the least distressing problem is that of gross motor skill, since by this age most have redirected their leisure activities into other more sedentary areas.

There are obvious differences in the type of activity the therapist will prescribe as part of a suitable programme compared with those designed for children. The sensorimotor requirements, however, for efficient writing, memory, coordination or reading are similar for both the 8-year-old and 18-year-old, although the method of acquiring them may differ.

When intervening with adults, it is important to appreciate that the pressures on their time are even greater than for teenagers, and that finding someone to help with a programme might be difficult. The need to prioritize treatment issues is paramount for these patients. Some will present also with a well-established personality disorder or blatant psychiatric condition, which will necessitate close consultation with their medical adviser. Clinical experience shows that those patients with a fully developed psychiatric condition gain little consistent improvement in their sensorimotor dysfunction with physiotherapy management.

Case Study 3

A 13-year-old from a country centre is referred because of severe writing difficulties, poor short-term memory, continuing reading problems and clumsy movements. He is in a special year 8 class at school which concentrates only on core subjects for the year in an attempt to make the reading, writing and mathematics functional for high school. Depending on his progress, next year he will go to a normal high school class. His family is supportive, but his parents are elderly; there is some friction due to this. He spends 3 hours each day travelling to school and home.

Consider the following:

- *Is this family suitable for a home programme?*
- *Do you need to consider other avenues of providing the therapy necessary?*
- *What might these include?*
- *If he had poor hand/arm proprioception, poor lumbrical control, poor sequential finger 'drumming' movements and poor*

pencil control, what exercises would you prescribe? How would they differ from those you might give to a 7-year-old?

Common Problems when Treating MCD

INADEQUATE OR SLOW IMPROVEMENT

Generally speaking children with MCD should show major improvement in function within 6 months of commencing treatment using a home programme with monthly review. In addition regular progress throughout this period should be demonstrable, at least in the areas being treated. If this is not forthcoming consideration must be given as to why the progress is slow. Reasons fall into three main groups: therapist based, diagnosis and child/family based.

THERAPIST-BASED REASONS

Good assessments require skilled specific assessment techniques, and sound knowledge of developmental stages as well as clinical experience of these children. If the physiotherapist is not experienced in carrying out developmental sensorimotor assessments, it is easy for some elements of the whole problem to be missed resulting in areas of difficulty not being addressed. If these underpin other areas receiving treatment then limited or transient gains may be seen.

Some therapists prescribe only broadly based or non-specific programmes, which may result in limited improvement and parent dissatisfaction. While younger children may need some broadly based activities, they must always be well planned, target particular areas of need, and progress to the more specific.

A problem noted with early global sensory motor programmes was that overstimulation resulted in overexcited and poorly controlled children and such non-specific programmes have been largely phased out. 'Sensorimotor' programmes now tend to be more achievement directed with specific aims in mind rather than having stimulation as the object.

If the physiotherapist concentrates too much on the cognitive level when underlying problems have not been effectively addressed, then limited gains or splinter skills may be the outcome.

CHILD/FAMILY-BASED REASONS

The child and family must respect the physiotherapist's professional skills and trust his/her judgement as to what their child needs. In turn the therapist must respect the right of the family to know, understand and approve what is being done. A good and open relationship between family/child and therapist allows the family to tell you exactly what is happening at home, rather than what they think you might want to hear. There are many normal situations which arise in any family which can interrupt the programme, and the therapist needs to know accurately which of the recommended activities are being done to gauge the effectiveness of the programme plan and to adjust it accordingly.

Some children become manipulative during therapy, imposing demands in return for cooperation. Putting the child and parent into direct confrontation should always be avoided. If confrontation occurs it may mean finding another person to carry out the programme or waiting until the child has a little more maturity and can cope better. As mentioned earlier some children will cope best if they own their programme, only needing a little support from parents.

Motor control of the child with MCD deteriorates faster than others when sick (e.g. upper respiratory infection) or under stress such as growth or emotional factors. Performance during such times can be variable and it is important that this is acknowledged by both parent and therapist. Explanations of such factors to the child often go a long way towards reducing anxiety.

DIAGNOSIS

Children with other sometimes progressive disorders or global developmental delay present as clumsy and assessment may appear to confirm MCD. Failure to progress as expected should alert the professionals involved to the possibility of another diagnosis.

CEASING TREATMENT TOO EARLY

Older children, teenagers and younger children with limited or specific problems may exhibit significant improvement in a short period of time, such as 4–6 weeks. Such rapid resolution of problems can be dramatic, but most children with a definite problem will need at least a short period of consolidation of gains or at least one more monthly review before discharge. The aim is to have as near normal and automatic function as possible, and too rapid withdrawal of treatment may lead to regression of gains achieved. Younger children with improved function may still need to be reviewed at critical periods when further rapid development of new skills normally occurs.

REFERENCES

Bairstow, PJ, Laszlo, JI (1981) Kinaesthetic sensitivity to passive movements in children and adults, its relationship to motor development and motor control. *Developmental Medicine and Child Neurology* 23: 606–616.

Bullock, MI, Watter, P (1978) A study of the effectiveness of physiotherapy in the management of young children with minimal cerebral dysfunction. *Australian Journal of Physiotherapy* 24(3): 111–119.

Bullock, MI, Watter, P (1987) A review of the histories of children with minimal cerebral dysfunction. *Australian Journal of Physiotherapy* 33: 145–149.

Burns, YR, (1992) *NSMDA. Physiotherapy Assessment for Infants and Young Children*, 48 pp. Brisbane: CopyRight Publishing.

Burns, YR, Watter, P (1974) Identification and developmental assessment of children with neurological impairment. *Australian Journal of Physiotherapy* 20: 5–14.

Burns, YR, Ensbey, RM, Norrie, MA (1989) The neuro-sensory motor developmental assessment Part I: Development and administration of the test. *Australian Journal of Physiotherapy* 35(3): 141–149.

Butler, T (1993) An investigation of the slump and straight leg raise neural tension tests in seven and eight year old normal children, and males with Minimal Cerebral Dysfunction. Honours thesis, University of Queensland.

Gillberg, IC, Gillberg, C (1989) Children with preschool minor neuro-developmental disorders. IV: Behaviour and school achievement at age 13. *Developmental Medicine and Child Neurology* 31: 3–13.

Hadders-Algra, M, Huisjes, HJ, Touwen, BC (1988) Pre-term or small-for-gestational age infants. Neurological and behavioural correllates at the age of 6 years. *European Journal of Pediatrics* 147: 460–467.

Hadders-Algra, M, Touwen, BC (1992) The long term significance of neurological findings at toddlers age. *Paediatric Grenzgeb* 28: 93–99.

Henderson, SE (1987) The assessment of 'clumsy' children: old and new approaches. *Journal of Child Psychology and Psychiatry* 28: 511–527.

Herrgard, E, Luoma, L, Tuppurainen, K et el. (1993) Neurodevelopmenatal profile at five years of children born at ≤ 32 weeks gestation. *Developmental Medicine and Child Neurology* 35: 1083–1096.

Hulme, C, Lord, R (1986) Clumsy children – a review of recent research. *Child: Care Health and Development* 13: 361–376.

Laszlo, JI, Bairstow, PJ, Bartip, J (1988) A new approach to treatment of perceptual-motor dysfunction previously called 'clumsiness'. *Support for Learning* 3: 35–40.

Lynch, MR, Raymer, ME, Elvery, JH (1992) The development of hand position sense. *New Zealand Journal of Physiotherapy* April: 15–20.

Powell, RP, Bishop, DV (1992) Clumsiness and perceptual problems in children with specific language impairment. *Developmental Medicine and Child Neurology* 34: 755–765.

Smyth, TR (1992) Impaired motor skill (clumsiness) in otherwise normal children: a review. *Child: Care Health Development* 18: 283–300.

Steele, C (1994) Anticipatory postural reactions in clumsy children. Master of Physiotherapy Thesis, University of Queensland.

van Dellen, T, Geuze, RH (1988) Motor response processing in clumsy children. *Journal of Child Psychology and Psychiatry* 29: 489–500.

van der Meulen, JHP, Denier van der Gon, JJ, Gielen, CCAM et al. (1991a) Visuomotor performance of normal and clumsy children. I: fast goal-directed arm-movements with and without visual feedback. *Developmental Medicine and Child Neurology* 33: 40–54.

van der Meulen, JHP, Denier van der Gonn, JJ, Gielen, CCAM et al. (1991b) Visuomotor performance of normal and clumsy children. II: arm-tracking with and without visual feedback. *Developmental Medicine and Child Neurology* 33: 118–129.

Watter, P (1982) Neurodevelopmental physiotherapy for MCD: its effect on educational progress. Master of Physiotherapy Thesis, University of Queensland.

Watter, P (1984) Assessment for neurodevelopmental physiotherapy for minimal cerebral dysfunction. In: Levitt, S (ed). *Paediatric Developmental Therapy*, pp. 153–163. London: Blackwell Scientific.

Watter, P, Bullock, MI (1983) Developmental physiotherapy for children with both minimal cerebral dysfunction and learning difficulties. *Australian Journal of Physiotherapy* 29(2): 53–59.

Watter, P, Bullock, MI (1987) Patterns of improvement in neurological functioning of children with minimal cerebral dysfunction. *Australian Journal of Physiotherapy* 33: 215–224.

Watter, P, Bullock, MI (1989) Minimal cerebral dysfunction in adults. *Australian Journal of Physiotherapy* 35: 239–244.

Weisglas-Kuperus, N, Baerts, W, Fetter, WPF et al. (1994) Minor neurological dysfunction and quality of movement in relation to neonatal cerebral damage and subsequent development. *Developmental Medicine and Child Neurology* 36: 727–735.

Williams, HG, Woollacott, MH, Ivry, R (1992) Timing and motor control in children. *Journal of Motor Behaviour* 24(2): 165–172.

Yokochi, K, Shimabukuros, S, Kodamam, M et al. (1993) Motor function of infants with athetoid cerebral palsy. *Developmental Medicine and Child Neurology* 35: 909–916.

Section H:

Dealing with Living

Prologue

YVONNE BURNS

Often the circumstances and / or types of impairment with which a child lives and grows can limit the range of opportunities and experiences or length of life able to be enjoyed. This does not mean that there can be no quality of life. The physiotherapist has much to offer in many of these situations. Sometimes, however, it is difficult for those who have grown up in a safe, stable, happy and healthy environment to envisage childhood in a vastly different context.

This section introduces a few challenging situations highlighting some of the differing roles, skills and philosophies which the physiotherapist may need to uphold. Severe and often multiple disability is an area where the physiotherapist can play quite an extensive, but often complex role with children, families and co-workers.

Working with infants, children and young people with acquired or congenital diseases or disorders which reduce life expectancy requires other special knowledge and attitudes. It is important to be able to accept anger and grieving, understand denial, recognize depression, encourage acceptance and provide appropriate support.

Social, psychological and physical factors which adversely affect the family structure and interpersonal relationships can interfere with the well-being of one or more of the children in that family and limit the child's ability to establish normal patterns of development. The after-effects of abuse and non-accidental trauma can be long-term. In many countries, unfortunately, the incidence of these types of problems is widespread and physiotherapists are often uniquely placed to help identify, prevent and also assist in the management of the problems.

In a world where poverty, unrest and outright war is widespread there are a number of other reasons why the growth, development and opportunities for independence of the child with special needs may be very limited. Whatever the challenges, whether a lack of professional, financial, physical or social resources, it is amazing what initiative, local knowledge and a clear idea of principles of therapeutic management can achieve.

23

Severe, Multiple and Long-term Disability

ANN WRIGHT

Effects of Specific Impairments
•
Assessment
•
Aims of Physiotherapy
•
Programme Management

Severe impairment in any area, be it physical, intellectual, visual or auditory, will have a marked impact on the developmental progress of a child. With a combination of such impairments, the impact on the child's life is compounded in a way that is much more than the sum of the individual impairments would have been. The child with limited function due to severe physical or neurological problems and poor understanding of and reduced ability to interact with their environment because of visual, auditory or intellectual difficulties has very special needs.

Most commonly, the underlying neurological deficit is as a result of cerebral palsy, acquired brain damage from trauma or infection, or one of a variety of genetically based syndromes. The manifestations of cerebral palsy and acquired brain damage are covered in detail in an earlier chapter, and will only be briefly mentioned here. Rather, the issues raised from the severe, multiple and long-term nature of this disability will be explored, with the focus on how the physiotherapist can contribute to the challenge

facing the child and their family of living life in the most positive way, despite their disability.

The first and most important step in responding to this challenge is to accept and respect the child as an individual. Despite the degree of disability, every child still has a dignity to be safeguarded, potential to be explored, and the capacity to experience and respond to people and their environment. Expectations and attitudes are important, as is a focus on abilities, rather than disabilities. All children can learn, grow and develop, although the rate of change for this population may be extremely slow, and the amount of change small. The ultimate aims of the professional's involvement in the child's programme is to maximize the potential for function, development, learning and enjoyment of life.

Extent of Disability

SEVERE DISABILITY
Severe impairment, especially if physical or multiple involves high support needs, for every aspect of daily life. These range from the physical in providing tools

437

and equipment for bathing, toileting, seating, mobility, transport and lifting as the child grows older, to the more complex areas of educational, social and emotional support. The implications for the child's family in terms of time, financial cost and quality of life are vast. That governments and the community must bear some of this responsibility has only recently been accepted.

MULTIPLE DISABILITY

Arguably the most profound disability resulting from multiple impairment, especially that involving hearing impairment and/or visual impairment is a lack of two-way communication, that is the ability to express needs and respond to people and the environment. Wyman (1986) notes that parents describe communication difficulties with their children with severe and multiple disabilities as being the most difficult and distressing problem. The eventual outcome of this difficulty for the child can often be extreme passivity and lack of motivation to attempt interaction.

LONG-TERM DISABILITY

The long-term nature of these impairments, combined with the lack of active movement and the oft encountered difficulties with maintaining appropriate motivation over time, mean that these children have a high potential for developing secondary complications. If not dealt with early enough, these will increase the child's disability and the difficulty for carers and professionals involved in looking after the child's needs and assisting their development. Most commonly, complications occur in the orthopaedic, respiratory and behavioural areas:

- Orthopaedic: muscle contractures, skeletal deformity, joint dislocation, fractures
- Medical: respiratory, malnutrition, gastrointestinal, skin lesions, obesity
- Behavioural: withdrawal, self-stimulation, antisocial behaviour

Some Key Issues

Passivity — lack of interaction with the environment

Making sense — awareness and interpretation of sensory input
Communication — receptive and expressive
Choices — decision-making, sense of control of own environment
Motivation — to act and interact, use of rewards and reinforcers

The programming needs for these children are complex and involve the close cooperation of a multidisciplinary team, with parents as major partners. It is the parents who usually know their child's abilities, responses and needs extremely well, and this knowledge is vital in determining priorities.

PASSIVITY

The problems of passivity are a common concern. Many of these children use little spontaneous active movement, tend not to interact with the people and the world around them, and lack the motivation to explore and actively act on their own environment. It is important to remember that a child will not be motivated to manipulate and interact with his environment if he does not know that it exists, or it is highly confusing and makes little sense to him. The difficulties that the child with severe and multiple impairment has in making sense of the world and beginning to respond to it are enormous.

AWARENESS AND COMMUNICATION

Development of meaningful communication is fundamental to successful interaction, and involves both the ability to be aware of the surroundings and other people's communications (receptive) and the ability to express needs, feelings or preferences (expressive). Early receptive communication involves the awareness of, and later interpretation of, sensory input (usually sound, touch or light). Early expressive communication involves prelanguage vocalizations, facial expressions or physical gestures. Appropriate responses from those around to the young child's early attempts at communication are an important factor in its continuation and expansion. Establishing a basis for this interaction is not only fundamental to the child's social and cognitive development, but is also the basis of their interest and motivation in active exploration, including participation in and response to any physiotherapy programme.

Rapid advances in technology are providing exciting opportunities to facilitate a child's communication and interaction with the environment, although sometimes 'low tech' alternatives are just as useful. It is important that the physiotherapist is both aware of and involved in the team decision-making in this fundamental area. Basically, the team needs to consider what stimuli the child is most responsive to (e.g. tactile, visual, auditory or multisensory), and what responses or motor output are under their consistent voluntary control, so that these may be used as a basis for interaction.

CHOICES

Over time, it is possible for the child with severe and multiple disability (SMD) to develop the extra handicap of learnt helplessness, if interactions and actions are always facilitated by others. In order to exert some control over their environment, the experience of choice and encouragement of decision-making is important. The team, including the physiotherapist, need to focus on means to encourage more active, exploratory, interactive behaviour, as children will always learn more by acting on the environment themselves. The challenge is in setting up situations from the earliest days, so that active and independent responses are required. Technology again offers wonderful opportunities for communicating choices and manipulating the environment, but 'low tech' situations such as Nielsen's 'active learning' equipment also offer such possibilities (Nielsen 1992).

MOTIVATION

Motivation is often a key factor in the success of a physiotherapy programme with these children. The rewards of activity itself, or even the pleasure of social approval may not be sufficiently motivating to overcome the difficulties (and sometimes fear) involved in movement.

With technological assistance, it is possible to devise switches to give immediate sensory rewards for a wide variety of active responses, limited in many cases only by the imagination of the therapy team involved in devising such switches. Vibration, sound, patterns of light, videos or the activation of a toy which may combine some of these can be used as rewards. With reinforcement, it is important that even a minimal response should be rewarded as the child's contribution to the current interaction, as success breeds interest and enthusiasm. Some of these children have a prolonged delay in the transmission of auditory or visual input as evidenced by EEG recording, and some time may need to be allowed for responses (Rushfirth 1984). When determining optimum conditions to help the child make an active response, it is important to only alter one small variable at a time (e.g. position or type of seating or switch), so that a systematic recording is available on which to base further decisions.

Consideration of these important issues takes time, patience and trial and error on the part of all who are involved with the child, including the physiotherapist, but it is time well spent in the long term. Too much input before the child begins to make some sense of the world, and establish some form of meaningful communication; or before establishing what the child is aware of, responds to, likes or dislikes, may mean withdrawal, or negative, unmotivated behaviour. This is neither conducive to the child's development nor the success of any therapeutic programme that has been instigated.

Effects of Specific Impairments

The interrelationship of these impairments, and specifically their impact on physiotherapy management, is easiest to understand by addressing each individually. A variety of combinations of impairments are encountered in this group of children, so that the problems and needs of each child must be considered on an individual basis. Because most children who are conventionally termed blind or deaf have some residual vision or hearing, the terms visual impairment (VI) and hearing impairment (HI) are used in preference.

Visual Impairment

Vision is the primary motivational force for movement, exploration and learning in the child (Levitt

1984, Jones 1988). Its presence facilitates the development of head righting, reaching, rolling, crawling and manipulation. The non-verbal aspects of communication such as eye contact and facial expression are important in the development of early two-way communication. Intact vision gives a permanence and security to the surrounding world, and encourages interaction with it through communication and activity. Even in isolation, visual impairment often results in developmental difficulties in gross and fine motor areas, as well as some other aspects of development.

COMMON DEVELOPMENTAL DIFFICULTIES

For a child with visual impairment, developmental difficulties will include:

- decreased motivation to explore by reaching and moving
- fear of movement, spatial insecurities
- absence of visual head righting
- poor development of body and spatial awareness
- slow development of postural and righting responses
- dislike of prone position, often slow to develop neck and shoulder stability
- tendency to fixate in stable positions such as sitting, with little rotation or movement
- less exploratory movement, therefore diminished sensorimotor experiences
- delayed gross motor milestones, may not crawl, slow to walk
- may be tactile defensive
- may be delayed fine motor manipulation, transfer, index poking and supination
- delayed development of some concepts such as causality and object permanence

The significance of visual impairment on a child's development will vary according to the severity and the underlying reason for it. In the population of children with severe physical impairment of neurological aetiology, there is a high incidence of visual disorders. A variety of deficits may be involved, such as refractive errors, retinal abnormalities, strabismus, oculomotor dyspraxia or cortical visual impairment. In this population, even moderate visual dysfunction will have a significant effect on the child's development and the approach taken to management of their physical difficulties.

CORTICAL VISUAL IMPAIRMENT

Vision impairment cannot be assumed to remain static, but can vary over time, with changes in arousal level, or even with alterations in the child's position or movement. Children with cortical visual impairment (CVI), once called cortical blindness and thought to be fixed and absolute, have now been shown to have visual abilities that fluctuate considerably, confirming what many people working with these children have long felt to be the case. Many of these children may gain improvement in their visual function over time (Good et al. 1994). The prognosis is dependent on the severity and time of the original insult, and the availability and type of intervention. If improvement in the first 2.5 years is obtained, further improvement may occur for up to 7 years. If no change, other than light perception or awareness of bright colours, as evidenced by stilling or blinking, is noted in the first 2.5 years, further improvement is unlikely (Crossman 1992).

The behavioural characteristics of children with cortical visual impairment will include the following (adapted from Crossman 1992):

- does not look blind
- lacks visual curiosity, and is visually inattentive
- visual abilities fluctuate considerably
- peripheral vision often more functional, tends to look away from visual interest
- attends better to moving objects
- sees better in familiar environments
- visually tires easily, spontaneously uses vision for short periods only
- identifies bright colour, particularly red and yellow, more easily than shape
- when moving, can be aware of and negotiate stationary objects
- in overstimulating environments, may tune into touch or hearing to the exclusion of vision
- appears to balance better when eyes are closed

VISUAL TRAINING

Visual function in a child with low vision from causes other than CVI, can also improve over time, as the functional use of residual sight can be enhanced through visual training. Needless to say, baseline assessment of visual function in this population can be very difficult. Michael and Paul (1991) suggest that visual training may be needed in order to get a true picture of the range of a child's functional visual abilities from assessment. Visual function may also deteriorate over time in the case of some genetic syndromes (e.g. Ushers) or in the presence of neurological deterioration (e.g. a tumour).

Visual training programmes are organized from a developmental perspective and incorporated into all aspects of the child's day as visual learning does not occur in isolation, but needs tactile and motor input to verify visual feedback. Knowledge of the principles involved in visual training is useful for the physiotherapist so that the child's ability to use residual vision optimally can be reinforced within the therapy programme. The fact that visual function varies in different positions is an especially important consideration when determining a physiotherapy programme. Abnormal tone and stereotyped movement patterns can affect oculomotor control, in the same way that it affects motor function elsewhere in the body.

PRACTICAL SUGGESTIONS

When interacting with a child with visual impairment:

- Explain or warn of your approach with a constant sign (voice or touch if deaf/blind).
- Make sure vision aids are used appropriately (clean lenses used in the correct position).
- The attainment of head righting and a stable sitting position is important, as it optimizes the child's ability to use their full visual field.
- It is better during physiotherapy to avoid holding the child's hands during movement activities, and not to place objects into their hands (their hands are their 'eyes', so to hold their hands is to blindfold them (Neilsen 1990)).
- Any sensory cues given to facilitate movement must be very clear and specific.
- Nystagmus which is common with low vision is often increased with stress.
- Unusual head positions may need to be accepted,

as the child may use these to obtain the best visual field, or the null point for nystagmus.

- Encourage appropriate use of vision during therapy activities, that is, to look, fixate or track (sometimes movement and vision control together may be too difficult.)
- When vision is necessary for a task and oculomotor control is a problem, be aware of the 'critical visual moment' of the task when vision will be required (Geniale 1991).
- Consider the effect of glare, colours and contrasts. For some conditions, it is easier to see in diffuse light. Black and white patterns, colours of red or yellow, or bright fluorescent colours, in simple shapes such as faces against an uncluttered, but contrasting background may be easier to see.
- The height or tilt of the work area may need to be raised to bring it as close to the eyes as the child chooses.
- Minimization of background noise is necessary, as the child will rely heavily on auditory feedback to give clues about their environment and their actions within it.

Hearing Impairment

The impact of a prelingual hearing loss on a child will vary greatly depending on the type (sensorineural or conductive), the pattern and degree of loss (as demonstrated on an audiogram), the child's other abilities or disabilities, and the stage at which the loss is diagnosed and intervention begun. Early use of appropriate auditory aids, and instigation of a two-way communication system via simultaneous signing and audition (total communication) is very important, not only for language and communication, but also for the child's social and cognitive development.

In a child with a severe and multiple disability, any hearing loss is often missed, or diagnosed very late. Lack of response to auditory cues is often assumed to be an intellectual impairment, or due to the severity of the child's physical impairment. Assessment of the degree of hearing impairment, necessary for the prescription of auditory aids, is often very difficult with this population. Even if not actually hearing impaired, the child with severe visual impairment and other disabilities may function with limited auditory awareness as he knows little of the world.

Because of the commonality of the vestibulocochlear nerve, with a sensorineural hearing loss of neurological aetiology, accompanying vestibular dysfunction is often present. This may be either peripheral dysfunction or a sensory processing difficulty. Either way, this may affect the child's physical development in the areas of righting responses to gravity, balance reactions and postural muscle tone.

PRACTICAL SUGGESTIONS

When interacting with a child with hearing impairment:

- The communication or signing system decided on should be reinforced by all.
- Check that hearing aids are turned on, batteries working and fitting well (i.e. not whistling). Daily testing is required as a lack of response may not be readily apparent.
- Background noise should be minimized. Unless a frequency modulated radio aid is used, the interference effect of background noise is amplified with aids on.
- Speak at a normal volume as hearing aids are adjusted to respond to normal speech.
- If total communication is used, make sure the child can see your hands and face clearly, and minimize the effect of glare.
- A stable head and seating position will optimize the child's use of hearing as well as vision. Their eyes are their ears, so that full use of their visual field including peripheral vision is important.
- Facilitation of independent head control and upright mobility can help children tolerate their hearing aids. Aids whistle when the child is creeping or rolling on the floor, and if a head support is needed, it can interfere with hearing.
- The position of vibrotactile aids when used for a profound hearing loss has to be considered so that auditory feedback is maximized with minimal interference to mobility. Common sites are on the sternum or on the wrist.

Dual Sensory Impairment

Children with dual sensory impairment are often labelled as deaf–blind. Because of difficulties in establishing effective communication systems with these children, accurate assessment of the degree of actual visual or hearing impairment is often not possible in the early years. Michael and Paul (1991) maintain that few of these children are totally deaf or totally blind. Up to 94% have some residual vision or residual hearing, but may not receive adequate early training in using these senses effectively.

If sensations from these primary 'distance' senses are impaired, the child has to rely on the secondary senses (tactile, proprioceptive, vestibular, olfactory and gustatory) for important additional sources of information about the environment. These do not necessarily improve in order to compensate, in fact some may also be dysfunctional if the child has additional disabilities. Obviously for a child with severe visual impairment, especially if combined with a hearing loss, interpretation of tactile information is vital for communication, either through some form of braille or deaf / blind signing, or use of a vibrotactile aid for a child with profound hearing loss.

When a child has either a severe hearing or visual impairment, even a mild loss in the other area will seriously affect his ability to function. A conductive hearing loss from a simple middle ear effusion will completely disorientate a child with severe visual impairment. Similarly, if glasses have been prescribed for a child with severe hearing impairment, the use of scratched or dirty glasses that do not stay in place will mean poor understanding of visual communication and thus motivation for interaction.

Intellectual Impairment

Intellectual ability is often an unknown factor in a child with severe and multiple disability, especially if this includes a dual sensory loss. As tests of cognition rely on some form of receptive and expressive communication, the true intellectual ability of these children may often be revealed by observation of their behaviour over many years as the child develops. It cannot be assumed in the early years that a lack of adaptive responses to the environment is due to severe intellectual impairment.

Progress in early stages of cognitive development is extremely slow for a child with SMD. Visual impairment will delay the development of object permanence and imitative learning. Hearing impairment can affect the development of causality or anticipation of events. Even severe physical disability alone may delay some conceptual developments, if the child cannot reach or manipulate the environment. Although with a widespread neurological insult intellectual ability may be severely impaired, it may also be within the normal range though delayed. Conversely, if a child does have a severe intellectual impairment, assessment of the degree of any visual or hearing impairment will be difficult and only take place over a period of time. Inconsistency of responses is a distinguishing factor of severe intellectual impairment (Rushfirth 1984).

Although determination of the degree of visual, auditory or intellectual ability is the primary function of other team members, as part of the team the physiotherapist must be aware of these underlying difficulties, and not make unfounded assumptions of either ability or disability in the early years of interaction with the child. Because the physiotherapist may be heavily involved with the child's physical development in the early stages, acute observation of the child's responses to touch, movement, light and sound may give valuable information to the team regarding these other abilities.

If a child has severe intellectual impairment, even with reasonable vision and hearing, their responses may still present a challenge for the physiotherapist in the assessment and management of any physical difficulties (Bertoti 1989). These children may react adversely to unfamiliar situations or people, so that a true picture of their function may be difficult to obtain, except by observation over time. They may dislike or fear the sensory experiences involved in touch or handling. They may have poor understanding of directions, or be unable to give adequate verbal feedback. Motivation and compliance with activities may be difficult to obtain if 'challenging' behaviour is present.

PRACTICAL SUGGESTIONS

When interacting with a child with intellectual impairment:

- Instructions whether verbal or signed should be clear and simple, involving only one step at a time.
- Repetition of the instruction or task in a different way, or broken down into parts may be required.
- Motivation is an important factor for continued activity. Behaviour modification principles may need to be applied (Rushfirth 1984).
- Appropriate reinforcements may be needed, such as vibration, controlled vestibular input, music, food or hugs. Take care that these do not reinforce inappropriate behaviour.
- More cooperation may be obtained in group situations, especially music and movement groups where the child may copy appropriate movements and behaviour.

Physical Impairment

In children with severe physical impairment, limited active movement may be due to sensory as well as motor dysfunction. This must be remembered by the physiotherapist in attaining the goal of voluntary movement. Lack of active movement, with the resultant deprivation of normal sensorimotor experiences and feedback will affect the development of body and spatial awareness. This will further exacerbate any sensory dysfunction that is a result of the original neurological insult.

SENSORY DYSFUNCTION

The existence of a general sensory modulation disorder, in which sensory registration and responsiveness can be viewed as a continuum with 'sensory dormancy', or hyposensitivity at one end and 'sensory defensiveness', or hypersensitivity at the other has been suggested (Royeen and Lane 1991). Under this description, it is possible to include not only tactile defensiveness, but also vestibular, auditory or visual defensiveness. Some children are defensive in all areas of sensory input, some in only a few. Certainly, this would describe commonly seen clinical pictures of children with severe and multiple disability who dislike touch, handling or movement through space, and who often react adversely to too much auditory or visual input. At the other end of this extreme are children with observable hyposensitivity to touch and sometimes to all forms of sensory input. Fluctuations in sensitivity within the one child are also clinically seen in this population.

As well as problems with modulation of tactile sensation, many children with severe and multiple disability also have poor tactile discrimination. Body awareness occurs initially through active exploration, such as hands to mouth, to midline, and later to feet. These activities will be very limited in children with severe physical problems, unless they are consciously encouraged when planning intervention, and as a result these children may have limited or bizarre body image (Rushfirth 1984). The mouth is one of the more precise tactile discriminators in infants, and knowledge about the qualities of objects comes from mouthing (Royeen and Lane 1991). Nielsen (1993) stresses the importance of midline mouthing for exploration in children with severe visual and multiple disability, and the need for assistance in its development if that stage has not been attained. Active exploration of the body and mouthing should be seen as only a stage of development to be eventually discarded. Because of the extreme slowness of development, however, in many cases this stage lasts for much longer than normal. A fear of the child getting locked into patterns of self-stimulation, could lead some clinicians to overlook the important developmental tasks of this stage.

Both tactile defensiveness and impaired tactile discrimination are important to assess and address in the overall management of a child with severe and multiple disability, because of the manner in which they interfere with all levels of interaction and hence learning as well as movement development.

INFLUENCE OF SEVERE PHYSICAL IMPAIRMENT ON OTHER SENSES

Severe physical impairment alone has implications for other areas of development, including optimal function of vision and hearing. In particular, the physiotherapist must be aware of the effect of the continued influence that primitive reflexes and difficulties with the development of head righting, inde-

pendent sitting or active movement will have on these areas.

Stereotyped Movement Patterns. These can have the same effect on oculomotor control as on other movements of the body (e.g. ATNR affects visual examination of objects held, TLR affects both head position and eye movement control). Lack of dissociation between head and eyes interferes with oculomotor control. For example, as the child extends their head to look, the pattern of extension is associated with elevation of the eyes, and vice versa when head is flexed, thereby limiting ability to use vision functionally (Geniale 1991).

Poor Head Control. The child who has difficulty maintaining head stability may have problems learning to fixate, follow or scan with the eyes. Lateral head supports can inhibit the use of visual field and hearing.

Inability to Sit Independently. Sitting allows a wider visual field. When moving around on the floor, hearing aids whistle or come out, and it is difficult to wear a vibrotactile aid.

Lack of Active Movement. Sensory feedback and interpretation may be dysfunctional. Difficulty interacting with the environment can limit exploration, experimentation and sensorimotor experiences. Lack of experiences may interference with body awareness, spatial relations and perceptual development.

Assessment

The importance and role of assessment has already been stressed in Chapter 7. The particular difficulties and concerns experienced when assessing the child with SMD will be covered briefly here. Assessment will be a team affair as an holistic picture of the child's abilities, needs and range of responses will be needed to prioritize goals and plan programmes.

The goals need to be achievable, yet offer some challenge. For example, Wyman (1986) emphasizes that although a child's achievements are dependent upon his/her physical and/or intellectual abilities, all children are capable of underfunctioning. This writer suggests that parental and societal attitudes and reactions can either limit or extend a child's achievements.

The goals that the physiotherapist sees as important may at various times in the child's life not be the primary concern of the family and the team. Many times, however, the physiotherapist who is sensitive to the overall concerns and needs of the child is able to adapt a treatment approach so that physiotherapy issues are addressed whilst meeting the primary concerns of the family.

The purpose of the assessment must be clear. Is the physiotherapist looking for typical performance or for optimal performance, that is the best that a child is capable of doing? Assessment of the child's typical performance in their usual environment is necessary to gain a true picture of their function, so that changes over time can be monitored and potential secondary complications can be identified and prevented.

Awareness of optimal performances can be useful in setting achievable goals. To assess this, attention will need to be paid to optimizing the child's chances of success, by normalizing tone as much as possible, positioning for maximal function, and arranging lighting and auditory conditions so that the child has the best chances of using their residual vision or hearing. The context of the situation, including whether the task has meaning for the child, is extremely important. Performances may also improve following appropriate sensory stimulation to increase arousal.

Probably the child's physical abilities are much easier to assess accurately than intellectual, visual or auditory abilities. Nevertheless, a comprehensive assessment of these children by the physiotherapist will require:

- a considerable period of time
- acute observation and problem-solving skills
- an understanding of appropriate means of communication
- an awareness of the impact of the child's other disabilities

Information from other team members will be vital to the physiotherapists assessment. The physiotherapist will likewise be an important contributor to the assessment of the child's visual, auditory and intellectual function. The results of these assessments will be more valid if the child is positioned so that the influence of abnormal tonal activity is minimized, and their ability to maintain a steady head position in the midline is maximized.

Suitable assessment tools need to be criterion based, and able to measure small degrees of change over time. Generally, a standardized tool developed for this population, as well as a number of useful checklists measuring function, motor and sensory criteria can be used (Jones 1988). As part of a physiotherapy neurosensorimotor assessment, evaluation of skeletal alignment, joint range and muscle imbalance are important areas to ensure prevention of secondary musculoskeletal disabilities.

Suitable assessment tools for children with severe and multiple disability include:

- Paediatric evaluation of disability inventory (PEDI)
- Pyramid scales: adaptive ability in severely handicapped persons
- Developmental assessment for the severely disabled (DASH)
- Gross motor function measure (GMFM)
- Carolina curriculum for infants and preschoolers with special needs
- Callier–Azuser scale for deaf–blind children

The recording of assessments will also enable progress and therefore the effectiveness of a programme to be measured over time. Anecdotal information in progress notes such as atypical displays of function or adverse responses and the circumstances involved are also vital to enable a full picture of the child to be formed and shared. Because of the long-term nature of this disability there will be many changes of professional staff and treatment approaches used, due to advances in professional knowledge and also the enthusiasm for 'new' treatment ideas. It is important for the child's continuing programme that what was successful or unsuccessful in the past has been noted. Past details of equipment and medical or surgical procedures must also be recorded in detail.

Aims of Physiotherapy

A physiotherapist's primary concerns usually centre around posture, movement and physical development. Functional goals of primary importance for the child with severe and multiple disability will be:

- Communication — awareness of and interaction with people and their environment.
- Activities of daily living — self-help activities and making easier the task of daily caring for the child by others.
- Exploration — exploring for enjoyment and to learn about themselves and the world in which they live, through fine motor manipulation and gross motor mobility.

All these functional goals have a significant motor component and the physiotherapist has an important contribution to make to their attainment. The physiotherapist's main contributions to improved functional abilities are described in Figure 1.

Stability

Enhancement of stability for optimal function can be gained through the use of therapeutic positioning and appropriate pieces of equipment.

THERAPEUTIC POSITIONING

This usually employs the following principles:

- inhibition of primitive reflexes and abnormal muscle tone
- attainment of postural stability
- enhancement of symmetry
- alignment of joints in optimum positions

No one position is ideal for every functional use, indeed a variety of positioning is vital as no child can be expected to stay in one position for prolonged periods of time, no matter how functional. If the child is not capable of independent movement, positions should be altered as frequently as possible throughout the day. Many variations of standing, sitting or floor play can be usefully employed for suitable function. Space precludes detailed examination of different variations, but Rushfirth (1984) is a useful source of flexible ideas for therapeutic posi-

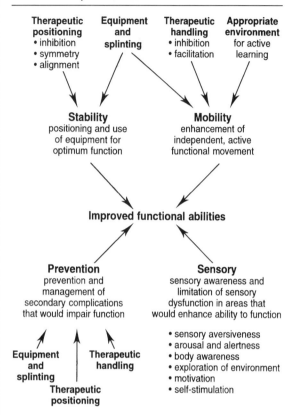

Figure 1 Summary of Physiotherapy Aims for the Child with Severe and Multiple Disabilities

tioning for a variety of different aims with this group of children. Maintenance of any stable and well-aligned positions usually involves the use of equipment for these children if their physical disability is severe.

SITTING

Sitting is often a position of maximum function for these children, and the attainment of a stable sitting position an important therapeutic goal. In a well-designed seating system abnormal tone is usually well-controlled. The use of available vision and hearing is optimal in this position, which usually enhances their ability to communicate and interact. Consequently, it is often tempting to let the child spend a lot of time in a stable seated position. The disadvantages of this include encouragement of flexor patterns which may limit function in the long term (particularly the ability to look ahead and reach out), possible hip and knee flexor contractures, and limitations of opportunities to further develop postural reactions and active movement. Once spasticity is inhibited, underlying postural tone may be low. In that case, the frequent use of stable seated positions can lead to deterioration of the ability to use and be aware of the trunk muscles for balance (Geniale 1991). Where some independent trunk and head control is possible, sitting in a variety of positions other than a conventional wheelchair, such as on an H or abduction stool, a tilt stool, a forward lean chair, or a wedge on the floor can promote independent balance and mobility goals.

STANDING

Standing is a position of great importance for this population. Weight-bearing through the lower limbs in an upright position assists the following:

- normalization of postural tone
- head righting
- skeletal development and prevention of osteoporosis
- respiratory development and function
- gastric, bowel and bladder function
- maintenance of hip and knee extension and a plantigrade foot
- proprioceptive awareness

Despite the extreme delay in reaching any motor milestones, it is important to introduce some form of supported standing as soon as possible, ideally in the second year of age. Children may demonstrate sensory defensiveness to weight-bearing, persistent abasia and earlier onset of deformity if the introduction of standing is delayed until other developmental stages such as sitting or creeping are reached (Rushfirth 1984, Fraser et al. 1990).

Active extension and head control may be successfully facilitated in standing, particularly in children with low postural tone who may find it difficult to maintain head control in supported sitting. The work surface can be raised and tilted, so that some weight can be taken through arms if further active extension is required for stability. For children whose oculomotor control is significantly affected by abnormalities in tone, a well-aligned upright position often allows better visual functioning than can be obtained in

either prone or supine, especially if the task is presented between waist and shoulder height (Geniale 1991).

Standing requires a plantigrade foot and almost full knee and hip extension. Although adaptations can be made for small variations in range from this ideal, care must be taken with abnormal forces through poorly aligned joints. Although not ideal, standing can take place on a subluxed or dislocated hip providing that adaptations are made for leg length difference, and there is no pain involved, which is often difficult to determine. Indeed if a child is a candidate for dislocation, standing is a better position than lying as it offers better control of hip position (Fraser et al. 1990). Apart from standing equipment and orthoses to support joints in extension, some children may need surgery to obtain a plantigrade foot.

Tilt boards and prone standers can also be used in standing. A slightly backwards tilt may be used initially when acclimatizing a child with no experience of the upright position and poor head control. Forwards tilt can be used to encourage head extension. Upright positioning can be used for children with gastro-oesophageal reflux (common in children with SMD) after a meal to supplement drug therapy. Positions used are upright sitting, inclined supine or inclined side-lying on the right side. Fraser et al. (1990) has noted the clinical usefulness of forward inclination at 30° on a prone stander.

FLOOR POSITIONS

Supine may not be a good position for function if a child has strong primitive patterns of movement, such as TLR or ATNR, although the effect of increased extensor tone may be minimized through the use of a wedge to raise the trunk and head or to maintain hip and knee flexion. If extensor tone or flexor weakness is not a problem, supine may be a useful stable position in which to encourage visual responses and eye–hand coordination. Ideally, visually interesting material should be presented in a position to encourage downward gaze and chin tuck to minimize extensor influences (Geniale 1991). It is a commonly used position in Nielsen's 'little room' for the exploration of spatial concepts for severely visually impaired, multiply disabled children (Nielsen 1992).

Prone is an important developmental position because of the facilitation of antigravity head righting, and later upper limb weight-bearing and shoulder stability, and trunk and hip extension. Prone is also a useful therapeutic position to counteract the flexion involved in sitting. Unfortunately, unless it is introduced at a very early stage, children with SMD, especially those with severe visual impairment or very poor head control, will often dislike and resist its use. Experience of the prone position at different angles on their mother's body during play as a baby is very important. Care must be taken in its use, however, that the commonly seen hyperextension of the upper cervical spine in the presence of weak neck flexors and the absence of chin tuck is not reinforced. Prone over a wedge requires less neck extension and frees arms to weight-bear or allows one to reach. If increased flexor tone in the presence of a strong TLR limits function, then a position with support under the shoulders and hips, leaving the abdominal area free, such as can be obtained over a parent's thighs, may be useful. Although important, Geniale (1991) cautions that the prone position should be used with care, as there may be other options for developing antigravity head control.

Side-lying can be a useful position to encourage symmetry with shoulders protracted and hands free to play together in the midline. Especially in the presence of a strong TLR, muscle tone may be more normal in this position, allowing weak flexor muscles to act. With appropriate positioning aids, it can help compensate for asymmetry associated with a strong ATNR or scoliosis. Supported four-foot kneeling can also be used to facilitate weight-bearing through limbs and tactile exploration through the feet and hands while experiencing a different position in space (Nielsen 1993).

Although the concerns of stability and mobility are closely linked as physiotherapy goals for these children, their relative importance for different children will vary. When tone fluctuates considerably, such as in a child with athetosis, independent movement will usually be available, but the lack of central stability is a crucial factor in allowing that movement to be functional. For a child with severe spasticity, fixation in a stable position through the use of equipment is often quite easily achievable. It is the lack of active movement that is the dilemma, and often achieving any reproducible volitional movement is a positive outcome, as it may enable the child to access their environment through the use of switching technology.

Mobility

Children learn best from doing. Their own active volitional movement has a more powerful effect on learning than any guided experience. Indeed, learning can be described as achieving knowledge through being active (Nielsen 1993). One of the most important aspects of the physiotherapy programme for these children is improving their ability to use movement to interact, explore and learn.

How can this best be achieved with this group of children? The physiotherapist can use skills of movement analysis to help set up an appropriate environment that will provide opportunities for activity, and can use facilitation skills that enhance the child's ability to use active volitional movement.

FACILITATION OF ACTIVE MOVEMENT

Active movement involves muscle contraction which gives proprioceptive feedback. It can be facilitated through appropriate handling and positioning techniques. When more normal movement patterns are facilitated following inhibition of abnormal tone, the child gains a sensory appreciation of these that they would otherwise not have experienced.

Neurodevelopmental treatment (NDT) forms the basis of handling techniques for children with abnormalities of tone and movement with a neurological basis. Inhibition alone is not sufficient to alter the child's movement patterns. The child must be an active participator in the process, and functional activities that are important to the child should be used. Thus handling techniques are incorporated into the child's own goal-directed movements to establish new motor patterns (Bly 1991). The aim is to use minimal amounts of handling, and reduce even that as soon as possible to allow more active control by the child. How effectively these motor patterns are generalized functionally is sometimes disputed (Palisano 1991). Emphasis should be placed on preparation for specific function and treatment in positions of function, and the programme arranged so that frequent opportunities to practice more normal movement during functional activities occur throughout the day.

Facilitation of active movement through NDT can also be applied to oculomotor control. To inhibit the effect of a strong ATNR on eye movements, the enhancement of symmetrical head position with chin tuck such as during active extension in standing, with the point of visual interest below the eyes is an example (Geniale 1991).

VOLITIONAL MOVEMENT

Volitional movement is more than just active movement, because it implies intent on the part of the child. This is important from a behavioural perspective because the child will be motivated if intent is involved to continue the activity and hence learn more about their world. From a neurological perspective, because of the intent and motor planning involved, sensory feedback and motor learning is enhanced.

The problem with movement that is not initiated by the child, is that they may be persuaded to attend to a task or be guided through an activity in which they have no interest. This experience provides little learning, less motivation to repeat, and over time leads to passivity (Nielsen 1993). Nielsen has demonstrated that given a wide variety of opportunities appropriate to the child's level of development, most children with severe visual impairments and multiple disabilities can learn actively to experiment and explore. If the child is not interested, more attention may need to be paid to observing what and how they do respond and then reacting appropriately to the child's cues. The child's position or environment may need to be adapted. Although the ultimate aim is to improve the child's ability to function, it is important to remember that apparently random exploration is also a vital step in development, and that not all movement needs to be specifically goal directed. When given sufficient opportunities and time to experiment and explore, the child can begin to compare and link experiences and learn what for them is the most practical way to succeed at a task.

The dilemma for the physiotherapist working with these children is that active volitional movement often involves the use of abnormal tone and stereotyped movement patterns. As the child becomes older, less importance is usually placed on the quality of movement, and more on function. Realistically, the child with SMD will never have normal patterns of movement. Indeed, in debates over the effectiveness of NDT it has been questioned whether normal movement patterns are always an appropriate goal (Van Sant 1991). When a child with abnormal tone that limits movement becomes interested and involved in exploring, they are often able to use active volitional movement to overcome partially the abnormal tone.

In children with SMD it is vital from the earliest days that any spark of motivation and intention to move and explore not be diminished in the push for equally important goals of developing more useful patterns of posture and movement. The skilled therapist knows when quality of movement can be compromised so that the child can experiment as they learn new movement patterns (Bly 1991).

INDEPENDENT MOBILITY

If the child has a severe physical impairment, independent ambulation may be unlikely. Independent mobility may be possible through the use of an electric wheelchair, or at an earlier age the use of a child's electric car. If a joystick control is too difficult, it can be adapted to single-switch use, controlled by a reproducible movement of the arm, foot or head. Reasonable use of vision and comprehension would be required, however, for success. There is ample evidence that independent mobility through these means is extremely important to the encouragement of curiosity, expression of personality, development of spatial awareness and is a lot of fun (Butler 1986, Trefler 1993).

If the predominant disability is visual and intellectual, with moderate physical impairment, independent ambulation may be possible. If the child is to have any ability or interest in using gait functionally, awareness of their body and of spatial relations is crucial (Nielsen 1992). Exploration with feet and hands in a 'little room' and opportunities to explore an area through floor play will be as important as using weight-bearing positions such as standing for play.

Mobility equipment may be needed to assist with balance, but should be used sparingly, as many of these children with potential for independent ambulation can become dependent on hands held for support.

Risk of Secondary Disability

Because of the high potential for developing secondary disabilities in children with long-term, severe and multiple disability, prevention and management of these are an important consideration in their management. Prevention requires knowledge of the commonly encountered complications, and how best to minimize their impact. Management usually involves monitoring through assessment, control where possible, and correction as required.

Physiotherapists, as team members, will be involved in prevention and management in all areas of potential complication during interactions with the child. Although they will have substantial input into the management of respiratory problems and the monitoring of skin condition, their primary role in prevention will be in the orthopaedic area. The physiotherapist is in a particularly good position to act as a liaison between the medical and educational teams involved with the child who, despite similarities in long-term goals, still may have a different perspective in terms of priorities and timing for intervention.

SKELETAL MODELLING

Most children with SMD have skeletal systems that are normal at birth (Fraser et al. 1990). Because the infant skeleton is primarily cartilagenous, normal muscle activity and weight-bearing through movement influences the shape and size of developing skeletal structures and joint alignment, through a process of modelling of bone (Cusick 1990). In children with abnormal neuromotor function, deformities develop during the growth process in response to abnormal neurological influences, abnormal patterns of movement and the resultant muscle imbalances (Cusick 1990, Fraser et al. 1990). Thus, biomechanical factors affect structure and function.

EFFECT OF DEFORMITY

Obviously, it is the influence of deformity on function, not the presence of deformity per se, that is the focus within this population of children. Deformities can affect function by:

- further limiting the potential for movement (e.g. kyphosis limiting forward reach)
- making positioning for function difficult (e.g. equinus preventing weight-bearing)
- causing pain (e.g. arthritic changes in joints under abnormal stresses).
- Causing medical complications (e.g. respiratory difficulties with scoliosis)
- increasing the difficulty for carers (e.g. adductor deformity affecting perineal hygiene)

Forces with particularly deforming potential are those involving obligatory reflex patterns, particularly where asymmetry is involved. The most common and functionally threatening deformities in children with strongly abnormal tone are:

- spinal deformities (scoliosis / kyphosis)
- pelvic obliquity
- hip flexion / adduction with possible subluxation / dislocation
- knee flexion
- foot equinus
- elbow and wrist flexion

All persons with SMD should be considered at risk of developing scoliosis, with incidence rates in this population quoted as high as 64%, and the frequency of spinal deformity directly related to the severity of neurological involvement (Fraser et al. 1990). The continued presence of a Galant reflex, particularly if asymmetrical was noted as being a precursor to scoliosis in this population (Fraser et al. 1990). Because scoliosis is usually postural and correctible at first, the use of positioning with modifications to counteract the asymmetrical and deforming forces, especially in seating systems, is vital. The use of a canvas corset, particularly in children with asymmetry whose truncal tone was low has been reported as being useful in delaying the onset of structural scoliosis until early teen years (Fraser et al. 1990).

Hip adduction, often combined with flexion is the most common hip deformity in this group of children. If the child is young, this will affect the formation of the acetabulum, and the tendency for posterior hip dislocation is high, particularly between the ages of 3 and 7 years (Fraser et al 1990). Although more rare, anterior dislocation, linked with hip extension deformity poses more difficulties as it prevents sitting if untreated. The link between scoliosis, pelvic obliquity and hip dislocation is well known, but which deformity is the precursor is disputed. Either scoliosis or hip subluxation may lead to pelvic obliquity and further deformity.

PREVENTION

Attention paid to prevention of further deformity is particularly important during the early years of growth, as most of the modelling of bone takes place in the first 7 years (Cusick 1990). Scarcity of research in this population makes it difficult to determine if it is possible to prevent deformities in the presence of strongly abnormal deforming forces with limited active movement. It seems that their development may be minimized or delayed by early intervention.

Prevention involves monitoring through biomechanical and neurological assessment. Frequent radiographs of the spine and hips should also occur through the growth years. Fraser et al. (1990) maintains that if the hip radiographs remain normal through 7 to 10 years of age, then the chances of hip deformities will be low. Although the progression of spinal deformities may slow or cease with skeletal maturation, in the population of children with SMD, skeletal growth may continue well into the 20s. Therefore, clinical and radiological monitoring of deformities should probably continue, though at less frequent intervals, throughout life (Fraser et al. 1990).

Maintenance of adequate range of movement has a place in prevention with these children. Although passive stretch has been used for years, there is little clinical documentation of its success in the prevention of contractures. In the presence of abnormal tone, minimization of tonal influences, followed by facilitated active movement, and supplemented by positioning for symmetry and function is more useful than passive ranging of movement. Therapeutic positioning and handling are important in prevention and ongoing control of deformities, particularly in the early years.

CONTROL AND CORRECTION

Splinting and casting may be used in this group to maintain range, particularly in the ankle. An ankle–foot orthosis (AFO) may sometimes be used in place of footwear for a non-ambulant child because of its ease of application as well as its maintenance of a plantigrade foot for standing.

Serial or inhibitory casting to increase range or improve lower limb movement patterns is less effective in this group unless the child is ambulant. Care must also be taken if it is used on a child with severe spasticity, that shunting of tone to already compromised joints does not occur.

If deformity is painful or severely limits function, surgery may be the only option. Surgery is not a lightly taken option, because of the high possibility of respiratory complications, the child's tolerance of casts and difficulties of their daily management, and the problems with adequate postoperative follow-up to maintain the gains made. Usually soft tissue releases are the surgery of choice. Although studies on the results of surgery in this population are rare, a retrospective study of soft tissue releases noted significant improvements in posture, ease of care and comfort, with no child being made worse (Louis et al. 1989). Early identification of subluxation and management with soft tissue releases can help prevent later hip dislocation (Fraser et al. 1990).

EQUIPMENT

The rationale for choice and prescription of appropriate equipment is dependent on careful assessment of the reasons why stability, alignment, mobility and function are being compromised. There is a wide range of equipment with adjustable modifications now available to suit most positioning and mobility goals in this population, especially in seating systems (see Chapter 11).

Regardless of the type of equipment chosen, regular monitoring by the physiotherapist is required to ensure the following:

- it is still achieving the goal for which it was prescribed (and whether that goal is still important)
- it is maintained in good condition (loose screws, battery terminals, weak points in orthotics)

- it is not a source of actual or potential harm (skin or circulation problems, brakes on chairs, potential falls)
- it is accommodating the growth of the child (adjustment as required, or plans for reordering)

Sensory Aspects

Although these children are often involved in a sensorimotor programme, its development and inclusion into the child's overall programme is often haphazard. Unless carefully planned and individually executed, the outcome for the child is probably, at best, fun; and at worst, highly confusing and even limiting to the child's ability to make sense of the world and to learn.

The development of the sensorimotor aspects of the child's programme begins with questioning of carers, and careful observation of the child to evaluate their responses to different sensory input, and their awareness of and interaction with their world. This information will affect how the physiotherapist interacts with and interprets the child's responses.

What may seem to us to be a stimulating environment may be for the child a highly confusing environment, particularly if it involves multisensory input. Some children have difficulty screening out irrelevant auditory or visual input, or could be considered auditorily or visually defensive as discussed earlier under sensory modulation disorders. They may be hyperresponsive, and have difficulty monitoring the intensity of sensory stimulation and modulating their response. Conversely what may seem to us to be adequate stimulation may need to be more intense for arousal or elicitation of an appropriate response. They may be hyporesponsive, and appear to have reduced perception of sensory stimulation, requiring more intense input for arousal or elicitation of a response (Kinnealy 1973).

Sufficient time in any sensory environment should be given for the child to respond and have adequate opportunity to experiment and explore at their own pace. Repetition of activities is a normal part of a child's play, and is especially important with these children to allow the development of such concepts as anticipation, causality and imitation (Rushfirth 1984, Nielsen 1993). The physiotherapist should not be in a hurry to alter programmes for the sake of variety, unless a negative response is noted.

Clarification of just how sensory input might be expected to help in achieving the overall functional goals for the child will then help in the design of the sensory motor aspects of the programme.

MANAGEMENT OF SENSORY AVERSIVENESS

Sensory aversion to touch or movement has a deleterious effect on the ability of the child to benefit from the physiotherapy programme, and needs to be addressed if present. Careful introduction of the child to a range of touch and movement experiences at an early age may avoid severe problems in this area.

Firm pressure is usually more easily tolerated than light touch. Initial management usually involves using firm encompassing pressure and compression, avoiding the particularly sensitive areas of the hands and face, sometimes combined with gentle vestibular input such as slow rocking, with its calming and integrative effect (Royeen and Lane 1991). Some of Sherbourne's (1990) relationship play activities involving firm, enveloping body contact have been adapted well to this group of children. From there, incorporation of weight-bearing, first through a static surface, then a more mobile one such as a trampoline can lead to further tolerance of other aspects of a sensory programme such as tactile play. Hydrotherapy may be usefully introduced at this stage also, for its tactile experiences as well as the movement possibilities in an antigravity situation.

When extending a child's tolerance of movement, a range of movement experiences need to be considered, as the child may react differently to varying speeds or direction of movement. It has been noted clinically that children improve in their ability to process and tolerate different types of vestibular input (angular or linear), depending on what has been used frequently (e.g. trampoline, hammock, therapy ball or rolling). Usually, a child who is fearful of movement experiences will tolerate movement more easily if it has some meaning for them, is under their control, or if they are in contact with the ground. This may be possible in the child whose visual or intellectual impairment is more severe than their physical, and this is often the group who are particularly averse to movement. Movement whilst firmly held by the mother may be more easily accepted in the early stages.

ALTERATION OF AROUSAL OR ALERTNESS

Tactile and vestibular input, presumably because of the input into the reticular activating system, can be useful clinically to alter arousal or alertness in children with SMD before other activities. Firm touch and slow rocking have a calming effect. Warm water as used in hydrotherapy can have a similar effect, as well as a reduction of muscle tone. Quick tapping of the muscles or faster vestibular input can increase arousal or alertness as well as antigravity muscle tone before activities requiring concentration. Geniale (1991) notes that an appropriate level of arousal and postural activity is actually a prerequisite to optimal visual function in children with severe physical and visual impairment.

DEVELOPMENT OF BODY AWARENESS

Passive touch, that is the touch of another, although not as effective as the active exploratory touch of the child's body with their own hand, is still useful, particularly in a child with severe disability. Teaching the child's mother baby massage in the early days can help with bonding, and if incorporated into handling or positioning techniques, can alter muscle tone.

The attachment of objects that have a visual, auditory or tactile interest to the wrists, chest or ankles of the child can be used in different ways to encourage body awareness. Midline hand play as encouraged in positions such as side-lying, can be made more interesting in a similar way. Many ideas to encourage hand-to-mouth play have been suggested by Nielsen (1992), such as the use of rubber gloves with the fingers filled with potato flour which makes a fascinating noise when rubbed or sucked.

With children who resist standing, active movements and awareness of the lower limbs may be improved through the encouragement of tactile play material attached to foot plates, or the walls of a 'little room' if it is used. Arbitrary movements may become intentional if auditory or tactile feedback occurs.

Figure 2 Nielsen's Little Room: a child actively exploring objects and space with his mouth, hands and feet. (Photographs courtesy of Fay Jennison)

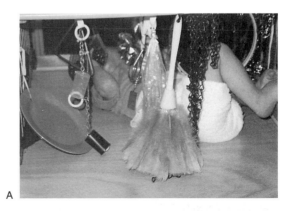

A

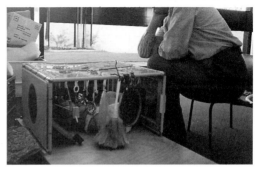

B

EXPLORATION OF THE ENVIRONMENT

The physiotherapist will be involved in setting up the environment to provide opportunities for active movement within it. One example of such an environment is the 'little room' (Nielsen 1992) where successful, self-initiated exploration by children with SMD can often be obtained through the use of suitable objects attached by elastic so they return to their original place when discarded. Because of the containment of the small space, spatial relationships can also be explored. Auditory feedback from manipulations is enhanced by the use of a resonance board and enclosure from the outside environment, making this an opportunity to encounter the concept of causality. By repetition of the same noise-making manipulation, the child with severe visual impairment may realize that his movements produced a response. Thus active learning can occur. See Figure 2.

Initial exploration, if vision is impaired will be through tactile or auditory means. Varying surfaces with differentiated textures and points and holes for fingers to feel are of particular interest. Common

Figure 3 Whilst using a variety of positions to develop postural stability, the physiotherapist can also encourage the child to explore the environment. (Photograph courtesy of Fay Jennison)

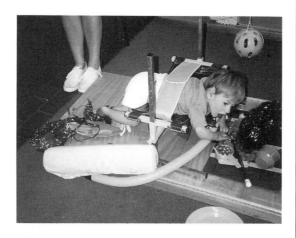

objects such as keys or crumpled paper, or home-made objects such as the 'scratching board' with its varying auditory feedback are often more interesting than plastic toys (Nielsen 1993). For a child with severe visual problems, a wide range of objects and activities that provide interesting tactile and auditory experiences may need to be provided to encourage exploration. Water and sand are obvious examples of tactile play, but exploration with different sized balls, food or grains may be well accepted. If selection of objects cannot be made visually, a great many may be picked up and discarded before activities of interest are found, a factor to be remembered when using toys to interest such a child in movement. See Figure 3.

MOTIVATION

As mentioned earlier, motivation is a key issue with these children, and sensory rewards will often be a successful reinforcement for activity where the activity itself or social approval is not. Switches can be used to turn on a toy which may provide any combination of vibration, light or sound as a reward for appropriate movement, such as head righting. The child's head can rest on the switch in prone, and turn the toy on when the weight is lifted off it. If head control is better in sitting, a switch can be devised so that when the child's head is almost upright the switch turns on. Time delays can even be introduced to encourage further holding of position, but only if this is within

the child's capabilities. The physiotherapist can work with the other team members here to devise appropriate sensory motivators.

Visual rewards and vibration are often highly successful in this population. It must be cautioned, however, that if a child enjoys visual reward, it cannot be assumed that it will be more motivating if this is linked to sound. If he is not able to integrate both, the child may withdraw and not respond at all. Although it is noted clinically that some of these children love and respond very effectively to music or voice, it is often only in a quiet one-to-one situation. Children with SMD may withdraw in a group environment where a lot of noise and confusion is commonly encountered.

SELF-STIMULATION

Much confusion and controversy exists over why children with SMD use self-stimulation as a pattern of behaviour. Even more exists as to what to actually do about it. The reasons are still basically hypothetical, and probably different for different children. Clinically, the important task is carefully to assess each child, and monitor the effect of any approach to evaluate its success. Evaluation of the status of the child's sensory responses may give clues to the reasons behind self-stimulatory behaviour, as may observation of the type of stimulation, and the situation in which it most occurs. Self-stimulation usually involves the overuse of a form of sensory input, such as vestibular (rocking, head banging), tactile (oral, sexual) or the visual 'blindisms' (light gazing, eye poking). It becomes a concern when it is so sustained that it limits other activities or exploration, or when its continuation is actually physically damaging to the child or to others (e.g. biting or banging). Two possible reasons that seem to correlate with what is seen clinically are to fulfil a need for sensory stimulus, or to withdraw from the world.

Reasons for self stimulation
1. To fulfil a need for sensory stimulus
- where the child has limited active movement and therefore little sensory feedback
- where the child is hyporesponsive to the usual amount of sensory input, and seeks more

2. To withdraw from the world

- where the child may feel there is an overload of stimuli in the environment, and be frightened or confused
- where the child is hyperresponsive to the usual amount of sensory input, and cannot integrate or interpret it
- where the child is acting out of frustration at an attempt to function
- where the child has an inability or disinterest in communicating with the world

Management possibilities

1. Providing a greater variety of sensory stimuli
- Consider the use of a multisensory room, such as a Snoezelen environment (Hulsegge and Verheut 1987). Notice if self-stimulation behaviour decreases after provision of more appropriate sensory opportunities.
- Vestibular experiences may be more difficult to provide than other types of sensory input for older severely disabled children. This can be a neglected area as they get heavier so that a hoist may be needed to make it available to the child with restricted mobility. Although vestibular input can be useful clinically, its rationale should be carefully planned.
- Care must be taken with this population of children who may be prone to epilepsy as it can be triggered through visual stimuli or the autonomic changes from vestibular input. There is a need to watch carefully for sympathetic signs such as blanching, sweating, change of pupil size or divergence of the eyes (Goven et al. 1984).

2. Limiting or ordering the environment
- This is particularly important if the child has combined visual and hearing impairment.
- Work in a quiet environment, so that any auditory input has a chance of making sense. Use one-to-one situations for therapy, and limit group work if there is a lot of background noise and visual input. Try working on a resonance board to maximize appropriate auditory feedback.
- If light gazing is a problem, work in a room with indirect light sources.

- With self-destructive behaviour such as hand biting, splinting may have to be used as a last resort, to limit full flexion but allow a possibility of sensory exploration with the hands and the ability to bring objects to the mouth for exploration. Maximize other forms of sensory experiences for the hands meanwhile.

Programme Management

Integration of the programme

As no aspect of a child's development occurs in isolation, so must the different aspects of their therapeutic programme be integrated. Not only can the physiotherapist have an effect on the child's social, cognitive and sensory development through interactions with the child, but also his/her role in enhancement of movement will permeate all other aspects of the child's development. When parents, therapists and educational personnel work together as a collaborative team to provide integrated services, the benefits for the child are greatly enhanced (Rainforth et al. 1992).

Programming Issues

To maximize effectiveness, the programme needs to be incorporated into everyday activities such as eating, dressing, sleeping and leisure. Some role release by all the professionals concerned is necessary to enable this. The physiotherapist can influence the team's awareness of and ability to use appropriate handling and positioning during everyday activities.

Although programming needs are complex, it is important to remember that a child with a severe and multiple disability is still a child, not just the recipient of a programme. No matter how well integrated, a programme must remain flexible and fun to cater for the child's developing personality, and the fact that sometimes he will behave differently, be uncooperative or just plain stubborn.

SETTING THE PROGRAMME

With the changes towards a more 'ecological' approach to the delivery of programmes for these children, physiotherapy will probably be delivered across a range of settings, changing as the child grows. Initially the home environment is often the ideal setting, with the focus later being primarily within an educational team setting. At various times, short periods will be delivered within the health setting, for acute respiratory reasons, orthopaedic surgery or for specialized orthotic and equipment prescription.

FOCUS OF THE PROGRAMME

Although the child's overall needs will always be considered, the major focus of the programme will change over time. The early years are of vital importance from the physiotherapy perspective. Because of the plasticity of the neural and musculoskeletal system at this stage, facilitating optimal quality of movement will greatly enhance functional outcomes for the child's future. Early introduction to a variety of positions and movement experiences, will enhance the child's potential for sensorimotor development. The most vital task for this stage, however, is learning to make sense of the world, and to interact with it, so that any spark of active involvement of the child in this process must be capitalized on, to avoid long-term passivity.

As the child grows older, independent function, educational programmes and social interaction assume more relative importance, and physiotherapy programmes will alter their focus accordingly. Although age-appropriate activities are to be encouraged, particularly for the way in which they influence interaction with other people, sometimes activities appropriate to the stage the child is interested in exploring are important. Even though the developmental pace is slower, more is often gained in this way. Equipment needs may also alter significantly through periods of rapid growth. If the child is unable to take weight through their feet or participate in transfers, the physiotherapist will also be involved in solving the problems of everyday handling and lifting as the child becomes larger. As well as information about appropriate lifting devices, this may include advice to the carer about their own fitness to cope with these tasks. During adolescence, future plans for how the child may function within the community, including the issues of independence from family, self-image, use of leisure time and the possibilities of supported employment need to be considered.

Role of Technology

The role of technology in the life of a child with severe, multiple and long term disabilities is only just emerging. For a child with such severe impediments to function, technology offers a window of opportunity for active participation with the world. Although initially daunting for some staff, equipment and solutions involving technology are now more easily accessible, in terms of price and specialized assistance available (Langley 1990, Wright and Nomura 1991). Physiotherapists need to keep abreast of the rapid changes within this exciting field, not only for the role it can have in enhancing movement, but also because the use of technology in the child's programme involves the entire team. Technology can be used from the very earliest days. Rather than waiting until a child is old enough to access an electric wheelchair or computer, the uses of simple switches can enhance the infant's ability to access fascinating toys, and can reinforce their earliest attempts at interaction.

If technology is used, the emphasis is, as always, on the child's needs and finding solutions to problems encountered. If a technological solution is found, it must always be re-evaluated over time to see whether it is still enhancing function. Thus technology is used as another therapeutic tool, not just because it is new or exciting. The solution may be as simple as a pointer to enable use of a typewriter, or as sophisticated as a single-switch scanning device to operate an electric wheelchair. A large variety of switches are commercially available to enable access to modified electrical toys or equipment. A switch can be devised in a variety of positions, to be used by an available physical movement that is under the child's voluntary control, and is repeatable at will. This can include hand, foot or head movements. Through the use of software programmes, a simple on–off switching device can allow access to any normally available computer programmes for fun and educational purposes.

Augmentative and alternative communication systems may involve the use of a variety of tools from a simple indication of yes or no with a physical movement or use of a communication board, to prepro-grammed or individually programmable synthetic voice devices, accessed by means of a single switch or scanning device. The ability to access switches, computers and communication systems has impor-tant long-term implications for residential and voca-tional options as adults.

Physiotherapists will be particularly involved in using technology for mobility in electric wheelchairs or commercially available electric cars or bikes. They may also use simple biofeedback devices that can give the child knowledge of or reward for appropri-ate movements. For this purpose, switches can be operated by pneumatic pads that respond to changes in pressure and are placed so that they are activated by movements such as rolling, weight-bearing through hands, weight-shift in standing or contact with the back of the chair in sitting.

Technology can be used as a tool to:

- motivate through interest or as reward for effort
- allow access to other equipment
- teach through biofeedback or cognitive means in the achievement of the functional goals of:

  - communication
  - social skills
  - self-help activities
  - fun and leisure
  - motor development
  - mobility
  - sensory function
  - cognitive learning

Therapeutic Approaches to Management

As mentioned throughout this chapter, physiothera-pists working with children with severe and multiple disability are able to draw from a variety of different approaches when planning the therapeutic pro-gramme. These are summarized next.

- Biomechanical: effect of structure on function, orthopaedic approach, use of orthotics, splinting and equipment for function (Cusick 1990, Fraser et al. 1990).

- Neurodevelopmental: inhibition of abnormal tone, facilitation of more normal postural responses and movements, handling in one-to-one situations (Levitt 1984, Bly 1991, Geniale 1991).
- Active learning: acting actively on the environment, setting up the environment to give visual, auditory and tactile feedback and a variety of experiences, development of spatial relationships (Nielsen 1990).
- Sensory: sensory awareness, facilitation of sensori-motor responses, multisensory environment to facilitate integration of senses (Goven et al. 1984, Jones 1988).
- Behaviour modification: importance of motivation, use of rewards for reinforcement, repetition to enhance learning (Rushfirth 1984).

In planning and re-evaluating a physiotherapy pro-gramme for such a child, the physiotherapist will need to be aware of the underlying premises and goals of differing strategies and approaches. There is no single approach that will meet the needs of the child over time, and the physiotherapist is often required to find a balance between apparent dichoto-mies. Possible controversies that will need to be considered are highlighted throughout this chapter and summarized below. These could be considered as differing, but not necessarily conflicting, approaches and strategies to be solved in a different way in different situations.

Possible dichotomies in approaches to management of children with SMD

multisensory environment ↔ sensory overload

age appropriate ↔ stage appropriate

facilitate movement ↔ set up the environment

positioning ↔ active movement to explore

equipment ↔ sensory freedom

The challenge in helping a child with severe, multiple and long-term disabilities to gain most from their life, is to combine the 'art' and the 'science' of physiother-apy in an eclectic manner that is driven by acute observation of and willingness to respond to the individual child's own cues.

REFERENCES

Bertoti, DB (1989) Physical therapy for the child with mental retardation. In: Tecklin, JS (ed.) *Pediatric Physical Therapy*, pp. 237–261. Philadelphia: JB Lippincott Co.

Bly, L (1991) A historical and current view of the basis of neurodevelopmental treatment. *Pediatric Physical Therapy* **3(3)**: 131–135.

Butler, C (1986) Effects of powered mobility on self-initiated behaviours of very young children with locomotor disability. *Developmental Medicine and Child Neurology* **28**: 325–332.

Crossman, HL (1992) *Cortical Visual Impairment, Presentation, Assessment and Management*, 75 pp. The Royal New South Wales Institute for Deaf and Blind Children, North Rocks Press: North Rocks, Australia.

Cusick, BD (1990) *Progressive Casting and Splinting for Lower Extremity Deformities in Children with Neuromotor Dysfunction*, 410 pp. Tuscan, Arizona: Therapy Skill Builders.

Fraser, BA, Hensinger, RN, Phelps, JA (1990) *Physical Management of Multiple Handicaps, A Professional's Guide*, 337 pp. Baltimore: Paul Brookes Publishing Co.

Geniale, T (1991) *The Management of the Child with Cerebral Palsy and Low Vision, A Neurodevelopmental Therapy Perspective*, 60 pp. North Rocks, Australia: The Royal New South Wales Institute for Deaf and Blind Children, North Rocks Press.

Good, WV, Jan, JE, Desa, L *et al.* (1994) Cortical visual impairment in children, a major review. *Survey of Ophthalmology* **38(4)**: 351–364.

Goven, P, Faber, T, Prins, S, Mangold, B (1984) *The Use of Sensory Stimulation in Teaching Mentally Impaired Students*, 244 pp. Springfield, Illinois: Charles C Thomas.

Hulsegge, J, Verheul, A (1987) *Snoezlelen, Another World: A Practical Book of Sensory Experiential Environments for the Mentally Handicapped*, 144 pp. England: Rompa.

Jones, CJ (1988) *Evaluation and Educational Programming of Deaf–Blind, Severely Multihandicapped Students, Sensorimotor Stage*, 295 pp. Springfield, Illinois: Charles C Thomas.

Kinnealy, M (1973) Aversive and non-aversive responses to sensory stimuli in mentally retarded children. *American Journal of Occupational Therapy* **27**: 464–472.

Langley, MB (1990) A developmental approach to the use of toys for the facilitation of environmental control. *Physical and Occupational Therapy in Paediatrics* **10(2)**: 69–91.

Levitt, S (1984) Severe visual handicap. In: Levitt S (ed.) *Paediatric Developmental Therapy*, pp 213–226. Oxford: Blackwell Scientific.

Louis, DS, Hensinger, RN, Fraser, BA, Phelps, JA, Jacques, K (1989) Surgical management of the severly multiply handicapped individual. *Journal of Pediatric Orthopedics* **9**: 15–18.

Michael, MG, Paul, PV (1991) Early intervention for infants with deaf–blindness. *Exceptional Children* **I**: 200–210.

Nielsen, L (1990) *Are You Blind? Promotion of the Development of Children who are Especially Developmentally Threatened*, 109 pp. Copenhagen: Sikon.

Nielsen, L (1992) *Space and Self. Active Learning by Means of a Little Room*, 112 pp. Copenhagen: Sikon.

Nielsen, L (1993) *Early Learning Step by Step. Children with Vision Impairment and Multiple Disabilities*, 168 pp. Copenhagen: Sikon.

Palisano, RJ (1991) Research on the effectiveness of neurodevelopmental treatment. *Pediatric Physical Therapy* **3(3)**: 143–148.

Rainworth, B, York, J, MacDonald, C (1992) *Collaborative Teams for Students with Severe Disabilities, Integrating Therapy and Educational Services*, 284 pp. Baltimore: Paul Brookes Publishing Co.

Royeen, CB, Lane, SJ (1991) Tactile processing and sensory defensiveness. In: Fisher, AG, Murray, EA, Bundy, AC (eds) *Sensory Integration, Theory and Practice*, pp 108–136. Philadelphia: FA Davis Co.

Rushfirth, S (1984) Physiotherapy for severely mentally handicapped children. In: Levitt, S (ed.) *Paediatric Developmental Therapy*, pp. 88–109. Oxford: Blackwell Scientific.

Sherbourne, V (1990) Movement for children and adults with profound and multiple learning difficulties. In: Sherbourne, V (ed.) *Developmental Movement for Children*, pp. 91–100. Cambridge: Cambridge University Press.

Trefler, E (1993) Powered vehicles for the very young, development through mobility. *Proceedings from the Australian Conference on Technology and Disability*, Adelaide, pp. 280–281.

Van Sant, AF (1991) Neurodevelopmental treatment and pediatric physical therapy, a commentary. *Pediatric Physical Therapy* **3(3)**: 137–141.

Wright, C, Nomura, M (1991) *From Toys to Computors, Access for the Physically Disabled Child*, 206 pp. San Jose: Wright.

Wyman, R (1986) *Multiply Handicapped Children*, 239 pp. London: Souvenir Press.

24

The Progressive Neuromuscular Disorders

AMANDA CROKER AND MARGARET MASEL

Problems in Infancy
•
Problems in Early Childhood
•
Problems in Middle Childhood
•
Problems in Adolescence

Progressive neuromuscular conditions can be categorized broadly according to the system in the body most affected by the genetic abnormality:

- muscle disorder – the muscular dystrophies
- anterior horn cell and peripheral nerve disorders – the muscular atrophies
- central nervous system disorder – ataxias
- metabolic disorder – leukodystrophies

Researchers are beginning to identify the specific genetic abnormalities which manifest as progressive neuromuscular conditions. There have been some exciting breakthroughs in the identification of gene products which are altered or missing as a result of the genetic abnormality. One major discovery has been dystrophin, the protein gene product that is absent in Duchenne muscular dystrophy and significantly decreased in quantity in Becker muscular dystrophy.

The focus for researchers is to find a way to introduce normal dystrophin genes into dystrophic muscles. Techniques such as myoblast transfer (injection of normal, pure myoblasts into dystrophic muscle) and

gene therapy (the introduction of artificially engineered normal genes) are currently under trial and may prove to be effective strategies in arresting these conditions (Karpati 1992). The presumed function of dystrophin in muscles is to provide a mechanical stability for the surface membrane of skeletal muscle fibres, and in the brain to control some synaptic plasticity.

Key features of the pathophysiology of muscle fibre necrosis are as follows (Karpati 1992):

- dystrophin has a role in the mechanical reinforcement of the plasmalemma, so it can withstand the normal contraction-induced strains
- lack of dystrophin may lead to focal breaches of the plasma membrane during contraction of muscle fibres which in turn initiates segmental necrosis
- large-calibre fibres (e.g. muscles of the trunk and legs) are more prone to necrosis
- regeneration of necrotic fibres is vigorous but aberrations of regeneration occur
- there is progressive muscle fibre loss and fibrous plus adipose tissue replacement

It is likely that very young children who have few symptoms will benefit most from these potential interventions. Until the researchers find a way to replace safely, effectively and efficiently the absent or reduced protein products of genes, children with these progressive neuromuscular conditions will continue to require effective physical management of their conditions, as well as appropriate emotional and psychological support for themselves and their families.

The age of onset of symptoms and life expectancy for children born with different types of progressive neuromuscular conditions varies considerably, and significantly influences the approach to intervention and management. An example of this variability is shown in Table 1 where the different forms of muscular dystrophy are compared.

The focus of this chapter will be the group of children where symptoms appear in early to middle childhood, who progress through to adolescence, but have a limited life expectancy. The issues for physical management and child and family support will be addressed through three stages: early childhood, middle childhood and adolescence. There is, however, a small group of babies born with severe disabilities and very short life expectancies and the issues within this group will be addressed first.

Problems in Infancy

Spinal muscular atrophy (SMA) is an autosomal recessive progressive neuromuscular condition, with classification of three types, depending on age of onset, severity of symptoms and life expectancy. The anterior horn cell is the area most affected. Type 1 SMA is characterized by severe generalized weakness at birth, or manifests before 6 months of age, with a very limited life expectancy usually due to respiratory failure (Evans et al. 1981). There are many issues which the family of a child born with SMA type 1 must confront. Coming to terms with the diagnosis and all its implications is a very stressful time and families should have access to social work and counselling support. The physiotherapist as a team member needs to be fully cognizant of the capacity of the

family to cope and the timing and appropriateness of advice and intervention is critical.

Issues for Physical Management

The physiotherapist may be involved in the diagnostic process. In some instances the distinction between severe hypotonia and severe weakness may not be obvious. During handling of the baby, the physiotherapist may be able to provide some sensory stimulation which positively affects the tone in the case of severe hypotonia. The same sensory stimulation would be unlikely to alter the muscle action in the case of severe weakness (SMA).

It is important for parents to develop confidence in handling their baby at this early stage, and managing the requirements of feeding, changing and bathing. Babies with severe weakness move very little, and have little protection or muscular support for their joints when handled.

Physiotherapists can offer parents helpful advice about positioning for sleeping, for wakeful periods, for bathing, changing and dressing and for feeding, and also handling (how to pick up and carry the baby). When positioning it is important to support the head and limbs and try to avoid clothing or blankets which apply pressure to joints. It is important not to place a baby with severe weakness in prone if they cannot use the face-clearing reflex to turn their head and breathe easily. The provision of equipment such as bath hammocks may be useful.

Respiratory physiotherapy management will be required if the baby has weak respiratory muscles and an ineffective cough and swallow. Gravity will assist the descent of the diaphragm and this may be achieved by raising the head end of the cot. Often there is a need to give advice regarding best position for swallowing and how to avoid choking and aspiration.

Parents may need to know how to remove secretions and saliva from the baby's trachea before discharge home from hospital. Suctioning may be necessary and portable suction units will be required.

The life expectancy for these babies may only be 1 or 2 years, however, attention should be given to

Table 1
The Different Forms of Muscular Dystrophy

Type	Hereditary pattern	Biochemistry	Age-onset	Rate of progression	Symptoms
Duchenne	1:3500 ♂ xP21 sex-linked recessive • males affected • female carriers • approx 1/3 new mutations	• faulty gene on X chromosome • dystrophin not produced in muscles, heart and brain • ↑ creatine phosphokinase (CPK)	early childhood	• steady • wheelchair usually by middle childhood	• pseudohypertrophy in some muscles • progressive weakness of pelvic and pectoral muscles • intellectual impairment
Becker	xP21 sex-linked recessive • males affected • female carriers	• faulty dystrophin production (3–30%) of normal (partial deletion of gene) • ↑ CPK	later than Duchenne mid–late childhood	• slower than Duchenne • often remain mobile into adulthood	similar to Duchenne but less severe
Congenital (Fukuyama type is well defined)	autosomal recessive	↑ CPK ↓ EMGs	birth or infancy	variable	• ocular involvement in some • hypotonia • generalized muscle weakness • CNS may be involved • joint contractures
Fascioscapulo-humeral (Landouzy—Dejerine)	autosomal dominant 1:20000	locus at chromosome 4q35 ↑ CPK (not as high as Duchenne)	usually early adolescence but variable	variable usually fairly slow	• muscles of the face and shoulder girdle affected first • foot dorsiflexors, proximal hip and distal arm and hand muscles can be affected
Myotonic	autosomal dominant	↑ CPK in some cases • gene produces an abnormal protein kinase (myotonin)	• variable • most common in early adulthood • less common in infancy and early childhood	• usually slow	• cataracts • testicular atrophy • frontal baldness • intellectual impairment • delayed relaxation of muscles after contraction • weakness of hands, feet and anterior muscles of the neck

Table 1 Cont.

Distal (2 types)	• autosomal dominant • autosomal recessive	↑ CPK	usually in mid-adult life (not childhood)	• slowly progressive	• small muscles of the extremities first involved • no neuropathy (as in peroneal muscular atrophy)
Limb girdle	autosomal recessive	may have slightly ↑ CPK	variable usually second or third decades of life	variable usually slow	proximal muscles of pelvis and shoulder girdle affected first
Ocular (several forms)	autosomal dominant usually	↑ CPK ↓ EMGs of skeletal muscles	usually in adulthood	slowly progressive	extraocular and swallowing muscles involved

Sources of information: Miyoshi *et al.* 1986, Knubley and Bertorini 1988, Mandel 1989, Bushby 1992, Karpati 1992, Personius *et al.* 1994.

appropriate developmental stimulation with significant modification of the environment to enable interaction. Switch-operated toys and other technologies may be useful.

Issues for the Family – Diagnosis

Communicating the diagnosis to parents is an important, but under-researched subject (Woolley *et al.* 1989). The manner in which it is imparted and the way it is experienced and responded to by others will have a long-lasting effect on the grief process and the coping patterns in families.

The task of telling the parents usually falls on the doctor. This is often the paediatrician who may have had a limited association with the family. The essential aim of medicine is to relieve suffering and here, in a way, there is a denial of that possibility. Because of this the doctor often feels inadequate and this can interfere with the ability to communicate. The parents are in shock and this adds to difficulties; comprehension is impeded so that even when the diagnosis has been conveyed in a clear, warm and honest manner parents frequently are not able to appreciate fully what has been told to them.

The physiotherapist will often be the next professional person to see the parents who will be looking for answers either not given clearly or not fully heard. Some parents will not want to know and will remain silent, afraid of confirmation of the truth. One mother of an infant with diagnosis of Duchenne muscular dystrophy, claims that the doctor did not tell her the diagnosis and that she saw it on the referral to the physiotherapist. She says the physiotherapist did not discuss it with her and that she looked it up at the library on the way home and then spent the next 3 days in a daze, unable to tell even her own family.

This example demonstrates the effects of shock and how this causes difficulty with communication and loss of coping ability in the parent, but it also shows how important the role of the physiotherapist is in the period when parents learn the diagnosis.

It will be important for the physiotherapist to communicate understanding and to try to gauge how much the parents have heard and how much more they want or need to know at that stage. The parents must know that the physiotherapist and the doctor are part of a team and as such will work together in the best interests of the child and family. The physiotherapist will be the professional person working most closely to the child and so parents will depend on him or her for ongoing information, support and treatment.

The quality of care given in the early stages is of crucial importance for long-term acceptance and management of the child's disability.

In a study by Woolley *et al.* (1989) of 50 families with children having life-threatening disease, all parents remembered vividly how the diagnosis was imparted to them and some, as was the case in the above example, were still preoccupied with this and tended to relive it at each stage of deterioration in their child's disease. In this same study most parents valued an open, direct, sympathetic discussion of the diagnosis in privacy and with sufficient time to take in its implications. They also stressed the importance of having other health professionals repeat and clarify the information given.

Problems in Early Childhood

The largest group of children presenting with symptoms in early childhood are boys with Duchenne muscular dystrophy (DMD). Kakulas (1988) described the early features of DMD as:

- the child falls easily as a toddler
- some muscle groups appear too well-developed (pseudohypertrophy)
- the spine is arched (lordosis)
- waddling gait and toe-walking
- difficulty arising from the floor and from a chair – Gower's technique
- climbing stairs is slow and awkward

There is, however, a group of boys who present initially with delayed communication skills and behavioural disorders. Dorman *et al.* (1988) described various studies which identified language disorders especially in younger boys with DMD.

The physiotherapist needs to be vigilant when performing neurodevelopmental assessments for young boys referred primarily for language/behavioural disorders. There may be very little evidence of the physical features of DMD at the commencement of assessment, but when fatigued the child may resort to using Gower's technique to stand up. The following case study illustrates this point.

Case Study 1

John was aged 2 years 6 months when referred by the family doctor to the children's hospital for a developmental assessment. His parents had become increasingly concerned because he did not appear to be developing any language skills, he was difficult to manage, and he was developing some obsessive habits. He was seen by a paediatrician, psychologist, speech pathologist, occupational therapist and physiotherapist. The physiotherapist observed generalized mild delay in sensory motor functioning, but it was not until about 30 minutes had elapsed, and the child was becoming fatigued, that the therapist noticed the child put his hand on one knee to give a final push when standing up. This was reported at the team meeting. The paediatrician tested creatine phosphokinase (CPK) levels and ordered a muscle biopsy. The diagnosis of Duchenne muscular dystrophy was confirmed. The family were referred to a specialized community agency who were able to offer therapy and social work support as part of an early intervention programme in conjunction with the education service.

Physiotherapy Assessment for Muscular Dystrophy

Neurodevelopmental, musculoskeletal, functional and respiratory assessments are important in identifying areas for intervention, and for providing baseline data to allow monitoring of the progress of the condition. Various protocols have been used to document the progression of neuromuscular conditions. Timed function tests and specific rating scales have been developed to document decline in function. Vignos *et al.* (1963) described an upper and lower extremity functional grading scale.

Vignos Classification Scales for Children with Duchenne's Muscular Dystrophy [Vignos *et al.* 1963, p. 92]

Upper-Extremity Functional Grades

1. *Can abduct arms in a full circle until they touch above the head.*
2. *Raises arms above the head only by shortening the lever arm or using accessory muscles.*
3. *Cannot raise hands above the head, but can raise a 180 ml cup of water to mouth, using both hands, if necessary.*
4. *Can raise hands to mouth, but cannot raise a 180 ml cup of water to mouth.*
5. *Cannot raise hands to mouth, but can use hands to hold a pen or pick up a coin.*
6. *Cannot raise hands to mouth and has no functional use of hands.*

Lower-Extremity Functional Grades

1. *Walks and climbs stairs without assistance.*
2. *Walks and climbs stairs with aid of railing.*
3. *Walks and climbs stairs slowly with aid of railing (over 12 seconds for four steps).*
4. *Walks unassisted and rises from a chair, but cannot climb stairs.*
5. *Walks unassisted, but cannot rise from a chair or climb stairs.*
6. *Walks only with assistance or walks independently in long leg braces.*
7. *Walks in long leg braces, but requires assistance for balance.*
8. *Stands in long leg braces, but is unable to walk even with assistance.*
9. *Must use a wheelchair.*
10. *Bedridden.*

Test–retest reliability of functional testing which included the Vignos scale was measured by Personius *et al.* (1994) and they found excellent reliability. Functional testing was also deemed the more relevant and important procedure in the view of the subjects of the trial (adolescents and adults with fascioscapulohumeral muscular dystrophy).

Manual muscle testing (MMT) and quantitative muscle testing (QMT) have also been researched to determine their reliability and usefulness in documenting progression. Varying degrees of intrarater and interrater reliability have been documented. For example, intrarater reliability for MMT also studied by Personius *et al.* (1994) was found to be 'almost perfect' and interrater reliability was 'moderate' or better. Furthermore, Florence *et al.* (1992) confirmed intrarater reliability of MMT grading of muscle strength in boys with DMD. These investigators found that the proximal muscles and muscle strength grades in the gravity-eliminated range had the higher reliability values. Joint contractures were identified as contributing to the less reliable grading of the distal musculature. Personious *et al.* (1994) suggested that the 'moderate' results for interrater reliability were due to differences in evaluator strength and the weight of the subjects' limbs (for the grades where resistance is applied).

Quantitative muscle testing (QMT) includes isometric force measurement which provides the most direct method of assessing the contractile activity in a particular muscle group. It has the advantage of maintaining constancy in muscle length, joint angle and velocity. This testing requires specialized equipment such as a force gauge.

Personius *et al.* (1994) found that muscles that were difficult to standardize between evaluators on MMT were reliably measured with QMT. Factors such as cooperation, motivation, attention and understanding of instructions are potential difficulties that make force testing more variable in children than in adults (Brussock *et al.* 1992).

Respiratory function tests such as forced vital capacity (FVC), forced expiratory volume in 1 second (FEV$_1$) (as measured on a vitalograph) provides information about the strength of respiratory muscles.

Evidence of respiratory muscle endurance may also be useful to measure (e.g. timed use of incentive spirometers).

The physiotherapist has to make a professional judgment about the use of assessment protocols, taking into account the age of the child, and their ability to follow instructions, the availability of equipment, the setting (clinic, home, school), the time available and the purpose (research or to provide a basis for intervention).

Issues for Physical Management

It is important with young children to facilitate normal developmental progress within the context of decreasing muscle strength. This may involve the modification of activities in order to keep the child as functional as possible. An example could be the substitution of a balloon instead of a heavier ball to develop ball skills and eye–hand coordination. A realistic home programme developed with the child and family should be provided. With increasing lordosis and toe-walking, there is shortening of structures across the anterior hips and posterior compartment of the lower leg. Positioning for play, reading or watching TV on a foam wedge on a daily basis may slow the development of these contractures.

Lying prone on a wedge can be followed by some gentle end-of-range pressure into hip extension and ankle dorsiflexion. As the dorsiflexors weaken, the use of ankle–foot orthoses (AFOs) may assist with balance and gait. The effect of hinged or fixed AFOs on the overall posture, especially their effect on the lordosis, hip flexion and position of centre of gravity will need to be assessed. Mobility for some children may not be enhanced or prolonged with the use of AFOs. In fact, balance may be more difficult if the ankle joint is suddenly fixed and extra movement of the hips is required to keep the centre of gravity over the base.

Games and activities which involve maximal respiratory function should be encouraged. If the child is in an early intervention, child care, preschool or primary school programme the physiotherapist will need to liaise with other team members to ensure that the child's programme meets their physical and developmental needs.

Issues for the Family – Counselling

Counselling for the parents must begin early after the diagnosis has been imparted to them; it should be available for the child when he or she is old enough to understand and to siblings and other extended family members throughout the life of the child and for parents and the siblings after the death of the child.

The grief expressed by parents of children with life-limiting disease is often described as chronic because it is present in some form for the entire life of the child. It may become anticipatory grief as the child's death approaches and then bereavement grief after the death. This grief must be seen as a healing process and a healthy expression of loss, but it will be painful for the parents and they will experience a variety of reactions to it before they come to acceptance. The outcome will depend on many factors inherent both within the family and in the social network which surrounds the family and also on the quality of the professional help available.

It is important for all therapists to have an understanding of the grief process and to be able to enlist help when necessary. They should look at models of 'phases' theory of grief; these provide one with a general framework with which to see how parents reorganize their world following the diagnosis of their child's illness. The stages will include shock, anger, protest, despair, detachment and acceptance. These will not often be seen in a linear fashion; some may be missed, some may be repeated, but most parents will experience many of them and they must be recognized as part of the grief process. Fixation on one of more of the phases can result in pathological grief and debilitation for one or more family members which in turn will have serious repercussions for the child.

All health professionals must be able to:

- accept anger in parents even if directed at themselves
- understand guilt feelings in parents
- recognize denial and understand parents' search for 'magical' cures

- recognize detachment and parents' apparent lack of interest at times
- recognize depression that is prolonged
- encourage parents to come to acceptance so that they can remake their lives

In larger centres the physiotherapist will be part of a team and will refer parents for counselling and practical help, but in smaller areas this may not be possible and the physiotherapist will often be the person involved in these issues. So besides being skilled in the speciality of physiotherapy, the therapist should have a working knowledge of the emotional, social and practical needs of the family.

Support can be provided by:

- advising parents to seek genetic information; this must be early as neonatal detection allows early identification of carriers and the birth of other affected children may be averted
- assisting in grief and loss expression
- helping to assure family cohesiveness and cooperation
- ensuring that issues of practical help are addressed

It may fall on the physiotherapist to become an advocate for parents so that they receive all appropriate support; to this end an optimal programme is developed for the child in the context of that particular family.

Problems in Middle Childhood

By this stage the increasing muscle weakness is starting to have a considerable impact on mobility, self-care and educational functions. The child realizes that there are significant limitations on their physical abilities.

Issues for Physical Management

The maintenance of appropriate activity levels, and the minimization of joint contractures will assist in the prevention of premature loss of function. Programmes and equipment to maintain postural alignment should be provided. This may include prone lying on a wedge for a particular activity each day.

Weight bags over the buttocks and lower legs may assist in keeping length in the hip flexors and hamstrings. Night splints for the ankles and wrists may be necessary, and standing frames are useful in maintaining alignment and providing compressive forces through the bones to minimize osteoporosis and possible fractures. The introduction of assistive devices such as wheelchairs and keyboards needs to be timed appropriately.

The physiotherapist needs to work closely with the family in a positive, but realistic, way in the pursuit of options for extending the ability to walk. Information should be provided regarding the possibility of interventions such as tendon releases where this could significantly prolong the child's ability to walk. Consultations with orthopaedic surgeons may need to be arranged. There are always advantages and disadvantages associated with surgical intervention and families often need a great deal of support in making these decisions.

Postural alignment should be monitored regularly especially with respect to the development of scoliosis. Once the child becomes a wheelchair user this is virtually inevitable.

In view of a decreasing activity level, increasing scoliosis and weakening respiratory muscles it is not surprising that the child is more likely to have retained secretions and the tendency to develop infections requiring physiotherapy. The home programme needs to be updated appropriately and carers will need advice about manual handling and back care.

Functional electrical stimulation (FES) has been tested in a few studies to examine the potential beneficial effect on muscle strength. Scott et al. (1986) claimed that the results of their study, in which FES was applied to tibialis anterior muscles, showed that muscles of children with DMD could be influenced to increase considerably their maximal voluntary contraction (MVC) with the application of chronic low frequency stimulation. The best results were obtained with younger boys who were still able to walk and had <20° fixed equinus deformity of the ankles. The fibres actually changed from fast twitch to slow twitch which have better endurance features. The results were explained as being possibly due to slower deterioration of the existing diseased muscle fibres and better and more rapid growth of regenerating fibres and/or hypertrophy of existing relatively healthy fibres.

The use of FES needs to be considered in the light of the current knowledge relating to contractile activity causing focal breaches in the plasma membrane of dystrophin-deficient muscle fibres (especially in the larger calibre fibres of the trunk and legs) (Karpati 1992). The benefits of FES to ankle dorsiflexors versus the judicial use of ankle–foot orthoses in assisting with gait and mobility would need to be carefully considered. The feasibility of intervening with FES if the child is attending a mainstream school setting would also be a consideration.

Issues for the Family

Issues for physical management are a big factor in the life of the child with a progressive life-limiting disease. The members of the team should aim at gaining the optimal function for the child within the scope of his or her physical limitation, and with much careful consideration of the family's commitment, or ability to participate in the programme. Russman (1990) advocates the use of an interdisciplinary approach in which each team member is not only skilled in a speciality, but also has a working knowledge of and a respect for the skills of other team members. The whole team should work together to develop a programme which encompasses the entire needs of the child and family. If there is open, clear communication between team members, the therapist will know the difficulties and limitations within the family and so will be able to set a programme to fit the family. At times it will be necessary to reduce therapy in order to help protect the family cohesiveness.

The following case illustrates this point:

Case Study 2

A physiotherapist who had worked in this area for some time adopted a child with severe physical disabilities. She realized how much she had expected of parents when devising programmes. As a parent herself she learnt about limitations on time, energy and emotional resilience and she saw the complex trade-offs inherent in rules, the value of which she had never previously questioned. For example, as a professional she would have recommended against the toe-walking which endangered the child's vulnerable ankles; as a mother she saw how he benefited socially, emotionally and intellectually from continuing to walk. She said also she would forego therapy at times in favour of trips to the park. It is the rare professional who has the chance to stand in parents' shoes, but this does show the need to be flexible in treatment.

Middle childhood to early adolescence is a very difficult time for the child and the family. Deterioration continues and wheelchair dependancy approaches. For many families there is a feeling of loss of hope and they may begin looking for 'magical cures' apart from the medical stream. If there is a close relationship with the therapist and good team co-operation these alternative programmes can be explained so that they know what is really involved. It is the wise therapist who accepts the right of the family to pursue these programmes in the knowledge that it is part of the grief process, but who will be ready to receive the child back into the normal stream without recriminations.

Coordination

Because these children often have long, slow deterioration, it is important for parents to know that one member of the team is available to coordinate services from the time of diagnosis onwards. This person needs to be able to enlist the appropriate help at times of crisis and to span the points of changing service interventions. When Woolley *et al.* (1991) conducted a survey with 41 families who had children with Duchenne muscular dystrophy, they found that two issues were paramount. Firstly parents frequently emphasized the difficulty in identifying sources of help and secondly they spoke of the

immense task of obtaining and orchestrating help in a way that still left them feeling in control of their own lives — lives already complicated and stressed by the impending loss of a child.

In 34 families of the same study where a special cornerstone carer relationship had evolved with one or more professionals, parents felt less bewildered by the diverse help available. They were able to use help as needed, but could maintain their preferred way of caring for their child. Figure 1 shows the services encountered by one family who had a 14-year-old boy with Duchenne muscular dystrophy. Although the paediatrician and the general practitioner play a very important role in the child's life and are usually more stable in their position, neither can take on the key role in coordinating the many services. Furthermore, these children only occasionally require acute medical intervention. Ideally the coordinating role should be shared by the therapist working most closely with the child and the social worker who has constant contact with the family.

Key workers must be responsible for ensuring that changes in personnel are made as smoothly as possible. Termination must be done in a way that causes the least trauma to the child and his family. Plenty of notice must be given and the successor introduced and supported. This will help to lessen the devastation that a break in a long and caring relationship can cause.

Problems in Adolescence

Adolescence is a period of psychological change which allows for new adjustments to face adult life and to reorganize experiences of childhood. It is a time of emotional, physical, sexual, intellectual and philosophical changes. For the young person with a life-limiting disease, there are many barriers to these alterations and adjustments.

It is essential that therapists working with these young people have a knowledge of the nature of adolescence and of the dynamic process which occurs. They will then be aware that for their patients who are deteriorating physically and facing death there is a feeling of failure to evolve into adult life in the full sense. The erosion of hope of normality and its effects on the

Figure I Services Encountered by a Family with a Child who has Duchenne Muscular Dystrophy

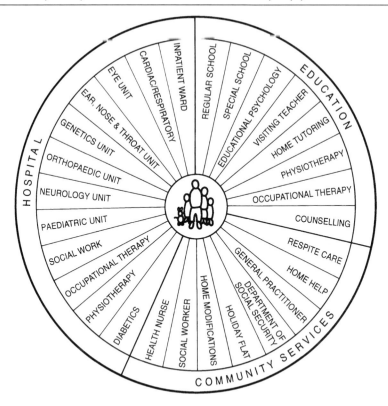

family will have a wide-ranging effect on all people involved in their life. Hilton *et al.* (1993) states that, over time, the adolescent lives in a smaller world as physical limitations preclude participation in many family, educational and social activities.

Therapists must be able to discuss issues openly and invite the young person to question treatment and prognosis and to ventilate fears, concerns and anger regarding his or her fate. They must learn to take seriously the normal adolescent concerns like acne, masturbation or delayed secondary sexual characteristics. It is often the therapist's help with these normal issues that will lead into a stronger relationship between the two. A young man with Duchenne muscular dystrophy spoke to his physiotherapist about his gynecomastia and told him of the comments made by his able-bodied school friends. The physiotherapist was able, after consultation, to allay his fears, and this began a relationship between the two which enabled the young man to explore his sexuality and to accept to a certain extent his limitations.

By adolescence the boy with muscular dystrophy will usually be an electric wheelchair user. Adolescents with spinal muscular atrophy type II and those with congenital muscular dystrophy are also often electric wheelchair users by this stage.

Issues for Physical Management

The programme of prone lying and passive range of motion to joints, to assist with contracture management, needs to be adapted as the physical condition changes. If the child's hips develop significant flexion contractures, their position will require support. Standing frames are usually no longer tolerated, although a tilt table may be useful in providing some weight-bearing at a semi-inclined position. The major issues at this stage tend to be scoliosis management and respiratory management.

SCOLIOSIS

A number of studies in the early to mid 1980s documented the progression of spinal curvature in boys with DMD and concluded that scoliosis developed inevitably, that bracing and modular seating had little effect on its development, and that early spinal fusion was the best course of action.

A study by Seeger (1984) found that there was a mean scoliosis angle of 10° for boys less than 10 years and 75° for boys over 16 years. When the curve becomes greater than 40° there is decreased sitting tolerance and loss of function, the arms are needed for sitting balance, pain is present and the vital capacity of the lungs decreases significantly (Hsu 1983). The adolescent growth spurt contributes to the rapid progression of scoliosis.

Early surgical intervention is desirable while pulmonary function is adequate. Some families, however, may choose not to proceed with surgery. Bracing or special seating may provide trunk support to leave hands free for activity. Wheelchair seating modifications may still be necessary following scoliosis surgery. Lateral supports can assist with upright posture and a tilt mechanism may offer some relief from buttock pressure periodically.

RESPIRATORY PROBLEMS

The effects of scoliosis on respiratory function can hopefully be minimized with spinal fusion. However, increasing muscle weakness will continue to compromise respiratory function. Some studies have shown that weight loss and nocturnal hypoxia may add to the process. For example, Rochester (1986) found that normal subjects with body weights 71% of the ideal, had respiratory muscle strength <40% of normal and that hypercapnia occurred when the strength reduced to 33% of normal.

The effects of respiratory muscle training in DMD were examined by Martin et al. (1986) and found that endurance could be improved, but not strength. A possible explanation was that the slow twitch fibres responsible for endurance were more likely to suffer disuse atrophy and thus be amenable to training.

The occurrence of hypoxemia during sleep in DMD has been found in a number of studies. In rapid eye movement (REM) sleep there is supraspinal inhibition of the skeletal muscles, including those used in breathing, with reliance on the diaphragm. If the diaphragm is weak and the effect of gravity elimi-

nated (as in lying) then hypoxia may occur and multiple arousals with sleep fragmentation can occur. Daytime symptoms of fatigue, irritability, memory loss etc. may result.

There have been trials of intermittent positive pressure ventilation via a nose mask which have helped to maintain O_2 saturation, restored normal sleep patterns and decreased daytime symptoms (Ellis 1987, Smith et al. 1988). Some hospitals have sleep clinics where sleep patterns and respiratory function can be monitored. This can provide useful information in deciding upon intervention.

Prolongation of Life

Twenty years ago there was very little to offer adolescents with terminal neuromuscular diseases, but now with surgical and medical advances the whole approach must be re-examined and these young people given some say in the medical decision-making. Life prolongation has become an important issue in the treatment of these young people. Hilton et al. (1993), in an article on end-of-life care in Duchenne muscular dystrophy, cite four sets of considerations to be observed when measures are being taken to extend the life of these young people. They are mainly concerned with mechanical ventilation, but these considerations are pertinent to all aspects of treatment to prolong life, for example, major operative procedures.

1. Medical Indications. Health professionals must know the patient's current condition, the prognosis with or without further intervention, and which options are feasible for that person. They must be familiar with all recent treatments and obtain consultations with others when appropriate.

2. Patient Preferences. These must be considered. The principle of self-determination requires that these young people be involved in discussions and decisions about treatment at whatever level they can. They must be given the choice to have family members present at some or all of the meetings.

3. Quality of Life of the Patient. This is important when he or she is not able to make decisions and this will have to be done by others. Decisions on quality of life would be made by looking at the physical, psychological, social and cognitive dimensions of the young person's life.

4. Effects of External Factors which may impinge on decision-making should be considered. These would include family, legal, cultural and social factors; for example, home mechanical ventilation may not be possible without adequate family support even when it is the patient's preferred choice.

Decisions about the continuation of treatment are always difficult and the therapist who has been giving the treatment will often be the pivotal person. However, if there has been honesty in communication and in addressing sympathetically but realistically the diagnosis, prognosis and therapeutic options and anticipated outcomes, there would have been the best possible transition from corrective to palliative to terminal management.

Anyone working with these young people must also understand when and how children perceive death. By 9–10 years children begin to understand that death is a universal process; by 16 years they begin to grasp the concept of their own mortality (Buhlmann and Fitzpatrick 1987). This conclusion is based on a study involving healthy children and it is thought that a child with a life-threatening disease may have an earlier perception of his own mortality. Justin (1988) studied 170 healthy teenagers to gauge their feelings about death. The study revealed that 35% of the group had discussed death with their family or friends. When asked about their feelings if they were terminally ill, 93% said they would want to know the truth about their condition, 86% said they would want to be included in decision-making and 85% said they would want life supports turned off if there was no hope. Although this survey was done with well children, it seems probable that affected children would have similar feelings.

Dying

Although the individual reactions of a terminally ill adolescent may vary, the phases of dying as described by Kubler-Ross (1973, 1985) and others are applicable

and can be a helpful guide to the coping state. The phases of denial, anger, bargaining, depression and acceptance do not often occur in a linear fashion. In fact one or more may be missed or the patient may become 'stuck' on one. Denial may last from a few days to the end of the dying process. A young person's denial may be an attempt to protect his family as occurred with a young man who did not tell his mother of the approaching death of his school friend who was suffering from the same disease. As the seriousness of the condition becomes more obvious, denial changes to anger and depression. The stage of bargaining is really an attempt to postpone. The patient knows from experience that there are rewards for good behaviour and the bargaining may be with God or with the therapist. The wish is usually for an extension of life but later will be for a period without pain or discomfort. When the inevitability of death is fully realized, most patients will undergo a process of bargaining and then acceptance to some extent.

Some adolescents will discuss their dying openly with family, close friends and valued health professionals while others will remain silent. Some will choose to protect their parents by not speaking of their fears, but instead will talk to someone who has worked closely with them. This may be the therapist and if he or she can tolerate listening to the adolescent's feelings about dying, the moments are privileged ones. It is a time to share, to listen and to communicate that they will not be abandoned and that they will be kept free from pain. Helping an adolescent and the family make a tragic situation more tolerable and meaningful is challenging, but rewarding.

They may want to discuss such issues as how death will come, and who will be with them; some will ask about their final resting place. One young man asked for cremation because he said his body had deteriorated so much in life. Another said he wanted to be buried so that his parents and sister would visit him. These are difficult things to discuss, but if the therapist understands that it will lighten the young person's load to be able to share this with a special person, it will somehow make the situation easier to endure. Pazola and Gerberg (1990) rightly call this privileged communication.

The planning of the funeral is a personal thing and most parents will want to do this. However, very often they need gentle guidance and some framework to allow choices. Parents may discuss these issues with the therapist; it is the wise and caring person who will direct them to the best possible help without appearing to avoid the issue. A physiotherapist, whose care with a young man with spinal atrophy had spanned many years, not only assisted the parents with his funeral but gave a eulogy that would have helped the family in their search for resolution of their grief.

Attendance at the funeral by team members who have worked closely with the young person is helpful and can be therapeutic both for parents and for themselves. The family will see it as a tribute and a token of love and support. Many parents have expressed their gratitude to see staff at the service. One mother spoke of the physiotherapist's tears at her son's funeral — 'I realized that he also loved my boy' she said.

It is imperative that persons working in this area will have examined their own feelings and will have come to grips with their own mortality. They must be able to encourage expressions of grief even if it causes pain and they must be able to seek help for themselves in their own grief. There is much wisdom in Shakespeare's words '. . . the grief that does not speak whispers the o'er-fraught heart and bids it break . . .' (Macbeth Act IV, II 209–210).

In general our society does not handle death well, but as therapists working with terminally ill children, adolescents and their families it is essential to be able to communicate well with the young person; this will help him or her to disengage from life with the most dignity possible. Sister Frances Dominica (1987), who has worked for many years in the area of care for terminally ill young people, has summed up this sharing relationship. She says 'being alongside these families you absorb some of their grief . . . but you also share some of the good things . . . enjoying a swift growth of friendship, bypassing the obstacles of class, creed, colour, age, education etc. . . . having all one's sensitivities heightened . . . and you recognize and reverence the beauty in every man, woman and child because tragedy lifts the mask of pretence and truth is revealed' (p. 110).

REFERENCES

Brussock, CM, Haley, SM, Munsat, TL et al. (1992) Measurement of isometric force in children with and without Duchennes muscular dystrophy. Physical Therapy 72: 105–114.

Buhlmann, U, Fitzpatrick, SB (1987) Caring for an adolescent with a chronic illness. Primary Care 14: 57–68.

Bushby, KMD (1992) Recent advances in understanding muscular dystrophy. Archives of Disease in Childhood 67: 1310–1312.

Dominica, F (1987) Reflections on death in childhood. British Medical Journal 294: 108–110.

Dorman, C, Hurley, AD, D'Avignon, J (1988) Language and learning disorders of older boys with Duchenne muscular dystrophy. Developmental Medicine and Child Neurology 30: 316–327.

Ellis, E (1987) Respiratory muscle function and nocturnal hypoxia. Proceedings of Australian Physiotherapy Association National Conference, Hobart.

Evans, GA, Drennan, JC, Russman, BS (1981) Functional classification and orthopaedic management of spinal muscular atrophy. Journal of Bone and Joint Surgery 63: 516–522.

Florence, JM, Pandya, S, King, W et al. (1992) Intrarater reliability of manual muscle test (Medical Research Council Scale) grades in Duchenne's muscular dystrophy. Physical Therapy 72: 115–122.

Hilton, T, Orr, RD, Perkin, RM et al. (1993) End of life care in Duchenne muscular dystrophy. Pediatric Neurology 9: 165–177.

Hsu, JD (1983) The natural history of spine curvature progression in the non-ambulatory Duchenne muscular dystrophy patient. Spine 8: 771–774.

Justin, RG (1988) Adult and adolescent attitudes toward death. Adolescence 23: 429–435.

Kakulas, BA (1988) Observations on the pathogenesis of Duchenne muscular dystrophy in the light of recent progress in molecular genetics. Australian Paediatric Journal 24 (suppl. 1): 4–8.

Karpati, G (1992) Recent advances in Duchenne/Becker dystrophy. Proceedings of the American Neurological Association Meeting, pp. 23–33.

Knubley, W, Bertorini, T (1988) Congenital muscular dystrophy with cerebellar atrophy. Developmental Medicine and Child Neurology 30: 378–390.

Kubler-Ross, E (1973) On Death and Dying, 260 pp. London: Tavistock Publication.

Kubler-Ross, E (1985) On Children and Death, 279 pp. New York: Collier Books.

Mandel, JL (1989) Dystrophin — The gene and its product. Nature 339: 584–586.

Martin, AJ, Stern, L, Yeates, J et al. (1986) Respiratory muscle training in Duchenne muscular dystrophy. Developmental Medicine and Child Neurology 28: 314–318.

Miyoshi, K, Kawai, H, Iwasa, M et al. (1986) Autosomal recessive distal muscular dystrophy as a new type of progressive muscular dystrophy. Brain 109: 31–54.

Pazola, KJ, Gerberg, AK (1990) Privileged communication — Talking with a dying adolescent. American Journal of Maternal Child Nursing 5: 16–21.

Personius, KE, Pandya, S, King, W et al. (1994) Fascioscapulohumeral dystrophy natural history study: standardisation of testing procedures and reliability of measurements. Physical Therapy 74: 253–263.

Rochester, DF (1986) Respiratory effects of respiratory muscle weakness and atrophy. Annual Review of Respiratory Disease 134: 1083–1086.

Russman, BS (1990) Rehabilitation of the pediatric patient with a neuromuscular disease. Pediatric Neurology 8: 727–740.

Scott, OM, Vrbova, G, Hyde, SA et al. (1986) Responses of muscles of patients with Duchenne muscular dystrophy to chronic electrical stimulation. Journal of Neurology, Neurosurgery and Psychiatry 49: 1427–1434.

Seeger, B (1984) Orthotic management of scoliosis in Duchenne muscular dystrophy. Archives of Physical Medicine Rehabilitation 65: 83–85.

Shakespeare, W (1962) Macbeth. In: Muir K (ed.) *The Arden Edition of The Works of William Shakespeare*. London: Methuen and Co.

Smith, PE, Calverley, PM, Edwards, RH (1988) Hypoxemia during sleep in Duchenne muscular dystrophy. *American Review Respiratory Disease* 137: 884–888.

Vignos, PJ, Spencer, GE, Archibald, KC (1963) Management of progressive muscular dystrophy in childhood. *Journal of the American Medical Association* 184: 89–96.

Woolley, H, Stein, A, Forrest, GC *et al.* (1989) Imparting the diagnosis for life threatening illness in children. *British Medical Journal* 298. 1623–1626.

Woolley, H, Stein, A, Forrest, GC *et al.* (1991) Cornerstone care for families of children with life-threatening illness. *Developmental Medicine and Child Neurology* 33: 216–224.

25

The Abused or Neglected Child

KARIN SHEPHERD

Historical Perspective

•

How Common is Child Abuse and Neglect?

•

What is Child Abuse and Neglect?

•

Who Abuses?

•

Multidisciplinary Team Approach

•

Role of the Physiotherapist and Family

•

Health Care of Abused and Neglected Children

•

Prevention

Whereas mankind owes to the child

the best it has to give ...

he shall be entitled to grow and develop

in health – to this end special care

and protection shall be provided

From the Declaration of the Rights of Children

(United Nations 20/11/1959)

Physiotherapists involved in the care and treatment of children and adolescents will undoubtedly encounter many families where abuse and neglect issues are pertinent. These issues will need to be addressed if the child and family are to receive appropriate professional care. Paediatric physiotherapists, given their training, close physical contact with young children, and their advocacy role with families, are ideally placed to help identify children who may be at particular risk. They are also uniquely placed directly to assist families by providing practical advice and support, which may help reduce the risk of child abuse itself, and to assist families in coping with the effects that child abuse and neglect may have on them and their child. Therapists treating children following abuse need to be particularly alert to the special requirements of this group. An understanding of child abuse and neglect is critical to good paediatric physiotherapy practice.

Historical Perspective

In terms of human rights children in the western world have made striking progress in the past 200 years. They have come from being virtually regarded as non-persons, to being seen as citizens with rights of their own. As the health and financial well-being of adults in western society has increased, so, in parallel, has the well-being of children, albeit somewhat more slowly.

In 1860 in Paris, Ambroise Tardieu, a specialist in pathology, described multiple fractures and other injuries in children that were inflicted by parents (Tardieu 1860). This appears to be the first report of skeletal injury as a manifestation of maltreatment of children. In 1874 Mary Ellen, a child living with step parents in New York, was subjected to cruel treatment and it required the Society for the Prevention of Cruelty to Animals to intervene on her behalf as there was no Society for Prevention of Cruelty to Children. Mary Ellen was removed to a safer home (Kempe 1974). Soon after came some improvement in the legal status of children with child labour laws and the introduction of universal and free education. The rediscovery of skeletal injuries in children inflicted by caregivers occurred during the 1940s and 1950s and led to the formal description and definition of the 'battered child syndrome' by Kempe *et al.* in 1962.

Sexual abuse of children was once regarded as an uncommon phenomenon despite attempts in the latter half of the nineteenth century by three French physicians Tardieu, Bernard and Brouardel to expose the problem. Child abuse reporting laws, together with the women's movement in the late 1960s and the early 1970s helped set the scene for increasing both public and professional awareness of child sexual abuse. Official reports began to escalate in the United States throughout the 1970s, a pattern repeated in Australia in the 1980s.

Over the past 20 years rapid growth in our knowledge of the epidemiology, consequences, and management of child abuse has occurred in combination with increasing public awareness and concern.

Knowledge in this complex area continues to evolve and there remain many areas of controversy in both the theory and management of childhood abuse.

How Common is Child Abuse and Neglect?

Abuse and neglect of children and adolescents is common in the Australian community, and is recognized as a major public health problem in both Australia and overseas. Figures from the Australian Institute of Health and Welfare compiled from all Australian state and territory child welfare authorities in 1991, show nearly 50 000 cases of suspected child abuse and neglect were reported and investigated. Of these about 45% were substantiated and in another 7% of cases the child was assessed as being 'at risk' (Angus and Wilkinson 1993). This represents a combined rate of 4.9 per 1000 children aged 0 to 16 years, or in other words approximately 1 in 200 children will either be at risk of abuse or actually suffering abuse. It seems likely that these figures considerably underestimate the actual number of abused children.

In the USA each year over one million children and adolescents are reportedly victims of child abuse, and approximately 2000 die from injuries or complica-

Table 1
Child Abuse and Neglect — Characteristics

Physical abuse or non-accidental injury (Schmitt 1987)
Injury to the skin, bruises, lacerations, abrasions and burns including cigarette burns; soft tissue injuries; intra-abdominal and intrathoracic injuries; fractures and other skeletal injuries; shaken baby syndrome; Munchausen's syndrome by proxy, including poisoning; drowning

Neglect
Lack of adequate supervision, hygiene, clothing and shelter; refusal or delay in obtaining health care; neglect of educational needs; and lack of adequate food. Neglect also involves failing to provide adequate nurturing; exposure to ongoing domestic violence; allowing easy access and misuse of drugs; and permitting criminal behaviour

Psychological or emotional abuse
Excessive parental demands that place expectations on children beyond their capabilities; instilling fear or terrorizing; rejection of the child with belittling and constant criticism; isolating the child by preventing participation in social activities or friendships, locking up the child alone; and the psychological impact from physical abuse (Garbarino 1989)

Sexual abuse
Sexual abuse is the exploitation of a child for the sexual gratification of the perpetrator and includes fondling, voyeurism and exhibitionism, oral sex, masturbation of the victim or the perpetrator; attempted or actual penetration of the vulva, vagina or anus; child pornography and prostitution; and ritualistic sexual abuse

tions relating to maltreatment or neglect, 90% of these fatalities occurring in children under 5 years of age (McClain *et al.* 1993). Research indicates the sexual abuse remains a significant community issue with 27% of women and 16% of men in the USA reporting sexual abuse as children (Finkelhor *et al.* 1990).

What is Child Abuse and Neglect?

The term 'child abuse and neglect' includes non-accidental injury/physical abuse and excessive punishment, emotional/psychological abuse, emotional neglect/deprivation, and sexual abuse/exploitation (see Table 1).

There is no universally accepted definition of child abuse, and child abuse is at times narrowly defined as maltreatment resulting in death or severe injury to a child whilst other definitions include any act of omission or commission that causes the child unnecessary injury, suffering or danger. The core issue in child abuse is the victimization of the child by someone in a position of power or authority over the child. The pathological relationship between the child and the abuser is central to our current understanding of abuse, as it is this relationship, in combination with the physical effects of abuse, which compromises the child's ability to reach fully their physical, developmental and emotional potential.

Child abuse or neglect is usually not an isolated incident of non-accidental injury, emotional torment, neglect of basic necessities or sexual abuse. It is often an escalating pattern of behaviour occurring over a period of time, the effects of which are cumulative. For this reason early identification and appropriate intervention are essential.

Infliction of injury per se rather than the degree of trauma that results must be the determinant for intervention. Small bruises on a young baby's face may be the only indication that the infant has been grabbed and shaken by an adult and while the bruising itself may appear to be inconsequential, the consequences for the child given the mechanism of injury can be very significant (e.g. subdural haematoma) (Figure 1).

Figure 1 Small bruises on a baby's face may indicate abusive shaking, which can cause subdural haematoma

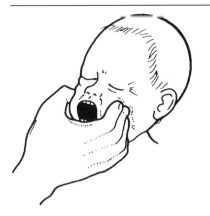

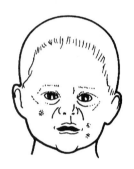

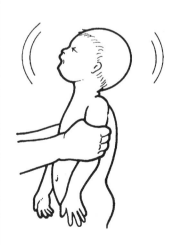

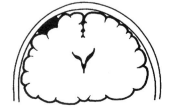

Table 2
Factors Contributing to Child Abuse and Neglect

Individual influences
A past history of abuse or rejection; poor self-esteem or problem-solving abilities; alcohol and drug abuse; poor health; unrealistic expectations of children; belief about the superiority and/or rights of adults over children; and belief in harsh physical punishment

Family influences
Communication and problem-solving abilities, including the presence of domestic violence and excessive secrecy within families

Community influences
Inadequate provision of public transport and health services; difficulty in obtaining health and education services, particularly for children with behavioural or mental health problems; housing difficulties; isolation whether due to physical distance, poor social skills or cultural isolation

Cultural influences
The tolerance of Australians and other western societies towards violence and sexuality; attitudes about the individual worth of children in society; and beliefs about the balance between parental and children's rights

There is no single cause for any of the four various types of child abuse. It is also unusual for one single type of abuse to be present in a child's life so that sexual abuse is often associated with psychological abuse as the child is intimidated or threatened, and physical abuse may be associated with psychological abuse including verbal abuse and so on. Research over the past two decades has repeatedly suggested that child abuse requires an environment where several factors including individual, familial, societal and cultural combine (see Table 2).

Finkelhor (1984) described four preconditions necessary for sexual abuse to occur:

1. The abuser must be motivated to abuse children or to be sexually aroused by children.
2. The abuser must overcome their own internal inhibitions or moral standards.
3. The child must be available to the abuser so that external inhibitors such as protective parents or normal family boundaries are overcome.
4. The abuser must overcome the resistance of the child by pressure, seduction or coercion.

Being a parent is a difficult job, and parents', own upbringing as well as their family environment influences their ability to raise children to adulthood with the ability to love and trust others, to have good self-esteem, to be able to deal rationally with problems, and in turn to become effective and nurturing parents for the next generation.

Figure 2 Fatal head injury in a 2-year-old allegedly from a fall of 15' from a balcony during play — investigation revealed that the home was lowset; a cricket bat was implicated as the source of the impact

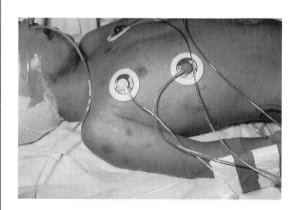

Non-Accidental Trauma

Physical abuse constitutes a significant risk to life (see, for example, Figure 2). Statistics regarding injuries in children are difficult to ignore. Fatalities from child abuse now occur seven times more frequently than death from meningitis (Waller *et al.* 1989). Approximately 10% of injuries in children under the age of 5 years seen in hospital accident and emergency departments are non-accidental, and children under 18 months of age are at the highest risk. Eighty percent of abuse fractures but only 2% of accidental fractures occur in this age group (Worlock *et al.* 1986). The most common cause of death from all head trauma in children under 2 years remains abusive head injury

Figure 3 A, Mechanism of injury – bruising to the back may be associated with anterior abdominal force resulting in intra-abdominal injury. B, 20-month-old child presenting with bruising to the back and perforation of the upper small intestine. A physiotherapist treating an elderly patient following a hip fracture heard this child's whimpering through the (fortunately) thin wall in the unit of flats, enquired next door and brought the child and mother directly to the accident and emergency department of the local children's hospital where resuscitation was required. The injury to the abdomen was estimated to have occurred some 24–48 hours earlier.

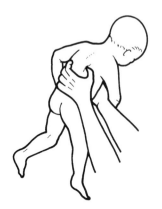
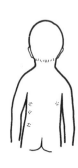

A

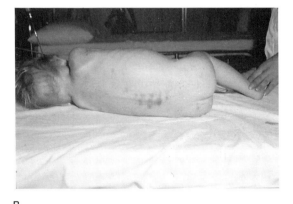

B

(Bruce and Zimmerman 1989). Shaking young children is particularly dangerous and can result in subdural haematomas (Figure 1). Asphyxiation of infants has a high associated morbidity.

Lesser degrees of head injury result frequently in neurological deficits and diminished developmental potential. The child may be left with intellectual impairment, seizure disorders, spastic diplegia or quadriplegia, learning difficulties, personality changes and behavioural problems.

Skeletal injuries are also common in physical abuse, particularly in children under the age of 18 months (Merten *et al.* 1983). Fractures may involve all bones but spiral fractures of long bones in preambulatory children are of particular concern, as are fractures of the ribs, sternum and ends of the clavicle, vertebral spine and metaphyseal injuries. Children with long bone fractures require ongoing medical supervision to ensure the limb attains adequate length and alignment. Given that children may be in and out of foster placements, and that some parents may avoid medical follow-up (the hospital may be the place where the diagnosis was made), physiotherapists involved in the ongoing supervision of the child have an important role.

Intra-abdominal trauma occurs more commonly than is often realized and may be difficult to detect. See, for example, Figure 3.

An unusual but increasingly recognized form of non-accidental trauma is Munchausen's syndrome by proxy (Rosenberg 1987, Meadow 1991). In this condition a parent, usually a mother, either fabricates or induces illness in a child and then seeks medical care for this. This condition often has a high morbidity and a chronic course. It can be difficult to diagnose unless a suspicion is raised when current medical symptoms, which cannot be reasonably explained, give rise to concern. To add to the problem, the ensuing medical treatment and investigations in themselves frequently increase the morbidity.

Child Neglect

Neglect encompasses a wide variety of acts of omission in the care of children (see Table 1). Children subjected to chronic neglect will commonly present clinically with poor nutrition, previously described as 'failure to thrive'. Non-organic failure to thrive is an obsolete term as it is now recognized that the cause of the growth failure is malnutrition. Malnutrition not only jeopardizes the child's growth but impairs immune competency, and contributes to both short- and long-term significant deficits in cognition, language and the acquisition of appropriate social skills (Frank and Zeisel 1988). Poverty is a significant risk factor (Walravens *et al.* 1989). Infants with difficult feeding behaviours which may be caused by medical conditions such as neurological disease or gastro-oesophageal reflux and families with poor organizational skills may increase the risk. Intervention, to be effective, must be multidisciplinary, and continued beyond the immediate nutritional crises. Children may present when neglect results in repeated accident or injuries, including poisoning, or where medical or dental care is below the level accepted within the community. Such chronic neglect can be a factor in the determination of developmental delay, impaired language acquisition, poor school performance and behavioural problems.

Psychological Abuse

Psychological abuse is often difficult to identify early in its course simply because it does not leave any physical injury. It is likely that it is not until the child shows signs of severe emotional problems or behavioural difficulties that it may be recognized. Some children constantly seek attention and may lie or steal, or become destructive or violent. Others may become withdrawn or depressed. Younger children may show no discrimination between adults and will attach equally with a stranger as with a parent. The harm of verbal abuse has been highlighted (Garbarino 1989). Children find it difficult to defend themselves against verbal abuse given their own language development. Criticized children are found frequently to criticize themselves and children who are blamed frequently blame themselves for their own abuse. Women who are physically abused or neglected by husbands or partners are more verbally abusive in turn towards their children (Ney 1987). It seems that it is harder to convince parents not to express irritation and frustration by blaming, humiliating or criticizing their children than it is to convince parents not to deal with their children in physically violent ways.

Sexual Abuse

Defining childhood sexual abuse is difficult. Within the legal context the definition would include rape, indecent assault and incest. While the medical consequences of sexual abuse such as injury, venereal disease and pregnancy are important, consideration of these in isolation fails to recognize the extreme importance of the psychological aspects of the sexual abuse. Sexual abuse has been defined as the involvement of dependent and developmentally immature children and adolescents in sexual activities that they do not fully comprehend, are unable to give informed consent to, and that violate the social taboos or family roles (Schecter and Roberge 1976). The most important aspect of this definition is the inclusion of a child's inability to give informed consent. It is not uncommon still for the child to be accused of 'leading the adult on' or looking 'older than her years'. Clearly sexual abuse involves the abuse of power and a betrayal of trust of someone who is smaller and weaker. Because children are generally taught to trust and obey adults, when sexual abuse does occur, it is very difficult for the child to tell what has happened from fear, or shame, or from confusion about what has happened, particularly if the offender is a member of the family or someone the family trusts. Many abusers are carefully attuned to children, and cultivate their trust, curiosity and need for attention, establishing a close rapport with a child over time, gradually undertaking the process of victimization (Berliner and Conte 1990). Recognition of sexual abuse often requires a high index of suspicion. Children may present giving either a history of sexual abuse, or with a number of physical signs which could be due to sexual abuse, or with disturbed behaviours which may also be indicative of abuse (Heger and Emans 1992).

The child's direct statement describing sexual abuse remains the most definitive historical indicator of abuse. Any complaint by a child of abuse should be taken seriously and the complaint investigated even if there are no physical signs or behavioural indications. However, statements such as 'children never lie' and 'children always lie', are equally fictitious. Investigation of sexual abuse requires a multidisciplinary approach that involves medical evaluation, mental health assessment and investigation by child protection and police authorities. The aim of this coordinated investigation is to protect the child from making multiple repetitions of the complaint, and at the same time ensuring an accurate assessment.

Although the long-term impact of sexual abuse on any individual remains difficult to predict, it is clear that victims of both child and adolescent sexual abuse are at increased risk for a number of emotional and interpersonal problems as well as psychiatric disorder. Sexually abused children exhibit more sexualized behaviour than non-abused control groups. Long-term problems can include difficulties with intimate relationships, sexual relationships, anxiety, depression, eating disorders, sleep disturbance, post-traumatic distress disorder, multiple personality disorder, suicidal and self-injury risk, and too often failure to protect their own children from sexual abuse (Finkelhor and Browne 1988).

Allegations of sexual abuse during child custody proceedings are commonly reported and 4–9% of these cases are shown to be false, despite concern that the majority of allegations within the Family Court setting are falsified (Paradise *et al.* 1988). As very young children are often involved in divorce and custody related cases, substantiating sexual abuse in these children is made even more difficult. Children with developmental difficulties are also potential victims of sexual abuse and some studies report significantly higher rates of abuse than in the non-handicapped population (Tharinger *et al.* 1990).

Who Abuses?

Most children are abused by someone whom they know and with whom they have an ongoing relationship. Sadly children are more in danger from someone they know and trust rather than from a stranger, despite media focus on this small group of abusers. Parents including stepparents, defacto parents and foster parents were the abusers in 64% of cases which were substantiated in Australia (Angus and Wilkinson 1993). Physical or inflicted injury usually happens in a moment of anger when a parent or caregiver loses control. It is rarely premeditated, although it may be limited to the home (e.g. domestic violence). Some adults who experienced harsh punishment as children repeat the pattern either because they know no other way of disciplining their children or else they believe 'it didn't do me any harm'. Both men and women are equally involved in causing physical abuse, and boys and girls are equally affected. The pattern is different in sexual abuse when the perpetrators are usually male, although women and juveniles have also been impli-

cated. Of sexual abuse victims 75% are girls, with the majority abused by parents or caregivers. Boys who are sexually abused will be abused mainly by someone outside their immediate family home. 'Sex tourism' by Australian citizens involved in child pornography or prostitution has recently concerned the Australian community who recognize we have a responsibility not only to our own children but to those of other nations.

Multidisciplinary Team Approach

The first consideration in the management of suspected child abuse must be the immediate well-being of the child.

Effective intervention in the field of child abuse is the result of the collective wisdom of many professionals involved in the process of assessment and management. Each discipline may hold one piece of the puzzle and until these pieces are joined a full understanding of the child's experience, the degree of risk present and the needs of the family cannot be appreciated. It is dangerous to assume that the practitioner working alone can adequately determine the risk or understand family dynamics or intervene effectively. Limited treatment resources, in particular, impair the ability of child welfare authorities to provide adequate treatment and support for the family. However, a multidisciplinary assessment enhances the likelihood of a more comprehensive approach, so that intervention when it occurs is justified, coordinated and effective. Medical and developmental information about the child can be critical in understanding the nature of the risk, the nature of the injuries and the treatment requirements of the child.

Child welfare authorities and police have a statutory obligation to investigate allegations of child maltreatment and take action necessary to assess risk and help secure the child's safety. In Queensland, Australia, Suspected Child Abuse and Neglect Teams have been established state-wide with medical practitioners required to work with police and welfare authorities to provide multidisciplinary assessment and intervention. Protection of the child may require court-ordered state care of the child, either short-term until the situation can be more fully assessed, or longer term in foster care, following a court's appraisal. When considering foster care, child protection agencies consider other family members and may recruit foster parents from the child's own ethnic community. While some children are not able to return home safely, the majority of children are able to be returned to the home following a period of intervention. Treatment and rehabilitation of the family aimed at reducing high-risk parental behaviours and attitudes, assisting the family's functioning and improving the child's physical and developmental health remains the goal. Depending upon the nature of any offence committed against the child and evidentiary requirements, criminal charges may also be brought against adult caregivers responsible for the assault. The focus of child protection work, however, is on the safety of the child rather than on identifying the adult responsible.

Role of the Physiotherapist and Family

While few health professionals would dispute that abuse and neglect of children have detrimental effects, there is often a reluctance on the part of the health professional to become involved with the child or family when child abuse is part of the clinical picture. This lack of involvement is seen in the very low rate of reported child abuse by medical practitioners (despite mandatory reporting) and other health professionals, and results in treatment and follow-up programmes being seen as the responsibility of the social worker within the welfare system. No one person or agency is able to understand or meet the needs of abused children, and it is important that health professionals contribute their knowledge and perspective so that child protection agencies can better carry out their own duties. Health professionals may be concerned about the accuracy of the diagnosis, and doubtful as to whether notification to the appropriate child welfare department will actually help the child or merely disrupt what seems on the surface to be a functional family. At a personal level,

some health professionals claim they lack the knowledge to assist, or may be concerned about the time and effort needed if they become involved, or may not wish to become involved in potentially adversarial situations. They may fear that reporting child abuse will lead to the immediate removal of the child on the one hand, or that the complaint will be dismissed lightly on the other.

It is often helpful to establish a relationship with local child protection services including those medical practitioners with expertise in child protection so that the physiotherapist understands better the alternative interventions which are possible and is then more able to contribute to discussions regarding the safety and health needs of the child.

Most parents, even those who are abusing, wish the best for their child. Dealing honestly and in a non-judgemental manner with parents makes it clear that we are concerned for the whole family and we can establish that we are willing to be supportive and will not desert the family. It is usually best for health professionals to explain sensitively to a family why they are concerned about the child's safety, and what actions they need to take because of this. In young children with injuries, action to safeguard the child may have to be immediate; for example 'I am really worried about the bruises on Katie's cheek. Bruises in little babies 3 months of age can be serious and I would like you to go and see your doctor about them — I can give her a ring, or perhaps you would rather take Katie to the hospital — what do you think?' Few parents would refuse to take the child for medical attention, and in this small minority notification to child welfare authorities would be the next best step. Medical practitioners, nurses and physiotherapists may be the first to note injuries which would otherwise be out of sight when children are undressed during treatment (see Figure 4)..

If appropriate action is not taken by the health professional it is unlikely that the circumstances of the injury will be investigated. In other situations a consultative approach with other colleagues including medical practitioners and local social workers is best and may help clarify concerns and ensure that any intervention is justified and coordinated. In particular, situations involving neglect, emotional abuse and

Figure 4 Abuse injuries may be hidden by clothing

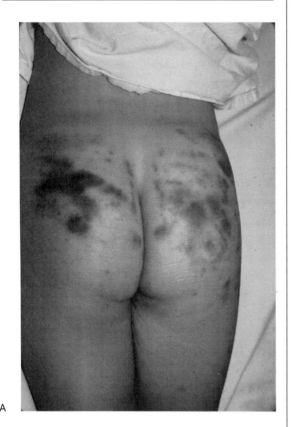

A

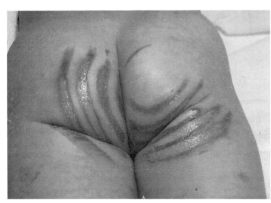

B

suspicions of sexual abuse do not require acute intervention and benefit from a full review of all the known concerns. While training in child abuse in most disciplines is inadequate, excellent educational seminars, reading matter and training courses are now widespread and freely available.

An important consideration is whether or not notification actually assists the child or simply causes emotional turmoil to the family. It should be recognized that abuse itself never benefits the child and that if nothing is done it is unlikely that the abusive behaviour will stop. In all Australian states, except Western Australla, doctors are required by law to report to the relevant authorities any reasonable suspicion of abuse or neglect. While physiotherapists may not have a legal obligation to notify, like medical practitioners in Western Australia, they could be seen to have a moral obligation to help protect those who may have no other advocate.

Health Care of Abused and Neglected Children

Children who have suffered physical abuse, injury or trauma clearly require immediate health care for these injuries. Many will also benefit from longer term rehabilitation programmes, for example, following significant head injury. It is not always as obvious that many other children with neglect or lesser degrees of injury also suffer significant developmental disorders. Many studies have demonstrated the extent to which neglect in particular impacts adversely on children's language development and social skills. Abused children have been shown to achieve significantly lower means on the WISC-R scale, to score lower on reading and language skill tests, and to be viewed by both teachers and parents as having more abnormal behaviour (Oates et al. 1984). These developmental problems may be masked by the child's behaviour if the child is either overly compliant or socially aggressive, or be overlooked due to the focus on the child's injuries or parental difficulties. These children are often more difficult to like and to relate to. They may be unkempt or dirty, they may be slow to engage in play and may approach unfamiliar adults tentatively with limited eye contact and poor cooperative play. Many are impulsive or demonstrate a fragmented or disorganized approach to play. Others may be relatively silent due to poor verbal skills and others may demonstrate rigid stereotyped repetitive play. Accurate assessment can thus be a challenge. Older children are often impressively independent with self-care skills, caring in turn for younger siblings who are often unable to self-feed, dress or toilet as expected for age.

In addition to meeting the needs of the parents for 'parenting' and support and providing appropriate rehabilitation for the child, health professionals need to be alert to any ongoing risks to the child. Until parental needs for nurturing and acceptance are met it is unlikely that the parents in turn will be able to meet the needs of their children. Undue focusing on the child's deficits or problems may further frustrate and isolate a parent. Children who have been abused or neglected frequently require developmental rehabilitation. This is often best achieved in a situation of play such as a daycare or kindergarten setting, where the focus is on the child's self-esteem and interaction with peers, rather than focused primarily on a specific cognitive, language or motor deficit. Abusing families frequently lack the social skills needed to access health and educational systems and obtain appropriate services for their children. Keeping appointments for their children is often a problem. A pre-appointment friendly phone call often assists. The physiotherapist will need to be more available (e.g. taking phone calls at inconvenient times) and to be aware of the family's practical difficulties – insisting on an 8.30 am appointment for a family who live some distance from public transport, have other children to take to school, or who live some distance from the therapy centre will guarantee failure to attend. We need to ask about these aspects directly, as many parents are not skilled at advocating for themselves.

Physiotherapists can also assist a positive outcome by liaising with other members of both the treatment team and the children protection team, and can help interpret health and developmental information to the case coordinator so that the needs of these children receive adequate priority.

Prevention

The dramatic increase in the number of children reported to welfare authorities over the last decade for investigation of abuse or neglect has forced not only the Australian community but also Commonwealth and State governments to take some action. Despite a high level of expenditure on child protection programmes the current response is not sufficient.

The growing arguments in favour of preventing child abuse are obvious and overwhelming. All agree that children have the right to grow up safe and protected without the painful experience of being abused and without having to deal with either the short- or long-term consequences of that abuse. Preventing child abuse makes sense not only because it is indefensible to wait until abuse has occurred before we respond, but also because it is increasingly shown that prevention is an achievable and cost-effective option.

Prevention of child abuse can be tackled at a number of levels. Tertiary treatment including early identification and reporting, evaluation and treatment, and associated legal actions have been discussed. Secondary prevention aims at preventing abuse or neglect at the time of the potential event by targeting high-risk groups who may benefit from education programmes, daycare facilities, financial counselling or other assistance. There has been increasing recognition during the 1990s that primary prevention, particularly a system of universal health visitation of families is a cost-effective and efficient mechanism of promotion of the health and well-being of children. Primary preventative programmes appropriate for young children have been introduced into many schools and community organizations to teach children how to recognize potentially abusive situations and how to respond assertively. This training has certainly resulted in more open discussion between parents, teachers and children, and the most effective programmes today are emphasizing the building of specific skills including assertive behaviours, decision-making and communication skills.

All health professionals including physiotherapists have unique opportunities to help prevent child abuse by helping families at various stages throughout a child's life. The first opportunity may come during the pregnancy when factors such as a history of childhood abuse in the parent, mothers who are adolescents or who present late in the pregnancy or those who have drug and alcohol addiction, may then be referred for appropriate social support or counselling. Often forewarning mothers-to-be of the possibilities of depression and tiredness, will make it easier for parents to seek help should managing the baby present more difficulties than they can handle. More importantly parents can be warned about the risks of shaking or throwing babies as many parents are unaware of this. Forewarning parents of the hazards associated with different developmental stages can help reduce accidental injuries resulting from children rolling from couches, accidents in baby walkers, burns and scalds, etc. Physiotherapists are also in a unique position to model directly to parents alternate ways of gaining the child's attention and cooperation during therapy sessions, and by avoiding themselves any acts of verbal or physical aggression or coercion. It is important to be aware that parents who have abused their children retain the right to determine their own priorities and be treated with professional courtesy.

REFERENCES

Angus, G, Wilkinson, K (1993) *Child Abuse and Neglect in Australia 1990–1991.* Australian Institute of Health and Welfare Series No. 2, Canberra: Australian Government Printing.

Berliner, L, Conte, JR (1990) The process of victimisation: the victim's perspective. *Child Abuse and Neglect* 14: 29–40.

Bruce, DA, Zimmermann, RA (1989) Shaken impact syndrome. *Pediatric Annals* 18: 482–484, 486–489, 492–494.

Finkelhor, DH (1984) *Child Sexual Abuse: New Theory and Research,* 260 pp. New York: Free Press.

Finkelhor, DH, Browne, A (1988) Assessing the long term impact of child sexual abuse: a review and conceptualisation. In: Walker, LE (ed.) *Handbook on Sexual Abuse of Children – Assessment and Treatment Issues.* New York: Springer.

Finkelhor, DH, Hotaling, G, Lewis, IA et al. (1990) Sexual abuse in a national survey of adult men and women: prevalence, characteristics and risk factors. *Child Abuse and Neglect* 14: 19–28.

Frank, DA, Zeisel, SH (1988) Failure to thrive. *Pediatric Clinics of North America* 35: 1187–1206.

Garbarino, J (1989) The psychologically battered child: toward a definition. *Pediatric Annals* 18: 502–504.

Heger, A, Emans, J (1992) *Evaluation of the Sexually Abused Child. A Medical Textbook and Photographic Atlas,* pp. 244. New York: Oxford University Press.

Kempe, CH, Silverman, FN, Steele, BF et al. (1962) The battered child syndrome. *Journal of the American Medical Association* 181: 17–24.

Kempe, CH (1974) The Mary Ellen case is noted in Ch. I, History of child abuse and neglect. In: Kempe, CH, Helfer, RE (eds) *The Battered Child.* Chicago: University of Chicago Press.

McClain, PW, Sacks, JJ, Froehlke, RG et al. (1993) Estimates of fatal child abuse and neglect, United States 1979 through 1988. *Pediatrics* 91: 338–343.

Meadow, R (1991) Neurological and developmental variants of Munchausen syndrome by proxy. *Developmental Medicine and Child Neurology* 33: 270–272.

Merten, DF, Radkowski, MA, Leonidas, JC (1983) The abused child: a radiological reappraisal. *Radiology* 146: 377–381.

Ney, PG (1987) Does verbal abuse leave deeper scars: a study of children and parents. *Canadian Journal of Psychiatry* 32: 371–378.

Oates, RK, Peacock, A, Forrest, D (1984) The development of abused children. *Developmental Medicine and Child Neurology* 26: 649–656.

Paradise, JE, Rostain, AI, Nathanson, M (1988) Substantiation of sexual abuse charges when parents dispute custody or visitation. *Pediatrics* 81: 835–839.

Rosenberg, DA (1987) Web of deceit: a literature review of Munchausen syndrome by proxy. *Child Abuse and Neglect* 11: 547–563.

Schecter, MD, Roberge, L (1976) Sexual exploitation. In: Helfer, RE, Kempe, CH (eds) *Child Abuse and Neglect: The Family and the Community.* Cambridge: Ballinger.

Schmitt, BD (1987) The child with non accidental trauma. In: Helfer, RE, Kempe, CH (eds) *The Battered Child,* 4th edn. Chicago: University of Chicago Press.

Tardieu, A (1860) Etude medico-legale sur les services et mauvais traitments exerces sur les enfants. *Annals de Hygiene et de Medicine Legale* 13: 361.

Tharinger, D, Horton, CB, Millea, S (1990) Sexual abuse and exploitation of children and adults with mental retardation and other handicaps. *Child Abuse and Neglect* 14: 301–

Waller, AE, Baker, SP, Szocka, A (1989) Childhood injury deaths: national analysis and geographic variations. *American Journal of Public Health* 79: 310–315.

Walravens, PA, Hambridge, KM, Koepfer, DM (1989) Zinc supplementation in infants with a nutritional pattern of failure to thrive: a double blind controlled study. *Pediatrics* 83: 532–538.

Worlock, P, Stower, M, Barbor, P (1986) Patterns of fractures in accidental and non-accidental injury in children: a comparative study. *British Medical Journal* 293: 100–102.

26

The Disabled Child in Countries with Minimal Rehabilitation Resources

GEERTRUIDA BEKKER

The Situation in Countries with Minimal Resources

•

Socioeconomic Conditions of the Disabled Child

•

Physiotherapy in CBR

•

Hansen's Disease (Leprosy)

This chapter attempts to provide some insight into how disabled children live in developing countries or similar situations. It focuses on new developing roles for physiotherapists to assist in improving the quality of life of disabled children. The process of adapting physiotherapy techniques to the local situation is also highlighted. Furthermore, this chapter explores the physiotherapy management of Hansen's disease (leprosy), as this is not an uncommon disease in countries with minimal rehabilitative resources.

The Situation in Countries with Minimal Resources

In 1980, approximately 80% of all disabled children lived in the developing world (Rehabilitation International/UNICEF 1981). In 1990, 5.5 million children with moderate and severe disabilities lived in developed countries versus 31 million in less developed countries (Helander 1993).

According to the United Nations Population Divi-

sion, 33% of the population in developing countries was urbanized in 1991. This figure, however, varies considerably from country to country. In the least developed countries, 19% of the population live in urban areas and in Latin America 71% (UNICEF 1993). In these urban areas less than 5% of persons with disabilities have access to rehabilitation services (CBM 1993). The population living in rural areas is almost totally deprived of any rehabilitation services. This presents a poor prospect for disabled children in developing countries receiving rehabilitation services — a situation caused by the lack of resources in general, such as food, work (money), schools, health services. Furthermore, there is often limited government attention for rehabilitation services, because of other priorities and/or low government funds. It is true that disability affects fewer persons than general health problems do. Likewise solving health problems will prevent a lot of people from becoming disabled.

The disabilities presented to rehabilitation personnel in developing countries are generally more severe and chronic. Many mild conditions and impairments are often not considered to be a problem until it seriously starts to interfere with normal functioning.

Prevalence of Disability

Thorburn (1994) states that in considering the size of the disability problem, one must first distinguish between overall prevalence of different types or categories of disability and the incidence of the main causes of disability. Clearly the former will vary according to the latter.

The prevalence or magnitude of handicaps will not only reflect disability prevalence, but also the attitudes and barriers to rehabilitation and participation of disabled people in the community (Thorburn 1994). A common problem is the lack of standardized disability definitions and reliable statistics on incidence or prevalence of disability. Rehabilitation International (1981) indicate a prevalence of childhood disability and impairments of 10%. The WHO (1981) mentions 7–10% for all age groups and that at any given time 1.5% of the total population is formed by disabled persons that could benefit from rehabilitation. Results of surveys in 55 countries indicate prevalence rates from 0.2% to 21% (Helander 1993).

The causes of disability vary considerably depending on the level of development of the country (Thorburn 1994), part of the country, or population group within a country. For example, infectious diseases depend largely on the level of hygiene and/or availability of vaccinations; nutrition and stimulus deprivation depend on educational and economical factors; perinatal anoxia on the available assistance during birth; traumatic, toxic and genetic factors on the level of public education and attitudes.

Whilst in more developed countries fewer people become disabled, these disabled people live longer. In countries with minimal resources the opposite is true. More people, especially children, become disabled, but many do not survive. Thorburn (1994) mentions that when health care improves, more severely disabled children survive longer and although the actual incidence of different causes may decline, the prevalence may not change and the number requiring rehabilitation increases.

Rehabilitation Services

Rehabilitation was defined as follows by an expert committee of the World Health Organization (WHO 1981):

...includes all measures aimed at reducing the impact of disabling and handicapping conditions, and at enabling the disabled and handicapped to achieve social integration. It entails the combined and coordinated use of medical, social, educational as well as vocational measures for training or for retaining the highest possible level of functional ability.

GOVERNMENT MEDICAL AND ALLIED HEALTH SERVICES

Most governments in developing countries try to equip physiotherapy departments in their largest hospitals, situated in the largest urban areas. A common problem is the lack of physiotherapists to manage them, and the lack of funds and know-how to equip and manage them or to maintain the equipment installed. The positions for occupational and speech therapists are often even harder to fill. Other medical specialist or rehabilitation specialist services are part of the normal package being offered by the government hospitals, but these also depend on the availability of specialists.

PRIVATE MEDICAL AND ALLIED HEALTH SERVICES

Private rehabilitation services also are mostly concentrated in the large cities in developing countries. Some of the professionals working in these private services are government personnel trying to get some extra income to complement their usually low government salaries.

COSTS

Government services are generally offered free or for a small fee. Private services are expensive, but considered to offer a better service. Medicine that is not available in the hospital can be purchased from nearby private or government owned pharmacies at relatively high prices compared with the costs of living.

SPECIAL EDUCATION SERVICES

An almost total lack of government involvement concerning the special education services can be observed in developing countries. Often non-governmental organizations (NGOs) or disability associations are taking on the task of educating disabled children. They target disabled children who have reached school age, and are able to attend. The number of children benefiting is very limited due to, amongst other things, financial constraints. Disabled children finishing primary school face the problem that few secondary education institutions will accept them. Not many services are offered for children from 0 to 6 years, despite the fact that more and more governments recognize the need for early stimulation. The existing early stimulation projects only serve a small part of the population.

Rehabilitation in the Community

PROFESSIONAL OUTREACH SERVICES OR EXTENSION SERVICES

In more and more countries the need for a better spreading of rehabilitation services is recognized. This has led to professionals reaching out from where they are based by travelling periodically to remote areas to offer their services. This approach confronts the need to train local persons to supervise and continue the therapy with the participants and their family between the visits of the professional team. The available professionals and travelling time determine the extent of this outreach. The trained volunteers often have little time and their supervision is difficult. Unless the outreach team is multidisciplinary, this approach tends to reach only a group of persons with one category of disability and likewise to deliver one type of intervention.

COMMUNITY-BASED REHABILITATION

Another form of rehabilitation service, often not well understood by established professionals, is community based rehabilitation (CBR). The World Health Organization has been describing and stimulating the development of CBR services and with this in mind has produced a manual since 1981. This manual describes rehabilitation methods used by communities in various countries — a result of the realization that stimulating communities to rehabilitate their disabled members had potential in the light of 'Health for all in the year 2000'.

CBR as defined by Helander et al. (1989) is a term used for situations where resources for rehabilitation are available in the community. There is a large-scale transfer of knowledge about disabilities and of skills in rehabilitation to the people with disabilities, their families and members of the community. There is also community involvement in the planning, decision-making and evaluation of the programme.

In many countries new CBR projects have been started in different forms since the first publications on CBR. Some have been created by the local community through a bottom-up approach, others were set-up through a top-down approach by government or other organizations. They can also be managed by a local steering team, or by an outside organization using local personnel. Some projects work with volunteers, others pay salaries, some train local leaders or interested parties (e.g. parents of disabled children), others may train a combination of all of these. Certain CBR projects are situated in urban areas, others in rural areas. Whereas some deal with all disabilities and all ages, others will concentrate on one or few disability categories and/or age groups.

All the different CBR projects have a common need for a regular professional evaluation of their participants. CBR tries to complement the work of the few professionals, not to replace it. In other words, improving the effectiveness of the professional input. New clients in a CBR project will receive an initial professional assessment. In some projects this is compared with the assessment and proposed programme plan elaborated previously by a CBR worker (to what extent depends on his/her training). A final programme is decided upon together by all involved (client, parent, CBR worker, professional).

The CBR worker will follow this proposed programme during regular (often weekly) visits to the client at home. S/he will do this through a process of modelling and teaching a family member and/or the client new activities to be carried out daily. A clear common-sense explanation during the training of CBR workers by various professionals will enable the CBR worker to plan and manage an individualized programme in line with the long-term objectives set by the assessment team after each evaluation. The level of this training often depends on the educational level of the CBR worker. A special education teacher will need to equip the CBR worker with teaching techniques that can be applied to both client and family member.

Socioeconomic Conditions of the Disabled Child

The Urban Situation

Disability does not recognize socioeconomic boundaries. A high incidence of impairments and disabilities that could have been prevented under better conditions, however, is observed amongst people living in marginal conditions. The majority of persons residing in the large urban and suburban areas of developing countries live in marginal conditions. Even though water and electricity are available, salaries are low, often making it necessary for both parents to look for work to make ends meet. There is a high level of unemployment and public transport is expensive for this group of the population.

Living conditions are even worse for the new arrivals in the cities. People squat wherever they can find a piece of land large enough to build a shelter using whatever material is cheap and/or available. Water supply, electricity, roads, schools, clinics, garbage removal, etc. are non-existent. Although these marginal communities become part of the city, they are often physically far removed from the centre, where services are concentrated.

Not surprisingly, a high mortality rate is found among (severely) disabled children in such marginal areas. The use of rehabilitation services for the surviving children means regular trips to the centre, paying the fare for mother and child, often walking large distances with a child that is growing heavier and buying a meal. Although one might have suspected that living in the

city brought the benefit of using the existing services, only the most determined, with a regular income, manage to continue visiting the rehabilitation services.

Furthermore, cultural beliefs can delay the process of seeking help from modern medicine. In some countries, for example, where the people believe in voodoo and spirits, the disability is often seen as a spirit or a spell holding the child in its power. In such cases the parents are likely initially to look for a cure by the local medicine man. Modern medicine will be a second choice.

The Rural Situation

The situation for the disabled child in the rural areas of developing countries is even worse. Some countries have a better developed primary health network than others, but for rehabilitation services they have to travel to the large cities. The majority of the people are farming families, who can hardly make ends meet. The quality of their land is often poor because of deforestation and erosion. Water is drawn from rivers or wells and is often contaminated.

Furthermore, being a farmer does not necessarily mean offering a balanced diet to the family. Cultural beliefs, like one in northern Nigeria (subSahara) that suggests feeding your child an egg will make him a thief, when other cheap sources of protein are unavailable to the family, can be very damaging.

Important factors to take note of when going to work in areas where minimal resources for rehabilitation exist:

- existing governmental and non-governmental services for networking
- statistics on disability incidence and prevalence per age group and per disability category
- information on main causes of disability
- information on the quality of the primary health care
- demographic data to decide on the area where a programme will have the greatest impact — reach more children
- the socioeconomic condition of the target group
- cultural factors affecting food, religion, social

contacts, or other factors influencing nutrition, attendance or compliance

- the availability of public transport and its affordability
- general attitude of the target group — passively receiving the offered aid or a willingness to become part of the solution
- availability of local counterpart(s) to be trained to spread the workload

Physiotherapy in CBR

Physiotherapy plays its specific role in conjunction with other health disciplines involved in rehabilitation, such as occupational therapy, speech therapy, special education and social work. Within the context of CBR or outreach services this role does not change. What changes is the way it is offered to the disabled child and his family — through the CBR worker representing various specialists. The CBR worker does not pretend to be all of these specialists, but is in this position out of necessity to help the professional(s) involved with the supervision of the daily programme to be carried out in the home.

Roles of the Physiotherapist

TRADITIONAL ROLE

Working in a general hospital, rehabilitation centre, chronic care centre or private practice, the physiotherapist is in direct contact with the child and caregiver on a regular basis, often up to three times per week. In countries with minimal resources, however, appointments might vary between twice weekly to monthly or two-monthly visits. This already indicates less direct control over the therapy while putting more responsibility in the hands of the parent or caregiver. It implies the need to give more explanation to the parent. In some situations the parent is asked to find accommodation for a couple of weeks in order to visit a few times per week to learn the techniques to be applied at home once they return.

SPECIALIZED PHYSIOTHERAPIST

In a specialized hospital or rehabilitation centre (for example, a leprosy hospital), different diseases or conditions will be encountered, such as leprosy, poliomyelitis, clubfeet, rickets, bone tuberculosis, exceptional neurological and orthopaedical disorders, to name but a few. Their specific management needs to be studied during a special course and/or practical period in a centre where these diseases and disorders are treated.

TRAINER

The role of the physiotherapist as a trainer has developed to make the best use of their scarcely available expertise in the light of the large number of patients needing physiotherapy. Possible persons to be trained include:

- assistants in the various physiotherapy departments to assist with the treatment of the less complicated patients
- nurses to use physiotherapy techniques while handling and caring for their patients
- CBR workers (local health worker or other person in professional outreach programmes) to be trained in the use of techniques and approaches that are applicable in the home situation

An important part of the CBR training is to explain which situation needs a referral or an early evaluation. This training could be given over a period of time, while the CBR worker is already working and putting the first principles into practice.

SUPERVISORY ROLE

In the regular or specialized physiotherapy departments, physiotherapists may be involved in the supervision of physiotherapy assistants. They may also have a supervisory role for workshops, such as shoe, metal and wood workshops, so as to assist in the fabrication of special aids. In this situation these special aids may have to be designed also by the physiotherapy department, due to lack of other professionals.

Within the context of CBR, ideally the physiotherapist should regularly evaluate the clients. This can be established either by visiting the community or receiving the parent, client and CBR worker in the physiotherapy department at regular intervals. The community visits can be realized by holding prescheduled consultations in a local public building, for example, clinic, community centre or church. To make the visit worthwhile for all persons involved, a team of professionals (preferably including a paediatrician specialized in developmental disorders) can plan to meet one day in a community and evaluate various participants. The participants scheduled for an evaluation will depend on the type of specialists visiting that day.

COORDINATOR OF A CBR PROGRAMME

A physiotherapist may take on the role of coordinator of a CBR programme. Without additional training this can be difficult. Requirements for a coordinator includes:

- knowledge of the disabilities that are presented by the children on the CBR programme
- a minimal but practical knowledge of the needed input and assessments of medical or paramedical rehabilitation professionals
- managerial skills to plan and coordinate work schedules, training, referrals, evaluations of participants, staff appraisal and disciplinary measures, supervision, staff meetings, screening of new personnel, support of parent associations, public education.
- good interpersonal communication skills
- teaching skills using simple language
- knowledge of available teaching materials and their translation in the local language
- knowledge of evaluation methods to plan adequate record-keeping for monitoring and evaluation
- conviction of the importance of CBR in order to obtain cooperation of other professionals

Thought Provokers

1. What kind of disabilities do you expect to encounter in children in countries with a high level of analphabetism, malnutrition, poor vaccination coverage and inadequate maternity services?
2. What aspects of physiotherapy do you think are applicable to these conditions in CBR?
3. Will you be able to explain these to persons with only primary school education, so that they will be able to understand and apply it? How?
4. If you are asked to take on one of the above described roles:
   - will you need additional training?
   - would the role fit your character and personality?
   - would you be able to live in a situation where vast differences between the life styles of the rich and the poor exist (being rich, or at least of middle-class level in the eyes of the target group)?

The first diploma course for teachers and planners of community-based rehabilitation in developing countries was started by the Institute of Child Health in London (UK) in 1985/86. One of the aims of the course was to enable the participants to start up similar courses in developing countries in order to promote CBR services. This course offers a good foundation for future CBR coordinators. It is not available to newly graduated physiotherapists, but to persons with previous rehabilitation experience in developing countries.

Other courses have since started in various developing countries. Some organizations like the Christoffel Blindenmission (CBM)/Christian Blind Mission International (CBMI) have developed a special CBR training for new coworkers going to work in CBR projects, and for project personnel of CBM-supported projects in Africa. Some CBR projects offer a period of in-service training for new CBR coordinators.

Adaptation to the Local Situation

Investigators suggest that up to 70–75% of the rehabilitation problems encountered can be solved at community level (Helander et al. 1989, Thorburn 1994). The complicated problems will need to be referred to centralized services, but the follow-up after the intervention, if not too complex, will again be managed better at community level.

The professional needs to be aware of the living conditions of the families with which the local volunteer or CBR worker are dealing. This teaching process, not surprisingly, is undertaken most effectively in the

Figure 1 Balance Boards and Rolls. Adapted from David Werner (1987)

Balance Boards

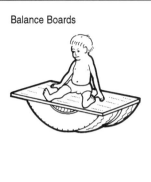
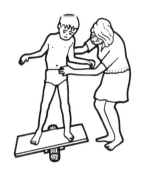
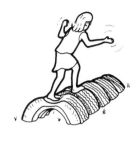

Rolls

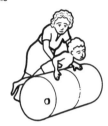
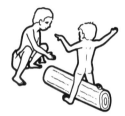
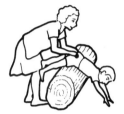

community. It is paramount that the process of problem-solving (how to apply principles and techniques in the local situation) should be part of the training.

SOME PRACTICAL SUGGESTIONS

When the usual physiotherapy equipment is not accessible use whatever materials are available in the home. These are normally cheap and in ample supply. Look around for materials being used by local craftsmen for construction, furniture, etc.

Sometimes the child needs to spend more time on the ground in homes or local centres. In situations where, for example, there is a dirt floor, or no space left inside, newspapers folded in strips and plaited into square mats can be used beneath a piece of cloth, tarpaulin or canvas. Simply add more plaited mats to enlarge the work space.

Towels, newspapers or periodicals can be used for temporary support or splinting purposes fastened with strips of cloth or string. Furthermore, pillows, empty milk powder tins, beach ball, mother's lap, low wall, wooden board over stones, branch (stick) or little hump in the ground can be adapted for exercise balls or balance boards (Werner 1987). See Figure 1.

For aids to be made out of wood or iron, check what local materials and techniques are available. Develop designs with parents and local craftsmen. For example, in Nigeria we used concrete-reinforcement iron rods to make calipers. Sometimes a prototype has to be produced by the CBR worker or a handy friend to show the craftsman the idea, when he does not understand drawings.

Think of trying out other materials for certain aids. In Nigeria and in Jamaica we use parts of PVC pipes for back splints or cock-up splints, even for providing support in corsets. Furthermore, in many countries large reinforced cardboard boxes are used to make corner seats. Old belts or strips of cloth can be used for straps. Some of these and many more ideas can be found in some of the books mentioned in the next section.

Early Intervention and CBR Programmes

Many guides and handbooks have been developed for use in home or community programmes. Table 1 compares various aspects of four useful books/

Table 1

Comparison of Some Material Useful for CBR

	DVC	WHO	PEEP	GEMS
Intended use by	Disabled persons; parents; health and rehabilitation personnel	Community members interested in planning and implementing and evaluating a CBR programme	Home teachers; teachers	Any person concerned with promoting movement development of young children
Character work	Work and reference book	Manual with guides and training packages	Developmental check-list with activity cards	Check-list of motor development with activity cards
Age range and type of target group	Children with disabilities	Disabled persons of all ages	Children with delays in normal development 0–6 years	Children with delays in motor development 0–2 years
Assessment tools for possible progress monitoring	Mental, social and physical development chart	Play activities	Infant stimulation and socialization; language cognition; self-help and motor development check-lists	Motor developmental check-list
0–2 years	68 behaviours	42 behaviours	294 behaviours	215 behaviours
2–5 years	18 behaviours	24 behaviours	239 behaviours	
5–6 years	21 ADL-behaviours and quality of activities check-list	23 ADL-behaviours	91 behaviours	
Older	See 5–6 years	Same 23 ADL-behaviours		

DVC, disabled village children (Werner 1987); WHO, training in the community for people with disabilities (Helander *et al.* 1989); PEEP, portage early education programme (Cameron and White 1987); GEMS, guide to early movement skills (White *et al.* 1994). ADL, activities of daily living.

guides and highlights how they are complementary to each other. All four incorporate ideas for intervention for movement problems or motor development. None of these books/guides has been written for specific professionals, therefore no jargon is used. That by Werner (1987) is diagnosis oriented, but presents a helpful disability guide and an extensive glossary. Helander *et al.* (1989) is more disability oriented and presents some training packages specific for children; other packages only partly concern children.

The lack of criteria for improvement is one of the drawbacks in methodology of CBR evaluations (Jaffer 1993). Two of the works, Cameron and White (1987) and White *et al.* (1994), can remedy this lack of criteria for improvement for preschool children. For example, Cameron and White (1987) offer a structured check-list of 624 childhood behaviours. The 63 behaviours in the motor development area for 0–2 years can be replaced by those of White *et al.* (1994). These two check-lists used together will help develop stimulation ideas for disabled children in all developmental areas. When only one agent of rehabilitation is involved with a family, such an approach is preferred above concentrating on one aspect of development only. It is advisable to seek training for the correct implementation of the PEEP and the GEMS. Both make use of a measurable weekly programme for progress monitoring.

Table 2 compares additional aspects of the manuals

Table 2

Overview of Information Presented in Disabled Village Children (Werner 1987) and WHO Manual (Helander *et al.* 1989)

	DVC	WHO
Early identification procedures for:		
● movement problems	disability guide	short screening test
● problems of balance/coordination	various	none

● visual problems	for: child > 3 months
	    child > 4 years
	    child with intellectual disability
		for: child 3 months–3 years
		    child > 3 years

● auditory problems	for: child > 4 months;
	    young children
		for: child < 6 months
		    child 6 months–3 years
		    child > 3 years and adults

Disability information	- disability guide to different
	  diagnosis
	- causes, consequences, prevention
	  and intervention
	- case histories, photos, drawings
		- consequences, prevention and
		  intervention
		- drawings

Rehabilitation aids	12 chapters; detailed on different types of aids	in most training packages (less variation)
Community involvement	12 chapters on village involvement, social integration and rights	roles of community rehabilitation committee, disabled persons and schoolteachers

by Werner (1987) and Helander *et al.* (1989). It shows their usefulness in teaching early identification procedures and providing information on disabilities.

Because the majority of the children on CBR programmes that need physiotherapy input are likely to have cerebral palsy, a comparison of three books dealing with this subject can be found in Table 3. These books (Finnie 1975, Levitt 1982, Wolf-Vereecken 1993) are useful in training CBR workers and disseminating information to parents in addition to information found in Werner (1987).

SERVICES FOR THE PRESCHOOL CHILD

Infants and preschool children who cannot make use of institutional rehabilitation services may be reached by outreach services or CBR services started in their communities. Because body and nervous system are still developing it is important that services are

established that encourage development in all developmental areas.

SERVICES FOR THE PRIMARY SCHOOL-AGE CHILD

School-age children with disabilities that are in need of intervention and can attend the local school, should be encouraged to do so, while they could still receive physiotherapy through the continuation of visits from or to the CBR or extension worker. The main problem faced by the child is that often the school refuses to admit him when he cannot walk or is not toilet trained. Assistance with trying to get the child placed in the local school becomes part of the job description of the CBR or extension worker.

Those children attending special education institutions might benefit from the rehabilitation services of the institutions if they exist. Otherwise they can still continue to benefit from CBR or outreach

Table 3
Comparison of Three Texts on Children with Cerebral Palsy (CP)

	Levitt (1982)	Finnie (1975)	Wolf-Vereecken (1993)
Intended use by	physiotherapists	parents of children with CP	rehabilitation and health workers with low educational level
Illustrations	photos + line drawings	clear line drawings	photos
Strengths	• clear treatment procedures encouraging normal development in stages of supine, prone, sitting, standing (walking) • description of common problems for each stage followed by treatment suggestions and daily care and separate physiotherapy suggestions	• simple clear language • section on handling, positioning, carrying	• separate chapters on: spastic quadriplegic, hypotonic and athetoid, hemiplegic and diplegic children • handling in the neonatal period • separate chapters on normal and abnormal development of neonate and infant
Groupwork	yes	no	yes
Hand function development	treatment + table 0–5 years	fundamentals	Table 0–12 months
Play	no	yes	yes
Glossary	none	yes	yes

services. If the children live in an institution the situation becomes more complicated. CBR and outreach services need a person to supervise daily the activities carried out by the child in between the visits. Even though the child is older, the need persists for continual guidance and encouragement to improve skills.

School-age children who are low functioning will continue to benefit from CBR or outreach services at home or in local centres until they are able to go to school (if ever). The children of this age group becoming permanently or temporarily disabled might pass through the established medical and rehabilitation system and either receive physiotherapy there or be referred to an existing CBR or outreach service. Many of them will not reach this system and not receive any assistance. These young people are likely to develop more severe permanent disabilities.

PROGRAMMES FOR 13- TO 18-YEAR-OLDS

Disabled children who finish primary school should be encouraged to continue their studies at a secondary institution, if possible and appropriate. If none of the family has ever continued with secondary education, it could be inappropriate. It may be more likely for them to start working, so they should be encouraged to do so and be given the opportunity. When still in need of intervention, the CBR worker or outreach worker might continue a programme with them. There will be less need for supervision by a third person, the older and more responsible they are. Assistance could be offered in finding an appropriate placement, where the disabled youngster will be accepted with their limitations.

The 13- to 18-year-olds who are unable to go to or finish primary school, but are able to complete simple or complex but structured tasks, could be trained to be useful for their family or community by an extension or CBR worker. Members from the community need to be involved in order to offer opportunities, expertise and supervision where possible. The focus of physical rehabilitation should be placed on activities of daily living and on enhancing the special skills needed. Ideally employment should follow once a disabled youth can be trained for a job.

For the youngsters of this age group living in institutions, intervention by a CBR or outreach worker could be effective once the youngster can take responsibility for his own treatment. Furthermore, low-functioning adolescents living at home can benefit from CBR or outreach services, even if only to motivate and support the family to maintain mobility for personal care.

Hansen's Disease (Leprosy)

Hansen's disease is a chronic infectious disease of man caused by *Mycobacterium leprae*. It mainly affects skin and nerves, causing depigmented or red patches with loss of feeling in the skin, raised nodules and/or neuritis of one or more of the nerves listed below with signs of nerve damage (in order of frequency).

ulnar
– sensory loss and dryness of ulnar half of hand
– Vth and IVth PIP joint clawing through weak or paralysed intrinsic hand muscles

posterior tibial
– sensory loss of foot sole
– claw toes due to weak or paralysed intrinsic foot muscles

common peroneal
– loss of sensation on lateral side leg and dorsum of the foot
– dropfoot or weak dorsiflexion/eversion

median
– sensory loss and dryness of radial half of hand
– Ist, IInd and IIIrd PIP joints clawing through weak or paralysed intrinsic hand muscles, with loss of abduction and opposition of the thumb

facial
– lagophthalmos (inability or weakness of eye closure)
– (very uncommon) loss of facial expression and inability to close the lips, through involvement of buccal, mandibular and cervical branches

trigeminal
– loss of feeling of the cornea and the conjunctiva

radial
– (rarely involved) wrist drop due to extensor and supinator paralysis

Hansen's disease normally develops and cures slowly except in epidemical situations. The incubation period is usually 2–5 years, but can be as much as 30 years (Summers 1993). It is not easily spread, but repeated close contact with persons with the untreated multibacillary type has proven to be a factor. Only 3% of a population presents a spectrum of low immunity to leprosy and could develop the disease (Summers 1993). The type of leprosy a person develops depends on their level of immunity. Patients can be classified as having:

- paucibacillary leprosy with few mycobacteria present and a relatively high immunity, or
- multibacillary leprosy with many mycobacteria present and a very low immunity to leprosy

The WHO recommend that multiple drug therapy (MDT) should be taken for 6 months by paucibacillary patients and for 2 years by multibacillary patients to cure the disease (Wheate and Pearson 1990, Summers 1993). Multibacillary patients are no longer contagious after a few days on the MDT.

Leprosy is not often found in very young children because of its long incubation period. Children with Hansen's disease are far outnumbered by adults. Despite this it would be a good practice to screen schoolchildren annually in leprosy endemic areas.

Physiotherapists are mainly concerned with the complications of nerve damage that can result from a neuritis caused by an immunological reaction of the body to either the leprosy bacteria or the treatment. The nerves are mainly affected where they appear close under the surface of the body. McDougall and Yawalkar (1989) indicate that leprosy does not damage the central nervous system. How Hansen's disease can lead to loss of fingers, toes and other amputations is explained in Figure 2.

Figure 2 Mechanisms Causing Disability after Nerve Damage from Leprosy. Adapted from Bryceson and Pfaltzgraf (1979)

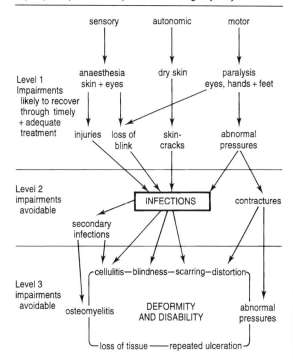

It is estimated that 2–3 million individuals in the world are physically and socially disabled as a result of leprosy (Nordeen 1992). Furthermore, Shah *et al.* (1993) indicate that approximately 25% of patients not treated at an early stage of the disease develop anaesthesia and/or deformities of the hands and feet.

Prevention of Disabilities

In leprosy hospitals usually the physiotherapy departments are involved in the recording of disabilities and provide health education classes where they teach the patients life-time injury avoidance habits. ILEP (1993) indicates five major prevention of disabilities (POD) components:

1. early case detection and effective treatment with MDT
2. preservation of nerve function
3. preservation of vision
4. training patients in self-care
5. the provision of protective footwear

Action to be taken to preserve nerve function and vision includes:

- clear and complete disability records on admission and every check-up thereafter
- early diagnosis of neuritis followed by correct drug treatment within 6 months of the onset of the anaesthesia, weakness or paralysis
- physical therapy during drug therapy for neuritis
- splinting to rest the involved body part during inflammation
- maintaining joint motion
- strengthening of muscles once neuritis has subsided

Training patients in self-care is necessary to prevent (more) secondary impairments and subsequent disabilities. Life-time injury-avoidance habits to be daily carried out at home are as follows (Watson 1986a,b):

- think-blink for insensitive eyes or lagophthalmus
- protect insensitive eyes against dryness and dust by shielding eyes from sun, wind and dust
- watch insensitive hands during activities for daily living and protect them where necessary, e.g. use of gloves or potholders for cooking or drinking hot liquids
- use provided protective footwear, avoid long walks with insensitive feet and take small steps
- daily inspection for injuries of insensitive areas with emphasis on earlier injured sites
- early and correct wound care
- daily skin care for dry skin
- daily exercises to prevent weak or paralysed muscles causing contractures
- Check for and report early signs of any newly inflamed or reinflamed nerve

Musa the Hausa boy

Eight-year-old Musa stayed home from school when he developed a smelling ulcer under his right foot. He had started to walk strangely some months ago – lifting his right foot higher than his left. The father of his friend Elisha, a cured leprosy patient, suspected leprosy. This was confirmed by the leprosy inspector. After spending 6 weeks at the leprosy centre, his ulcer had healed, sensation had come back in his foot sole, but he had to wear a dropfoot strap. Musa wore this strap every month when he went to see the leprosy inspector to collect his treatment, but stopped wearing it otherwise, because his classmates made fun of him. A few months after finishing the 6 months of drug treatment, the leprosy inspector ran into Musa and discovered he did not wear the strap. He arranged for Musa to get a tendon transfer of the tibialis posterior muscle. After the operation Musa came home walking normally without a strap. He could even run normally again. He soon forgot how difficult it had been at first to lift his foot after the plaster was removed.

Tendon transfers in combination with life-time injury avoidance can also prevent secondary impairments. Tendon transfers are frequently undertaken in an attempt to restore functional activities such as ankle dorsiflexion, metacarpophalangeal flexion and interphalangeal extension and blink. The physiotherapist's role preoperatively for tendon transfers includes optimal correction of contractures and isolating and strengthening the muscle tendon which is to be transferred.

Postoperatively there is the need for restoring joint motion, teaching new muscle action to become an integral part of restored functions, and continuation of life-time injury-avoidance habits when necessary.

For those patients with deformities of the hand, and no or minimal loss of fingers, several splints described by Shah (1992) can be applied to improve and/or assist hand function:

- gutter splints to decrease fixed clawing of the fingers
- finger loop splint if the fingers can be actively (partially) straightened in supported lumbrical position
- opponens loop splint for ape thumb deformity or mild thumb web contracture
- adductor band for abduction deformity of little finger only

Bryceson and Pfaltzgraf (1979) suggest that when surgery is indicated at all in leprosy it is an admission of failure to educate the public and patients about the importance of early diagnosis and adequate therapy; in the medical management of leprosy and its complications, and of in teaching of how to live with anaesthesia.

Record-keeping is important in leprosy and special assessment forms have been developed because of the particular features involved. Examples are found in various publications from the Leprosy Mission International or ILEP.

Hansen's disease and AIDS

McDougal and Yawalkar (1989) indicate that because the acquired immune deficiency syndrome (AIDS) depresses the immune response, there is a possibility that its spread will cause deterioration of the type of leprosy in individuals already infected with Hansen's disease, and result in larger numbers of people in leprosy-endemic communities developing the disease.

Thought Provokers

1. How would you teach a 7-year-old child:
   - daily injury inspection
   - how to protect his insensitive hands
   - to wear a dropfoot strap or other splints despite others making fun of him?
2. How will involving his family help?
3. If you had two insensitive hands, how much would you have to adapt your life in order to avoid injuring your hands?

REFERENCES

Bryceson, A, Pfaltzgraf, RE (1979) *Leprosy*, 155 pp. Edinburgh: Churchill Livingstone.

Cameron, RJ, White, M (1987) *The Portage Early Education Programme, A Practical Manual, Checklist and Activity Cards*. Windsor: NFER-NELSON.

CBM (1993) *Concept Paper on Education and Rehabilitation, internal consultants policy statement*. Germany: Christoffel Blindenmission e.V.

Finnie (1975) *Handling the Young Cerebral Palsied Child at Home*, 337 pp. New York: Dutton.

Helander, E (1993) *Prejudice and Dignity*. New York: United Nations Development Programme.

Helander, E, Mendis, P, Nelson, G et al. (1989) *Training in the Community for People with Disabilities*, 656 pp. Geneva: WHO.

ILEP (1993) *Prevention of Disability, Guidelines for Leprosy Control Programmes*, 45 pp. London: ILEP.

Jaffer, R (1993) Monitoring and evaluation of community based rehabilitation – need for a participatory approach. In: Finkenflügel *The Handicapped Community*, pp. 51–64. Primary Health Care Publications 7. Amsterdam: VU University Press.

Levitt, S (1982) *Treatment of Cerebral Palsy and Motor Delay*, 267 pp. Oxford: Blackwell Scientific.

McDougall, AC, Yawalkar, SJ (1989) *Leprosy, Basic Information and Management*, 44 pp. Basle: CIBA-GEIGY.

Noordeen, SK (1992) Elimination of leprosy as public health problem. *Leprosy Review 63*: 1–4.

Rehabilitation International (1981) Childhood disability: its prevention and rehabilitation. Report to the Executive Board of UNICEF. E/ICEF/L.1410 In: *UNICEF Assignment Children 53/54*: 43–75.

Shah, A (1992) *Prevention and Correction of Claw Hand by Splintage — A New Approach to Deformity Care*. Training and Education Series 1, 24 pp. Bombay: Hindustan CIBA-GEIGY.

Shah, A, Yawalkar, SJ, Ganapati, R (1993) *Modulan Grip-aids for Rehabilitation in Leprosy*. Training and Education Series 2, 35 pp. Basle: CIBA-GEIGY.

Summers, A (1993) *Leprosy for Field Staff*, 116 pp. UK: The Leprosy Mission International.

Thorburn, MJ (1994) Childhood disability in developing countries: basic issues. In: Thorburn, MJ, Marfo, K (eds) *Practical Approaches to Childhood Disability in Developing Countries: Insights from Experience and Research*, pp. 15–43. Tampa: Global Age Publishing.

UNICEF (1993) *The State of the World's Children 1993*. Oxford: Oxford University Press.

Watson, JM (1986a) *Essential Action to Minimise Disability in Leprosy Patients*, 32 pp. Brentford: The Leprosy Mission International.

Watson, JM (1986b) *Preventing Disability in Leprosy Patients*, 116 pp. Brentford: The Leprosy Mission International.

Werner, D (1987) *Disabled Village Children*, 674 pp. Palo Alto: The Hesperian Foundation.

Wheate, HW, Pearson, JMH (1990) *A Practical Guide to the Diagnosis and Treatment of Leprosy in the Basic Health Unit.*, 38 pp. Wuerzburg: German Leprosy Relief Association and ILEP Steering Committee on Teaching and Learning Materials.

White, M, Bungay, C et al. (1994) *Guide to Early Movements Skills, A Portage-based programme promoting the first stages of motor development* (Checklist, Activity Book and Instruction Booklet). Windsor: NFER-NELSON.

WHO (1981) *Report of the WHO Expert Committee on Disability Prevention and Rehabilitation*. Technical Report Series 668. Geneva: WHO.

Wolf-Vereecken, MJ (1993) *Cerebral Palsy Children in Africa, Early Identification and Intervention*, 197 pp. Amsterdam: TOOL.

Index

Number in **bold** refer to tables; numbers in *italic* refer to figures.